Interdisciplinary Handbook of Trauma and Culture

Yochai Ataria • David Gurevitz
Haviva Pedaya • Yuval Neria
Editors

Interdisciplinary Handbook of Trauma and Culture

Springer

Editors
Yochai Ataria
Department of Neurobiology
Weizmann Institute of Science
Rehovot, Israel

Haviva Pedaya
Department of the History of Israel
Ben Gurion University
Beer-Sheva, Israel

David Gurevitz
The Interdisciplinary Center Herzelia
Herzelia, Israel

Yuval Neria
Columbia University Medical
Center and the New York State
Psychiatric Institute
New York, NY, USA

ISBN 978-3-319-29402-5 ISBN 978-3-319-29404-9 (eBook)
DOI 10.1007/978-3-319-29404-9

Library of Congress Control Number: 2016939236

Printed on acid-free paper

This Springer imprint is published by Springer Nature
The registered company is Springer International Publishing AG Switzerland

To Adi, who is my home in the chaotic darkness, my citadel in a strange and alienated world.
Yochai

To my beloved children Matan and Yuval.
For Rachel, with Love.
David

To all those who shared with me their wanderings.
To Yochai.
Haviva

I am grateful to my wife Mariana, and my children Michal, Oren, and Maya. Without the love and strength you have given me, my scientific work was not possible.
Yuval

Acknowledgements

The editors are grateful to Mikael Rubin for his exhaustive editorial work, and to Peter James and Ari Lev Plat for their editorial assistance.

Contents

Part II Theory of Trauma

Part III Case Studies of Collective Trauma

Contributors

Dan Arav, Ph.D. School of Media Studies, The College of Management Academic Studies (COMAS), Rishon LeZion, Israel

Yochai Ataria, Ph.D. Department of Neurobiology, Weizmann Institute of Science, Rehovot, Israel

Ory Bartal, Ph.D. Department of History and Theory, Bezalel Academy of Arts and Design, Jerusalem, Israel

Bracha Lichtenberg Ettinger, Ph.D. Marcel Duchamp Chair and Professor of Psychoanalysis and Art, European Graduate School (EGS), Saas-Fee, Switzerland

Kirby Farrell, Ph.D. Department of English, University of Massachusetts, Amherst, MA, USA

Saul Friedländer, Ph.D. Chair in Holocaust Studies, History Department, UCLA, Los Angeles, CA, USA

R. Ruard Ganzevoort, Ph.D. Amsterdam Centre for the Study of Lived Religion, Faculty of Theology, Vrije Universiteit Amsterdam, Amsterdam, The Netherlands

David Gurevitz, Ph.D. The Interdisciplinary Center, Herzelia, Israel

Katharine Reiner van der Hoorn, M.A. Columbia University Medical Center and the New York State Psychiatric Institute, New York, NY, USA

Emily Joyner, M.A. Columbia University Medical Center and the New York State Psychiatric Institute, New York, NY, USA

Robert Lemelson, Ph.D. Department of Anthropology, University of California, Los Angeles, CA, USA

UCLA Semel Institute of Neuroscience, Los Angeles, CA, USA

Foundation for Psychocultural Research, Pacific Palisades, CA, USA

Ruth Malkinson, Ph.D. International Center for the Study of Loss, Bereavement and Human Resilience, University of Haifa, Haifa, Israel

Allen Meek, Ph.D. School of English and Media Studies, Massey University, Palmerston North, New Zealand

Maya Neria, B.A. Middlebury College, Middlebury, VT, USA

Yuval Neria, Ph.D. Columbia University Medical Center and the New York State Psychiatric Institute, New York, NY, USA

Haviva Pedaya, Ph.D. Ben-Gurion University of the Negev, Jewish History Department, Elyachar Center for Sephardi Heritage, Ben-Gurion University, Beer-Sheva, Israel

Ari Platt, B.A. Columbia University Medical Center and the New York State Psychiatric Institute, New York, NY, USA

Anne Rothe, Ph.D. Department of Classical and Modern Languages, Literatures, and Cultures, Wayne State University, Detroit, MI, USA

Mikael Rubin, M.A. Psychology Department, University of Texas at Austin, Austin, TX, USA

Simon Shimshon Rubin, Ph.D. International Center for the Study of Loss, Bereavement and Human Resilience, University of Haifa, Haifa, Israel

Lisa Saltzman, Ph.D. Professor and Chair of History of Art and the Andrew W. Mellon Foundation Chair in the Humanities, Bryn Mawr College, Bryn Mawr, PA, USA

Frank Seeburger, Ph.D. Department of Philosophy, University of Denver, Longmont, CO, USA

Erel Shvil, Ph.D. Columbia University Medical Center and the New York State Psychiatric Institute, New York, NY, USA

Dennis Sobolev, Ph.D. Department of Hebrew and Comparative Literature, University of Haifa, Haifa, Israel

Srdjan Sremac, Ph.D. Amsterdam Centre for the Study of Lived Religion, Faculty of Theology, Vrije Universiteit Amsterdam, Amsterdam, The Netherlands

Teresa Stoppani, M.Arch., Ph.D. School of Art Architecture and Design, Leeds Beckett University, Broadcasting Place, Leeds, UK

Seinenu M. Thein-Lemelson, Ph.D. Institute of Personality and Social Research (IPSR), University of California, Berkeley, USA

Eliezer Witztum, M.D. Division of Psychiatry, Faculty of Health Sciences, Ben-Gurion University of the Negev, Be'er Sheva, Israel

Koji Yamashiro Faculty of Humanities, Hebrew University of Jerusalem, Jerusalem, Israel

Ayelet Zohar, Ph.D. Art History Department, Tel Aviv University, Tel Aviv, Israel

Introduction

Yochai Ataria, David Gurevitz, Haviva Pedaya, and Yuval Neria

Previous scholars who discussed the evolution of mental trauma as a research field identified its origin as related to the nineteenth-century railway accident (e.g., Farrell 1998; Leys 2000; Luckhurst 2008). They connected trauma with modernity, since one of the most important characteristics of the modern age has been railway transportation (Thacker 2003). Seltzer (1997), for instance, suggested that the "modern subject has become inseparable from categories of shock and trauma" (p. 18). Essentially, such scholars defined mental trauma not merely as a by-product of the industrial era but rather went a step further, suggesting that if railways are indeed the icon of modernity then mental trauma stands at the very core of this era, as a constitutive phenomenon that has shaped the structure of its cultural discourse.

The association between trauma and culture, however, has much deeper and long-standing roots. The stories of Cain and Abel, the Binding of Isaac, the Binding of Ishmael (after his laughter), and the Crucifixion of Jesus can all be viewed as traumatic events that stand at the core of the monotheistic culture. In this sense, trauma itself lies at the heart of Western culture. Bearing this in mind, this book seeks to remap and expand the relationship between trauma and culture.

When attempting to describe the multifaceted relations between trauma and culture two questions seem to lie at the core of such an effort: First, in what ways traumatic events are represented in specific cultures? and second, in what ways collective traumas may shape the structure of culture?

The current volume has three parts. The first part is focused on represenations of trauma in culture. The second and the third parts of the book focus on the different ways collective trauma may shape the structure of cultures. While the second part of the book attempts to discuss theoretical aspects of trauma-indcued cultural changes, the third part presents a number of case studies of collective trauma.

In the first part, Geurvitz (Chap. 1) examines the relationship between trauma and literature, illustrated by an analysis of the works of Franz Kafka and Cormac McCarthy. The following three chapters discuss various associations between trauma and the media. First, Meek (Chap. 2) describes the development of cultural trauma as a concept over the past 100 years and how this idea came to be linked with visual media. Arav (Chap. 3) then seeks to shed light on the moving image in general, and television in particular, as a major factor in the establishment of the contemporary culture of trauma. Lastly, Rothe (Chap. 4) argues that melodrama is the dominant narrative mode for representing experiences of victimization and suffering, discussing how kitsch and sentimentality are encoded at the paradigmatic mode of reception. In the fifth chapter, Sobolev examines the relationships between modernism, literature, and trauma; this essay stresses the uniqueness of Hopkins' hermeneutics of trauma and emphasizes the existence of a shared hermeneutic repertoire for dealing with trauma. Further, Saltzman, in the sixth chapter, explores the unique relations between trauma and representation by attending to a set of cultural works including architectural, artistic, and literary—all inspired by the tragic events of 9/11 2001. The seventh and the eighth chapters both deal with representations of World War II in Japanese culture: while Bartal (Chap. 7) examines how the memory of the nuclear holocaust is treated in Japanese comics and animation, Zohar (Chap. 8) explores the *kamikaze* projects of Koizumi Meiro and the manner in which he portrays the trauma of the perpetrator in Japan. The final two chapters of the first part focus on artistic topics: Stoppani (Chap. 9) aims to explore the trauma of architecture and Ettinger (Chap. 10) seeks to define art as a transport-station of trauma and, in so doing, characterize artistic work in terms of processing and representing trauma.

The second part of the book explores theories of trauma and culture more broadly. In the first chapter, Seeburger (Chap. 11) argues that philosophy is forced to confront what can be viewed as its own defining trauma. From such a perspective, the very history of philosophy can be told as a tale of trauma. Following this, Rothe (Chap. 12) critiques the trauma theory presented by scholars such as Ruth Leys, Wulf Kansteiner and Harald Weilnböck. In particular Rothe analyses the transformation of the concept of trauma from signifying the psychological aftereffects of extreme violence into a metaphor for a stipulated postmodern crisis of signification. As such, it argues that trauma theory is both nonsensical and irresponsible. In the next chapter (13) Ataria examines the notion of bearing witness through a comparison of two Jewish writers: the Italian Holocaust survivor Primo Levi and the French novelist Georges Perec. The next two chapters examine the relationship between trauma and Monotheism. Pedaya (Chap. 14) analyzes the act of walking as a basic reaction to trauma and adversity. The projection of trauma in exploring space is examined through its manifestation in Jewish time perception, particularly the Messianic concept of time and its progression as developed by the Kabbalists—born out of the Spanish Expulsion. The strong affinities between walking as dispersion and collecting, with its internal identity construction, illuminate the modern conceptions of both Benjamin and Freud. Following this, Yamashiro (Chap. 15) discusses one of the most important questions regarding monotheistic religions: can we rewrite the birth, development, and death of the monotheistic religions as traumatic history? This chapter represents a starting point for such an attempt. Ataria (Chap. 16) then seeks to examine the notion of manhood following the Vietnam War, presenting what can be considered to be the trauma of the white man in the USA. Ettinger (Chap. 17) conceptualizes the *Laius Complex*, articulating and offering a critique of the paternal subject's (the analyst's) desire to scarify the son—based upon an impulse that can reach a degree of *Laius delirium*—which is projected on the analyzed ("son") in a psychotic countertransference. Lastly Rubin, Neria, and Neria (Chap. 18) explore the complex relationships between trauma and fear, examining how they intertwine in the context of their most relevant psychopathology—posttraumatic stress disorder (PTSD).

The third part of the book presents a number of case studies of collective trauma. Friedländer (Chap. 19) critically discusses key cultural patterns by which Israelis process memories of the Holocaust. Joyner, Neria, and colleagues (Chap. 20) examine sociocultural aspects of the emotional responses to the 9/11 2001 attacks. Following this, Ruard and Sremac (Chap. 21) examine the unique relationships between male wartime sexual trauma, masculinity, and posttraumatic spirituality. Farrell, in the fourth chapter (22), examines the Sandy Hook school rampage in Newton Connecticut and the radical firearms advocacy that followed, which can be viewed in the context of traumatic aftermath. In the following chapter (23), Witztum, Malkinson, and Rubin address conceptual issues regarding traumatic bereavement and culture in Israel. Lastly, in the final chapter (24), Seinenu Thein-Lemelson and Robert Lemelson explore the relationship between the personal experience of trauma and larger cultural and political processes that can shape individual outcomes through an examination of two historic national tragedies in Southeast Asia: one in Burma and the other in Indonesia.

References

1. Farrell, K. (1998). *Post-traumatic culture.* Baltimore: Johns Hopkins University Press.
2. Leys, R. (2000). *Trauma: A genealogy.* Chicago and London: University of Chicago Press.
3. Luckhurst, R. (2008). *The trauma question.* London: Routledge.
4. Seltzer, M. (1997). Wound culture: Trauma in the pathological public sphere. *October, 80*, 3–26.
5. Thacker, A. (2003). *Moving through modernity: Space and geography in modernism.* Oxford: Manchester University Press.

Part I

Representations of Trauma

1 Literature as Trauma: The Postmodern Option-Franz Kafka and Cormac Mccarthy

David Gurevitz

1.1 Postmodern Literature and Trauma: Intersecting Paths

This chapter deals with the relationship between the discourse of trauma in contemporary society and the contribution of literature to its conceptualization. It seeks to demonstrate the ways in which posttraumatic thinking is similar to literary writing and its interest in writing as trauma, and how the posttraumatic mind drove the work of Franz Kafka in "In the Penal Colony" and Cormac McCarthy in *Blood Meridian: Or the Evening Redness in the West*. The aim of this discussion is not merely to identify traumatic themes in these authors' work, but to describe reading, writing, and deciphering the text as reflective processes that depict themselves in posttraumatic terms.[1] It is my contention that the mechanisms of breakdown and dissociation, lacuna and loss, memory lapses and forgetting, utterance and silence, similarity and difference, forgiveness and atonement, desire and impotence, disintegration, fragmentation, and ecstasy—all central features of posttrauma and posttraumatic discourse—are also key terms in the postmodern poetics of contemporary literature. In other words, the postmodern approach is, in fact, a critical confrontation with the traumatic nature of the literary experience itself. Analysis of the works of the two authors will show the paradoxical allure of trauma as an intense experience, despite, and perhaps because of, the acute suffering it entails.

The discussion below begins with theoretical aspects of the cultural discourse of trauma, followed by the parallels between posttraumatic discourse and traumatic discourse in postmodern literature. The conclusions are then applied to the analysis of two major works of literature, one from the early twentieth century and the other more recent, in which the contribution of the authors, Franz Kafka and Cormac McCarthy, to the contemporary discourse of trauma is examined.[2] As I will

[1] The traumatic body is created when its skin (both physical and metaphorical) is penetrated. The fissure allows for the transformation and devastation of the inner organs on the physical and mental levels. Trauma and its clinical, media, and cultural meanings have been discussed extensively. See, Agamben (1998), Alexander (2004:1–30, 2012), Badiou (2002), Blanchot (1995), Caruth (1995), Derrida (2001), Dineen (1999), Douglass and Vogler (2003:1–53), Elsaesser (2014), Herman (1992:175), Kleinman and Kleinman (2009:288–303), LaCapra (1998), Laplanche and Pontalis ([1967] 1973:214–217), Leys (2000), Loftus (1996), McNally (2003), Rothe (2011), Seeburger (2013), Spiegel (1986:61–78), and Young (2007:21–48).

[2] If space allowed, it would also be interesting to examine the aspect of trauma in the works of Thomas Pynchon, Primo Levi, David Foster Wallace, Michel Houellebecq, and others, all of whom deal, *inter alia*, with the social effects of the link between trauma and paranoia in contemporary society.

D. Gurevitz, Ph.D. (✉)
The Interdisciplinary Center, Herzelia, Israel
e-mail: davidg51@netvision.net.ilv

Y. Ataria et al. (eds.), *Interdisciplinary Handbook of Trauma and Culture*,
DOI 10.1007/978-3-319-29404-9_1

attempt to demonstrate, despite the differences in mentality and culture, and the distance of time, both writers address the issue of trauma in a world of nihilistic and unexplained evil, an evil that threatens to impose a rule of postapocalyptic death. The chapter ends with a look at the fundamental structures that help create the postmodern poetics of contemporary literature.

Kafka and McCarthy serve as the cornerstones of this discussion. Close analysis of their work will reveal the ways in which literature writes trauma into society. This postmodern literature, which rejects the utopian project of modernism, no longer conceives of language as a mechanism of redemption. Instead, it is depicted as a tool of oppression, working relentlessly to silence and alienate. Literature now focuses on the very moment of traumatic crisis, a moment represented both on the thematic level of the work and on the reflective level of its creator. Through the act of writing, this moment becomes an event that is already indicative of the world "after the Fall," after the end of time. The compulsive repetition that characterizes the pathology of the traumatic experience is thus reflected in literature.

The postmodern "shift" illustrated by the works of Kafka and McCarthy occurred in a specific historical context. In the mid-twentieth century, the discourse of extermination (Auschwitz) thrust itself into the humanistic and rational messages, and optimistic myth of European enlightenment, like an uninvited and unnerving guest. Faced with the supremacist, mythical, and racist discourse of Nazism, modernism found it difficult to continue to represent the values of enlightened society (Bauman, 2013).[3] The postmodern reaction[4] framed modernism as the late, traumatic, presence of progress in the heart of the twentieth century. This contention led to a new historization of modernism: not as a utopian site of freedom by virtue of faith in science, morality, and art, but rather as a dystopic place depicted as the circles of hell.

The same period saw the emergence of a new posttraumatic philosophy: "post-Auschwitz" humanity, suddenly confronted with the impossible task of finding an explanation for the atrocities and expressing what the mind refused to take in, was forced to acknowledge the unbridgeable, incommensurable,[5] gap between the universality

[3] Modernism refers to an inclusive cultural and ideological approach from the Renaissance to the first half of the twentieth century. It lauded the heroic nature of the "new," while turning its back on the traditional values that dominated past history. The proponents of modernism stressed faith in reason and science, opposed ideologies of political oppression, and saw art as a potential path to human redemption. As an art movement, modernism refers to literature and fine art from the second half of the nineteenth century to the mid-twentieth century. The issue of the end of modernism has been the subject of considerable controversy. See, for example, Blumenberg (1985), Bradbury and McFarlane ([1976] 1991), Calinescu (1987), Giddens (2013), Greenberg ([1961] 1993), Habermas ([1985] 1987), Hall (1992), and Kolb (1986).

[4] Postmodernism is critical of modernism, focusing primarily on criticism of the redemptive attitudes (both political and aesthetic) of modernism and enlightenment. It follows three major avenues: (1) Questioning the concept of the autonomy of knowledge and the ability of science to reach the truth, (2) deconstruction of the unified subject or text in which it appears in favor of a hybrid subject that makes room for cultural and ideological differences, and (3) deconstruction of the representation of language: the text says "more" and "less" than the speaker intended and language can no longer be said to represent reality. Through the act of writing, language reveals the balance of power between the elements existing within it. For a definition of the postmodern condition, see, Baudrillard (1983), Bollas (1995), Derrida ([1967] 1976), Dews (1987), Docherty (1993), Huntington (1998), Jameson (1991), Lyotard (1984, 1993), Rabinow (1986), Silverman (1990), Spence (1984), and Wheale (1995). Analysis of the postmodern elements in the works of Kafka and McCarthy reveals the world in a state of uncertain ontology dealing with a posttraumatic reality that has been normalized in the language and culture.

[5] Incommensurability is a term from the philosophy of science that denotes that two scientific systems cannot be judged by the same standard, even if there is no logical contradiction between them. It is impossible to "translate" one system of thought into the other. On the cultural level, the traumatic experience involves, among other things, the inability to find a common standard of measurement between the language of the victimizers and that of their victims (Lyotard, 1984). Incommensurability is a major issue in Kafka's "In the Penal Colony": there is a total divide between the normative human language of the Traveler observing the killing in the colony, and the ideological "magical" language spoken by the unseen agents of the regime. The foolish attempt to translate from one to the other drives the violence and grotesque evil in the story. A similar situation is depicted in McCarthy's *Blood Meridian*, where it is impossible to find a common denominator between the sublime language of evil spoken by Judge Holden and the somewhat naïve human language of his protégé, the Kid.

and rationalism of "civilized society" (presumably including language as a universal and rational foundation shared by murderers and their victims) and the appalling personal/magical dimension of a "sublime" language reserved for the murderers alone (Lyotard, 1988a). The experience of Auschwitz therefore marked a crisis in language itself, as indicated by Adorno famously questioning whether it was at all possible to write poetry after Auschwitz. Could language carry the burden of semantic and emotional pain after one had been exposed to the filth, degradation, abuse, obliteration, and impotence manifested by the concentration camps? The sad conclusion: language can no longer serve as a universal safety net to be spread out in time of existential distress.

According to Jean-Francois Lyotard (1988b), this crisis of language and culture gives rise to the notion of the "differend," or the dispute that ensues when the discourse of one side cannot be reconciled with the pain in the discourse of the other. A differend emerges when the need to give expression to the dispute becomes urgent. Theorizing the gap makes it possible to release the silenced voices that are not heard in the dominant discourse. Thus, repressed memory, the memory that has been erased and forgotten by the language of the majority, can be recovered. Acknowledging the differend therefore means acknowledging one's own pain and that of others, the inability to say what one wants to say, and the inability to express the inexpressible. Insofar as the differend relates to that which cannot be expressed through language, it also appertains to the sublime Lyotard (1990)[6]. It is the moment at which the distant voice (utterance) that exists beyond one's own linguistic habits is represented as alien and seemingly indecipherable. Paradoxically, it is through this profound encounter with that which cannot be said that one can sense the rejected, the denied, and the "other." If the traumatic experience of Auschwitz reflects the distant and inexpressible echo of the ontological gap denoted by the term "differend," then it also represents the traumatic symptom of a wound that cannot be presented or discussed, along with healing. In other words, the boundaries of the trauma are pushed to the limit where the horror silences the victim and the witness, while at the same time it generates a therapeutic process that holds out for the possibility of symbolic recovery in the world that has collapsed.

It is no coincidence, therefore, that a key concept in postmodern discourse (the differend) closely resembles an issue in the posttraumatic discourse of literature. Both fora speak of the need to find new paradoxical ways to talk about the crisis and the immeasurable suffering and to attempt to express the inexpressible, or as Celan put it, "the snow of that left unspoken."[7] Both

[6]According to Kant's *Critique of Judgment* the "sublime" and the "beautiful" are two categories for defining aesthetic pleasure. The beautiful is an emotional and mental experience arising from rational judgment and aimed at producing pleasure without any purposefulness. The sublime lies beyond the intellectual category of the beautiful because it deals with aesthetic emotion whose object is the infinite, the oceanic, the inexpressible, etc. Thus, the sublime reaches outlying regions whose borders cannot be defined and are consequently dangerous places in which the subject is enveloped in the immeasurable, the thrilling, and the infinite. As the sublime relates to the inexpressible, it is also a sign of our powerlessness to comprehend and "write" reality. In the works of Kafka and McCarthy, the sublime indicates an indecipherable sphere whose essence is associated with both the beauty and the evil in the world. It represents the postmodern category of the "unpresentable," as well as the parallel experience of the fractured effectiveness of the distorted traumatic text that repeatedly punishes the subject.

[7]With a variable key:

With a variable key you unlock the house in which drifts the snow of that left unspoken.

Always what key you choose depends on the blood that spurts from your eye or your mouth or your ear.

You vary the key, you vary the word that is free to drift with the flakes.

What snowball will form round the word depends on the wind that rebuffs you.

Paul Celan, *Von Schwelle zu Schwelle*. © 1955 Deutsche Verlags-Anstalt, München, in der Verlagsgruppe Random House GmbH. English translation © Michael Hamburger, taken from *Poems of Paul Celan* (Third edition, 2007).

Here, "the snow of that left unspoken" fills an abandoned house which the speaker seeks to open with "a variable key," a sort of impromptu skeleton key that opens doors onto the emptiness and frost inside. This is a metaphor for the frozen death of the negative language that speaks of the "unspoken." The word drifts with the flakes and a snowball forms around it, connoting the moment at which it becomes devoid of meaning.

seek to release the voice of the "other" (whether internal or external), who is a victim of the post-trauma. Another procedure that similarly strives to deal with the lacuna at the heart of posttraumatic discourse is suggested by the deconstructivist philosopher, Jacques Derrida (Arav & Gurevitz, 2014; Derrida, 2001).[8] According to Derrida, there is an enduring tendency for violence in Western philosophy which he terms "logocentrism." Characterizing Western thinking from Plato to Marx, logocentrism is a commitment to logos (i.e., authority, speech, the divine, meaning), which entails a search for the source, the core, the one coherent meaning. It therefore pushes out alien, hybrid, or "impure" elements that are inconsistent with the ideology of a dominant authoritative center. Commitment to such a "presence" is challenged by oppositionary forces that seek to tear it apart, similar to the disintegration of the self on the mental level. The whole, integrative presence is eradicated by the posttraumatic experience. The release of the myriad voices running through the mind of the trauma victim is part of a painful process of recovery that requires willingness to feel pain as one acknowledges the violent, inexplicable, and devastating nature of the world. This nature is revealed in different types of writing, such as archival writing, whose sole purpose is to provide a response to the crisis of time and disintegrating, fragmented memory (Derrida [1998], 2002).

According to psychoanalyst Jacques Lacan, traumatic recognition of the crisis in language parallels recognition of the "real." Lacan (1977) defines the real as one of three orders, the others being the imaginary and the symbolic. The real relates to the most painful experience, the time and place of the trauma. It includes perilous regions where the subject is drawn to the extreme, which offers infinite pleasure, but also anxiety, humiliation, and madness. These are the magical regions of the unimaginable, the inexpressible, etc. In other words, the real relates to the trauma, except that the trauma plays out in the heart of everyday experience. That is, the real reflects the ongoing presence of the trauma in daily life and language, which is embodied by the symbolic order as well. Thus, the language of the culture as a whole, which gives presence to the "big Other,"[9] also contains unrecognized elements of the real, the subject's traumatic regions. From this perspective, trauma is an integral part of "normal" perceptible experience and reflects the culture's social life and ideologies. This conceptualization adds a further dimension to the collaboration between postmodern (and post-structuralist) discourse and the cultural discourse of trauma. The innovative nature of Lacan's theory lies in the bold manner in which he positions trauma as part of the repressed, subconscious experience, the product of the desolate symbolic order of culture. His approach allows for a novel view of trauma as the main subject of cultural endeavors, thereby serving as a convenient platform for the analysis of the traumatic elements, those that threaten our very lives, in contemporary literature.

It is clear, therefore, that postmodernism perceives the world, and language, as sites of trauma. Ironically, we can see that the breakdown in the unity of the world and the subject, one of the foundation blocks of postmodernism, is comparable to the posttraumatic experience as described in philosophy, psychology, psychoanalysis, the media, and literature (Felman & Laub, 1992).

[8] The connection between Derrida's deconstructivist philosophy and the discourse of trauma seems only natural. Derrida describes language as a mechanism constantly rejecting the initial meanings of the text. The text contains elements of fragmentation, erasure, ruptures of memory, schizophrenia, and ecstasy. These elements, which undermine the consistency of the text, depict it in traumatic terms. For the link between Derrida and poststructuralism and the discourse of trauma, see, Berger (1999), LaCapra (1998), and Stolorow and Atwood (2014).

[9] The "big Other" refers to absolute otherness that cannot be assimilated through identification. It is impossible to integrate or connect with this radical otherness. It is like an inaccessible father figure that may take the shape of constructions such as the law, the absolute, truth, ideology, and so on. The unconscious inherent in language is the discourse of the "big Other." In Kafka's story, the secret sentence inscribed on the body of the condemned signifies the inaccessibility of the law. In McCarthy's novel, Judge Holden fills the symbolic function of the "big Other," whose violence, both evil and sublime, controls the helpless subjects over whom he rules (Lacan, 1988).

Exposing the trauma reveals the mental and moral price we pay in an effort to maintain the optimistic illusion of modernism and enlightenment (Gray, 2013). Indeed, postmodernism arose in opposition to the belief in the all-encompassing, redemptive unity proposed by modernism. The totalization[10] of the world, a product of this way of thinking, did not allow for heterogeneity, for the multiple voices inhabiting the subject to find expression. Absolutist thinking prevents us from discerning the repressive mechanism silencing other voices that are not part of the redemptive and revolutionary message of modernity. In contrast, the posttraumatic messages in postmodern discourse enable us to trace the symptomatic presence of these voices in contemporary literature.

While the paradoxical representation of the traumatic wound in the postmodern era may come in a variety of forms, all of them, in essence, turn pain into a social commodity (Rothe, 2011). The horrific apocalyptic scenarios that have already played out (such as 9/11) have made trauma a sensational commodity of popular culture sold by the media (Ibrahim, 2011). Literature written (and read) today must therefore contend with the decline of public suffering, with it having become part of the normalized discourse that has converted catastrophe (emotional turmoil, pain, atrocity, "filth") into a legitimate consumer product. Its function is no longer to appall, but on the contrary, to preserve and comfort (Alexander, 2004). What, then, is the role of postmodern literature, which seeks on the one hand to describe the vicious cycle of pain, and on the other to offer new ways to subvert the evil that created it, particularly in an era when the options for social criticism are limited? One of the aims of this chapter is to identify these options.

To conclude, the literary works examined here each strives, in its own manner, to voice criticism of the decline and fall of the world, of language, and of the meaning of suffering, and thereby to contribute to the understanding of posttraumatic discourse in contemporary society. The flight of Icarus and Daedalus, a master craftsmen from Greek mythology, may serve as a metaphor for this condition. The efforts of this pair ended in disaster when the wings Daedalus fashioned for his son could not withstand the destructive and vengeful heat of the sun, a symbol of light, knowledge, and human rationality. When Icarus flew too close to the sun, the wax in his wings melted, plunging the son of the architect/inventor/artist into the sea, where his head hit the bottom and he was killed. This traumatic flight, a naïve yet explicit analogy for both the heights that modernism can reach and its potential to crash, appears again and again in contemporary postmodern literature, which presents the uncompromising, incessant presence of the cultural trauma that has been intensified by commercialization. The depiction of "falling" heroes whose reality is a state of trauma and defeat, and the conversion of language itself into a site of trauma, represent the new trends in the trauma discourse in literature in recent decades. This literature thus presents the "ground zero" of faith, an ongoing dialog with itself and its own death, as a value system. Through the analysis of the works of Kafka and McCarthy below, I will attempt to map the avenues taken by art to cope with the massive presence of traumatic, recurring, and meaningless evil in the contemporary world.

1.2 Franz Kafka's "In the Penal Colony": Trauma, Writing, Body, Play

Any discussion of language as trauma must look to Kafka as its first source or anchor. Stories like "The Judgment," "A Report to an Academy," "AHunger Artist," and "In the Penal Colony" all deal with a single obsession: the desperate

[10] The term "totalization" refers to a hegemonic process in which the dominant ideology forces itself on the interpretation of a political, philosophical, or literary text. Poststructuralist critique, which gave birth to this term, seeks to counter the trend of focusing on the universal unifying nature of the text, arguing in favor of identifying the ruptures within it which allow for minority voices to be heard. In the works of Kafka and McCarthy, the totality of the text can be seen to break down, offering a rare peek at the force striving to enforce totalization on the subject.

attempt to decipher and depict a world of intrinsic and impersonal violence that absurdly connects the victimizers and their victims in a meaningless universe. This condition denies the possibility not only of redemption, but also of comprehending the meaning of the suffering imposed on the victims. The only thing that is certain is that humanity is constantly on trial, awaiting sentence, and can expect neither divine mercy nor the security net provided by knowledge. Indeed, a basic premise of this postmodern pessimism is that it is no longer possible to trust in political, moral, or artistic redemption of the sort previously proposed by the "European way of seeing things" and the spirit of enlightenment.

The story "In the Penal Colony," written in 1919, occupies a unique place in Kafka's work, as it describes a collective trauma that takes place under a colonial, totalitarian regime in which both the victimizers and the victims have a role to play. They are brought together in a wondrous and appalling, almost "sublime," manner around the killing machine that operates in the penal colony, torturing its victims to death by inscribing their sentence on their body. The intricate sadistic device enables the victim to "understand" the sentence by following the "blood writing" carved into his body (which he cannot actually see). This raises the question of the possibility of indirectly deciphering a mysterious text that is hidden from the condemned and most likely not entirely clear to the executioner himself, who is obeying a higher system, a vague enigmatic regime that employs the machine and functions in Lacanian terms as the "big Other," an authority inaccessible to the "self" and to all those involved in the killing. Thus, the execution is performed by a sophisticated apparatus that carefully "programs" the torture of the victim and culminates in his death (at the end of a meticulously crafted 12-h "artistic" performance that causes unimaginable pain), after which the corpse is thrown into a pit dug in advance.

In a certain sense, the death of the victim can be said to be rational in that the killing is orchestrated by a strict capitalist economy, which links the tortured body and the measure of suffering produced, to the quality of the machine, with all its intricate and precisely calibrated parts. It operates with great efficiency, turning out the industrial products for which it was designed: the dead bodies of victims manufactured by the inscription of "blood writing" (the sentence). Through his death, the pain of the condemned man strapped into the machine creates the "law," the mysterious supreme power whose commands the machine obeys. This reading of the story (Fracchia, 2008, pp. 37–38) evokes a comparison between the capitalist processes of production involved in the legal torture of the condemned (which testifies to the power of law) and similar descriptions in Marx's *Capital* ([1867] 1992), in which capitalist production is given manifest physical form, with exploitation and injustice of the workers "carved" into their bodies. Just like Kafka's killing machine,[11] "capital" inscribes its ideological messages on the worker's body. Thebody is brutally yoked to the capitalist system of production for one purpose alone. Through physical pain, the hegemonic messages of class, or the "law" working in its name, are inscribed on the wretched workers chained to the logic of the deadly machine.

To set aside this Marxist interpretation of Kafka's story for a moment, the death of the condemned can also be seen as a ritual, the end product of an "old custom" practiced in the colony from time immemorial. Here, violence occupies a "sublime" sphere beyond the goal of profit-making oppression the execution was meant to promote (as per the Marxist interpretation). In other words, the killing is a special event that cannot be "understood," whose meaning cannot be represented by a decipherable text. As noted above, this reality of an incomprehensible message is shared by the Condemned Man

[11] The Marxist interpretation of the story sees the killing machine as an allegory of the exploitation of the worker by the capitalist system (Scarry, 1985: 246–248). Marx used the metaphor of capitalism "carving" its ideology onto the back of the worker to describe its manner of exploitation. This metaphor, which characterizes Marx's writing in the mid-nineteenth century, sounds particularly Kafkaesque. In Kafka, as well, the tortured body is a physical body that resists any form of "writing," or abstract verbal expression of the message.

and the Officer, as well as by the outside observer dubbed the Traveler, a traveling dignitary who has been asked by the New Commandant to offer his opinion of the legalized killing in the colony being carried out before his eyes. This reality is a precise replication of the scheme of trauma, the inability to understand a life-threatening event, and thus the inability of the victim, witness,[12] or victimizer himself (the Officer) to describe or represent it. This lacuna is expressed in Kafka's text as the inability of the traveler/observer/witness to decipher the sentence written in the drawing he is shown, which is soon to be inscribed on the body of the victim. The same failure is demonstrated when the Officer offers the Traveler the grotesque explanation, spiced with black humor, that the illegible, highly embellished script spells out the ludicrous text, "Be just."

The trauma depicted by the "just" act of killing does not derive only from the horrific evil, whose form may have changed over the generations but which still continues to claim lives, but also from the inability to understand the ontological scheme that puts it in action, the "divine" absolute evil behind it. The lack of understanding is also reflected in an intertwining of the spheres: the rational sphere describing a legalized (albeit controversial) procedure, an impersonal "industrialized" capitalistic execution; and the semimagical sphere of artistic violence verging on the total, the divine. Given the shocking lack of a clear boundary between them, the two spheres complement each other in a sickening, uncanny (Freud, [1919] 2003) manner, despite the fact that, ontologically speaking, they are opposites. At the hybrid moment in which the rational and the irrational (the presentable and the unpresentable, respectively) come together, we find ourselves facing a new ontology that engenders a harsh deconstruction of the very possibility of understanding and interpreting the radical economy of suffering imposed by the all-powerful and arbitrary "big Other." This enigmatic economy establishes and maintains the principles of normalcy in the world portrayed in the story.

In this situation, there is real danger that the appalling rite of suffering will become a nihilistic and formalistic ritual whose absurd demonic survival is an end in and of itself. The purpose of the event appears to be to sanctify the meaningless violence despite the changing identity of the victims over time. Thus, the overriding aim of the procedure is not to pass judgment in a "trial" conducted on the bloody body of the condemned, but to perpetuate the official practice of the "artistic" killing project for generations to come. What this implies is the consecration of form over content: unfathomably violent formalism takes the shape of an artistic event.

Indeed, Kafka stresses the artistic aspects of the killing machine (the "device" or "apparatus"

---

[12] An integral part of the question of representing trauma relates to the collapse of reliable witnesses, whose function is to testify to the trauma and insert it into the historical memory of a society. This issue has received considerable attention, e.g., Felman and Laub (1992), LaCapra (1998), and Laub (1995). It is regarded as a significant problem, since, as Felman and Laub explain, "to bear witness is to take responsibility for truth" (1992: 204). The question is whether the posttraumatic witness is capable of taking on this responsibility, since the testimony of the survivor is generally regarded as unreliable, based on an imagined narrative, biased by personal memory, or influenced by present fantasies, all of which fundamentally alter the construction of the traumatic narrative in the mind. Another problem with the survivor's testimony is that it is by nature fragmented and incomplete, attesting less to what occurred and more to the emotional pathological response to the event as a result of the suffering experienced by the witness. Even the testimony of the outside observer to a traumatic event is considered suspect since it raises pointed questions about the circumstances that enabled this individual to survive, and how those circumstances affect the reliability of the report. Furthermore, the "crisis of witnessing" that distinguishes contemporary critical discourse is associated with the construction of memory and testimony by agents of memory such as cinema and television, which contribute to producing the visual image of truth as part of the "rhetoric of truth" disseminated by the media.

In Kafka's story as well, the issue of the Traveler's testimony is critical to understanding the meaning of evil in the text. It is because he anticipates that the Traveler will present the New Commandant with damning testimony that the Officer takes the drastic step of submitting his own body to the machine in a masochistic and impossible desire to become one with the source of power of the "big Other." Moreover, the witness's hasty retreat from the valley of death does not necessarily ensure that the "enlightened world" he represents will immediately take a stance against the dictatorial regime in order to end the reign of terror in the penal colony.

as the Officer calls it) and of the execution itself, carried out as a carefully choreographed ritualistic performance. The structure of the machine is described in aesthetic detail: "It was a huge affair The Bed and the Designer were of the same size and looked like two dark wooden chests. The Designer hung about two meters above the bed; each of them was bound at the corners with four rods of brass that almost flashed out rays in the sunlight. Between the chests shuttled the HARROW on the ribbon of steel." (Kafka, [1919] 2002, p 100). The heart of the device, the "harrow," equipped with glass needles that carve the sentence in blood on the body of the victim, is also described formalistically. The machine is encased in glass, like a museum exhibition case that enables visitors to enjoy the aesthetic object. The brass rods of the apparatus gleam, and the harrow is shaped like a human body and was designed by a master craftsman to ensure that the excruciating process will produce the greatest possible physical effect.[13] At the end of the meticulously contrived torture, the dead body falls in an "incredibly soft flight" into the pit. The entire procedure is described as the coordinated operation of rollers that drive the harrow and carve the murderous sentence into the flesh of the condemned. Everything seems to be aimed at maximizing the atrocity, hierarchically, functionally, and aesthetically. To use the term coined by Deleuze and Guattari (1985), it is a "desiring machine" intended to generate the greatest amount of general desire possible. It is a system of production whose output is excitement and desire, even if its nature is pain and death. The pronounced aestheticization of the machine serves to underline the fact that it is an all-encompassing system shared by both victims and victimizers, the two groups described by Deleuze and Guattari as the "mechanics," an integral part of the machinery.[14]

In addition to the aestheticization of the apparatus and its depiction as an omnipotent "desiring machine," the inscription on the body of the condemned also abounds with aesthetic elements. "The script itself runs round the body only in a narrow girdle; The rest of the body is reserved for the embellishments." (Kafka, [1919] 2002, p 105), the Officer explains. They are empty decorations and embellishments that in no way help to decipher the text carved into the body. This "secret" message, hidden within an elaborate, artistic, "calligraphy," is only legible to the Officer, who operates the machine. The total absurdity of his testimony, which attributes the execution to a minor disciplinary infraction of the Condemned Man—he offended his superiors—merely magnifies the atrocity. Similarly, at the pinnacle of its popularity, the execution carried out through lethal writing was an imposing ritual, a spectacle performed "in front of hundreds of eyes," including wide-eyed children, all enthralled by the aesthetic workings of the machine and drawing immense pleasure from the mute suffering of the condemned, denied even the right to scream by a lump of felt stuffed in his mouth.

Clearly, then, Kafka centers his description around the aesthetics of violence, expressed in the death/pleasure desires of the spectators, the Officer (who functions not only as executioner, but also as absurd judge), and the victim alike.

[13] The apparatus, or the killing machine, can serve as an allegory of the mechanics of power. The upper section, the inscriber, is the supreme power with its mysterious ideology that shines down from above and demands that its orders be carried out by the lower ranks. The middle rank, the harrow, is responsible for operations. Made of a series of glass needles, it carves the "blood writing" of the sentence into the body of the condemned. The lowest section, the quivering bed to which the condemned is strapped, represents the metaphoric possibility of "sleep": the man's subconscious directs him against his will to absorb repressive ideological power gleaming down on him. This power normalizes and creates the subjects under it.

[14] According to Deleuze and Guattari (1985), desiring is not generated by the principle of lacuna; it is not movement toward the object in which it is represented. Instead, desiring is a machine activated by the "positive" and productive. The desiring machine produces an infinite series of sensations. In Kafka, the breakdown of the machine stems from its "strong degree of unity," as the authors explain at the end of the first chapter of their book. Thisunity, into which "the man enters completely," may halt the random movement of desiring, and consequently, the machine itself falls apart.

Indeed, throughout the process, the victim cooperates in his annihilation, in some strange way even appearing to find joy in the pain. Everyone is drawn into the aesthetics of the horror. The Officer, for example, realizing that the Traveler's report may be damning and may put an end to what he refers to as his "life's work," immediately releases the lucky Condemned Man and takes his place under the harrow. And then something wondrous happens: the machine cooperates fully with the new body within it: "The officer, however, had turned to the machine. It had been clear enough previously that he understood the machine well, but now it was almost staggering to see that how he managed it and how it rise and sink several times till it was adjusted to the right position for receiving him; attached only the edge of the Bed and already it was vibrating;" (Kafka, [1919] 2002, p 118). The collusion between violent evil, represented by the machine at work, and its changing victims is symptomatic of the reality portrayed in the story. It is the depiction of a horrific interface between the human body and mechanized evil, which is inhuman and uncontrollable. The instrument of murder (or the murderer) and the victim have become one. The former murderer (the Officer, decked out in a fancy uniform with silver braids and tassels) is now the new victim, offering himself willingly to ensure that the ritual of execution in the modern valley of death, this "ancient rite" of human sacrifice, will survive forever. The Officer's suicide is indicative of his nearly psychotic devotion to the "big Other." It is an attempt to identify with the inaccessible source of divine/satanic power, which he construes as the "law." The result is the destruction not only of the man, but also of the machine. In an extreme act of lawlessness, it leaves behind the controlled violence that characterized its normal operation and becomes a formless instrument of murder that annihilates both itself and its naïve and fanatic victim, who wanted only to "unite" with it.

Similarly, the aesthetic sphere in the story eagerly works hand in hand with the sphere of pure violence. Here, too, there is a perverse symbiosis that maintains the ritualistic atrocity which must continue, regardless of the "human flesh" that feeds the killing machine (the regime), whose hunger is never satiated. The repetitive operation of the machine is compulsive. Rather than processing, or "understanding," the early symptom, preserved in the ritualistic memory of the killing rite, the Officer (and the machine) prefer to configure this symptom of the past (the repressed memory) as a pattern of behavior in the present. The machine/officer (they exist in symbiosis) perpetuate the type of "Repetition compulsion" described by Freud ([1914] 1958). The machine turns the unprocessed symptom in the memory into the object of perverse ecstasy for the present self. It appears to be beyond human control, becoming the metaphysical embodiment of the repressed traumatic evil that cannot be contained, represented, identified with, or "worked through" in order to comprehend the world through the tragic experience of pain.

The breakdown of the machine, in an act of self-destruction, can be seen as acknowledgement of the failure to deal with the repressed memory at the core of the past history of the murderous law that administers the penal colony. Consequently, the secret "artistic message" inscribed on the body of the condemned is also incomprehensible, and the text the Officer "deciphers" for the Traveler (and witness to the killing) contains an element of grotesque, sarcastic evil. "Be just," he spells out, seemingly asking the foreigner to exercise fair judgment in regard to his horrendous "life's work." Since his efforts appear doomed to failure in light of the damning report expected from the Traveler, he opts for an absurd suicide in order to preserve the existence of the violent ritual in the colony. As we have seen, however, this "voluntary" act is not a solution, but a problem: it intensifies the psychotic symptom by "acting out" the compulsive repetition, thereby causing the entire system to collapse in on itself.

The Officer's choice of suicide might be interpreted in a different manner as well, not only as a crucial turning point in the story, but also as symptomatic of a body rebelling against the law to which it is supposedly subject. Unlike the first body, that of the condemned prisoner, which surrenders itself to the bloody sentence, the second sacrificial body, that of the Officer, resists the inscription of the sentence in its flesh. The act of writing, however indecipherable, does not occur, and the Officer's death is not described as a just or lawful process (an "execution"), but as "murder, pure and simple." His body thus rebels against the very act of writing, it protests against the will of the law to bring it under its control, to write it into the legitimate representations of society. From this perspective, the subject can be created only through the codes inscribed on its body. That is, only the act of writing enables the narrativization of the body (Grosz, 1995, p. 33). This rebellious body, which Lyotard refers to as an "aesthetic" or "infant" bodily mode (Lyotard, 1989; Neal, 1999), resists being written as a story, refuses to be represented in the culture. It is primitive and heterogeneous, an outlaw seeking freedom and denying signification. It exists within the traumatic presence of the symptom, here and now, and is not represented by the (legalized) "writing" of the sentence. Its rebellion is apparent from the very beginning, as the mechanism of law is incapable of "digesting" it.[15] As a result, the entire system spins out of control, leading to the apocalyptic destruction of the apparatus and creating a situation of sublime horror that can no longer be represented within the confines of the law. Thus, through a radical act of self-sabotage, the "aesthetic body," expressing the poetic protest of terror, overrides the lawful body (on which the sentence was meant to be inscribed) and reopens the issue of legalized killing in the penal colony.

This raises the question of how we are to understand the hasty retreat of the Traveler from the site of terror, the penal colony, whose landscape is reminiscent of hell in Dante's *Divine Comedy*. Does his escape indicate the moral bankruptcy of the enlightened world, demonstrated by the fact that this representative of the liberal "European way of seeing things" cannot face the horror of the real when the sentence is not carried out through the symbolic experience of inscribing the text on the victim's body? Or perhaps the opposite is the case, perhaps his escape is to be read as ironic identification with the broken machine, with the law that has suffered a fatal blow? The machine itself appears to have decided to "take the gloves off" and stop maintaining the illusory façade that it is engaged in the artistic, "aesthetic" representation of the atrocity. Instead, it takes it to new apocalyptic heights. "Out of alignment," it breaks down and becomes nothing more than a meat grinder, leaving intact the traumatic message of an age of "sound and fury" that is beyond the modernistic hope of redemption.

Or could it be the opposite? Could the magnification of the horror, represented by the machine self-destructing, paradoxically be meant to offer a ray of hope for change, the possibility that the dictatorial/colonial reign of terror will destroy the ontological underpinnings of its own evil regime? As is often the case in Kafka's works, here, too, the answer appears to be "all of the above." Kafka's texts preclude any attempt to interpret them, to clarify and comprehend the meaning of the terror. "The horror! The horror!", Kurtz's last words in Joseph Conrad's *Heart of Darkness* (1902) as well as the concluding line of Francis Ford Coppola's *Apocalypse Now* (1979), can also serve to connote the bankruptcy

[15] Lyotard's interpretation of "In the Penal Colony" relates to the contrast between the rebellion of the primitive, anarchistic aesthetic body, which is not represented, and the obedience of the body inscribed by society and recognized by the law. "Law," here, refers to the way in which the human body becomes part of the community and society, the way in which the law conceptualizes and generalizes the body so that it will be understood, subject to judgment and punishment, etc. According to Lyotard, the law does not recognize the natural body before it is established in the dominant cultural discourse. Indeed, the writing cut into the body of the condemned in Kafka's story is a clearly visible text, since constantly washing away the blood is a vital part of the operation of the apparatus. However, when the Officer decides to commit suicide and places himself in the machine, he becomes a resistant aesthetic body that does not submit to the authoritative and controlling writing of the law. Given this fact, it is not surprising that the law "went wild," that the killing machine lost its power and could no longer write the social law (the sentence) on the body of its victim. For this interpretation, which links Kafka with the postmodern philosophy of Lyotard, see Curtis (1999).

of the "comprehensible world" in Kafka's story, as well as the entire history of the penal colony. Its mechanism of legalized murder is halted when the most extreme violence is directed not at the body of the victim, but at the method of punishment itself. Ultimately, the system of internal destruction, the mechanism of self-annihilation which is built into the apparatus, has the final say.

The parties that are witness to the twisted scene of horror are therefore given the impossible task of interpreting its meaning. The reality seems to freeze both the reader and the Traveler in a state of traumatic paralysis in which the history of the customary punishment in the penal colony is wiped out and sinks into oblivion. Trauma becomes the fate of the Traveler, the observer/judge who represents normative humanity still nostalgic for a world in which terms like "law," "justice," "guilt," and "defense" are not just empty words used as a villainous caricature of enlightened values. This "European" world offers no more than a restrained response to the traumatic ritual played out before its eyes. The"enlightened witness" makes do with a visit to the grotesque grave of the Old Commandant. Despite his opposition to the ancient rite of execution, he flees the colony precipitately, like Jonah fleeing Nineveh without considering the consequences of his departure (Jon. 1). In other words, the supposedly wise judge, who condemns the "evil judge," the Officer who commits suicide by submitting his own body to sentencing, cannot necessarily bring about a historic change in the annals of the penal colony, and chooses instead to leave the tainted landscape behind as quickly as possible.[16]

The hurried departure of the Traveler, the "honorable" enlightened observer, is more readily understandable if we consider the difficulty of deciphering the meaning of the sentence administered by the killing machine as it cuts wounds/words into the body of the condemned. "You've seen that it's not easy to figure out the inscription with your eyes," the Officer explains to the puzzled Traveler, "but our man deciphers it with his wounds." The question is whether the victim does indeed decipher the symbolic message through his real pain. One possibility is that he does not, that, in fact, no one can comprehend the text: not the victim; not the observer, who needs it to be spelled out for him in order to judge the degree of humanity of the penal colony's method of punishment; and not even the Officer, who can seemingly read the script but conveys it in a biased context of self-interest or a ludicrous context devoid of any logic. He reports that it says "Be just," implying that it means for the Traveler to "be just" in passing judgment on the enigmatic event.

This is an indication of the severe problem of communication in the story. The Officer speaks French, a language no one else, including the Condemned Man, is familiar with; the text carved into the body of the condemned is illegible and undecipherable; and the various sides have no way to refer to the incommensurable gap in interpretation, that is, they are totally incapable of defining the "differend." All of them appear to be obeying the radical authority that holds sway (the"big Other"), which remains mysterious and indeterminate. In the colony's form of punishment, all sides are party to a performative act of naked power that reifies its existence before the crowd of cheering awestruck spectators watching the "blood economy" through which the colonial regime "reveals" itself to its native subjects. Its lethal public presence, demonstrated on the body of the condemned, instills an awareness of horror. The function of the practice, as Foucault (1977) shows in *Discipline and Punish: the Birth of the Prison*, is to make the occasion a public spectacle in which the punishment is "absorbed" into the flesh of the offender, while

[16]The hasty departure of the Traveler, who is a witness to the horrific acts in the penal colony, might be compared to the behavior of witnesses called upon to contend with trauma in the works of Camus. *The Plague* portrays a situation of absurd traumatic evil with which the people in the city are struggling. The witnesses to the evil, Jean Tarrou and Dr. Rieux, fight the plague and ultimately bring it to an end. *The Fall* depicts a different situation. Here, a "judge-penitent" who happens to see the suicide of a young woman cannot fulfill his moral duty as a witness. He avoids testifying, unwilling to face evil and rise up against it.

at the same time enhancing control over the populace by turning the machine's theater of horrors into an "ideological state apparatus" (to use Althusser's term) that normalizes the subjects' thinking and thereby precludes any subversive notions (Cumberland, 2013, p. 207).

The pronounced aesthetics of the design of the chilling process adds to the blinkering of the masses: extravagant aestheticization of the apparatus of naked power makes it possible to control the specious thinking of the oppressed. In contrast to modernism, which employs the aesthetic sphere in its efforts to create a better political and moral world, exposing the contemptible stratagem of its use to promote oppression (Benjamin, 1986), postmodernism contends that art joins with the meaningless violence of the crazed apparatus, collaborating with it and glorifying it. In this traumatic version of art, it takes no positive initiative to counter violence by means of what Benjamin dubs the "politicization of art," that is, revealing the aesthetic artifice and identifying the political interests it serves. Consequently, the only option available to art is to lie. The aesthetic calligraphy embellishing the text on the body of the condemned in Kafka's story is empty decorations that serve merely to accentuate the naked, total, random violence they hide.

It goes without saying that "In the Penal Colony" also relates to "writing" per se. Writing fulfills two functions in the story: it phrases the text of the sentence; and it carries out that sentence by the very act of being written. Writing is thus a performative event that reifies the meaning of the text on the naked body of the victim. It is stripped of its abstract symbolic dimension and becomes an undertaking that physically implements its intent, an action (Butler, 1993) that cannot be undone or appealed. This is an expression of its inherent power. Writing ends in death, that is, the completion of the text is synonymous with the death of the victim. The text is therefore lethal, the work of a sophisticated killing machine of words that merges the various linguistic functions together and channels them all toward the Lacanian "real," where there is only anxiety, madness, abjection (Kristera, 1982),[17] and death (Canfield, 2003). Symbolic language remains unreadable, flawed, and incomprehensible to all parties. The Traveler cannot decipher the script and the condemned man only comes to understand it when it kills him. Moreover, the various sides do not understand each other's language and are incommensurably unfamiliar with their manner of speaking. They do not recognize the "differend," which could open a window onto a deeper philosophical apprehension of the pain of the "other" or the crisis of language, an insight that might unite them.

Thus, the text collapses because of its incomprehensible arbitrariness, without the users being able to recognize the "différance" (a term coined by Derrida) that undermines the "logos" and nullifies sensible meaning. Once again, language is seen to be a central site of breakdown, analogous to the fractured body of the condemned. Even in death, this body remains undefined, unknowable, unsignified by social codes, or in other words, meaningless. The terminal violence of the text is therefore fundamental and primal. It is a violence of unexplained justification that turns abuse into both a generative and a preserving act through

[17]The concept of "the abject" is drawn from Julia Kristeva's "Powers of Horror: An Essay on Abjection" (1982). It refers to the element of baseness, contempt, filth, and degradation in human experience, the primitive narcissistic nature of the organism, associated with amorphic bodily fluids, in its prelinguistic phase. The "abject" is the sense of panic communicated by the body before it becomes a "self." The humiliating presence of the void, the presence of the other in what could have been the self, arouses horror. The situation depicted in Kafka's story might also be said to present the human body as it loses the self, as if it were in the first phase of bodily fluids and other degrading metabolic functions. The condition created by Kafka's killing machine could be seen as a supreme effort to demean the body and display it in total, horrifying breakdown and regression. For this interpretation of "In the Penal Colony," see Muller (2006). Similarly, in McCarthy's novel the body seems to break through its boundaries. The Judge's body is carnivalesque, demonstrating excess by its unrestrained physicality. Through its grotesque proportions, the carnival body illustrates the conjunction between humor and horror. See Covington (2011) and Stinson (2007).

which naked power controls the totalitarian reality portrayed in the story.

The ontological dimension of writing as an absurd act of murder (similar to the sentences carried out in other stories by Kafka and in Camus's *The Stranger*) is accentuated even more by the use of the aesthetic terms of "play" to describe the inscription on the body. Playing is an intense aesthetic activity that highlights the imaginary nature of the event, which is limited to the autonomous world in which the "rules of the game" apply. These rules are explicitly distinct from the laws and behavioral codes in the real world (Huizinga, 2014). In Kafka's story, however, the writing steps outside the borders of the autonomic aesthetic because it is lethal: the script kills. This is a game of death, not an autonomous flight of imagination characteristic of humanity, but a loss of humanity behind a veil of meaningless artistic embellishment. The "writing"[18] cannot be understood in terms of either the autonomous aesthetic world or the world of justice established by law. The text is a surrealist caricature of the sentence that does not even pretend to reflect transparency of the legal proceedings. The procedure begins with the presumption of guilt, or as the Officer explains, "guilt is always beyond a doubt."

[18]In his early book *Of Grammatology* ([1967] 1976), Derrida introduces the term "writing" (écriture) as a central concept of deconstruction. It deals not with representations of the world, but rather creates a world of multiplicity that stresses the signifier, not the signified (i.e., the idea or definitive meaning). It therefore continually rejects meanings, expressing the flow of the text that denies rigid conceptualization. Applying this concept to Kafka's story raises the question of whether it is the multiplicity of hybrid meanings carved in blood by the writing on the body of the condemned that makes it impossible for the parties to the ritual to decipher the text. This would not appear to be the case, as here the writing literally kills. The condemned man understands the script only through his pain, which cannot be represented in words (i.e., symbolically). The meaning of "pain" cannot be comprehended, but only felt in a semiconscious state, which is, in essence, traumatic. If for Derrida writing frees because it recognizes the fragmentation and breakdown of meaning, for Kafka writing leaves its victim in a state of desperation. Screaming in pain, he is entirely immersed in a physical reality of suffering that cannot be understood, deciphered, etc.

The fractured, incomprehensible text is thus a traumatic event that cannot be represented or deciphered by language. From the start, it foregoes its communicative function, breaking down before our eyes just as the machine carrying out the sentence breaks down, just as the tortured body of the condemned breaks down. Along with them, the legitimacy of the "source," the baseless "logos" of the speakers and writers (the inscribers), the agents of power and authority over the body of the victim, breaks down as well. This senseless violence prevails over all the participants in the narrative event: the third-person narrator, who is evidently not omniscient and does not "understand" the story he is telling; the condemned who does not understand the sentence until its violent completion; and the reader, who is shocked by the lack of any indication of an explanation for the event or a "solution" heralding future remedy of the absurd violence. Nor are the witnesses to the traumatic event capable of understanding it on the symbolic level or of issuing a public warning against it. As Felman and Laub (1992) demonstrate, there are no witnesses to the evil that generates trauma. The only witness who might have carried the memory of traumatic evil outside the penal colony, the Traveler, who was apparently given a mandate by the New Commandant to appraise the justice and legitimacy of the execution ritual, has trouble finding the "way out" of the horrific spectacle described in the story. Although he states firmly that he is "opposed to this procedure," he cannot stop it. Ironically, it is his implied humanitarian intervention that causes the Officer to switch roles and go from executioner to victim in an absurd and desperate attempt to restore the killing power of the crumbling machine and promote the obsessive notion that the execution ritual must continue for all eternity, whatever the cost.

The testimony of the witness, the last human barrier to the atrocity, collapses because it immortalizes the death scene and makes it even more absurd. In addition, it is hard to ignore the fact that the Traveler hastens to depart from the penal colony, and we are told nothing of his future plans, what he means to do, and whether he has any intention of taking the issue further, that is, informing the world of the injustice and horrific acts whose logic he has been unable to determine. Thus, at the end of the story the reader is left with the trauma, not knowing if it will be reported to the untainted, "enlightened" world, which in any case is powerless to deal with it firmly. The only hint we are given of any resistance are a few bizarre mysterious words regarding a prophecy that the Old Commandant will rise from the grave and lead his followers in a preposterous rebellion against the "aesthetic of violence" that has taken over the colony and the world.

One final issue regarding the breakdown of writing relates specifically to the writing of Kafka and its traumatic dimension. Writing is presented in the story as an act of self-violence, a murderous inscribing machine that destroys itself and its creator, leaving him with no illusions as to the heroic status of the writer as the redeemer of the world. Can we not see an analogy here between the avoidance of representing and deciphering the text inscribed on the body of the condemned and Kafka's avoidance of any attempt to decipher the demonic, traumatic world around him?[19] If the analogy is true, and the killing machine is merely a brutal metaphor for the self-destructive "text machine," can writing serve as an instrument of release from the trauma or does it simply perpetuate it? In other words, although literature can report on the traumatic nature of reality, it is sabotaged by the absurdity of writing itself. The allegory of the undeciphered text of evil might therefore be seen as ars poetica revealing the infirmity of Kafka's writing. Literature can reach only to the edge of "negative dialectics" (Adorno, 1973); it can report on the abyss of the text, on the unfulfilled desire to uncover the traumatic secret inherent in writing itself, but it cannot present the positive synthesis that emerges at end of the conflicted act—the meaning of writing.

1.3 Cormac McCarthy: The (Traumatic) Intoxication of Dirty Death

> "This you see here, these ruins wondered at by tribes of savages, do you not think that this will be again? Aye. And again. With other people, with other sons" (McCarthy, [1985] 1992, p. 141).

Despite the difference in time between "In the Penal Colony," written at the start of the twentieth century, and Cormac McCarthy's *Blood Meridian: Or the Evening Redness in the West*, from the end of the century, there is a strong connection between them. Kafka writes about the terrifying landscapes of European reason during World War I; McCormac writes about the nightmarish landscapes of America's historical memory of the Mexican-American war and its aftermath in the mid-nineteenth century. Kafka relates to the collapse of justice grounded in Kantian reason in an absurd, violent world in which it takes the form of punishment and death rituals; McCormac regards the murderous ritual of killing off the Native Americans in the regions along the border with Mexico (the classic setting for Westerns) to be the birth of violence as a fundamental American experience. Furthermore, the works of the two authors reveal a basic common denominator: a perception of the violent manner in which language traps us in a meaningless traumatic reality, and the corresponding proposition that the dialectics between violent ritualistic evil and the futile yearning for redemption delineates

[19] In his early book *Of Grammatology* ([1967] 1976), Derrida introduces the term "writing" (écritures) as a central concept of deconstruction. It deals not with representations of the world, but rather creates a world of multiplicity that stresses the signifier, not the signified (i.e., the idea or definitive meaning). It therefore continually rejects meanings, expressing the flow of the text that denies rigid conceptualization. Applying this concept to Kafka's story raises the question of whether it is the multiplicity of hybrid meanings carved in blood by the writing on the body of the condemned that makes it impossible for the parties to the ritual to decipher the text. This would not appear to be the case, as here the writing literally kills. The condemned man understands the script only through his pain, which cannot be represented in words (i.e., symbolically). The meaning of "pain" cannot be comprehended, but only felt in a semi-conscious state, which is, in essence, traumatic. If for Derrida writing frees because it recognizes the fragmentation and breakdown of meaning, for Kafka writing leaves its victim in a state of desperation. Screaming in pain, he is entirely immersed in a physical reality of suffering that cannot be understood, deciphered, etc.

the narrow borders of humanity in the contemporary world.

Like Kafka, McCarthy centers his story around a killing machine, in his case, a war machine. And here, too, violence does not appear as the opposite pole to rational justice, but as an integral part of it. In Kafka's story, the Officer is judge and executioner, and ultimately willing victim as well. The same can be said of Judge Holden in McCarthy's novel. Both works tell a tale of continuous death rituals conducted by their "judges" with dubious zeal. And at the core of both are strategies of colonial punishment/abuse carried out on the bodies of the natives (the condemned in "In the Penal Colony" and Native Americans in *Blood Meridian*). The two writers describe a mechanism of colonial power that involves performative abuse which appears on the body as a public testament to guilt, and compels the natives to submit to the excessive violence of the colonizer.[20] Shockingly, the works of Kafka and McCarthy also highlight the disturbing link between murderous violence and beauty. Both describe a powerfully aesthetic world created out of war and death, a world in which the aesthetics of violence creates social unity.

The two authors also portray trauma as a primal force. In their worlds, trauma has generative power; although destructive, it is a potent life force as well. In *Blood Meridian*, it is in a constant state of acting out, expressed in the feverish activity of the killing machine operated against the Native Americans. It thereby embodies the full potential of capitalist logic, which exploits trauma[21] for its own benefit. The trade in Indian scalps finances the American irregulars, the violent movement of settlers westward is motivated by imperialist aims as well as economic advantages, and so on. Although the horror of death is set in different historical and geographical landscapes in the two works, they describe a similar transhistorical experience: the yearning of representatives of civilization for the sadomasochistic sublime of death, the desire to rise above limited human language and reach the treacherous mythical heights where violence is normalized and becomes an intrinsic part of the thinking and consciousness of victimizers and victims alike. Forboth Kafka and McCarthy, the encounter with the breakdown of language is an impassable barrier. Language becomes the place where the horrible, and even the "pornographic," meet the wondrous and infinite. This barrier is used to create a caricature of the modernist project of freedom (Dacus, 2011).

Blood Meridian presents the journey of a character known only as "the kid" through a series of atrocities in the borderlands as he rides along with his savage mentor and spiritual guide, Judge Holden. As in all classic Westerns, the final battle is waged between the innocence of the kid and the satanic evil of the Judge (Benson, 2011). This struggle, which has a religious, ritualistic nature, takes place in the mythical space of the genre, a squalid saloon replete with whores, drunks, and a dancing bear dressed in a crinoline, who is shot to death on stage. The description of the saloon corresponds with the picture of hell in the tradition of the Yuma Indian tribes: a place of games and dancing among the dead (Peebles, 2003, p. 240). Indeed, the whole scene is set in a saloon of horrors, where lethal temptations have the final word.

[20] For a postcolonial interpretation of "In the Penal Colony," see Boehmer (1993), Cumberland (2013), Kohn (2005), Lemon (2011), McClintock (2004), Walder (1998), West (1985), and Zilcosky (2003). The mechanism of colonial oppression, which imposes and "writes" the history of the trauma on the bodies of the natives, appears both in Kafka and in McCarthy. In Kafka's story, it is a penal colony run by a reign of draconian punishment directed toward criminals breaking colonial laws. In McCarthy's novel it is the colonial history of America and the appalling acts carried out by the settlers on Native Americans in the mid-nineteenth century. Both works express harsh criticism of the brutal apparatus of oppression of the colonizer, which shapes the mentality of the oppressor and oppressed alike.

[21] Capitalist logic is behind the murderous mechanism in both works. In Kafka, the killing machine represents industrialization of the execution rite. The purpose of its operation is to ensure the survival of the totalitarian capitalist regime, which exploits technology for the political oppression of the population. In McCarthy, the gang's killing raids on the Indians are also designed to further capitalist aims by taking over the territory and resources of the natives.

At the end of the story, the kid's death in the deadly arms of the Judge in an outhouse signifies the ultimate degradation of humanity and the unquestioned victory of the "dirty" and demonic over the alternative possibilities of catharsis and redemption. In this state, all that is left are the remnants, or "excretions" of the body. The traumatic reduction of existence to anal matter is an expression of the crisis in reality and the breakdown of the language used to describe it: language itself becomes "befouled" when it depicts the collapse of the human body into a pool of excrement.

Paradoxically, the devastation brings together the divine and the contemptible, the "pure" and the "impure," the humorous and the demonic, creating a "dark revelation"—one of many on the road to the shaping of America's traumatic history (LaCapra, 1998).

> Far out on the desert to the north dust spouts rose wobbling and augured the earth and some said they'd heard of pilgrims borne aloft like dervishes in those mindless coils to be dropped broken and bleeding upon the desert again and there perhaps to watch the thing that had destroyed them lurch onward like some drunken djinn and resolve itself once more into the elements from which it sprang. Out of that whirlwind no voice spoke and the pilgrim lying in his broken bones may cry out and in his anguish he may rage, but rage at what? And if the dried and blackened shell of him is found among the sands by travelers to come yet who can discover the engine of his ruin? (McCarthy, [1985] 1992, p. 106)

There is no explanation for the extreme violence in the book. The dervishes fly in the air, but their flight is "mindless." There is rage at this human defeat, but is there anything to address it to, anyone to blame? Total ruin is a fact "on the ground," but what is the theological principle that justifies it? Once again we are faced with the absolutist rule of chaotic death, the "dirty death" that generates trauma, whose dark logic does not go beyond the fierce desire to turn living by the sword into a crazed universal human ideal. The main effect of this tale of devastation is obliteration—the obliteration of threatening nostalgia, of history, of memories, of the piles of ruins that reconstruct the vision of destruction in the same place at a different time. This principle, which echoes the compulsive repetition of death and prevents historical time from flowing on, marks the borders of the trauma depicted in the novel.

> "It makes no difference what men think of war, said the judge. War endures. As well ask men what they think of stone. War was always here. Before man was, war waited for him. The ultimate trade awaiting its ultimate practitioner" (McCarthy, [1985] 1992, p. 245).

As with Kafka's killing machine, here, too, the ritualistic presence of war and violence are enduring primal elements that invariably find man guilty. And here, too, the killings are the work of an "ultimate practitioner" of his trade, a master artisan, again linking death and beauty. The opinions voiced by the learned "judge" (whether the character is meant to be a caricature of a satanic man ironically labeled "judge" or a former judge turned mass murderer), which contain echoes of a Nietzschean pantheism and proto-fascistic notions, are not mere theoretical musings. Throughout the story, he puts them into action through atrocious acts that verge on pornographic perversion. He abuses the scalped Indians, sadistically throws two pups into a river, and plays judge and executioner for infirm raiders or horses that jeopardize the future of the apocalyptic campaign of killing to which he is committed, as if he is obeying the command of some mysterious dark master. His depraved acts, which trigger the heights of his philosophical teachings, are especially chilling and heinous because they are also the favorite pastimes of this "great ponderous djinn" (McCarthy, [1985] 1992, p. 88). His broad education is troubling as well. He is well-versed in paleontology, astronomy, mineralogy, natural philosophy, ontological theories on the nature of being, and more. Yet this man, who is in the habit of lecturing knowledgeably about the nature of man and the world, is also a despicable monster who leads a gang of degenerate murderers. McCarthy paints the sinister portrait of a pedophile, a psychopath (reminiscent of Chigurh in his novel *No Country for Old Men*) whose mental disorder and murderous philosophy go hand in hand in horrifying harmony with the "humanism," aesthetics, education, macabre sense of humor, intelligence, and fondness for rhetoric that he displays to a band of mad death-defying outlaws as they make their way through life in total darkness.

This darkness is accentuated by the fact that he is a "judge," supposedly an agent of the law, whose knowledge of history and progressive education is turned into a sickening caricature and whose legal expertise becomes a cynical lever for his ruthlessness. The figure of a violent savage judge might be expected to surprise us. However, if we consider Walter Benjamin's "Critique of Violence" (1986), we may realize that violence lies at the foundation of the metaphysics of law, as it is both a generative and a preserving principle. Turning a judge into a violent judge exposes the sublime, uplifting, dark moments when the law is seen to be stripped bare, primal, baseless, an unrestrained, uninhibited expression of pure primitive violence, before it is covered over by forests of symbols designed to hide the pre-legitimized abyss from which it sprang (Dorson, 2013). The distinct constitutive violence of the law also resounds through "In the Penal Colony." There, too, the rite of execution by killing machine is construed as a substantive organizing principle of the life of the society itself, explaining the attempt to preserve it for generations to come.

The character of the learned psychopath is fully revealed in his perverse vision of the "suzerain," the ultimate power that defines existence. As the judge explains: "Only nature can enslave man and only when the existence of each last entity is routed out and made to stand naked before him will he be properly suzerain of the earth" (McCarthy, [1985] 1992, p. 195). What distinguishes the suzerain, according to the demonic judge, is that he is the supreme ruler who "rules even where there are other rulers." He seals fates; he is the Minister of Death. This is precisely how the judge behaves throughout; he is responsible for a series of violent and sadistic events described by McCarthy (similar to Kafka) with a distant objectivity. After a while, this style of writing ceases to appear menacing to the reader.

The radical nature of the process becomes clearer if we turn our attention to the virtuoso manner in which the sadistic and suicidal violence that radiates from a band of wandering pilgrims/mercenaries is blended with the sublime inspiring beauty of the colors of the desert, the rocks painted red with blood in the sunset, etc. These cinematographic spectacles, which we are accustomed to seeing in Westerns, are given new meaning by McCarthy.

> They rode on and the sun in the east flushed pale streaks of light and then a deeper run of color like blood seeping up in sudden reaches flaring planewise and where the earth drained up into the sky at the edge of creation the top of the sun rose out of nothing like the head of a great red phallus until it cleared the unseen rim and sat squat and pulsing and malevolent behind them. (McCarthy, [1985] 1992, p. 43)

With the elements of extraordinary beauty fused with elements of harsh phallic violence, the world is seemingly created anew. Man is condemned to a life in which the sexual, violent, and "masculine" intrudes disturbingly into an already threatening mix of the sublime and the horrifying. We are sucked into a surreal aesthetic. Like the lost pilgrims, we are captivated by a violent beauty. This reality, described in a baroque, ritualistic, repetitive style, declares the creation of a new world with a dark "suzerain" as overlord. Its aesthetic can be seen in the strangely deadly and poetic desert landscapes, which serve as liminal regions[22] between the human and the bestial, between indifferent nature and the caravans of lost people seeking to bring about a traumatic

[22] *Blood Meridian* is set in a specific area, the borderlands between the USA and Mexico. The borderland, however, is not solely geographical. It is also expressed in other fictitious spaces, such as the border between the human and the bestial, between the judge's exceptional intelligence and his animalistic drives, which turn his learned theories into dark parodies of themselves. A liminal reading of the novel would see it as a series of rites of passage and radical training rituals. It would point to the dangerous region of the borderline as a space the undermines the conventional binary distinctions between civilization and lawlessness, between natural and human, between symbolic and real, between the historical tale of the Glanton gang that operated in the region in 1849 and the mythicization of history which turns it into a primordial and enduring campaign of violence beyond the history of human civilization. See Andreasen (2011), Engebretson (2011), Rothfok (2004).

change in history. It is an arid intermediate space constituting a heterotopia, [23] as Foucault (1986) defines it: a zone comprised simultaneously of two worlds, two time systems, or two symbolic systems. This heterotopia is the site of a clash between the social/historical space and the perverse fictional space; it presents the outrageous and imaginary in relation to the corresponding acceptable and real. Thus, the borderlands where the horrors take place are at one and the same time the historical space of documented American history and the twisted apocalyptic space portrayed through the demonic character of the judge. The same is true in Kafka's story, in which the real and fictional boundaries of the penal colony are depicted as an exotic heterotopian space where the normalized and legal meets the perverted and sick, with the two clarifying and critiquing each other.

The unconventional aesthetic accorded both the fictional space and the judge who fashions himself as its overlord creates a new form of radical and depraved authority, which has precedents in the history of ideas. Carl Schmitt, a German intellectual known as the "crown jurist of the Third Reich," similarly contended that the power of the ruler stemmed from his ability to decide questions of life and death, to suspend routine life and declare an enduring state of emergency ([1922] 2006). In effect, this state of emergency is a political heterotopia. By declaring such a condition, the law exempts itself from universal application and from preserving the basic rights it is meant to uphold in order to ensure public safety for a given period. In *Blood Meridian*, this is also the theory of the maniacal judge, who speaks of a ruler whose "authority countermands local judgments" (McCarthy, [1985] 1992, p. 195). Here, the extraordinary circumstances, the "state of emergency," are embodied in the disturbing fusion of violence and beauty. It is the permanent state of the world in the novel, a world without judge or justice, without law, without the principle of restraint deriving from the social charter in rational society.

[23] For a heterotopian reading of *Blood Meridian*, see Holmberg (2009).

This atavistic world is dominated by the electrifying, seductive, and petrifying power of death, which serves in the works of both Kafka and McCarthy as the supreme criterion for authority. In *Blood Meridian*, the ruler worships war and death, seeing them as the primal generative force. Similar to the fascist views in the novels of Ernst Jünger, such as *Storm of Steel* (1929), death is regarded as the foremost source of human exaltation, which is achieved in the aesthetic sphere in which play meets war. As the judge explains:

> Games of chance require a wager to have meaning at all. Games of sport involve the skill and strength of the opponents and the humiliation of defeat and the pride of victory are in themselves sufficient stake because they inhere in the worth of the principals and define them. But trial of chance or trial of worth all games aspire to the condition of war for here that which is wagered swallows up game, player, all. (McCarthy, [1985] 1992, p. 246)

War is thus the supreme principle of the conflict, the progenitor of all existence. The universal conflict, expressed on both the micro and macro levels, gives birth to the existence that shapes mankind. Indeed, the judge's "war games" uphold the Heraclitean tenet, "we must know that war is common to all and strife is justice, and that all things come into being through strife necessarily" (Fragment B80). Aestheticizing war by turning it into a game triggers a dangerous process which makes violence legitimate because it is "beautiful." This beautiful game ends in death. The very term "war games," which exists in many languages, implies a consummate aestheticization of the violence and killing native to every war (Benjamin, 2008).

The "war game" the judge is attempting to explain involves a wager, and the ultimate wager is, of course, for life or death. As the sick parody of an aestheticist of the humanistic tradition, he continues to unravel his philosophy.

> Suppose two men at cards with nothing to wager save their lives. Who has not heard such a tale? A turn of the card. The whole universe for such a player has labored clanking to this moment which will tell if he is to die at that man's hand or that man at his. What more certain validation of a man's worth could there be? This enhancement of the game to its ultimate state admits no argument

> concerning the notion of fate. The selection of one man over another is a preference absolute and irrevocable…This is the nature of war, whose stake is at once the game and the authority and the justification. Seen so, war is the truest form of divination…. War is the ultimate game because war is at last a forcing of the unity of existence. War is god. (McCarthy, [1985] 1992, pp. 246–247)

According to the judge, decisions of life and death subsume all "lesser" considerations, "moral, spiritual, natural" (McCarthy, [1985] 1992, p. 247). They are supreme decisions regarding all things causal, rational, and deterministic. And these decisions can be made at the toss of a coin. In other words, the judgment is made by blind luck. Once the coin lands the man's fate is sealed, without any rational explanation for the decision. Indeed, the judge is ready to toss a coin at anything and everything: he purchases two pups by tossing a coin at a Mexican boy and then pitches them into the river with theatrical sadism (McCarthy, [1985] 1992, p. 189); he performs a coin trick before the astonished eyes of Brown, one of the lost pilgrims riding toward hell, and "the coin returned back out of the night and crossed the fire with a faint high droning and the judge's raised hand was empty and then it held the coin" (McCarthy, [1985] 1992, p. 243). Thus, he devotes his life to two things: a portrayal of the world as an eternal war game designed to produce a random and contingent "unity of existence"; and the desire to prove that evil, death, and ritualistic beauty are inextricably interwoven.

It is clear, that for the judge, the trauma, that is the impossibility of separating the aesthetic from the horrific, is a generative element at the very foundation of life.[24] Both here and in Kafka's story, the judge (and executioner) oversees a ritual of death that resembles an ancient rite of human sacrifice to blood-thirsty gods of unknown identity. And in both cases, the "last man standing" (the Traveler in Kafka and the kid in McCarthy) is helpless to stop the terror rising out of the apocalyptic ruins of the world. The merging of the act of devastation with the act of artistic creation makes this situation untenable. It leaves the reader face to face with the deranged potency of evil, an evil clad in a seductive and perverse beauty that is eternal, indifferent, and irredeemable.

1.4 "Beyond Good and Evil": Trauma as Generative

The works by Kafka and McCarthy illustrate amajor posttraumatic trend in contemporary discourse. In the punitive worlds they describe, there is no attempt to recover from or remedy the trauma. Furthermore, in both stories the trauma furthers ideological colonialist needs and is thus an integral part of the political unconscious of modern and contemporary capitalism. In the postmodern world, the ritualistic recurrence of trauma can no longer lead to change or recovery. It does not even raise awareness of the differend, that is, of the differences that prevent one side from comprehending the language of suffering of the other. The strategy of resolving conflicts by cognitively processing the pain and open wound (i.e., the trauma) is no longer available. When trauma cannot be processed, or "written," it cannot be overcome. It becomes a wild fantasy that generates reality in the present. An ontological crack is thus opened in the foundations of the contemporary world, which adopts evil as an experience of ecstasy and empowerment that is much more potent than the passive and feeble experience of good. Evil and suffering are perceived as primal elements that delineate the borders of a nihilistic outlook.

Our historical memory is based on precisely this evil. The memory of evil is repressed and becomes incapable of recognizing the roots of its influence on the present. Since evil is not

[24] By way of generalization, it could be said that much of McCarthy's work deals with the traumatic. *The Road* (2006) is a postapocalyptic tale of the survival of a father and son after the destruction of the familiar world; *No Country for Old Men* describes a posttraumatic reality through the character of its antihero, the psychopathic murderer Chigurh; and *Blood Meridian* portrays the personal trauma of the kid amid the violence-ridden borderlands and the genocide of the Native Americans, as well as the national trauma of shaping American identity and the fundamental violence of the American political subconscious (Benson, 2011).

spread out before us for all to see its deformities, it cannot spark a process of admission of guilt/atonement/forgiveness. The only thing that remains of the demented memory is unbridled ecstatic writing with its enigmatic violence. We must admit, however, that the two authors exert considerable effort in attempting to "tell the trauma," despite the fact that the narrator (especially in *Blood Meridian*) is in danger of being bewitched by its allure and fascination, without any real ability to free himself and offer an option of cleansing, reparation, and absolution (Collado-Rodríguez, 2012).

If trauma exposes the concealed wound and shatters the wholeness of the subject and the coherent unity of the world, then in the postmodern era fragmentation as a cultural condition is a given. This fits neatly into the capitalist discourse dealing with the banalization and normalization of the traumatic fantasy as part and parcel of its "commercial realism." As McCarthy puts it, compulsive war and trauma create the unseen "unity of existence." In contrast to the modernist outlook, which sees trauma as an instrument of wisdom and an opportunity to redefine human destiny, in the postmodern world we are enveloped in radical fatalism and pessimism that lays bare the perilous seductiveness of trauma—the total collapse of the enlightened scientific/moral rationalism of the West and the conversion of trauma into a sickening cultural and marketing strategy of extreme potency.

It is due to this potency that the traumatic symptom becomes the source of narrative intensity and pleasure. The narrator in "In the Penal Colony" relates the ritualistic events with an emotional indifference that does not hide the "pleasure of telling," evidenced, for example, in the dramatic climax of the story when the Officer decides to sacrifice himself on the altar of the mad machine that unexpectedly spins out of control. At the same time, it is clear that he does not find redemption in the narrative pleasure. "Writing" as an indecipherable trap is also a major feature of his story. It is no longer a redeeming and comforting act, but continues down its own demonic path. Similarly, it is hard not to notice McCarthy's captivation with himself as he continuously aspires to an aestheticization of his traumatic material that is sublime and "dirty" at one and the same time. Here, too, hybrid literature seems unable to unravel the web of internal contradictions and relegates to the writer the task of redeeming the world. Although it makes concerted efforts to draw close to these impossible borders, it never makes it to the promised land. As both writers are drawn into their own enticing and terrifying narratives, they document a society in a manic state of acting out. The ironic escape from the trauma comes from reframing it as a new source of growth and narrative power characterized by a high degree of self-awareness.

If, on the personal clinical level, "adapting to trauma" signifies recovery from the disorder, on the cultural level we are confronted with a reality that defines trauma as part of the new social order it serves. Here, trauma is no longer outside the symbolic order of the culture, but within it; it is no longer the language of the "other," but our own language which has been normalized, internalized, and undergone a new process of medicalization and representation that includes the blind power it entails. Formulating trauma as a fundamental element of a rational society has far-reaching effects. It seeks to position the pain and masochistic pleasure of the traumatic experience as an integral part of the social and media fabric. The appeal of the extreme, the historical sublime, the horrifying, and the "real" (e.g., videos of ISIS's atrocities) in contemporary culture are all illustrations of this new reality. Lack and lacuna, absence and emotional dissociation, the breakdown of language and communication, loss and repetitive memory—all characteristic of post-traumatic syndrome—are thus also the basic elements of postmodern poetics today.

This poetics is diametrically opposed to the primary ideals of modernism and enlightenment: optimism, hope, rationalism, redemption through art, etc. The two examples discussed above indicate that this sort of redemption is no longer possible. Rather, they fuse the aesthetic and the demonic to describe a condition of being drawn in by the power of the traumatic experience without any attempt to resist it. They depict the postmodern reality in which trauma is part of Western rationalism and capitalism. The pleasure/pain principle of trauma has become a generative element, a cultural recipe for creating and maintaining the balance of power in society. The "escape to trauma" as an experience that shapes the real is now shared by all, even if we seek to deny this premise in our conscious day-to-day activity. A critical view of contemporary society therefore demands recognition of trauma as a basic ingredient of our emotional and cultural reality, a tangible element underlying the unity of our social world. This recognition, demonstrated with extraordinary virtuosity by Kafka and McCarthy, is a painful expression of the politics and poetics of trauma in contemporary literature.

References

Adorno, T. W. (1973). *Negative dialectics* (Vol. 1). New York: Seabury Press.

Agamben, G. (1998). *Homo sacer: Sovereign power and bare life*. Stanford, CA: Stanford University Press.

Agamben, G. (1999). *Remnants of Auschwitz: The witness and the archive*. New York: Zone Books.

Alexander, J. C. (2004). Toward a Theory of Cultural Trauma. In J. C. Alexander, R. Eyerman, B. Giesen, N. J. Smelser, & P. Sztompka (Eds.), *Cultural trauma and collective identity* (pp. 1–30). Berkeley: University of California Press.

Alexander, J. C. (2012). *Trauma: A social theory*. Cambridge: Polity Press.

Andreasen, L. V. (2011). *Blood Meridian* and the spatial metaphysics of the West. *Southwestern American Literature, 36*(3), 19–30.

Arav, D., & Gurevitz, D. (2014). Trauma, guilt, forgiveness: The victimizer as witness in the cinematic and televisual representations of conflict inIsrael. *Media, War & Conflict, 7*(1), 104–120. doi:10.1177/1750635213515098.

Badiou, A. (2002). *Ethics: An essay on the understanding of evil*. Berkeley: Verso.

Baudrillard, J. (1983). The ecstasy of communication. In H. Foster & J. Baudrillard (Eds.), *The anti-aesthetic: Essays on postmodern culture* (pp. 126–134). Port Townsend, WA: Bay Press.

Bauman, Z. (2013). *Culture in a liquid modern world*. Cambridge: Polity Press.

Benjamin, W. (1986). *Reflections: Essays, aphorisms, autobiographical writings*. New York: Schocken Books.

Benjamin, W. (2008). *The work of art in the age of mechanical reproduction*. London: Penguin.

Benson, J. (2011). An ironic contention: The kid's heroic failure to rebel against the judge's hypermasculinity in *Blood Meridian*. *Southwestern American Literature, 36*(3), 70–86.

Berger, J. (1999). *After the end: Representations of post-apocalypse*. Minneapolis: University of Minnesota Press.

Blanchot, M. (1995). *The writing of the disaster, trans. A. Smock*. Lincoln, NE: University of Nebraska Press.

Blumenberg, H. (1985). *The legitimacy of the modern age*. Cambridge and London: MIT Press.

Boehmer, E. (1993). Transfiguring: Colonial body into postcolonial narrative. *NOVEL: A Forum on Fiction, 26*, 268–277.

Bollas, C. (1995). *Cracking up: The work of unconscious experience*. London: Psychology Press.

Bradbury, M., & MacFarlane, J. W. [1976] (1991). *Modernism: A guide to European literature, 1890-1930*. Harmondsworth, UK: Penguin books.

Butler, J. (1993). *Bodies that matter: On the discursive limits of sex*. New York: Routledge.

Calinescu, M. (1987). *Five faces of modernity: Modernism, avant-garde, decadence, kitsch, post-modernism*. Durham, NC: Duke University Press.

Canfield, J. D. (2003). The dawning of the age of Aquarius: Abjection, identity, and the carnivalesque in Cormac McCarthy's *Suttree*. *Contemporary Literature, 44*, 664–696.

Caruth, C. (1995). Trauma and experience. In C. Caruth (Ed.), *Trauma: Explorations in memory* (Preface). Baltimore, MD: John Hopkins University Press.

Collado-Rodríguez, F. (2012). Trauma and storytelling in Cormac McCarthy's "No Country for Old Men" and "The Road". *Papers on Language & Literature, 48*(1), 45–69.

Conrad, J. (1902). *Youth: A narrative, and two other stories*. Edinburgh and London: William Blackwood & Sons.

Covington, R. M. (2011). The subjection of authority and death through humor in *Blood Meridian*. *Southwestern American Literature, 36*, 60–69.

Cumberland, R. (2013). Inscribed bodies: The cruel mirage of imperialistic idealism in Kafka's "Penal Colony". *Papers on Language & Literature, 49*, 203–222.

Curtis, N. (1999). The body as outlaw: Lyotard, Kafka and the Visible Human Project. *Body & Society, 5*(2/3), 249.

Dacus, C. (2011). Borderline insanity: Modernity as a political problem in Cormac McCarthy's *Blood Meridian*. *Southwestern American Literature, 36*, 96–106.

Deleuze, G., & Guattari, F. (1985). Kafka: Toward a minor literature: The components of expression. *New Literary History, 16*(3), 591–608.

Derrida, J. (2001). *On cosmopolitanism and forgiveness*. London and New York: Routledge.

Derrida, J. [1967] (1976). *Of grammatology,* trans. G. C. Spivak. Baltimore and London: The Johns Hopkins University Press.

Derrida, J. [1998] (2002). *Archive fever*. New York: Springer.

Dews, P. (1987). *Logics of disintegration: Post-structuralist thought and the claims of critical theory*. London: Verso.

Dineen, T. (1999). *Manufacturing victims: What the psychology industry is doing to people*. London: Constable.

Docherty, T. (1993). *Postmodernism: A reader*. New York: Columbia University Press.

Dorson, J. (2013). Demystifying the judge: Law and mythical violence in Cormac McCarthy's "Blood Meridian". *Journal of Modern Literature, 36*(2), 105–121.

Douglass, A., & Vogler, T. A. (2003). Introduction. In A. Douglass & T. A. Vogler (Eds.), *Witness and memory: The discourse of trauma* (pp. 1–53). London: Psychology Press.

Eddins, D. (2003). "Everything a hunter and everything hunted": Schopenhauer and Cormac McCarthy's *Blood Meridian. Critique: Studies in Contemporary Fiction, 45*, 25–33.

Elsaesser, T. (2014). *German cinema—terror and trauma: Cultural memory since 1945*. New York and London: Routledge.

Engebretson, A. (2011). Neither in nor out: The liminal spaces of *Blood Meridian. Southwestern American Literature, 36*, 9–18.

Felman, S., & Laub, D. (1992). *Testimony: Crises of witnessing in literature, psychoanalysis, and history*. New York: Routledge.

Foucault, M. (1977). *Discipline and punish: The birth of the prison*. New York: Vintage.

Foucault, M. (1986). Heterotopias. *Diacritics, 16*(1), 22.

Fracchia, J. (2008). The capitalist labour-process and the body in pain: The corporeal depths of Marx's concept of immiseration. *Historical Materialism, 16*(4), 35–66.

Freud, S. (1958). *Remembering, repeating and working-through. Further recommendations on the technique of psycho-analysis II. Standard Edition*, 12: 145–156 (Vol 1915, pp. 117–140). London: Hogarth Press.

Freud, S. [1919] (2003). *The uncanny*. London: Penguin.

Giddens, A. (2013). *The consequences of modernity*. Hoboken, NJ: John Wiley & Sons.

Gray, J. (2013). *The silence of animals: On progress and other modern myths*. London: Macmillan.

Greenberg, C. [1961] (1993). Modernist. In C. Harrison & P. Wood (Eds.) *Art in theory, 1900-1990: An anthology of changing ideas*, Hoboken, NJ: Blackwell.

Grosz, E. A. (1995). *Space, time, and perversion: Essays on the politics of bodies*. New York: Routledge.

Habermas, J. [1985] (1987). *The philosophical discourse of modernity*, trans. F. Lawrence, Cambridge, MA: The MIT Press.

Hall, S. (1992). *Understanding modern societies: An introduction*. Cambridge: Polity Press.

Herman, J. L. (1992). *Trauma and recovery*. New York: Basic Books.

Holmberg, D. (2009). "In a time before nomenclature was and each was all": *Blood Meridian's* neomythic west and the heterotopian zone. *Western American Literature, 44*(2), 140–156.

Huizinga, J. [1949] (2014). *Homo ludens*. New York: Routledge.

Huntington, P. J. (1998). *Ecstatic subjects, utopia, and recognition: Kristeva, Heidegger, Irigaray*. New York: SUNY Press.

Ibrahim, Y. (2011). Domestication of suffering: The politics of pity and communion through ICTs. *Empedocles: European Journal for the Philosophy of Communication, 2*(1), 137–150.

Jameson, F. (1991). *Postmodernism, or, the cultural logic of late capitalism*. Durham, NC: Duke University Press.

Junger, E. (1929). *The storm of steel, trans. B. Creighton*. London: Chatto and Windus.

Kafka, F. [1919] (2002). In the penal colony, trans. Edwin Muir and Willa Muir. In: The metamorphosis and other writings (pp. 97–122) New York and London: Continuum.

Kleinman, A., & Kleinman, J. (2009). Cultural appropriations of suffering. In U. Linke & D. T. Smith (Eds.), *Cultures of fear: A critical reader* (pp. 288–303). New York: Pluto Press.

Kohn, M. (2005). Kafka's critique of colonialism. *Theory & Event, 8*(3).

Kolb, D. (1986). *The critique of pure modernity: Hegel, Heidegger, and after*. Chicago: University of Chicago Press.

Kristeva, J. (1982). *Powers of horror: An essay on abjection, trans. L. S. Roudiez*. New York: Columbia University Press.

Lacan, J. (1988). *The ego in Freud's theory and in the technique of psychoanalysis, 1954-1955, Book II, trans. S. Tomaselli*. Cambridge: Cambridge University Press.

Lacan, J. [1966] (1977). *Ecrits: A selection*. New York: WW Norton & Company.

LaCapra, D. (1998). *History and memory after Auschwitz*. New York: Cornell University Press.

Laplanche, J., & Pontalis, J. [1967] (1973). *The language of psychoanalysis*, trans. Donald Nicholson-Smith. London: Karnac Books and the Institute of Psychoanalysis.

Laub, D. (1995). Truth and testimony: The process and the struggle. In C. Caruth (Ed.), *Trauma: Explorations in memory* (pp. 61–75). Baltimore: John Hopkins University Press.

Lemon, R. (2011). *Imperial messages: Orientalism as self-critique in the Habsburg fin de siècle* (Vol. 101). New York: Camden House.

Levinas, E. (2003). *Humanism of the other (Poller, N. Trans.)*. Chicago: University of Illinois Press.

Leys, R. (2000). *Trauma: A genealogy*. Chicago and London: University of Chicago Press.

Loftus, E. F. (1996). *Eyewitness testimony*. Cambridge: Harvard University Press.

Lyotard, J.-F. (1984). *The postmodern condition*. Minneapolis: University of Minnesota Press.

Lyotard, J.-F. (1988a). *Le différend* (Vol. 46). New York: University of Minnesota Press.

Lyotard, J.-F. (1988b). *Peregrinations: Law, form, event*. New York: Columbia University Press.

Lyotard, J.-F. (1989). Discussions, or phrasing "After Auschwitz". In A. E. Benjamin (Ed.), *The Lyotard reader* (pp. 360–392). Cambridge: Basil Blackwell.

Lyotard, J.-F. (1990). After the sublime: The state of asthetics. In D. Carroll (Ed.), *The states of theory: History, art, and critical discourse* (pp. 297–304). New York: Columbia University Press.

Lyotard, J.-F. (1993). *Toward the postmodern*. Amherst: Humanity Books.

Marx, K. [1867] (1992). *Capital, volume I*. Harmondsworth, UK: Penguin/New Left Review.

McCarthy, C. [1985] (1992). *Blood Meridian: Or the evening redness in the west*. New York: Vintage.

McClintock, S. (2004). The penal colony: Inscription of the subject in literature and law, and detainees as legal non-persons at Camp X-Ray. *Comparative Literature Studies, 41*, 153–167.

McNally, R. J. (2003). *Remembering trauma*. Cambridge: Belknap Press of Harvard University Press.

Muller, V. (2006). Abject d'Art. *M/C Journal, 9*(5). http://journal.media-culture.org.au/0610/04-muller.php.

Neal, C. (1999). The body as outlaw: Lyotard, Kafka and the Visible Human Project. *Body and Society, 5*(2–3), 249–266.

Peebles, S. (2003). Yuman belief systems and Cormac McCarthy's *Blood Meridian*. *Texas Studies in Literature and Language, 45*, 231–244.

Rabinow, P. (1986). Representations are social facts: Modernity and post-modernity in anthropology. In J. Clifford & G. E. Marcus (Eds.), *Writing culture: The poetics and politics of ethnography: A School of American Research advanced seminar* (pp. 234–261). Los Angeles: University of California Press.

Rothe, A. (2011). *Popular trauma culture: Selling the pain of others in the mass media*. New Brunswick, NJ, London: Rutgers University Press.

Rothfork, J. (2004). Language and the dance of time in Cormac McCarthy's "Blood Meridian". *Southwestern American Literature, 30*(1), 23–36.

Scarry, E. (1985). *The body in pain: The making and unmaking of the world*. New York: Oxford University Press.

Schmitt, C. [1922] (2006). *Political theology*, trans. G, Schwab. Chicago: University of Chicago Press.

Schopenhauer, A. (2012). *The world as will and representation [1818]* (Vol. 1): Courier Corporation.

Seeburger, F. (2013). *The open wound: Trauma, identity, and community*. Seattle: CreateSpace.

Silverman, H. J. (1990). *Postmodernism: Philosophy and the arts*. New York and London: Routledge.

Spence, D. P. (1984). *Narrative truth and historical truth: Meaning and interpretation in psychoanalysis*. New York: WW Norton & Company.

Spiegel, D. (1986). Dissociation, double blinds, and post-traumatic stress in multiple personality disorder. In B. G. Braun (Ed.), *Treatment of multiple personality disorder* (pp. 61–78). Washington, DC: American Psychiatric Press.

Steinberg, E. R. (1976). The judgment in Kafka's "In the Penal Colony". *Journal of Modern Literature, 5*(3), 492–514.

Stinson, E. J. (2007). "Blood Meridian's" man of many masks: Judge Holden as tarot's fool. *Southwestern American Literature, 33*(1), 9–21.

Stolorow, R. D., & Atwood, G. E. (2014). *Contexts of being: The intersubjective foundations of psychological life*. New York: Routledge.

Walder, D. (1998). *Post-colonial literatures in English: History, language, theory*. Hoboken, NJ: Wiley-Blackwell.

West, R. (1985). Authority, autonomy, and choice: The role of consent in the moral and political visions of Franz Kafka and Richard Posner. *Harvard Law Review, 99*(2), 384–428.

Wheale, N. (1995). *The postmodern arts: An introductory reader*. London and New York: Routledge.

Young, A. (2007). Posttraumatic stress disorder of the virtual kind: Trauma and resilience in post-9/11 America. In A. Sarat, N. Davidovitch, & D. A. Bogazianos (Eds.), *Trauma and memory: Reading, healing, and making law* (pp. 21–48). Stanford, CA: Stanford University Press.

Zilcosky, J. (2003). *Kafka's travels: Exoticism, colonialism, and the traffic of writing*. London: Palgrave Macmillan.

2 Cultural Trauma and the Media

Allen Meek

2.1 Introduction

In recent decades, cultural trauma has become a widely accepted form of collective identity in images and narratives transmitted through mass media and information networks. The iconic cultural trauma of the twenty-first century so far is the World Trade Center catastrophe of September 11, 2001. The idea of cultural trauma, however, can be traced at least back to Freud and has been associated with many events including the Holocaust, Afro-American slavery, the bombing of Hiroshima and Nagasaki, the Vietnam War, and the assassination of John F. Kennedy. Cultural trauma narratives tell stories about heroes and martyrs. By associating catastrophic events with heroic persons and acts, these narratives attempt to redeem unbearable losses and shameful acts: in short, they rewrite history.

In the late nineteenth century and first half of the twentieth century, psychological trauma was associated with biological degeneration, in the case of female hysterics, or cowardice, in the case of combat trauma. Today, trauma is no longer a shameful sign of weakness and those who identify with cultural trauma share the honor of the heroism associated with particular historical events. Cultural trauma narratives, however, often falsify the terrible facts of modern mass death in which most individuals are given no opportunity to act heroically. Moreover, by identifying with these narratives, individuals and groups have the opportunity to lend support for to acts of political and military retribution and the further destruction of innocent life.

This essay explains some of the complex relations between cultural trauma and modern media. The first section examines how a cultural trauma narrative about 9/11 fosters collective identification with the victims and how this can also falsify understandings of the larger political implications of the event. The next section explains the development of cultural trauma as a concept over the past 100 years and how this idea became linked with visual media. The essay then goes on to explain how the experience of shock is embedded in media culture and how the idea of cultural trauma becomes aligned with the perceptual habits and psychological reflexes of the media viewer. This section explains the historical relation between psychological research on trauma, the visual recording of human behavior, and the manipulation of viewer responses. Cultural trauma, then, is not just a popular narrative about identity but a new experience of collective identity in a technologically mediated society. The essay concludes with some further thoughts about the political implications of this mediated experience of trauma.

A. Meek, Ph.D. (✉)
School of English and Media Studies, Massey University, Palmerston North, New Zealand
e-mail: A.Meek@massey.ac.nz

Y. Ataria et al. (eds.), *Interdisciplinary Handbook of Trauma and Culture*,
DOI 10.1007/978-3-319-29404-9_2

2.2 Case Study: 9/11

On May 15, 2014 Barack Obama gave a speech at the opening of the National September 11 Memorial and Museum in which he related the moving story of the "man in the red bandanna": a young man who had risked, and ultimately lost, his own life to help others escape the burning South Tower of the World Trade Center. This young man, Wells Crowther, embodied the "spirit of 9/11: love, compassion, sacrifice." 9/11, proclaimed Obama, will always remain part of American identity: "We stand in the footprints of two mighty towers … Nothing can ever break us. Nothing can change who we are as Americans." Although he was not President at the time of the 2001 attacks, this was not the first time that Obama publicly invoked the trauma of 9/11. In his 2011 speech announcing the assassination of Osama bin Laden, Obama also vividly described the events of that September day. On this earlier occasion the evocation of the attacks had a different purpose: to justify a military intervention on foreign territory and, some would say, to justify an act of political retribution. In both speeches, the President's use of video to address the American people, whether "live" on television or on the Internet, made the trauma of 9/11 the basis of a common history and purpose and evoked a shared sense of grief and resolve.

The idea of trauma as a marker of cultural identity is not new in America. After the defeat in Vietnam, American psychotherapists working with war veterans developed the diagnostic category of Post Traumatic Stress Disorder (PTSD). Hollywood responded immediately with movies such as *Coming Home* and *Deer Hunter* that featured traumatized veterans home from the war. After the years of antiwar protest in which returning veterans had often been reviled by the public, these Hollywood narratives allowed the soldier's combat trauma to be shared with his loved ones, family, and, implicitly, the larger American community. This was the same period that the ABC miniseries *Roots* (1977) presented the story of African American identity emerging from the trauma of slavery, followed by *Holocaust* (NBC 1978) which first brought the Nazi genocide to the arena of mass entertainment. The 1960s had been characterized by the anguish of the Civil Rights and antiwar struggles and the assassinations of the Kennedy and Dr. King. If post-Vietnam identity invoked the specter of military defeat, shame at American atrocities, collective mourning, and depression then the Holocaust promised a return to a redemptive narrative in which the Americans acted as liberators and defenders of human freedom. The Hollywoodization of Vietnam and the Holocaust for the first time allowed audiences to identify with the position of the traumatized victim, even if that victim tended to belong to, or look like, mainstream America rather than Vietnamese or East European Jews—or African-Americans. This was not enough, however, to dispel the specter of military failure. The Gulf War of 1991 was proclaimed by President George Bush as a new demonstration of American strength and a victory that settled the score of the defeat in Vietnam.

Obama's narrative about "the man in the red bandana" exemplifies this process. A civilian, who had the great misfortune of working in the targeted building, managed to rescue some of his coworkers before being killed in the building's collapse. This is the kind of story that we expect to hear in news stories and Hollywood movies about disaster and war. The passenger who saves others during a plane crash, shipwreck, or an earthquake performs a spontaneous act of heroism. Soldiers who are killed in war, whether they act heroically or not, have sacrificed their lives for their country. But the bombing of civilians, the incarceration and genocide of populations in camps and killing centers, and the spread of urban terrorism, has changed the political status of victims of catastrophe. Giorgio Agamben (1998) has argued that these civilian victims fall into the category of *homo sacer* (a figure he retrieves from archaic Roman law) "*who may be killed and yet not sacrificed*" (p. 8). Civilians who are killed in modern war, genocide, and terrorism are dehumanized populations targeted for destruction: "collateral damage," "subhumans," "enemies of the state," etc. Turning those civilians who are killed into martyrs conceals the reality that most of the victims did not give their lives for their country or for their beliefs but were simply disposed of as part of a hostile military or political agenda.

Stories of heroism falsify the terrible fate of modern mass death. If we hear a story of heroic resistance or selfless courage in Auschwitz we know that it can never change the fact that millions were gassed. For this reason Agamben rejects the term "Holocaust" because it connotes sacrifice rather than mass killing. The "man in the red bandana" is a hero who is fashioned by political rhetoric to represent the victims of the 9/11 attacks, most of whom were not martyrs for a cause but objects of violent destruction. Narratives about particular individuals who gave their lives for others construct a community of victims around a sacrificial hero and thereby attempt to redeem catastrophe through a narrative of nationhood, shared values and beliefs, and caring for others.

At one level this is a straightforward process of political refashioning: an event that revealed a failure of national security, now becomes a symbol of the resilience of the American people. But it also shows an attempt to contain the traumatic impact of events that have the potential to cause social panic and political instability. Events that revealed the vulnerability of civilian populations are thereby transformed into monuments of collective strength. Instead of the WTC as an enduring symbol of economic power, its very absence becomes a monument to the spirit of American community that will endure forever. It is the job of political leaders to turn defeats into victories and construct powerful narratives about collective identity. What is new is that trauma has become an acceptable way to define that shared identity, rather than something that is shrouded in guilt, fear, and secrecy. Of course there are many—some of whom participate in the 9/11 Truth movement—who do see 9/11 as shrouded in guilt, fear, and secrecy. But there is now a widely held belief, after generations of psychotherapy, mediated catastrophe, and celebrity culture, that trauma is an acceptable and legitimate basis of identity.

As our lives have become increasingly saturated by communication technologies and information networks, our collective identification with "traumatic events" has apparently increased. Catastrophes cannot now be recalled without entire series of associated media images or "flashbulb memories" (Zelizer 1992, p. 5) from photojournalism, television news, and Hollywood dramatizations. Like traumatic memories, media images appear in sudden and often disconcerting ways in our daily lives, they impact us with their drama and immediacy, and they almost always show us events that are distant in space and time. Since the JFK assassination television has made the traumatic event the moment in which everyday schedules are suspended and viewers are captivated by dramas unfolding in real time. Does trauma, then, promise some authentic experience of community that is otherwise felt to be lacking in our lives? Trauma promises us a return to a shared understanding of history, breaking through the screen of visual information that has numbed our responses, and reengaging us in social life. It is because this promise wields so much symbolic power that we need to critically examine the claims that surround cultural trauma and its uses by academics, media professionals, and political leaders.

2.3 Cultural Trauma and the Media

The term cultural trauma appears to suggest the shared psychological experience of specific events. The idea of shared trauma, however, sits uneasily with the fact that different individuals and groups often respond to similar events and experiences in different ways. As Allan Young (2007) has shown, research reveals that most people do not develop trauma symptoms even when exposed to conditions sufficient to cause PTSD (p. 21). Cultural trauma implies not that everyone in a society had the same experience but that certain events have been given extraordinary status for a society. Just as a psychological trauma has long-term effects on individuals and communities, cultural trauma suggests social and political conflicts that remain unresolved, losses that are difficult to mourn, events that are difficult to represent or symbolize. When events achieve the status of cultural trauma, however, they *have* become symbols of the collective that mean more than the sum of collective psychological suffering. On the other hand, psychological trauma is never without cultural, social, and political dimensions, whether it be caused by child abuse, rape, war, genocide, colonization, ecological catastrophe, etc.: to be abused is to suffer the misuse of social authority and responsibility, violence is authorized by governments and political leaders, and natural environments are impacted by human behavior and technology.

Cultural trauma is composed of images and narratives that convey the impact and threat of catastrophe on large populations. Modern visual media play and important role in the transmission of cultural trauma images and narratives. The following sections explain some different aspects of this process:

2.3.1 The "Protective Shield"

Freud's account of the "protective shield" against shock in *Beyond the Pleasure Principle* (1920) explained how the conscious mind developed a "thick skin" to block out external threats by learning to anticipate them with acceptable levels of anxiety. Only when the shield was pierced by an unforeseen force did experience become traumatic. Freud's theory was adapted by Walter Benjamin in the 1930s to develop his own account of shock in modern urban societies. Photography and film, argued Benjamin (2003), function as shields that protect the psyche against the intrusive stimuli of modern life. The inhabitants of large cities learn to accept or avoid sights of social deprivation while going about their business, while in various forms of news and entertainment media an ordinary person might witness scenes of suffering and death on a daily basis. If these sights are too disturbing or distressing the individual will not be able to cope with the tasks and challenges of everyday life. Modern life requires psychological defenses for survival and trauma is experienced only when these defenses are suddenly shattered.

Media not only insulate us from shock, they also deliberately induce shock. News and entertainment media attempt to capture our attention with images that shock and surprise but they also allow us feel insulated from threats of actual violence and destruction. For many Americans the 9/11 attacks disrupted this safe distance and posed a new kind of threat: the destruction of civilians by bombs had always happened in other countries but now civilians were vulnerable to attack at home. For these reasons, media images of the 9/11 attacks may indeed have been traumatic for many people. If psychological trauma had been suffered by the entire population, however, this would have been more widely disruptive of social life. The continued functioning of normal social behavior and social institutions after 9/11 suggests that psychological defenses remained in place for most people. After 9/11 media played its role in both transmitting and containing the threat of psychological distress by repeating certain images and censoring others and by producing narratives of collective suffering, solidarity, and retribution.

2.3.2 Historical Trauma

Since Freud the analysis of psychological trauma has repeatedly been extended to larger claims about cultural beliefs and historical events. As early as *Totem and Taboo* (1913), Freud related trauma to the collective psychic repression of acts of violence in prehistoric society. Community was founded on a shared sense of guilt. In his final work, *Moses and Monotheism* (1930), Freud explained Judaism in terms of the trauma of monotheistic faith, which he argued made greater psychological demands than polytheism. This text could be seen as Freud's explanation of why the Nazis sought to be rid of the Jews: they wanted to free themselves once and for all from the burden of guilt imposed by the one God. Freud explained political violence in terms of a deeper "traumatic" social memory; i.e., societies attempt to release themselves from collective feelings of guilt and anxiety by expelling or killing "alien" individuals and groups. This conception of historical trauma reached its culmination in Theodor Adorno's (1973) often-cited postwar comments about the fate of culture "after Aschwitz." Adorno proposed that after human beings had been reduced to disposable "garbage" in the death camps, culture could no longer address timeless human values; after Auschwitz, culture had been traumatized by irreparable damage to the individual's sense of subjective meaning and purpose.

2.3.3 "Psychic Numbing"

These conceptions of media as a protective shield and political violence as an historical trauma come together in postwar America with reference to the bombing of Hiroshima, the Nazi death camps, and the Vietnam War. For the first time, the sense of an unconscious historical trauma merges with psychotherapeutic research on survivors of war and catastrophe and a critique of mass media. Robert Jay Lifton's (1967, 1973) studies of Hiroshima survivors and Vietnam veterans continued in the tradition of Freud insofar as they moved from individual case studies to broader claims about the psychic history of entire societies. He proposed that Americans were traumatized by guilt for bombing Hiroshima and for this reason failed to address the full implications of weapons of mass destruction. Lifton went beyond Freud when he addressed the role of mass media in constructing narratives about catastrophe that served as psychological defenses against disturbing historical realities. Photographs and film footage that documented the effects of the atom bombs dropped on the Japanese were confiscated by the American authorities and hidden from public view for decades. In place of these documents, Americans were presented with the image of the mushroom cloud as a symbol of technological power and a source of Cold War anxiety. After his work with Hiroshima survivors, Lifton went on to do psychotherapy with American veterans of combat in Vietnam, leading to the formulation and acceptance of Post Traumatic Stress Disorder as a diagnostic category. In the book that resulted from this research, *Home from the War* (1973), Lifton proposed that the televising of the war contributed to massive psychic numbing among the American public.

2.3.4 Testimony

In the 1990s, cultural trauma was taken up by literary criticism, leading to the emergence of trauma studies as a successful interdisciplinary paradigm in the academic humanities. Shoshanna Felman's and Dori Laub's *Testimony* (1992) was the first book to bring together discussion of literary texts, psychotherapy with Holocaust survivors, and film and video documents. Laub discussed therapy with Holocaust survivors and video testimony recorded and archived at Yale while Felman included a long essay on Claude Lanzmann's film *Shoah* (1985), which was composed entirely of testimony by survivors and witnesses and included no archival images. This book was a defining text for trauma studies and established a tendency to look for authentic representations of trauma in serious literature and film or in testimonial documents as opposed to mass media dramatizations. This influential book, however, itself participated in a larger trend in which the Holocaust assumed a new prominence in international popular culture.

2.3.5 Identity Politics and Moral Universals

Trauma has formed part of a philosophical critique of collective identity and violence but it has also come to signify a sense of cultural participation and belonging. The rise of trauma studies in the 1990s was preceded by the identity politics of the 1960s and 1970s: Civil Rights, antiwar, feminism, and Gay Liberation. The legacies of slavery, racism, war, domestic violence, and rape were central concerns of these struggles against social and political oppression. Struggle was articulated through speaking out, breaking the silence surrounding prejudice and abuse, and giving testimony to the suffering experienced by oppressed individuals and groups. This politics of grievance has often been subject to ridicule by the dominant culture and attacked as "political correctness." Cultural trauma has more recently been universalized in the work of theorists such as Jeffrey Alexander (2012) and Daniel Levy and Natan Sznaider (2006), who see the Holocaust as constitutive of new moral paradigms and transnational identities. Michael Rothberg (2009) has also shown how discourses about the Holocaust are historically interwoven with those about European colonialism and anticolonial struggles.

The legacies of racial violence, genocide, and war crimes have become highly significant in the contemporary politics of memory. International relations can be swayed by the acknowledgment of, or failure to acknowledge, responsibilities for past crimes, and injustices. Within nations, different ethnic groups and minorities seek recognition for sufferings experienced by previous generations. These struggles for recognition can be understood as therapeutic for communities that suffer from collective trauma; or as self-conscious constructions of identity seeking political gain; or even as reinscriptions of aggressive, xenophobic, and racist forms of identity that a deeper understanding of historical injustice would discredit. Dominick LaCapra has explained these different articulations of cultural trauma in terms of Freud's distinction between "working through" and "acting out": the subject of trauma must either come to a gradual recognition of the unconscious source of their suffering or be doomed to compulsively repeat the original scenario in new situations (LaCapra 1998). The influential writings of theorists like LaCapra, Alexander, and Rothberg have made cultural trauma a universal paradigm for understanding contemporary identity. There is a danger, however, that this universalization of trauma might prevent us from inquiring into the specific institutional and technological changes that have given trauma the cultural authority it assumes today.

2.4 Media, Medical Research, and Shock

Cultural trauma has become a way of articulating claims about historical responsibility for suffering and injustice. Because these claims often lead to what some call the "politics of blame," other discourses argue for cultural trauma—particularly in the case of the Holocaust—as a concern for all humanity. This universalizing rhetoric tends toward a liberal humanist perspective on history and politics and tends to ignore the ways that trauma is premised on a medicalization of social identity. Today, older theological or philosophical conceptions of suffering related to a sense of loss, injustice, and evil have been largely replaced by psychological and psychiatric understandings of human experience as driven by biological processes (Young 1977). The widespread use of the term "trauma" is symptomatic of this shift. Although psychological trauma is often understood as an analogy for a physical wound, the two concepts, as Allan Young has explained, are actually linked genealogically. The "discovery" of traumatic memory was based in the scientific observation of physical symptoms. The first cases of psychological trauma were caused by railway accidents and the impact of a physical shock that did not leave evidence on the body but instead was registered through a disturbance of the nervous system, giving rise to compulsive behaviors (Young 1977, pp. 246–247).

Evidence of the physiological damage caused by fear, or fright, further embedded psychological and emotional responses in biology. Trauma is biological, but its location in the nervous system makes it one step removed from the physical world: one can suffer psychological trauma without experiencing any overt physical injury. Modern media further removes trauma from the physical world by simulating the experience of violence and catastrophe and thereby allowing the viewer to experience a "virtual" trauma. Photography and moving images also allow us to witness threatening events at a safe distance. This is one reason why psychological trauma has been aligned with mediated experience in contemporary instances of cultural trauma.

In *The Empire of Trauma* (2009), Didier Fassin and Richard Rechtman explain that before the Vietnam War combat trauma was usually treated with suspicion and seen as cowardice. Since the official recognition of PTSD, however, the condition of victimhood as a legitimate form of identity has become widely accepted. Although many people may still see traumatized war veterans and even victims of rape and domestic abuse as social outsiders or deviants (and somehow deserving of their suffering), the idea that the defeat in Vietnam was traumatic for Americans or that the Holocaust is a trauma for all Jews is acceptable to many who identify with these national or ethnic groups. Fassin and Rechtman discuss the convergence of psychiatric therapy, political rhetoric, and media coverage in the adoption of trauma as the central paradigm for understanding 9/11. As they point out, there is a slippage between the sense of trauma as a psychological disturbance and its "metaphorical extension disseminated by the media" (p. 2) in which an entire nation can be said to have experienced a traumatic event. In the television coverage of the Vietnam War there remained unresolved tensions between the new freedoms of the news media, the military agendas of the state and public support for, or opposition to, the war. The narrative of Vietnam as a shared trauma for Americans was constructed later in Hollywood films such as *The Deer Hunter*. The spectacular nature of the World Trade Center catastrophe and the immediate evidence of American civilians as victims of terrorism, however, made it possible to impose a political consensus about the collective trauma suffered by Americans and the necessity of military response.

One way to better understand and perhaps move beyond this enshrining of victimhood is to excavate its origins in medical discourses, the politics of mass societies, and the development of technological media. Freud continues to cast a long shadow over cultural trauma: from his own speculations on the origins of society in collective violence, through Adorno's notion of Auschwitz as a trauma for Western culture, to Lifton's claims about psychic numbing in America. The danger in this line of thought is that it makes the psychological individual a model for understanding entire societies. Psychological trauma is often aligned with liberal humanist conceptions of politics and history that fail to consider the role of technological media in shaping individual and collective experience and identity. But if we take a step back from Freud to consider the earlier conception of trauma advanced by his mentor, Jean-Martin Charcot, we see a more direct convergence between medical research and technological media which became the basis of later forms of mass entertainment and politics. Cultural trauma is not aligned with mass media because it allows a collective empathy for, or identification with, the suffering of others. Rather it is because the conceptual origins of the "traumatic" subject are medical and technological, taking human life as an object to be recorded, analyzed, and manipulated. This medico-technological model of the human subject was carried over from the physiological study of trauma into research on the responses of media viewers, particularly with respect to the physiological impact of shock.

Many of the pioneers of photography and film were also engaged in medical and scientific research. For example, Charcot used photography to study the pathological symptoms of hysterical women. The hysteric seemed possessed by uncontrollable, compulsive gestures that could only be understood through close attention to the minutiae of her movements and behaviors, which were then interpreted as pathological symptoms. For this purpose the camera proved to be an invaluable tool. The gestures of hysterics were extensively documented in photographs, many of which were made available to the public in published albums (Didi-Huberman 2003).

Albert Londe, the photographer who worked at Charcot's clinic, was a friend of Etienne-Jules Marey, the inventor of *chronophotographie*, or time photography. Marey trained as a doctor specializing in research on cardiology and blood circulation, which he combined with an interest in the mechanical functions of hydraulics. He saw the human body as a machine and he set out to discover the laws that govern physiological processes (Braun 1992, pp. 11–13). This led him to the study of movement. But the intricacies of human movement were not visible to the human eye. Again the camera provided the technology that could record movement in all its microscopic detail. Marey's photographic studies decomposed movement into discrete gestures and transformed individual actions into graphic information. As with Londe's photographs of hysterics, Marey's studies of movement allowed the gestures and behaviors of individuals to be studied and form the basis of generalizations. The individual manifested the symptom of a general pathology or acted out the biological trait of the species.

As a scientist, Marey was interested in using the camera to analyze movement, not to produce an illusion of movement for the purposes of entertainment. Nevertheless, Marey's serial images of bodies in motion became the earliest filmed images to be screened for the public. The Lumière brothers were familiar with Marey's work and solved the problem of how to project moving images. Marey's greatest legacy, however, is the scientific management of labor. August Chauveau, who became the director of the Institute Marey after Marey's death, conducted studies on muscular fatigue. His pupil, Jules Amar, conducted further such studies on inmates of a prison in Algiers, requiring the prisoners to carry weights up to the point of exhaustion. In 1914 Amar published the results of his research in *The Human Motor*. The visual recording and study of human movement forms the basis of studies of industrial labor oriented toward maximizing production and profit. These studies were also extended to media viewers in order to direct their responses and behaviors as consumers.

The use of moving pictures for the purposes of managing both labor and entertainment are not unrelated but actually integrated in industrial mass production and consumption. In his study of this history of labor management, also called *The Human Motor* (Rabinbach 1990), Anson Rabinbach describes the attempt in the nineteenth century to "harmonize the movements of the body with those of the industrial machine" (p. 2). This view of the worker as an extension of the machine formed a central part of the productivist ideologies of Taylorism and Fordism, in which efficiency became understood as the domain of management, based on the analysis of the worker's movements removed from the site of production. The worker lost control of the pace and output of his/her activities. Skill and experience was now subordinated to surveillance and analysis. Centralized planning and control sought to quantify and standardize labor. Frank Gilbreth, who worked with Frederick Winslow Taylor, extended the research of pioneers such as Marey and Muybridge, through photographic studies of worker's movements. The visual records of skilled workers' gestures established standards for others to follow.

This attempt to monitor, control, and exploit human labor by recording and analyzing it as visual information is related to cultural trauma through the uses of shock. Ivan Pavlov's research on human reflexes showed that the administering of shock demanded attention but also numbed emotional and intellectual responses. Mass media drew on this research, using shock to capture audience attention. This also rendered audiences unresponsive, requiring continual intensification of visual and aural impact in order to achieve the required effect (Beller 2006). The manipulation of attention at work and through media images formed a new cultural experience conditioned by mechanical repetition and sudden shock. With the incorporation of visual experience in the organization of both labor and leisure in industrial societies, argues Jonathan Beller, the human subject encounters his/her self-image in a technological form. The responses and choices made by the worker-consumer are integrated through physiological research informing technological design and communication. This refashioning of human behavior is pioneered in industrial mass production and further refined by digital technologies and information networks.

For Pavlov, the nervous system was a "medium for the translation of signaled stimuli into responses" (Beller 2006, p. 123) and his experiments on dogs included electric shocks. As Allan Young explains, the victims of these experiments learned to associate pain with other environmental factors. Sensory stimuli associated with the memory of the shock later caused the victim to relive the distressing experience. The victim was thus conditioned to respond in two possible ways: by following routines that sought to avoid the upsetting stimuli, or assuming a completely passive attitude (psychic numbing). Young notes a third possible reaction, which he links with posttraumatic stress disorder: victims seek out circumstances that repeat the original trauma. The distressing memory produces endorphins that tranquilize the subject, leading to an addiction to the repeated behavior (Young 1977, pp. 257–258).

Media technologies are designed to capture human attention and this requires the individual to adapt his or her "protective shield" against intrusive sensory information. When this protective apparatus is breached the effect is "traumatic." Images that have a traumatic effect achieve a special status and become connected to other series of media images that hold the spectator in place as a member of an imagined community or social network. Shock becomes a primary way that individuals and groups define themselves, and thus fit "traumatic" narratives about cultural identity. Shock is part of the everyday experience of humans in technologically advanced societies, making media images an important feature of cultural trauma. The suffering of those who have suffered actual violence or abuse or who have experienced some catastrophic event has been aligned with collective identity through a media apparatus that administers and manages shock for a mass audience. The media audience's expectation of, and appetite for, shock transmitted by mass media and information networks has enabled the successful promotion of cultural trauma as a basis for membership in a political community and a shared experience of history.

2.5 The Politics of Mediated Trauma

Shock can form part of voyeuristic pleasure but can also foster identification with the position of victim. Media provides its own version of psychotherapy: by presenting images and stories that surprise and distress viewers and by integrating them into narratives about collective identity the media supply both the trauma and the treatment. In this, the entertainment industries can be understood to follow the model set by the medical establishment. In *Manufacturing Victims* (Dineen 1999), Tara Dineen argues that the "Psychology Industry" exploits human suffering to produce victims as the objects of diagnosis, treatment, and, ultimately, profit. She writes of three methods by which this process is achieved: psychologizing, pathologizing, and generalizing. Psychology translates experiences into theoretical constructs and applies these constructs to people through labels (such as "traumatized") and then generalizes them to the point that extreme experiences of violence become confused or equated with more mundane forms of distress (p. 27). She argues that Lifton's interpretation of the experiences of Hiroshima and Holocaust survivors follows this pattern of producing theoretical abstractions (such as "the survivor") that then become generalized and applied in different situations. Dineen's criticism is persuasive to the extent that cultural trauma narratives take a specific individual's or group's experiences and translate them into moral universals. However, if we take into account the role of technological media and shock in fostering identification with cultural trauma, Lifton's account of psychic numbing can be understood as useful and insightful.

For over a century modern visual media has been shaping certain kinds of responses and expectations which have gradually been integrated into broader cultural and political processes. Catastrophes, political upheavals, and economic crises attract intense media coverage fostering mass anxiety and leading to demands for the restoration of social order and stability. In such situations, public figures, intellectuals and media commentators construct trauma narratives which seek to make sense of disruptive and disturbing experiences for large groups of people. For this reason such situations also offer important opportunities for political leadership and new political initiatives. What Frank Furedi (2004) has called "therapy culture" has tended to replace narratives of political engagement or protest with those that emphasize emotional and psychological vulnerability. Moments of catastrophe and crisis allow mass media to construct moments of national consensus and communities of mourning. Through ritual performances such as commemorative ceremonies and funerals, the media orchestrates a collective and communal emotional response.

Images of human suffering are commodities that circulate in competitive media markets. The iconography of violence and pain in commercial media tends to falsely universalize human suffering because it is unable to reconcile the moral ambiguity surrounding exploitation for profit, on one hand, and the need to inform the public on the other. Those who suffer are also pathologized, their experiences turned into trauma narratives that circulate as a form of symbolic capital in various medical, legal, political, and mediated contexts (Kleinman & Kleinman 2009, p. 295). What is often left out of these professional discourses is any acknowledgement of the ways that the "victim" understand their own experience. These "traumatized" populations are denied political agency and become objects of pity, charity, or worse, idle curiosity.

Since the end of the Cold War, humanitarian interests have become the new justification for Western military interventions that receive intensive media coverage and are seen by governments as opportunities to give a public display of high moral values and aspirations. Media representations construct other nations in crisis as chaotic scenes of suffering and violence without meaning, except for their evident need for rescue by the West. Philip Hammond (2007) has proposed that these humanitarian interventions are examples of "Western narcissism and the search for meaning" (p. 49), in which the West attempts to recover its sense of moral purpose and legitimacy by way of catastrophes suffered by others: "their" suffering is "our" therapy. Hammond's critique of Western humanitarianism can be extended to the widespread acceptance of cultural trauma narratives. The visual consumption of violence and catastrophe creates an expectation of shock and horror. The absence of political analyses that can make sense of this spectacle of suffering and destruction contributes to the numbing and emotional disengagement of the viewer. The viewer experiences a loss of meaning. Cultural trauma narratives fill this vacuum by allowing the viewer to identify with the position of victim and translate their own cultural and political disorientation into membership in a community.

But doesn't the preoccupation with cultural trauma and the Holocaust follow a similar logic? The Holocaust has become a symbol of "absolute evil" in modern societies where there is increasing fragmentation of shared moral values. The universality imputed to the Holocaust also relativizes the ongoing crimes and injustices perpetrated by other modern states, particularly the liberal democratic societies in which the Holocaust has achieved such cultural prominence. As Anne Rothe (2011) puts it: "redemptive narratives serve to transform the pain of others into politically anesthetizing mass media commodities" (p. 15). The Holocaust, narrated in popular forms such as novels, films, television dramas, children's books, and comics, has begun to function as a master narrative of victimization allowing for, or encouraging, widely divergent individuals and groups to identify themselves with the roles of victim or benevolent savior.

The "events of September 11" have become an iconic example of the ways that spectacular and dramatic media images played a role in defining America as the victim of hostility, envy, and malicious attack. The impact and authority of these images also overshadowed the more complex history of conflict and violence from which the attacks emerged. Fatima Naqvi (2007) asks why Western societies, who remain in positions of economic and military dominance, tend to represent themselves as victims (p. 1). With the breakdown of many social structures that in the past defined cultural belonging and status, identification with the victim may appear to promise an alternative legitimacy. Victimhood is an affirmation of social belonging. In an age when visual media provide a limitless supply of images of human suffering, the overwhelming majority of which happens outside Western societies, their claim to victimhood takes on a particularly hollow ring. While images and dramatizations of the Holocaust may allow contemporary audiences to identify with the position of innocent victim, images of starvation, genocide, and torture in distant parts of the world confront the West more directly with its responsibility for perpetuating, directly or indirectly, violent oppression.

Often the application of psychological concepts to cultural criticism has been focused on the role of modern visual media as the mode of transmission. In academic trauma studies, this has meant trying to determine the most authentic means to convey the reality of historical experiences through images and stories. But these approaches have tended to ignore the cultural and technological transformations that have made trauma a central narrative in modern societies. Our understanding of historical trauma needs to address the ways that mediated forms of shock open up new spaces for rearticulating and repositioning collective identity. Cultural trauma allows a society to assume the role of victim, displacing the guilt associated with perpetrating violence against others. It also allows populations to be defined as subjects of therapy or actors in a collective psycho-drama. Meanwhile, the suffering of other populations remains silent and invisible.

References

Adorno, T. (1973). *Negative dialectics*. New York: Continuum.

Agamben, G. (1998). *Homo sacer: Sovereign power and bare life. Trans. Daniel Heller-Roazen*. Stanford, CA: Stanford University Press.

Alexander, J. (2012). *Trauma: A social theory*. Cambridge: Polity.

Amar, J. (1920). *Human motor; or the scientific foundations of labour and industry*. New York: Dutton.

Beller, J. (2006). *The cinematic mode of production: Attention economy and the society of the spectacle*. Hanover and London: UP of New England.

Benjamin, W. (2003). On some motifs in Baudelaire. In H. Eiland & M. W. Jennings (Eds.), *Walter Benjamin: Selected writings volume 4, 1938-1940* (pp. 313–355). Cambridge, MA: Harvard University Press.

Braun, M. (1992). *Picturing time: The work of Etienne-Jules Marey (1830-1904)*. Chicago: University of Chicago Press.

Didi-Huberman, G. (2003). *Invention of hysteria: Charcot and the photographic iconography of the Salpêtrière*. Cambridge, MA, London: MIT Press.

Dineen, T. (1999). *Manufacturing victims: What the psychology industry is doing to people*. London: Constable.

Felman, S., & Laub, D. (1992). *Testimony: Crises of witnessing in literature, psychoanalysis and history*. New York: Routledge.

Furedi, F. (2004). *Therapy culture: Cultivating vulnerability in an uncertain age*. London and New York: Routledge.

Hammond, P. (2007). *Media, war and postmodernity*. London and New York: Routledge.

Kleinman, A., & Kleinman, J. (2009). Cultural appropriations of suffering. In U. Linke & D. T. Smith (Eds.), *Cultures of fear: A critical reader* (pp. 288–303). London and New York: Pluto Press.

LaCapra, D. (1998). *History and memory after Auschwitz*. Ithaca and London: Cornell University Press.

Levy, D., & Sznaider, N. (2006). *The Holocaust and memory in the global age*. Philadelphia: Temple University Press.

Lifton, R. J. (1967). *Death in life: Survivors of Hiroshima*. New York: Random House.

Lifton, R. J. (1973). *Home from the war: Vietnam veterans: Neither victims nor executioners*. New York: Simon & Schuster.

Naqvi, F. (2007). *The literary and cultural rhetoric of victimhood: Western Europe, 1970-2005*. Hampshire, New York: Palgrave.

Rabinbach, A. (1990). *The human motor: Energy, fatigue, and the origins of modernity*. Berkeley, Los Angeles: University of California Press.

Rothberg, M. (2009). *Multidirectional memory: Remembering the Holocaust in the age of decolonization*. Stanford: Stanford University Press.

Rothe, A. (2011). *Popular trauma culture: Selling the pain of others in the mass media*. New Brunswick, NJ, London: Rutgers University Press.

Young, A. (1977). Suffering and the origins of traumatic memory. In A. Kleinman, V. Das, & M. Lock (Eds.), *Social suffering* (pp. 245–260). Berkeley, Los Angeles, London: University of California Press.

Young, A. (2007). Post-traumatic stress disorder of the virtual kind: Trauma and resilience in post-9/11 America. In A. Austin Sarat, N. Davidovitch, & M. Albertstein (Eds.), *Trauma and memory: Reading, healing, and making law* (pp. 21–48). Stanford: Stanford University Press.

Zelizer, B. (1992). *Covering the body: The Kennedy assassination, the media, and the shaping of collective memory*. Chicago: University of Chicago Press.

3 Television: A Traumatic Culture

Dan Arav

3.1 Introduction

From its inception, the moving image has been a major component in the assimilation of the culture of trauma into everyday life.[1] Today, by means of the veteran medium of television and its contemporary digital derivatives (YouTube, Instagram, etc.,), individuals in Western society are, more than ever before, exposed to trauma in its various and sundry forms, both on the individual and the collective levels.

It should be noted that the link between the traumatic experience and the medium of television exists only in the cultural-aesthetic sphere. In point of fact, according to the common viewpoint found in both scientific and cultural discourse, when it comes to reality, the traumatic experience and the medium of television are positioned precisely at opposite ends of the equation. Trauma is defined as an anomalous occurrence that takes place outside the symbolic order, making it an experience that is difficult, if not impossible, to report on, bear witness to and become engaged in. In contrast, the popular format and content of the medium of television consistently claim to be an accurate, reliable, and complete reflection of reality (Fiske, 1987, pp. 17–37). Television realism is based on an ongoing attempt to blur and conceal the means by which the message is transmitted. More than anything else, television seeks to incorporate into the hearts and minds of the viewers the belief that the reality visible on the screen is ostensibly "the thing itself" without any mediation, shaping or personal or ideological factors involved in the process. "The view of television realism is often expressed by the metaphors of transparency or reflection—television is seen

[1] Both the moving image and trauma as a concept are the products of modernity and of the Industrial Revolution. Recognition of trauma on both the scientific and the public levels is, as noted, tied to the strong relationship with the emergence of the railroad and the numerous railroad accidents since its inception. As railroad accidents began to introduce spectacular images of destruction and disaster into the public imagination that are not related to the battlefield, the medical profession began to encounter psychological symptoms among the survivors. Like other scientific developments, the cinema, whose origins date back to the late nineteenth century, is an expression of progress—a machine harnessed for the sake of investigating the world and human beings. If we so desire, we can find an anecdotal connection between railroad accidents, which epitomized the post-traumatic condition, and the documentary film by the Lumière brothers, *The Arrival of a Train at a Station* (1896). The images from this first film to be screened commercially aroused anxiety in the hearts of its viewers, who in their imaginations transformed the train rushing across the screen into a horrifying reality from which they had to flee.

D. Arav, Ph.D. (✉)
School of Media Studies, The College of Management Academic Studies (COMAS), 7 Yitzhak Rabin Blvd., Rishon LeZion 7502501, Israel
e-mail: aravdan@gmail.com

Y. Ataria et al. (eds.), *Interdisciplinary Handbook of Trauma and Culture*, DOI 10.1007/978-3-319-29404-9_3

either as a transparent window on the world or as a mirror reflecting our own reality back to us" (Fiske, 1987, p. 18). Trauma, then, appears to be the exact opposite of television. In effect, what can be said about trauma is that it denies realism and persistently refuses to find any relationship between the signifier and what it signifies "in reality." This tension between the television medium and trauma appears to be what has given rise to the entire complex of associations and reciprocal relations between the two.

In contemporary culture and particularly Western culture, the moving image constitutes a major channel for leisure and entertainment. As a means directed at mass consumption, the television medium is umbilically tied to market logic. It is widely considered to be an aesthetic form characterized by contemporary capitalism and as a medium that acts to reinforce the prevailing political-economic system. In effect, television operates in two dimensions: On the one hand, to generate interest, excitement, identification, and ongoing attention as responses from its audience, televised content must present an unstable reality marked by innovation, conflict, and crisis. On the other hand, and at the same time, for both aesthetic and ideological reasons the text presented on television constantly strives for closure: for solutions to the dramatic plot and for a return to order even if this is only an illusion.[2] This duality is diffused over the role of television trauma. Television as a medium that strives to capture attention mediates trauma to the masses. At the same time, as a medium that works out of and in the name of the prevailing order, television strives in various and sundry ways to process and normalize collective trauma.

This chapter, then, seeks to map the various expressions of the traumatic experience as they are manifested on television and to consider the major role played by this experience in contemporary television discourse. This chapter is unique in that it positions trauma not only as a popular phenomenon represented in various ways on the screen, but also as a central concept used to decipher the logic behind the operation of the medium itself. The focal point of the chapter lies in the following distinction: On the one hand, it views the culture of trauma as a cultural product shaped primarily by television, while on the other hand it perceives the television medium as a major means of working through trauma, on the personal level and in particular on the collective level.

In an attempt to consider all the associations between trauma and television, I have divided the topic into two arenas for discussion:

1. *Television as a form of traumatic utterance and as a generator of trauma.*

   This discussion is based upon the deterministic technological tradition that sees the development of technology as the first and foremost factor in shaping the development of society. It is also based on the doctrine of philosophers such as Bruno Latour (1992) and others, who contend that the contemporary media experience has been established by a unique and independent pattern based on the incorporation of the world of machines into the human space. Accordingly, the discussion focuses on technology per se and on the unique aesthetic attributes of television as machine and identifies how these are associated with trauma. This leads to a discussion of televised content and of how the media represents "Trauma" events and a consideration of what is, in fact, televised trauma.
2. *Television as a mechanism for working through trauma; posttraumatic memories on television.*

   Here, the discussion focuses on an attempt to consider the extent to which modern media influences the traumatic experience within the individual and in the public sphere. What role does television play in "marketing"

[2] Researchers who see the medium of television as a transparent means of promoting the values of the dominant culture tend to see the text as "closed," a text whose interpretation is in line with the prevailing values. Alongside these are those who stress the "openness" of the text and its freedom to be interpreted in different ways by different groups and in different contexts.

trauma and in assimilating it into the public imagination? And how, if at all, has technology been harnessed to work through individual and collective trauma? The possibility of seeing the medium of television as a platform for rehabilitation and recovery, or at least for working through trauma, is examined by means of several aesthetic mechanisms that serve the medium in its operation. Central to this notion are the practices of testimony and reconstruction. The practice of testimony is implemented on television as an inherent part of diverse television texts, ranging from the news and documentary broadcasts to reality shows, talk shows, and commercials, thus marking the medium itself as a mechanism for testimony. The act of televised reconstruction (or televised reenactment) aims at producing an agreed-upon version of reality while exploiting the unique technical possibilities offered by this medium. One method that stands out in this aesthetic-technological process is the use of slow motion, which is discussed in detail. Ultimately, slow motion and other major aesthetic mechanisms seem to lead to a nostalgic aestheticization of trauma and in fact to concealing its threatening essence. This is the stage at which the trauma of television subjugates itself to the economic logic on which the television medium is based and to the consumers' built-in expectations of pleasure. This is the stage at which trauma turns into a commodity, to a paradoxical territory of objects marked by a mixture of terror and entertainment.

3.2 Television as a Form of Traumatic Utterance and as a Generator of Trauma

Traces of symbolic trauma are inherent in every television text. In effect, television is a traumatic form. If trauma can still be defined as an experience that is formulated as the result of an encounter with that which has deviated from the human experience, with that which radically does not conform to what is expected, the medium of television—"the preeminent machine of decontextualization" (Doane, 1990, p. 225)—can be seen as an effective and sophisticated mechanism that constantly strives to produce trauma.

In essence, this decontextualization can be seen as the core of the traumatic mechanism of television. Every televised representation, whether realistic or metaphorical, contains the potential for trauma. Yet this statement must be clarified as follows: Trauma cannot be identified with televised conflict. While the television text is based on the ongoing structuring of artificial conflicts, trauma is precisely the outcome of the inability to represent conflict. While television conflicts are solved by adopting a coherent, organized, and binary position, trauma in effect denies the binary concept and the basic ability to normalize conflict by means of an organizing principle.

Time, and specifically the time a television consumer spends watching the screen, is television's ultimate commodity. As the first and foremost mechanism of capitalism, the television medium seeks to produce an ongoing viewing experience that will "nail" the television viewer to the screen while creating a continuing experience of decontextualization. Hence, media consumers (of television and the Internet) appear to surf or hop from channel to channel without any connection to space, time, or genre. Narrative, coherence, and rationality often have no significance in the consumer's viewing experience. The result is a random bricolage of pieces of television. The culture critic Raymond Williams (1974) stressed the notion of flow. According to him, the textual content moves from one image to another in an incessant flow of its own. This flow can be seen on the shopping channels and on CNN and MTV. John Ellis (1982) conceives of this as segmentation, contending that television does not represent textual development, but rather a rapid turnover of segments that have been formulated into blocks of images. Neil Postman (1985) maintains that the television text lacks causality, that it is a text without a beginning or an end, and that its major message is inherent in the words "and now to ...." The logic of the broadcast schedule and the way it is presented require that the viewing experience be shaped according to a narrative flow, even if it lacks coherence, to make it difficult for the viewer to "escape" to other channels.

The television text, the medium's basic formative approach, can be compared to the traumatic condition. In essence trauma is anomalous; it deviates from the flow of time and from causality. Like the traumatic experience, an experience that blurs the boundaries between present and past, television is also a paradoxical experience. Its flow is discontinuous and sporadic. Its fragmented, nonlinear text lacks causality, undermining continuity, and normal routine. Nevertheless, it is important to recognize the two as distinct one from the other. Trauma is an event that is difficult, if not impossible, to contain within the narrative of life. In contrast, the principle underlying the television medium is based on setting out a series of small shocks, which are sufficiently regulated so as to keep viewers alert but not so shocking as to disturb them.

Considering that television is totally embedded within a clearly capitalist context and that broadcasting organizations across the globe are powerful corporations, the medium functions as an anchor of conformity. As a medium operating within and in the name of the system, television acts to preserve and reinforce the status quo. The authoritative text produced in the television workshop proposes a resolution or annulment of the conflict, even if only symbolically and thus strives for an illusionary return to maintaining order. Commercials, sports events, news items, and in essence all television texts are organized around a dramatic format and use a rhetoric of conflict that simultaneously strives for resolution. Hence, every (television) conflict is in essence an introduction to the required lesson, to the desired solution (even if only partial) and to a soothing catharsis. Its appearance signals that additional conflicts will arise and be solved, and so on and so forth.

Television's intensive focus on terrorism and disasters seems to have reached its peak in the coverage of the collapse of the Twin Towers in September 2001. Images of this incident, which has been described as the greatest event in television history, provided the background for the rapid development of a new research field focusing on trauma generated by watching television (Ahern et al., 2002, 2004; Bernstein et al., 2007; Pfefferbaum, Pfefferbaum, North, & Neas, 2002). Special interest in this field was generated not only by the extreme nature of this event, its dimensions and its position at the core of America's sense of power. The way this incident was mediated to the public—through a live and developing broadcast to millions of people worldwide glued to their television sets—has led researchers, many from the behavioral sciences, to wonder whether television indeed constitutes a venue for trauma. Is exposure via the television screen to disturbing events, such as incidents of mass terrorism, likely to be traumatic? (Eth, 2002; Putnam, 2002).

It should be noted that most of the studies in the above field have discovered some sort of association between level of exposure to television during broadcasts of catastrophes and disasters and an increase in the prevalence of posttraumatic syndrome. Yet this relation is not direct. Usually another individual factor is needed that loads watching television with the potential for trauma. It should be remembered that exposure is not only measured by the amount of time devoted to watching but also by the quality of the exposure, by the degree of the viewer's involvement and by various other personality factors that can have an impact on this issue.

One way or another, the role of television in the Twin Towers disaster and other shocking incidents generated renewed awareness of the way in which television helps in positioning trauma, in packaging it as content that can be duplicated and recycled in various ways and intensities and in vigorously marketing it. Awareness of the role of television in shaping public memory as a traumatic memory has also increased.

3.3 Television as a Mechanism for Working Through Trauma; Posttraumatic Memories on Television

As in other discussions considering the nature of the television medium, the matter of working through the trauma also entails two quite contradictory approaches. The first sees television as a medium that does not at all facilitate working through trauma, while the second assigns television a central role in working through trauma, while imbuing it with personal and collective meanings.

3.3.1 Television: An Endless Repetition

According to the first approach, television causes the human experience to atrophy. It does not permit structuring the collective past by means of overcoming the individual past because it isolates the subject from authentic experiences. Thus, instead of private and individual moments, television recycles stereotypical versions of the past, a past that does not belong to anyone in particular. "Instead of experience and memory, television's past, whether funny or not, evokes laughter and distance; it is a dissociated, dated history, out of synch with the present, with nothing, now, to do with us—it is over and thus, paradoxically, ahistorical and nostalgic" (Mellencamp, 1990, p. 242). Television in effect traps the viewer in a region that is devoid of time, in which authentic experiences are not possible. It merely produces in the present, "a celebration of the Instantaneous" (Doane, 1990, p. 222). Mellencamp sums this up as follows: "TV triggers memories of TV in an endless chain of TV referentiality" (Mellencamp, 1990, p. 242).

Indeed, Mellencamp claims that television synchronizes memories of television, ending with the atrophy of experience. This is the reason that representations of trauma on television do not have a disturbing impact on the viewer; in effect they are not a direct confrontation with the event but rather a repetition of it. Thus, even the compulsive repetition of horrifying images plays a role in flattening and erasing the trauma. This form of television processing is essentially antihistorical and always belongs to the present. It may not be an exaggeration to claim that this endless repetition is likely to be reminiscent of the repetition compulsion that is often the fate of trauma victims (Arav, 2004).

By its very nature, television is a medium based upon repetition: repetition of what is known and safe, of what is "obvious" and of what "we've already seen." Clearly, despite television's promise of new development and renewal, in practice the medium is inexorably tied to circularity and repetition.

Psychoanalysts like Freud and Lacan devoted a significant amount of thought to the concept of repetition. In their view, repetition has one goal: to not remember. Repetition serves a fixed goal: the transition from knowing to not knowing. What the subject repeats is the trauma itself (Freud, 1914).

Freud referred to the repetition of a traumatic experience as the "repetition compulsion." In his early writing Freud interpreted this repetition as an attempt to control the traumatic event. Later and in contrast to other theoreticians, Freud did not make do with this explanation and formulated the concept of the "death drive." According to Freud, repetition is an instinct, "an urge in organic life to restore an earlier state of things" (Freud, 1920, p. 36). "Repetition compulsion" overrides all conscious intentions and objects vigorously to change. In his view, the explanation of repetition as an attempt to gain control over the trauma does not give expression to what he called the "demonic" character of the repeated experience.

However, other psychoanalysts claim that repetition is a spontaneous attempt to assimilate a traumatic event. Russell, for example, believes that "what is reproduced is what the person needs to feel in order to repair the injury" (Russell, 2006, p. 610). Caruth (1995), in contrast, diminishes the centrality of repetition in structuring the trauma and places the stress on forgetting. According to her, only by means of and within inherent forgetting can the experience be felt from the outset. What is recorded in the victim's brain is not only what he or she sees but in effect both things: the memory of the event itself and the distortion the event undergoes by means of remembering the trauma. Lacan associates repetition with the symbolic order. According to him, the repetition compulsion results from displacement of the original and initial impulse of some signifier. The repetition brings back to consciousness the signifier upon which the instinct was displaced, while repressing its initial content (Lacan, 1977, p. 50). In contrast, the philosopher Gilles Deleuze considered repetition an expression of difference (Deleuze, 1995). In his view, every act of writing is in effect repetition, but this is a form of writing with a difference. In a situation in which the only raw materials are the set of signs already existing in language, the original has no meaning. History, therefore, is always a reconstruction of the past.

It appears, then, that the notion of repetition is central to the very nature of the television medium. The format of the "rerun" is based primarily on constant repetition, as is the concept of an "open studio" or continuous live broadcast: repetition of what is already known, of a collection of the most dramatic images that can be found. For shocking events of all sorts, repetition becomes the essence. Does the uncompromising repetition of peak events (the explosions of the Columbia and Challenger space shuttles, the Twin Towers disaster in New York, the tsunami in Southeast Asia) turn the event into a visual spectacle, a show seen as something that can be controlled? It can be claimed that repetition creates a sense of continuity and control when confronting a violent event. Yet, against the backdrop of the television medium's ability to provide context (that is, to present events in their full historical complexity) on the one hand and in view of the compulsive repetition of the chain of images on the other, it can also be claimed that television practically erases the event. It closes off its viewers in an area lacking pain and time, where they cannot confront and work through the past.

Converting remembering into repetition is not, as noted, a major line of thinking in Freud's discussion of the response to trauma. In his view, repressing events from past memory causes these repressed memories to take the form of actions. Disregarding these memories leads to expression as acting out these conflicts rather than remembering them (Freud, 1914). According to Lacan, this "acting out" is not only derived from the failure to consciously remember the past, but also from the inability to communicate this failure to the other. The refusal of the other to listen to the subject causes the subject to give up on verbal communication and to channel his failure toward acting out. The subject is not conscious of this acting out. By actively turning the object outward, it becomes an alternative disclosure of the cause, of the repressed memory. Thus, acting out is a fraudulent unconscious pattern of action that compulsively repeats itself and is defensively turned upon the other.

3.3.2 Working Through Television

The second approach is concerned with the encounter between trauma and television. It considers the process through which television reworks the raw material of news into a structured narrative format as a process that essentially resembles the notion of working through. The therapeutic situation engenders the granting of meaning and the generation of structure as the attribute that individualizes the work of the therapist. Working through is a critical interpretive process that enables the subject to acknowledge the existence of repressed elements and to release himself from the suffering entailed in the mechanism of repetition. Ellis (1999) claims that television, in striving to explain and to provide additional information and perspectives regarding the raw material of the news, seeks to grant greater stability to images of disorder. Television refocuses and reframes, turning the items it contains into a narrative. According to Ellis, working through is a diverse process that takes place in a variety of programs and content fields, including talk shows, soap operas, documentary films, dramas, and feature films (Ellis, 1999). In practice, the link between the process of working through on television and the traumatic experience appears to be fully manifested in two major clinical/television practices: testimony and reconstruction.

3.4 Testimony

The developing discourse regarding the role of testimony and the status of eyewitnesses has become a major part of contemporary discussions of trauma and posttrauma. "To testify is (thus) not merely to narrate but to commit oneself, and to commit the narrative, to others, to take responsibility—in speech—for history or for the truth of an occurrence, for something which, by definition, goes beyond the personal, in having general (not personal) validity and consequences" (Felman, 1991, p. 39–40). Testimony is discourse in practice, the pledge to tell, to generate a speech act as tangible proof of the truth. The ability of testimony to exist relies upon the presence of an event and on a later, though reliable, report after the event. Yet 70 years after the Holocaust and in view of the traumatic history of the second half of the twentieth century, recognition of the crisis in testimony is growing. Researchers such as Felman and Laub see trauma as an epistemological crisis that extends beyond individual therapy and points to the difficulty accessing our historical experience (Felman & Laub, 1992). Laub ties this crisis to the question of the witness and testimony. According to him, the Holocaust led to "the collapse of testimony," for the history of the Holocaust ostensibly took place "without any witnesses." Its terrible circumstances made it impossible to be "part of the event" and to survive as well, so that the historical commandment "to bear witness" could not be carried out (Laub, 1995).[3]

In opposition to this dual viewpoint focusing on the tension between the commandment to testify and the crisis of testimony, the testimony of television is positioned as a major component of the practice customary in this medium. An "eyewitness" is a key actor and a basic component of the television text. Moreover, the television text claims the status of a testimony that carries unequivocal proof of factual truth. In essence, it can be said that in view of the massive use of eyewitnesses on television and considering the perspective that sees the text itself as testimony, discussion of the role of the witness and consideration of the status of testimony in culture have become extremely relevant and urgent.

Like the status of the eyewitness in legal practice—which is based on investigating the truth—media, and in particular the moving image, sing the praises of eyewitness testimony: the one who was out there "in the field" and who saw the events with his or her "own eyes." This close and direct contact, and yet, at the same time free of any real involvement in the event, is captivating to a medium that proudly waves the flag of reality. The growing trend toward using testimony "from the field" can be seen as part of the conventions of the news genre, which seeks—through its format—to signify control and the return of order. The witness provides his version and thus reorganizes the shattered reality into a more or less coherent story that binds the exceptional event into the symbolic order. And indeed, testimony given directly to the camera can be seen in news broadcasts, documentary films, historical feature films, police reconstructions, reality shows, commercials, and other formats as well. Witnesses are everywhere. They all contribute to creating the illusion of direct knowledge of reality, without any externality interests.

In view of the power of personal and ostensibly unmediated testimony, often given in revealing and moving close-up photos, considerations regarding the validity of eyewitness testimony are often pushed to the side. What, in effect, is the witness giving testimony about? Does being present at an event actually bring someone closer to the "truth"? Or does being there, close to what is happening, conceal the "big picture" from the witness and limit his or her understanding of the event? And what about the validity of testimony given after some time has gone by? The idea that time is liable to blur and weaken the witness's

[3]Another expression of the crisis in testimony brought about by the Holocaust is inherent in the representation plane: the absolute philosophical distance between the language of the murderers and the language of their victims (Agamben, 1999; Lyotard, 1983, 1989), the inability to talk about death while using customary language and the claim that Auschwitz is "an historical fact" even though it has no place in the language—all these make historical testimony virtually impossible, for it demands breaking through rational thought itself.

memory is pushed to the side. Is it even possible to consider testimony as "authentic" in view of the fact that testimony is mediated by other testimonies and representations of the event? And what is the fate of testimony when it is given a second and third time? Does repeating the testimony guarantee that the story will be preserved, or does it lead to change? In particular, to what extent is the testimony subject to the representational regime, to the set of preliminary expectations built by its representational context? How are general and market interests involved in the process? None of these questions are apparent to the television viewer.

Even more problematic criticism of the reliability of eyewitness testimony has been raised by the post-Freudian school of thought, which has gained prominence in recent years. This movement has challenged the view of individual memory as something sacred and immune and has rejected the very existence of repressed memory. For example, the American researcher Elizabeth Loftus (Loftus, 1996; Loftus & Kitchum, 1994) stresses the structuring of memory by means of information acquired after the fact. According to her, memories of events that are perceived as difficult when they occur will be easily recalled. If indeed the testimony of an eyewitness is likely to be based, in whole or in part, on implanted memory, it may be that the media also behaves in a similar manner. An eyewitness, like the general public, is exposed to versions of the past that are vigorously marketed by the media, seen here as a powerful creator of false and implanted memories.

Television, then, is deeply involved in the question of the status of testimony today. In effect, the medium has played a major role in undermining the status of the witness and of testimony as a major element in the effort to establish a collective memory. Today "the aesthetics of testimony" appears to be replacing testimony itself. Before our very eyes the genre of testimony and confession is being transformed into ritual and media convention. When the witness becomes a permanent resident on the television screen, his testimony, rather than testifying to an event, in essence testifies to a new cultural condition. In this new era, testimony is tantamount to truth, and personal confession is the passionate object of the confessor and of the audience as well. In this medium, whose underlying principle relies on the illusion of the intimacy it generates among its recipients, generates "easy conditions" for the witness. These conditions transform the testimony into an object of temptation, a basic component of the economics of televised images. The witness and the medium of television are engaged in a relationship of symbolic exchange. By virtue of appearing on television, the witness is glorified. In the eyes of the viewers he is seen as someone whose testimony is important. Television also benefits from this relationship. In appearing on television, the witness enhances the halo on which the broad acceptance of television is based: the direct and unmediated contact it sells, the strong belief that television testifies to what "really" happened.

3.5 Reconstruction, Reenactment

In essence, the photographic image contains within itself a reconstruction of the past. Every photograph testifies to what already was, bears witness that the event occurred (Barthes, 1980). Every testimony, photographic or otherwise, is a text of reconstruction. The trauma victim can also be seen as someone who carries within himself a reconstructed version of the past—one that is partial, complex, and inaccessible.

To reconstruct is to create anew. Reconstruction is the renewed construction of some order of things, usually of what has gotten out of control and requires repair. Reconstruction assumes that it is possible to discover the true reason, to recreate the approximated order of things, to reliably, and accurately revive the past. In effect, both on the personal and on the social level, reconstruction—in the media, in law, in art, and in other fields of endeavor—can be seen as an agreed upon social ritual relying on sophisticated technology and intended to stimulate a sense of faith and control over reality. It is also a ritual, entailing an effort to restore the social order.

In being faithful to its "obligation" to provide viewers with a reliable and accurate picture of reality, the medium of television frequently offers them artificial reconstructions. When the natural order, that is the ongoing supply of images from an event, is disrupted, when there are no "real" pictures from the scene of the event, the medium employs simulations, by means of hyperrealistic technologies and familiar aesthetics, that transform the reconstruction into an undisputable picture of the truth. A central aesthetic component of televised reconstruction is slow motion. This deviation from the "normal" pace of life, i.e., the representation of time at a slower pace, creates an effect of conspicuousness, distinction, and deviation (Madsen, 1973, p. 185).

Slow motion thus simultaneously serves to realize two goals of television: One is the attempt to take things out of context—removing an event from the ordinary order of events in order to signify it as exceptional. The other is the restoration of order—the moderation of the event and the slowing down of its visual (moving) images in order to break it down and examine it, and thus to moderate it and return it to the symbolic order (Arav, 2004).

Slow motion has two ostensibly contradictory dimensions. Alongside the extreme sense of realism that stresses the medium's "investigative" abilities, slow motion, which suspends cinematic time for the sake of imaginary and unrealistic time, also provides an almost contradictory feeling: the sense of artificial reality, expropriated from the precise context of time and place. Hence, in addition to its investigative and disassembling role, slow motion serves to enhance and glorify the moment by generating a flood of feelings of longing and fond remembering.

From this, it should be understood that slow motion is an aesthetic form that corresponds with—and perhaps even dictates—the symbolism of trauma. Images in slow motion have already been assimilated into the public imagination as an aesthetic platform for the representation of an extreme event experienced on the personal or public level. Thus, when the victim of a trauma describes the instigating event, more often than not he or she will describe it as an experience absorbed by his or her senses in slow motion.

Televised representations of horrific events will often appear to be slowed down. That which is extreme and deviant more often than not is represented as an artificial, unnatural, and fantastic form of reality. Hence, the extreme aestheticization of the process or event that generates the trauma (the collapse of the Twin Towers shown over and over again in slow motion) is intensified to the point of transforming it into a purely aesthetic experience that attracts attention by virtue of its performative qualities, which have been enhanced by the medium. The viewer's yearning for these aesthetic images signifies the beginning of a process in which what is traumatic seeps into what is nostalgic and entertaining.

3.6 Nostalgia

The exhaustive blending of the private and the public, between repetition and reconstruction, between eyewitness reports and the commercialization of testimony, penetrates and influences the content and form of collective memory. Currently the place occupied by trauma seems to be taken over by nostalgic sentiment. The pattern of acting out, as described above, that is derived from the inability to provide a representation of the object (in this case, the traumatic experience) and is based upon the element of repetition, is found in the sense of nostalgia based on the repetition of what is known, a fitting framework for its operation. If acting out aims at an excess sense of vitality that denies the wound and the unprocessed pain, nostalgia transforms the reality of the past into something alive in the present. Like acting out, nostalgia also refuses to work through the past in order to transform it into a meaningful memory. The mechanism of nostalgia focuses on excess activity, on virtual activity in the present, as a substitute for the inability to remember. The nostalgic image produces a sentimental substitute whose entire mission is to deny the fact that this is a matter belonging to the past. Addiction to nostalgia creates a sense of excess vitality and, with respect to reality, thus withholds from the individual any thoughts of denial or criticism.

The notion that television speeds up the transformation of traumatic memory into a type of melancholic nostalgia certainly has major psychopolitical significance. The repeated and nostalgic representation of war through the ritual of fixed media images can be seen as a process of denial that operates continually and efficiently to blur the factor generating the collective trauma, i.e., the state of ongoing war. It may be that the disturbing association between traumatic experience and an exhibitionist, nostalgic television culture instills within us dangerous illusions, because of the idea that the discourse of trauma will lead us to redemption and serenity. It is precisely the popularization of the use of the concept of trauma that is what covers up the condition of political helplessness and despair.

3.7 The Moving Image as a Clinical Means

We cannot conclude this essay without wondering at the use of the moving image as a possible practice in therapy with the victims of certain types of trauma. The television archives and the medium's diverse techniques are often turned into therapeutic tools by the therapist in order to confront the patient with the trauma-generating experience (Moore, Chernell, & West, 1965).

In order to achieve emotional relief intended to release the individual from the memory of the traumatic experience, Freud introduced the concept of abreaction, a therapeutic method based on recalling and reenacting the traumatic experience in a controlled environment. Abreaction is designed to lead the patient to undergo the emotional experience which was suppressed in the original incident, which thus leads to catharsis. When the victim experiences crying, anger, a desire for revenge, and the like, the emotion that accompanied the traumatic experience is released and the memory of the traumatic experience is moderated and can be contained. Freud believed that abreaction could be achieved through hypnosis, which ensures suspension of the patient's defenses. Later he claimed that the ordinary psychoanalytic process based on conversation and free association could also result in the patient achieving abreaction.

Thus, if, as argued above, watching television is liable to arouse trauma, at the same time the medium is likely to serve as a means of abreaction. Watching a televised documentary or feature film focusing on an incident similar to the one generating the trauma is likely to flood the trauma victim with the repressed emotions and to bring him to catharsis. This can take place in the therapeutic space or under any other viewing conditions.

At this point the circle is closed. Television as a medium and an instrument mediating the private and public spheres blurs and shapes the traumatic experience as a televised commodity subject to the medium's constraints of content, format, and socioeconomic context. On the other hand, under the sponsorship of the television medium, a shocking private event is transformed into a public spectacle and is ultimately returned to the individual in the form of a televised reconstruction intended to heal him.

3.8 Conclusion

This chapter has attempted to describe the central mechanisms that integrate trauma into the contemporary television culture. The traumatic experience—an experience that ostensibly cannot be conceptualized—is translated into the prime raw material for producing attractive content. Major practices of the televised text, among them testimony and reconstruction, emerge as essential in the establishment of the contemporary culture of trauma.

The question of the extent to which television is likely to function differently remains open. The basic rules of the medium, its customary regime of images and its economic logic will not change in the near future. Television's promise to provide a clear picture of reality and the public's yearning for a "happy end" and for closure and order—even if these are merely an illusion—will continue to accompany contemporary society for many years to come.

References

Agamben, G. (1999). *Remnants of Auschwitz: The witness and the archive (D. Heller, Trans.)*. New York: Zone Books.

Ahern, J., Galea, S., Resnick, H., Kilpatrick, D., Bucuvalas, M., Gold, J., et al. (2002). Television images and psychological symptoms after September 11 terrorist attacks. *Psychiatry, 65*, 289–300.

Ahern, J., Galea, S., Resnick, H., & Vlahov, D. (2004). Television images and probable posttraumatic stress disorder after September 11: The role of background characteristics, event exposures, and perievent panic. *Journal of Nervous & Mental Disease, 192*(3), 217–226.

Arav, D. (2004). Trauma in slow-motion: Historical reconstruction on television. In H. Bresheeth, S. Sand, & M. Zimmermann (Eds.), *Cinema and memory: A dangerous relationship?* (pp. 217–233). Jerusalem: The Zalman Shazar Center for Jewish History. Hebrew, Kolnoa Ve-Zikaron: Yacasim Mesucanim.

Barthes, R. (1980). *La Chambre Claire*. Paris: Editions de l'Etoile, Gallimard, Le Seuil.

Bernstein, K. T., Ahern, J., Tracy, M., Boscarino, J. A., Vlahov, D., & Galea, S. (2007). Television watching and the risk of incident probable posttraumatic stress disorder: A prospective evaluation. *Journal of Nervous & Mental Disease, 195*(1), 41–47.

Caruth, C. (1995). Trauma and experience. In C. Caruth (Ed.), *Trauma: Explorations in memory*. Baltimore and London: The Johns Hopkins University Press.

Deleuze, G. (1995). *Difference and repetition*. New York: Columbia University Press. Original work published 1968.

Doane, M. A. (1990). Information, crisis, catastrophe. In P. Mellencamp (Ed.), *Logics of television. Essays in cultural criticism* (pp. 222–239). Bloomington: Indiana University Press.

Ellis, J. (1982). *Visible fictions: Cinema, television, video*. London: Routledge.

Ellis, J. (1999). Television as working-through. In J. Gripsrud (Ed.), *Television and common knowledge* (pp. 55–70). London and New York: Routledge.

Eth, S. (2002). Television viewing as a risk factor. *Psychiatry, 65*(4), 301–303.

Felman, S. (1991). *In an era of testimony: Claude Lanzmann's Shoah* (Yale French studies, pp. 39–81). New Haven, CT: Yale University Press.

Felman, S., & Laub, D. (1992). *Testimony: Crises of witnessing in literature, psychoanalysis, and history*. New York and London: Routledge.

Fiske, J. (1987). *Television culture*. London: Routledge.

Freud, S. (1914). Errinern, Wiederholen und Durcharbeiten. (Weitere Ratschläge zur Technik der Psychoanalyse, II). *Internationale Zeitschrift für ärtztliche Psychoanalyse, 2*, 485–491. Remembering, repeating and working-through, SE, 12: 147–156.

Freud, S. (1920). *Beyond the pleasure principle*. New York: Norton.

Lacan, J. (1977). In A. Sheridan (Ed.), *Seminar, Book XI, the four fundamental concepts of psychoanalysis*. London: Hogarth Press and Institute of Psycho-Analysis (Original work published 1964).

Latour, B. (1992). Where are the missing masses? The sociology of a few mundane artifacts. In W. Bijker & J. Law (Eds.), *Shaping technology/building society: Studies in sociotechnical change* (pp. 225–258). Cambridge: MIT Press.

Laub, D. (1995). Truth and testimony: The process and the struggle. In C. Caruth (Ed.), *Trauma: Explorations in memory* (pp. 61–75). Baltimore and London: The Johns Hopkins University Press.

Loftus, E. (1996). *Eyewitness testimony*. Cambridge, MA: Harvard University Press.

Loftus, E., & Kitchum, K. (1994). *The myth of repressed memory: False memories and allegations of sexual abuse*. New York: St. Martin's Griffin Press.

Lyotard, J. F. (1983). *Le differend*. Paris: Editions de Minuit.

Lyotard, J. F. (1989). Discussions, or phrasing "after Auschwitz". In A. Benjamin (Ed.), *The Lyotard reader* (pp. 360–392). Cambridge, MA: Basil Blackwell.

Madsen, R. P. (1973). *The impact of film. How ideas are communicated through cinema and television* (p. 185). New York: Macmillan Publishing Co.

Mellencamp, P. (1990). TV time and catastrophe, or beyond the pleasure principle of television. In P. Mellencamp (Ed.), *Logics of television. Essays in cultural criticism* (pp. 240–266). Bloomington: Indiana University Press.

Moore, F. J., Chernell, E., & West, M. (1965). Television as a therapeutic tool: "O Wad Some Power the Giftie Gie Us". *Archives of General Psychiatry, 12*(2), 217–220.

Pfefferbaum, B., Pfefferbaum, R. L., North, C. S., & Neas, B. R. (2002). Does television viewing satisfy criteria for exposure to posttraumatic stress disorder? *Psychiatry, 65*(4), 306–309.

Postman, N. (1985). *Amusing ourselves to death: Public discourse in the age of show business*. New York: Penguin.

Putnam, F. (2002). Televised trauma and viewer PTSD: Implications for prevention. *Psychiatry, 65*(4), 310–312.

Russell, P. (2006). Trauma, repetition and affect. *Contemporary Psychoanalysis, 42*(4), 601–620.

Williams, R. (1974). *Television: Technology and cultural form*. New York: Shocken Books.

4 Popular Trauma Culture: The Pain of Others Between Holocaust Tropes and Kitsch-Sentimental Melodrama

Anne Rothe

4.1 Introduction

The representation of what Susan Sontag (2004) has famously described as the pain of others is not restricted to postmodern trauma theory and the select examples from the literary and filmic canon that constitute its limited empirical corpus as most scholarship in literary and cultural studies would still suggest.[1] According to the alternative paradigm proposed here, it is precisely the question trauma studies scholarship has left out that ought to be explored: namely, how the ubiquitous notion of trauma functions in contemporary culture. And since collectively shared ideas and cultural trends in imagined communities are generated and disseminated through the interaction of mass media products and the vast audiences that consume them, the representation of victimhood and oppression, violence, and suffering—which are considered inherently traumatizing experiences without differentiation[2]—has to be analyzed precisely in popular culture artifacts.[3]

According to Bruno Latour (1987), a concept succeeds based on its degree of associative power to bind otherwise heterogeneous ideas, i.e., the extent to which it functions as a discursive knot. Expanding Latour's argument from the natural sciences to representation at large and popular

[1] Caruth (1995), Caruth (1996), and Felman and Laub (1992) are the inaugural texts in trauma theory. Their exclusive focus on canonical literature and film has become paradigmatic in trauma studies scholarship. See, for instance, Horwitz (2000), King (2000), Whitehead (2004), Robson (2004), Kaplan (2005), and Nadal and Calvo (2014). Only Roger Luckhurst (1998) has acknowledged the ubiquity of depictions of trauma, victimization and suffering in popular culture and sought to integrate them into an analysis of the subject in canonical representations. However, in his monograph (Luckhurst, 2008), he focuses on analyses of trauma in the literary and filmic canon. See also Rothe (2011) for a more extensive discussion of popular trauma culture.

A. Rothe, Ph.D. (✉)
Department of Classical and Modern Languages, Literatures, and Cultures, Wayne State University, 487 Manoogian Hall, Detroit, MI 48202, USA
e-mail: au8313@wayne.edu

[2] As the idea of trauma widely disseminated through the mass media reflects little of the PTSD concept beyond the vague notion that it describes a psychological reaction to an experience of extremity, the cultural history of the psychiatric concept will not be discussed here.

[3] Since postmodern trauma theory, which emerged in 1990s American literary studies by way of a questionable expansion of Yale deconstruction and psychoanalysis into a general theory of representation, ignored popular culture as a source for empirically verifying the mostly speculative arguments and, moreover, the reception of such specialized academic discourse is limited to the discursive space of the academic ivory tower, trauma theory scholarship bears no relation to my notion of popular trauma culture and will therefore not be discussed here. For detailed and convincingly argued epistemological and ethical critiques of trauma theory see Leys (2000), Kansteiner (2004), Kanseiner and Weilnböck (2008), and Weilnböck (2008). See also my own critique of postmodern trauma theory in chapter 12.

Y. Ataria et al. (eds.), *Interdisciplinary Handbook of Trauma and Culture*,
DOI 10.1007/978-3-319-29404-9_4

culture in particular, I suggest that the trauma concept functions as a discursive knot in contemporary Western and especially American popular culture due to its vast associative powers of generating connections between disparate ideas. As I have argued in *Popular Trauma Culture* (Rothe, 2011), when American collective memory transformed the Holocaust from an event in European history into a metaphor for evil, it generated the narrative paradigm—the basic plot structure and core set of characters—for representing such vastly diverse experiences as child abuse, Holocaust survival, war combat, terminal illness, and addiction recovery.[4]

This chapter will be structured as follows: After tracing the emergence of trauma culture's exemplary plot paradigm and cast of characters in American Holocaust discourse, I will explore the transition from the victim to the survivor figure as the preeminent protagonist and the transformation of witness testimony into victim talk. Subsequently, I will discuss melodrama as the dominant narrative mode of representing experiences of victimization and suffering in trauma culture and the kitsch sentimentality they encode as their paradigmatic mode of reception. This chapter concludes with a discussion of consuming trauma kitsch as fantasies of witnessing in a dubious search for late-modernity's holy grail of authenticity.

4.2 Holocaust Tropes

Popular trauma culture emerged when the genocide of European Jewry became a core constituent of American collective memory because its dominant mode of emplotment as good-versus-evil melodrama provided the narrative paradigm that would subsequently be employed for the ubiquitous representations of pain and suffering, victimization, and oppression in the mass media. The Holocaust became such a prominent component of American memory because it could be politically appropriated. Cast in quasi-religious terms as the embodiment of ultimate evil, the ahistorical notion of Nazism provided the United States with an exculpatory screen memory that minimized the crimes perpetrated throughout American history. If the Holocaust is defined *a priori* as ultimate evil, the forceful seizure of the New World and the destruction of Native American life, slavery and segregation, the nuclear bombing of Japan, and the Vietnam War pale in comparison (Cole, 1999; Novick, 1999). And while a serious and sustained encounter with its own crimes "might imply costly demands on Americans to redress the wrongs of the past, contemplating the Holocaust is virtually cost free: a few cheap tears" (Novick, 1999, p. 15).

Moreover, when cast in the moral universe of melodrama, where good and evil are both absolute and hence clearly distinguishable subject positions, the Holocaust can provide the simple moral certainties sought in an increasingly complex and divided late-capitalist America. As Michael Berenbaum, the former director of the US Holocaust Museum noted, "people don't know what good or evil are, but they are certain about one thing: the Holocaust is absolute evil" (cited in Wieviorka, 2006, p. 117). The Holocaust thus not only allows Americans "to know the difference between good and evil," as Raul Hilberg put it,[5] but also functions as the negative foil against which America defines itself as its good and innocent Other (cited in Cole, 1999, p. 13). As such, the Holocaust enables Americans to celebrate and reinforce their traditional values by defining them as the antithesis of Nazism (Novick, 1999, p. 13) and therefore serves a core sociopolitical function in "the fundamental tale of pluralism, tolerance, democracy, and human rights that America tells about itself" (Berenbaum cited in Cole, 1999, p. 14).

[4]Nancy Miller and Jason Tougaw (2002, p. 4) noted in passing that the incorporation of the Holocaust into American national memory has "produced a discourse—a set of terms and debates about the nature of trauma, testimony, witness, and community." James Young (1988, p. 118) stated that it generated a new plot archetype. And Gary Weissman argued that although the Holocaust played no role in American history, it has become such a core component of US culture that the term not only references the genocide of European Jews but also its emplotment in American collective memory.

[5]Cited in Cole, *Selling*, 13.

Prefigured by the stage and movie adaptation of Anne Frank's diary, the Holocaust entered the American public sphere with the television broadcasts from the 1961 trial of Adolf Eichmann in Jerusalem. The trial not only introduced the significant notion that the genocide of European Jewry constituted a distinct event, separate from the Second World War, and a defining moment in twentieth century history but it also marks the advent of popular trauma culture.[6] It introduced stories of extremity into the public sphere via the mass media, expanded the subject position of witness and the genre of testimony beyond the legal realm, and replaced the victim, preeminently represented by Anne Frank, with the survivor, represented by the witnesses and subsequently by Elie Wiesel, as the core protagonist in Holocaust memory.

Information about the trial was not only widely disseminated via radio and newspapers, such as Hannah Arendt's famous reports for *The New Yorker*, subsequently published as *Eichmann in Jerusalem*, but also and especially through the new medium of television. Although it was the first trial filmed in its entirety, the American television broadcasts focused on the testimony of Holocaust survivors and thus both reflected and reinforced the significance attributed to the witness accounts by the prosecution who cast survivors rather than legal experts as core figures because the primary function of the trial was not to establish the defendant's guilt but to constitute a history lesson for the world (Wieviorka, 2006, p. 56). As most survivors had no knowledge of crimes for which Eichmann could be legally held accountable, they did not serve as eyewitnesses in the juridical sense but were ascribed the new social function and subject position of historical witnesses (Wieviorka, 2006, p. 80). Moreover, as they were accompanied by dramatic displays of raw emotions, survivors' narratives of persecution were far more suitable for televisual representation than complex juridical accounts of Eichmann's role in the so-called Final Solution. In fact, the scene shown most frequently on TV is indeed the most spectacular, namely when Yehiel Dinor, better known under his *nom de plume* of Ka-Zetnik as the author of the best-selling Holocaust novel *House of Dolls*, fainted when he testified (Wieviorka, 2006, pp. 80–81). As the televised witness testimony represented the Holocaust as spectacular stories of unimaginable horror and "the television audience of the world wanted only the moments when the surviving witnesses testified," (Wieviorka, 2006, p. 84) the dominant mode of reception successfully encoded was not the history lesson the prosecution had intended for the trial itself but rather the titillating spectacle of horror kitsch that would become paradigmatic for mass media representations of the pain of others in popular trauma culture.

Prior to the trial, all Holocaust victims, including survivors, were either absent from the public sphere or stigmatized as naïve and weak, because they had neither fled nor resisted. While the murdered victims were thus blamed as at least partially responsible for their killing, they were simultaneously cast as quasi-saints, redeemed by their suffering and unjust deaths. Survivors had experienced condescension because they had been humiliated like the victims but were not ascribed the status of sanctified innocents but were rather further stigmatized as ruthless collaborators who had only survived at another's expense (Novick, 1999, pp. 138–140). Only when the broadcasts from the Eichmann trial generated the subject position of the historical witness, which ascribed social significance to experiential knowledge of victimhood and suffering, were Holocaust survivors transformed from shunned pariahs into revered heroes and their survival came to signify perseverance and strength, success, and accomplishment (Wieviorka, 2006, pp. 86–88). Most immediately indicative of this transvaluation was the fact that both the prosecutor's and the judge's office in Jerusalem were "being bombarded with hundreds of requests from people who wished to testify" (Wieviorka, 2006, p. 86). In the United States, the trial moreover imbued the survivor with the Christian notion of sanctification and purification through suffering that had been restricted to the dead

[6] For discussions of the Eichmann trial as a cultural and media event see Wieviorka (2006) and Shandler (2000).

victims while also casting them as victors in the Social-Darwinist struggle for the survival of the fittest. The figure thus merged the role of saint and victorious hero.

Although the discursive shift from the ambiguous figure of the victim to the survivor as the preeminent Holocaust representative, when the latter was redefined in solely positive terms, was initiated in the realm of early Israeli political culture via the generation of the social role and subject position of historical witness at the Eichmann trial, subsequently, the transition was largely generated in American culture, most significantly by Elie Wiesel. Acting as "a self-appointed spokesman-of-sorts for the survivor generation" (Cole, 1999, p. 16), Wiesel is America's "emblematic survivor" (Young, 1995, p. 17) and, at least until the 1993 premier of *Schindler's List*, he was also its most important public interpreter. Wiesel casts the Holocaust as an incomprehensible sacred mystery of the negative sublime that could only be approached by the new priesthood of survivors. His divinations are dominated by paradoxes, particularly the notion that despite its uniqueness—an untenable axiom based on the analogy of Jewish religious chosenness rather than historical analysis—and supposed incomprehensibility, the Holocaust contains universally relevant lessons (Novick, 1999, p. 201). And seeking to transform the Holocaust from a source of shame into one of pride, he furthermore argued that unlike victimhood, survivorship comprised a status that was earned rather than imposed, and therefore constitutes an accomplishment (Fackenheim, Steiner, Popkin, & Wiesel, 1967, cited in Wieviorka, 2006, pp. 102–103). While some prominent survivors, most notably Primo Levi, have argued against transforming survivors into modern-day heroes, saints, and prophets, it was Wiesel's notion that they had achieved the ultimate in surviving their intended destruction, which imbued them with the pride of accomplishment, that became paradigmatic in American Holocaust discourse. While their prior collective demonization as ruthless collaborators was both unethical and historically inaccurate, elevating survivors to proud and accomplished heroes is likewise untenable not least because the redefinition was enabled at the expense of the non-surviving victims, who were discursively employed as the accomplished survivor's failed Other. In reclassifying surviving genocidal persecution from a source of shame into one of pride, Wiesel thus echoes the Social Darwinist notion of survival fitness (Chaumont, 2001, p. 228).[7] Nevertheless, Wiesel's untenable duality of the shame of victimhood and the pride of survival and hence the infusion of American Holocaust memory with Social Darwinism became paradigmatic. As the narrator of Tova Reich's satirical novel *My Holocaust* observed: "In this world if you survive, you win, and if you win, you're good. [...] If you don't survive, you lose. If you lose, you're nothing. [...]. Why had they survived? Luck, it was luck, they said. But they didn't believe it for a minute. It was the accepted thing to say, so as not to insult the memory of the ones who hadn't survived, the ones who, let's face it, had failed. [...] The real truth, they knew, was that they had survived because they were stronger, better—fitter. Survival was success" (Reich, 2007, p. 17).

Although the Eichmann trial was conceptualized as a large-scale history lesson, it did not define the Holocaust as a complex socio-political event but rather as the sum total of the individual testimonies given in the Jerusalem court and in front of the vast audiences of the Western media (Wieviorka, 2006, p. 71). It thus introduced the notion that the past is best understood via witness testimony, rather than the analytical and self-critical discourse of professional historians. This notion was reinforced by Elie Wiesel's ascent to America's preeminent survivor and "most influential interpreter of the Holocaust as sacred mystery" (Novick, 1999, p. 274) as he promoted the interrelated rise of the survivor to the preeminent representative and of the testimonial genre as the paradigmatic narrative for representing both the Holocaust and subsequently all other experiences

[7] Following Wiesel's logic, one could even argue that while the Nazis had cast the Aryan race *a priori* as the superior one, the Holocaust had shown that it was indeed the Jews, at least those among them who had passed the ultimate test of survival fitness, who were truly the fittest race.

of victimization and suffering. Hannah Arendt remarked in her critical commentary on the trial that most of the witnesses did not posses "the rare capacity for distinguishing between things that had happened to the storyteller more than 16, and sometimes 20, years ago and what he had read and heard and imagined in the meantime" (Arendt, 1963, p. 224). While this view became a dominant notion in Holocaust historiography,[8] it remained marginal in the public sphere because the mass media embraced the contrary idea that witness testimony constitutes the optimal resource for understanding the past. In fact, Wiesel's promotion of witness testimony was coupled with the demotion of critical scholarship. He not only declared that "any survivor has more to say than all the historians combined about what happened" (cited in Novick, 1999, p. 201) but even stipulated about "the scholars and philosophers of every genre," that "Auschwitz, by definition, is beyond their vocabulary" (cited in Weissman, 2004, p. 48).

Both the witness figure and the discourse of testimony have come to occupy such a prevalent position in Western culture since the Eichmann trial that Annette Wieviorka not only described this as the era of the witness but scathingly criticized the notion that witness testimony is increasingly replacing historiography as the primary discourse about the past. She considers this development to be most strongly promoted by the Shoah Visual History Foundation. Unlike the video testimonies collected for the Yale Fortunoff Archive, which were intended to supplement the necessary abstractions of Holocaust historiography, the Shoah Visual History Foundation claims to provide an "exhaustive picture of the life of Jewish communities in the twentieth century," a notion Wieviorka (2006, p. 116) criticizes as promoting "the substitution of testimonies, supposedly real history, for the history of historians." While she does acknowledge the therapeutic potential of testimony for reestablishing the survivors' dignity and validating their experience, which many had feared would not be believed, she emphatically asserts that "the concentration camp experience does not confer any prophetic talent" to the survivor (Wieviorka, 2006, p. 134). She even provocatively questions the social function of witness testimony and cites Holocaust survivor and psychoanalyst Anne-Lise Stern who likewise challenged the doctrine that testimony provides important lessons. "We are expected, we are urged to testify 'before it is too late,' Stern explains, "yet what knowledge do they hope to gain? What deathbed confession, what family secret, do they expect to hear? Where is all this listening to survivors leading, whether by those who have had little education or by those who are overeducated?" Aptly summarizing the ubiquitous Holocaust commodification, she answers: "Toward sound bites, I fear, which future generations will play with and enjoy. It's happening already" (cited in Wieviorka, 2006, p. 134). Similarly, Alexander von Plato (2007, pp. 151–152) has cautioned that Holocaust video testimonies will be considered footage because in today's media landscape "talking heads" have minimal entertainment value.

The function of such testimony sound bites is to authenticate the media product because in the era of the witness, it is no longer the historian who is employed to signify the factual accuracy of documentaries (Kansteiner, 2006, p. 324) but rather the witness, whose emotional testimony signifies the pseudoauthenticity of Reality TV that audiences have come to expect and consume *en mass* in pursuit of trauma culture's holy grail of authenticity. The new genre of survivor testimony thus rose to such discursive dominance in American culture that not only is the Holocaust misleadingly understood as the sum total of survivor testimonies (Wieviorka, 2006, p. 116), but it also generated the paradigm for representing diverse experiences of victimization and suffering in American culture.

[8] Lucy Dawidowicz (1976, pp. 11–12), for instance, argued that survivor accounts must be categorically excluded as primary sources for Holocaust historiography because they are not only based on imperfect observation and flawed memory but also "full of discrepancies" and "distorted by hate, sentimentality, and the passage of time" as well as by the inclusion of "hearsay, gossip, rumor, assumption, speculation, and hypothesis."

4.3 Figuring Trauma Culture

The subject positions and social roles of victim and survivor, witness and perpetrator constitute instances of what philosophers call human kinds and distinguish from natural kinds. Unlike natural kinds like, say, thunderstorms or bacilli, human kinds do not exist independently of our knowledge about them because "they come into being hand in hand with our invention of the categories labeling them" (Hacking, 1996, p. 236). Michel Foucault thus argued in the *History of Sexuality* that while male–male and female–female sexual acts existed prior to the invention of the category of homosexuality, the people engaging in them were not homosexuals. Analogously, the broadcast of witness testimony by surviving Holocaust victims from the Eichmann trial transformed the meaning of victimhood, introduced the subject positions of witness and survivor into the public sphere, and disseminated these newly generated human kinds widely. While people had of course suffered, died from, or survived both natural disasters and man-made catastrophes before, they neither thought of themselves nor were perceived by others in precisely these paradigmatic trauma culture categories. Furthermore, while our knowledge about natural kinds changes over time, the changing knowledge does not have any direct effect on them, only the human actions based on new knowledge does, such as killing bacilli with vaccines (Hacking, 1996, pp. 228–230). Human kinds, however, are directly impacted by the knowledge created about them because, as Ian Hacking (1991, p. 254) explains, "the available classifications within which [people] can describe their own actions and make their own constrained choices" create new ways for people to be. While "people classified in a certain way tend to conform to or grow into the ways they are described" Hacking (1995, p. 21) writes, "they also evolve their own ways, so that the classifications and descriptions have to be constantly revised." In other words, human kinds not only evolve as categories over time like natural kinds, because our knowledge about them changes, but also because something collectively agreed upon as a truthful statement will change the very individuals "about whom it was supposed to be the truth" (Hacking, 1991, p. 254), which generates a continuous interactive feed-back loop. In imagined communities, such new ways for people to be are not only generated through the immediate social interaction between individuals but also and especially via the interaction of consumers and media products. Hence, the subject positions of victim and perpetrator, survivor, and witness rose to cultural dominance in Western culture when the Holocaust entered the public sphere with the broadcasting of victim testimony from the Eichmann trial via radio and television.

When modernity transformed suffering from an ordinary experience into a psychopathology and separated it from the body in pain by transferring suffering into the psyche, it became a symptom of chronic illness. This entitled those who suffered to help but only if they fulfilled the social expectations of the victim role. Moreover, help is solely cast in the individualistic terms of therapeutic discourse, which depoliticizes victimization and thus reinforces the status quo that generated such experiences. Moreover, while contemporary Western culture largely pathologizes suffering, it also still honors the pre-modern Christian notion that the suffering caused by a body in pain purifies the soul and sanctifies the sufferer. This tradition has influenced American Holocaust memory and popular trauma culture at large to the extent that, despite the pathologization of suffering and the association of the victim position with such negative attributes as weakness and helplessness, when recast as survivor, the figure continues to be revered as a modern-day saint as suffering is invested with redemptive value and reinterpreted as sacrifice. The pseudo-religious reevaluation of victimhood as sacrifice is reflected in the public persona of Elie Wiesel as Christ figure (Novick, 1999, p. 274) and especially in the term "Holocaust," which, derived from Greek via Late Latin, signifies a burnt sacrificial offering, to name the genocide of European Jewry. The transformation of sufferers into a figure Joseph Amato (1990, p. 48) termed saint-victims became dominant in Western culture not only because of its roots in Christianity but also because of the ethical imperative that senseless suffering, particularly when gratuitously inflicted, is unjust. We thus attribute meaning to suffering and transform it into sacrifice in order to believe that, despite appearances to the contrary, the world is predominantly good and just.[9]

Trauma culture is moreover characterized by the conflation of suffering and victimhood as everyone who suffers is considered a victim. The quintessential trauma culture notion of "I suffer, therefore I am" can thus be extended as "I suffer, therefore I am a victim." However, the equation of victimhood and suffering constitutes a logical fallacy: While all victims suffer, not everyone who suffers is a victim, because some forms of suffering are not the result of victimization. A victim is someone whose suffering was caused, either intentionally or accidentally, by another (Giesen, 2004, p. 46). In other words, unlike the discursively wider notion of suffering, the concept of victimhood requires that the subject position of its Other, the perpetrator, be occupied. Hence, when we casually speak of, say, cancer or earthquake victims we essentially anthropomorphize the disease or disaster because the suffering was not caused by a human agency.[10] Although logically fallacious, the conflation of suffering and victimhood constitutes an ethically justified demand for equal recognition of all forms of suffering, whether caused by a perpetrator or not.

In the melodramatic universe of trauma culture, perpetrator and victim are understood as dichotomous subject positions and, cast as the embodiment of the absolute innocent and good, victims are ascribed the status of ultimate moral authority based on the notion that physical pain purifies the soul and sanctifies the sufferer. "As once the upper classes, especially the nobility, defined the good," Joseph Amato (1990, p. 157) writes, "now victims—the downtrodden, the oppressed, the humiliated—were equated with the good." From a strictly synchronic perspective, victim and perpetrator are indeed mutually exclusive social roles, such as torturer and tortured or child abuser and abused child. However, a diachronic perspective, say, the history of Stalinist persecution in the Soviet Union or the witch hunts of supposed communists in the United States under McCarthy, illustrates that one may be simultaneously victim and perpetrator or occupy these subject positions subsequently in either order and through numerous changes. As victims can become perpetrators and vice versa, these subject positions are not absolute and binary but relative and fluctuating. Conflating victims and perpetrators with absolute good and ultimate evil respectively—which became ubiquitous when Holocaust emplotment as suffering and redemption melodrama generated the paradigm for representing all victimization experiences in American culture—is thus misleading. While the infliction of gratuitous violence may well constitute our notion of absolute evil, we know at least since the introduction of the trauma concept by Jean-Martin Charcot, Pierre Janet, and Sigmund Freud more than 100 years ago that, contrary to the Christian notion, extreme suffering does not ennoble (Luckhurst, 2008, pp. 34–49). It neither imbues anyone with permanent innocence and righteousness nor instills in then a guaranteed life-long dedication to the fight against inhumanity, persecution, and oppression. Zygmunt Bauman (1998, p. 36) even provocatively argued that victims are not "guaranteed to be morally superior to their victimizers" and Joseph Amato (1990, p. 196), who shares Bauman's ethical critique of infusing victimization experiences with redemptive value

[9] This notion dominates the moral universe of many Holocaust survivors who find it intolerable to think that their suffering and survival were solely arbitrary and therefore retroactively attribute meaning and purpose to it.

[10] Giesen (2004, p. 46) argued that only if at least vague information about the quake and the risk to human lives had been available, yet no or insufficient warning was given, i.e., if the deaths and injuries are at least in part based on human action, is there term "victim" justified. His argument can be extended to individuals who suffer from the pain caused by physical illness. Only if the illness was caused and/or exacerbated, for instance through misdiagnosis and/or mistreatment, does a patient constitute a victim. While the fact that the author-narrators in so-called pathographies, auto/biographical narratives of terminal illnesses, particularly AIDS and cancer, claim victim status based on their suffering, constitutes a core example of the fallacious conflation of suffering and victimhood, it also reflects the need of all who suffer to see their suffering if not lessened then at least recognized.

and transforming victims into quasi-saints, even proposed that nothing "guaranties that today's victims won't be tomorrow's victimizers."

Trauma culture also altered our understanding of perpetration. Traditionally, "perpetrator" designated someone who—sanctioned and protected by sociopolitical and economic hegemonies—intentionally caused another to suffer by gratuitously inflicting physical pain. However, the vast bureaucracies of advanced capitalist societies have made the human agencies responsible for facilitating the socioeconomic contexts that generate large-scale victimization—through exploitation, unemployment, poverty, and the destruction of the environment in the so-called developed world and extreme poverty, starvation, and preventable diseases in the developing world—impenetrable and only rarely attributable to individuals. Consequently, the perpetrator role has been generalized and tends to be attributed to abstract entities like life, society, the government, or, for the politically left-minded, to the inherently inhumane economic order of capitalism. However, anthropomorphizing such abstract entities serves to hide the actual perpetrators, so that claims for recognition and compensation cannot be addressed to them, but are rather made to society at large. It also serves to ensure that the status quo that generated the insidious victimization inherent in the capitalist, patriarchal, ethnocentric, and hetero-normative hegemony remains unquestioned.

Global capitalist competition forces victims, who have little or no other resources to contend for power, to translate their suffering into a moral currency (Amato, 1990, p. 157). Consequently, the largely altruistically motivated discourse of testimony, which primarily seeks to prevent the victimization of others and/or commemorate non-surviving victims, increasingly degenerated into a rhetoric Martha Minow (1993) dubbed victim talk. It asserts that in order to right their wrongs and reestablish the equilibrium of justice, victims must be compensated for their suffering, whether through pecuniary reparation, like West Germany accorded Holocaust survivors, or via indirect benefits of preferential treatment, as granted by the American affirmative action program, thus defining victims not only as a wronged but an owed party. Infused with the pop therapeutic discourse of the self-help industry, victim talk also ascribes the status of the mentally infirm to victims. While telling personal stories of victimization can be therapeutically beneficial and in defining victims as legitimately ill, therapeutic discourse sanctions their need for help and support, it also defines them as chronically sick, permanently damaged, weak, and helpless people. As victim talk asserts that the psychic damages of victimization are irreparable and that suffering constitutes the dominant aspect of victims' lives, it asserts that victim status and its benefits are for life. As Joseph Amato (1990, p. 164) put it, "once you were granted membership into the official family of 'suffering victims,'" no good fortune—whether superior education, wealth, or other personal successes—will erase your victim role and hence your right for preferential status. Claims to the privileges of victim status established "in terms of the moral patrimony of past suffering" (Amato, 1990, p. 18) culminated in the notion that ancestral victimhood can be inherited, which is central particularly to secular Jewish identity. However, as Zygmunt Bauman (1998, p. 34) acerbically criticized the notion of so-called vicarious Holocaust victimhood, anyone "basking in the fame of his ancestral martyrs without paying the price of the glory" is "living on a borrowed identity—as martyrs by appointment, martyrs who never suffered."

Since in capitalism's market economy the inherently relative commodity value of any entity is determined by the ratio of supply and demand, establishing one's own right to the victim position and its moral capital requires denying it to others in order to keep supply low and demand high. As Michael Bernstein (1994, p. 85) put it, "once victimhood is understood to endow one with special claims and rights, the scramble to attain that designation for one's own interest group is as heated as any other race for legitimacy and power." In the victim talk world, people thus "exchange testimonials of pain in a contest over who suffered more" (Minow, 1993, p. 1430) and generate what Bauman (1998, p. 35) dubbed a "pecking order of pain" reminiscent of the rivalry among the tuberculosis patients in Thomas Mann's *Magic Mountain*, "who quickly established their own hierarchy of prestige and influence measured by the size of their pulmonary caverns." When testimony became victim talk, it quickly spiraled into infinite blame game cycles in which everyone seeks to outsuffer competing claims in order to assert their own preeminent position in what Peter Novick (1999, p. 195) described as the "Victimization Olympics." Consequently, American politics degenerated into "a competition for enshrining grievances," in which "every group claims its share of public honor and public funds by pressing disabilities and injustices" (Novick, 1999, p. 8) and even "the most banal causes adopt, exploit, and thus cheapen the moral rhetoric of suffering owed" (Amato, 1990, p. xxiii).

Victim talk rhetoric and the inflation of victim claims undermined the commodity value of victimhood's moral capital and engendered a change in signification, so that the victim figure was understood as simultaneously denoting a saintly hero and a weak loser in fight for the survival of the fittest. Alison Cole (2006, p. 17) argued that the victim became such a key concept in American culture precisely because of its "very susceptibility to diverse, indeed, opposing, interpretations, and applications" as they "facilitate contestation and render keywords pregnant with meaning." However, trauma culture is emplotted according to the simplistic good-versus-evil structure of melodrama, which requires unambiguous characters. In order to disambiguate the paradigmatic representative of trauma culture, the victim was increasingly replaced by the survivor, a transition that had been prefigured in American Holocaust discourse. Although the survivor is an inherently composite figure because it fuses such diverse discourses as Social Darwinism, Christianity, and Holocaust memory, it is solely defined in positive terms. And while the meaning of survival was vastly expanded metaphorically to signify that one's life was no longer dominated by the victimization experience rather than that one had defied a threat to one's life, it nevertheless became the ultimate achievement in trauma culture and increasingly replaced traditional notions of accomplishment and heroism.

4.4 Emplotting Trauma Kitsch as Melodrama

Represented as kitsch-sentimental melodrama, the pain of others was transformed into popular entertainment commodities in the mass media of television, commercial cinema, and popular literature. The kitsch concept originates in mid-nineteenth century German culture and has been explored in two distinct research paradigms: Mass culture theorists define kitsch as a style derivative and imitative of higher art styles which it reduces to banal, trite, and predictable formulas and stock motifs.[11] As a cheaply mass-produced product lacking craftsmanship and artistic refinement, they define kitsch as symptomatic of mass culture. Contrary, the popular culture approach proposes that kitsch objects reflect as much creativity as the products of highbrow culture and therefore the distinction between high and low art forms is without grounds (Binkley, 2000, p. 133). However, Sam Binkley (2000, p. 134) argued that kitsch should neither be understood as exhibiting the same innovative, avant-garde features as high art nor as its failed, inferior version but rather that it should be understood on its own terms because it exhibits its own distinct aesthetic: It celebrates banality and advocates continuity, conformity, and routine. It proposes simple moral truths, which are repeated over and over, thus reducing complexity by relying on well-rehearsed formulas, clichés, and conventions. Most importantly, kitsch relishes in sentiment and expresses "a joy in feeling itself, whether that feeling is elation, sorrow, or fondness" (Binkley, 2000, p. 142). The sentiment that kitsch artifacts both depict and evoke in consumers not only reduces the intricacy of human emotions and sweetens them with melancholy and nostalgia but it also manipulates the audience's emotive responses to indulge in the pleasure of their own sentimental arousal and thus represses a reception mode marked by critical distance (Binkley, 2000, p. 145). Last but not

[11] Clement Greenberg (1986, pp. 5–22), for example, dichotomizes kitsch and high art in his classic essay "Avant-Garde and Kitsch."

least, kitsch transvalues its aesthetically anti-innovative features to signify authenticity, modesty, sincerity and frankness, and—assuming a pseudo-democratic posture of naïveté and anti-elitism—asserts that it is both representative of the essence of human nature and universally comprehensible (Binkley, 2000, pp. 140–141).

Avishai Margalit (1988, pp. 215–216) argued that kitsch should not only be conceptualized as an aesthetic but as a moral category because it "distorts reality by turning the object (or event) represented into an object of complete innocence" and claims that the ontologically innocent are constantly being menaced by evil incarnate and therefore "have to be relentlessly protected from those plotting their destruction." The quasi-religious innocence ascribed to the victim-cum-survivor protagonist is central to the reception because it enables and even enforces the troublesome ease with which consumers align themselves with this subject position and dictates a particular, predetermined emotional response. Margalit (1988, p. 208) invokes the well-known reflections on kitsch sentiment as an economy of the second tear in Milan Kundera's *The Unbearable Lightness of Being*: Whereas the first tear signifies a genuine emotional response of sorrow, kitsch sentiment is expressed by the second tear. It does not emerge from direct involvement with the object of feeling but rather constitutes a derivative response, a meta-tear shed upon the perception of the first tear, allowing and encouraging the audience to relish in their own emotional arousal. Luc Boltanski (1999, p. 92) similarly describes the dominant mode of reception encoded in atrocity photographs as the "sweetness of being moved to tears" when "a certain joy is mixed with sadness" and analogously argued that there are two gazes for looking at the mediatized and hence distant suffering of others: The altruistic gaze, which gives rise to the genuine emotional response of sorrow that Kundera termed the first tear, is "motivated by the intention to see the suffering ended" (Boltanski, 1999, p. 92). And akin to Kundera's disingenuous second-tear response, Boltanski (1999, p. 21) writes that there is also "a selfish way of looking which is wholly taken up with the internal states aroused by the spectacle of suffering: fascination, horror, interest, excitement, pleasure." Unlike Kundera, who understands kitsch sentiment as derivative of the genuine emotional reaction, Boltanski thus considers the altruistic and the selfish mode of reception as mutually exclusive. Margalit (1988, p. 208) analogously reinterprets Kundera's notion of second-tear-jerking kitsch sentimentality. He argues that an artifact constitutes kitsch in its purest form when it evokes the second tear without the first and when the audience's emotional response is thus entirely disingenuous and narcissistic.

Kitsch's proclivity for formulas, tropes, stock plots, and set pieces generates familiarity but in turn also produces banality and therefore, as Andy Warhol wrote, "when you see a gruesome picture over and over again, it doesn't really have any effect" (cited in Sturken, 2007, p. 284). The dominant mode of reception encoded into the emplotment of mediatized others' suffering in popular trauma culture is thus the kitsch sentimentality signified by Kundera's metaphor of the second tear because in turning quintessentially political subjects into individual tragedies, or rather melodramas, it conveys the idea that the narcissistic indulgence in one's own sentimental response constitutes an appropriate reaction. While trauma kitsch narratives ostensibly represent an apolitical world, they actually remove the experiences of victimization, oppression, and suffering from the social, political, and economic contexts that enable or at least permit them and suppress the critically distanced mode of reception from wherein political action can arise. In other words, as they proclaim that no matter what happens, whether genocide or child abuse or lesser evils, there will always be a happy ending when good wins over evil, victims become survivors and perpetrators are punished, trauma kitsch narratives suggest that socioeconomic hegemonies need not be changed through political action. In conveying the message that teary-eyed sentiment is an adequate reaction, trauma kitsch reinforces the oppressive hegemonies of late-modern capitalism that have generated or at least enabled the violence and victimization, pain, and suffering over which mass media audiences have shed many a second tear.

Trauma kitsch elicits such an escapist and politically acquiescing mode of reception because it emplots all forms of injustice and oppression, violence and suffering as melodrama. According to Peter Brooks (1976, p. 14), in its "effort to make the 'real' and the 'ordinary' and the 'private life' interesting," melodrama infuses the realm of the quotidian with the sublime. However, in the post-sacred era, the sublime no longer signifies solely the sacred but also the supremely evil. Moreover, melodrama thrives on the simultaneity of extreme situations, events and emotions, and the ordinary world of the every day. It indulges in "strong emotionalism; moral polarization and schematization; extreme states of being, situations, actions; overt villainy, persecution of the good and final reward of virtue; inflated and extravagant expression; dark plottings, suspense [and] breathtaking peripety" (Brooks, 1976, pp. 19–20). Melodrama furthermore "represents both an urge toward resacrilization and the impossibility of conceiving sacralization other than in personal terms" (Brooks, 1976, pp. 16–17), which is why good and evil are personalized, i.e., they are embodied by characters lacking in psychological complexity because they represent allegorical absolutes. When "good and evil can be named as persons," Brooks (1976, p. 17) writes, "evil is villainy; it is a swarthy, cape-enveloped man with a deep voice." While evil is thus embodied by the figure of the Gothic villain, good is represented by the ontological innocence ascribed to Christian virginal virtue, which the Romantics merged with the nostalgic-utopian notion of innate childhood innocence into the Gothic figure of the maiden-in-distress. Trauma kitsch particularly evokes the tradition of Gothic melodrama which is "preoccupied with nightmare states, with claustration and thwarted escape, with innocence buried alive and unable to voice its claim to recognition" and "with evil as a real, irreducible force in the world, constantly menacing outburst" (Brooks, 1976, pp. 19–20). Analogously, in trauma kitsch, the violence gratuitously inflicted by a hypermasculine perpetrator—of which the ahistorical Nazi figure and the child-abusing father figure are the paradigmatic representatives in the American popular imagination—on an inherently infantilized and/or feminized ontologically innocent victim is juxtaposed to the realm of the quotidian and exists unrecognized as Gothic melodrama's dark secret of which the mundane world is, or at least pretends to be, ignorant.

Originating in postrevolutionary France, the genre of melodrama "expresses the anxiety brought by a frightening new world in which the traditional patterns of moral order no longer provide the necessary social glue" and thus reflects the insecurities and anxieties of the new post-secular age of the enlightenment (Brooks, 1976, pp. 19–20). Analogously, as the dominant mode of emplotment of victimhood and violence in the mass media today, melodrama echoes the trepidations and angst brought about by a world in which mundane life is increasingly experienced as a constant struggle for survival and thus as insidiously traumatizing. Anthony Giddens aptly described the infinitely complex institutions and practices of the late-modern world as disembedding because they "uproot individuals from the 'protective cocoons' that flood social interactions, cultural outlooks and experiences with cohesive meanings, and tie daily life to fundamental patterns of trust and reassurance" (Binkley, 2000, p. 135). As modern societies offer individuals "unprecedented choices in consumer goods, ethical outlooks, and life plans," the "routines, recurring practices, comforting cosmologies, and world views" of conventional life are shattered (Binkley, 2000, p. 135). They generate a sense of omnipresent but intangible threat thus undermining our sense of ontological security because life's uncertainties and existential questions are also no longer bracketed by the comforting conventions of the premodern world (Giddens, 1990, p. 17).

In merging the aesthetic conventions of kitsch and melodrama, the mass media representations of the pain of others in American popular culture pretend to maximally re-embed the late-modern individual. They counter "the excessive personal freedom, the uncertainty and the risk of modern social life [...] with a return to a sense of continuity, a 'closed system' [...] in which cultural forms are predictable, continuous and repetitive"

(Binkley, 2000, p. 149). Simulating premodern embeddedness, trauma kitsch reassures its consumers' threatened sense of ontological security by convincing them that what is to come will resemble the familiar and the world is predictable and safe. And in depicting the increasingly global, technocapitalist world by reducing its infinite complexity to melodrama's simplistic and highly moralistic good-versus-evil universe reassures consumers that all is well that ends well.

However, the re-embedding nature of depicting the pain of others as kitsch-sentimental melodrama is undermined by the fact that the vast majority of the plot casts ontological innocence as constantly threatened by seemingly omnipotent evil, which moreover lurks everywhere under the surface of mundane life. The simultaneity of overt optimism and covert angst is paradigmatic for melodrama as genre, as plot paradigm in Gothic novels, and as the dominant mode for emplotting the pain of others as politically anesthesiatizing "feel-good horror" stories (Reich, 2007, p. 99) in contemporary American popular culture. As audiences seek more and more reassurance that, despite appearances to the contrary, the world is predictable and all will be well, they look in all the wrong places. Despite the repetitively formulaic plots and their overtly optimist redemptive-happy endings, emplotting victimhood and violence, pain and suffering as kitsch-sentimental melodrama covertly reinforces the consumer's sense of omnipresent but intangible danger paradigmatic of trauma culture.

4.5 Consuming Trauma Kitsch

While many late-modern individuals experience their lives as existentially threatened and inherently traumatizing, they also find them mundane and banal, interchangeable and unoriginal, lacking meaning and a deeper purpose, in short, as inauthentic. As K.K. Ruthven (2001, p. 149) writes, "the concept of 'authenticity' appears to be extrapolated from the inauthenticities of everyday life as an imaginary and ideal alternative, just as the idea of paradise succeeds an awareness of paradise lost." And it is precisely "the reification of authenticity" that "results in an ontological fiction called the 'real thing'" (Ruthven, 2001, p. 169). As the desire for the "real thing" constitutes a pseudo-nostalgic longing for something that never actually existed, authenticity constitutes the ever-elusive holy grail of our late-modern era. Moreover, late-modern individuals turn less to such grand narratives as religion and political ideology than to mass-produced media commodities to satisfy that "'passion for the real,' that thirst for rapturous, authentic experiences" (Cole, 2006, p. 16). Contemporary Western culture is, moreover, permeated by what Richard Sennett (1977, p. 259) characterized as an ideology of intimacy wherein only the personal, emotional, and experiential are ascribed the status of being authentic and real. However, as ordinary life is considered mundane and hence inauthentic, authenticity is ascribed to personal experiences of extremity, or rather to its supposed vicarious experience via the reception of media representations. In other words, consumers oxymoronically ascribe the capacity to satiate a nostalgic longing for something designated as "real," "true" and "authentic" to the consumption experience of the pain of others emplotted as kitsch-sentimental tales of suffering and redemption.

However, it is not only the ubiquitous survival narratives of trauma-and-redemption kitsch in mainstream cinema, television, and popular literature but also the touristic engagement with sites of atrocity that are ascribed the quasi-mystical power to imbue consumers with the authenticity they feel lacking in their own lives.[12] Particularly Nazi concentration camps have become tourist attractions (Young, 1994). Dark tourism, as John Lennon and Malcolm Foley (2000) termed it, is becoming increasingly popular because places

[12] For a discussion of the popular literature genre of so-called misery memoirs and the representation of experiences of victimhood and violence on daytime TV talk shows as trauma kitsch and trauma camp, see Anne Rothe, *Popular Trauma Culture: Selling the Pain of Others in the Mas Media* (New Brunswick: Rutgers University Press 2011), pp. 83–135 and pp. 49–82, respectively.

of mass killings are ascribed the status of sacred sites. While visitors seek a quasi-religious experience of the negative sublime, they engage in the consumption relation characteristic of all tourism. In fact, as the sites of dark tourism enable the modern-day pilgrims to generate fantasies of witnessing traumas they did not suffer and supposedly gain "a trace of authenticity by extension" (Sturken, 2007, p. 11), they offer trauma culture's ultimate consumer product. While these modern-day pilgrims seek to enter a realm where past and present merge because it exists outside of quotidian time–space, Ruth Kluger scathingly criticized such sentimental journeys of trauma tourism in her renowned Holocaust memoir *Still Alive*. She not only rejected the sacralization of atrocity sites and insisted that they were empirically real places rather than imaginary spaces of some negative utopia but also proposed the notion of timescapes to signify the categorical difference of the same place at different times and consequently between its experience as a concentration camp on the one hand and a memorial and tourist site on the other (Kluger, 2003, pp. 67–68). Trauma culture thus gave rise to what Michael Bernstein (1994, p. 91) termed an ideology of the extreme and described as the belief that "the truth lies in the extreme moments which 'ordinary bourgeois life' covers over." However, ascribing life lessons and some mystical ultimate truth to consuming media representations of other's pain and suffering is both absurd and deeply unethical. Particularly deploring the American fascination with Holocaust horror, Bernstein (1994, p. 84, 89) thus emphatically rejected the notion of *in extremis veritas* and argued that our beliefs and values ought to be developed and tested in the routines of everyday life.

Similarly, Gary Weissman (2004, p. 137) critiqued the idea of turning the Holocaust and/or its representation into a mystery of the negative sublime that could reveal some ultimate truth about human nature as "a kind of existential sentimental education." Moreover, he emphatically rejected the epistemologically and ethically untenable analogy between the personal experience of the Holocaust and the consumption experience of its representation generated in American culture via the vast extension of the notion of "witnessing" from signifying the former to the latter. The ubiquitous metaphorical uses of "witness," "memory" and their respective derivatives—including "vicarious witnesses," "secondary witnesses," "retrospective witnesses," "witness's witness," "witnesses by adoption," "witnesses through the imagination," "postmemory," "prosthetic memory," "secondary memory," and "vicarious memory"—facilitates this blurring because their imprecise meanings merge "both the survivor's recall of lived experiences and the nonwitness's familiarity with Holocaust narratives" (Weissman, 2004, p. 92). Contrary to convention in Holocaust studies scholarship and commemorative practice, Weissman (2004, p. 5, 25) designates those who have neither experiential knowledge of the Holocaust, and hence know it only in mediated form, nor an immediate, familial connection to the genocide as "nonwitnesses." He argues that they are predominantly Jewish and that the Holocaust constitutes a core identity marker for them. The term, Weissman explains, stresses that anyone who did not experience it, "did not witness the Holocaust, and that the experience of listening to, reading or viewing witness testimony is substantially unlike the experience of victimization" (Weissman, 2004, p. 20). Stating what should be obvious, Weissman (2004, p. 20) argues, that while nonwitnesses "can read books or watch films on the Holocaust, listen to Holocaust survivors, visit Holocaust museums, take trips to Holocaust memorial sites in Europe, research and write about the Holocaust, look at photographs of the victims," they are not witnessing the Holocaust but rather consuming its myriad representations.

The untenable notion of defining a supposedly authentic secular American-Jewish identity by engaging in literal and metaphorical trauma tourism via "sites or texts where the Holocaust may be vicariously experienced" (Weissman, 2004, p. 4) can be extended to the media consumption of the pain of others at large in trauma culture's paradigmatic quest for authenticity. And since trauma kitsch emplotments of violence and victimhood as suffering and redemption melodramas not only promise that good wins over evil and we are thus safe despite the disembedding nature of late-modernity's institutions and practices, but they also offer a false sense of authenticity, they satisfy the late-modern individual's two most dire needs and are therefore produced and consumed relentlessly.

4.6 Epilogue: Survivors Made in America

Rather than ending this chapter in the traditional discursive mode of narrowing down the argument in a conclusion, I would like to open it up and propose new ideas that could be explored by briefly looking ahead at my next book project, which will trace the genealogy of the survivor figure in American culture. It is tentatively titled *Survivors Made in America: Intersections between Holocaust Memory, Social Darwinism and Popular Culture*. After exploring the survivor as a quintessentially American figure because it is a variation of that other ur-American figure of the self-made man, who not only overcame the impossible but did so without relying on others, I will analyze the ascent of the survivor figure in American Holocaust memory. In addition to the Eichmann trial, it was particularly the American translation of Wiesel's *Night* from the original French in 1959 and his subsequent rise to celebrity status that significantly impacted the genealogy of the American survivor figure. Comparing his memoir to the earlier, Yiddish version, I will argue that while Wiesel had previously cast himself as a victim forever inscribed by his memories, in *Night* he reinvents himself as the saintly and heroic survivor who could overcome the traumatic past that would become paradigmatic in American Holocaust memory. The Yiddish urtext has thus been out of print for decades and was never translated into any language because it contradicts Wiesel's public persona. I will moreover discuss Wiesel as a public figure and media event by analyzing select speeches, essays, interviews, documentaries, video testimony, newspaper articles, letters sent to him by readers, and last but not least two *Oprah Winfrey Show Specials* that featured Wiesel and his famous memoir.

In tracing the discursive journey of the survivor figure beyond American Holocaust discourse, I will explore its infusion with Social Darwinist ideas in postapocalyptic Hollywood disaster movies and Reality TV shows. In the dystopian universe evocative of the concentration camp that is depicted in screen representation of the postapocalyptic world, the survivor figure must neither give up the fight for survival by turning into one of the walking dead, i.e., a victim-cum-corpse that evokes both the figures of the Zombie and the *Muselmann*, nor must he succumb to the ruthless Social Darwinist ethics of every-man-for-himself, i.e., their survival must not come at the expense of another's life. Essentially, the paradigmatic Armageddon survivor is the ultimate American hero. Physically and spiritually strong and defiant, he embodies both the warrior and the savior. And unlike the figure of the Holocaust survivor, he saves not only himself but also others and, trumping even the Christ figure, exhibits such exceptional survival skills that saving others does not even require sacrificing himself.

The survivor figure largely sheds the aura of Holocaust sanctity and fully embraces the notion of the survival of the fittest on the ultimate Reality TV show *Survivor*. Although the genre is European in origin and *Survivor* is marketed toward an increasingly global media audience, it is an inherently American show as it reflects and in turn reinforces both conformity and individualism. While these two core American ideals seem incongruous, they coexist on the show as they do in US society. Conventionally good-looking participants minimally clad in the identikit of pseudonative gear advocate conformity. However, the team spirit overtly espoused is fake because the ultimate ideal promoted is ruthless individualism with Social Darwinist overtones as every participant seeks to be the last survivor and win the million. As being voted off by the audience in a natural selection process of sorts as well as enduring serious discomforts, to which participants nevertheless expose themselves voluntarily in a pursuit of quick riches, constitute the only danger, the show reflects the most radical semantic extension of the notion of survival to date.

In media products created for intergender audiences, the survivor is a decidedly masculine figure, self-reliant in his defiance of impossible odds, i.e., a survivor by nature. Only in narratives produced primarily for female audiences, particularly the interrelated discourses of popular feminism and self-help literature, is the figure female. However, unlike the male figure, the female one must undergo a metamorphosis by overcoming her supposedly inherent state of victimhood and be transformed from a weak and helpless victim into a strong and self-reliant survivor. In fact, the plot is structured around this transformation and despite the overt message of female empowerment in these texts, written primarily for and to a significant extent by women, many of whom consider themselves feminists, they instead reflect and reinforce traditional gender stereotypes. Not only is the paradigmatic survivor figure defined as inherently male in traditional gender terms but the supposed normalcy and rightness of masculinity is furthermore reinforced because the transformation process advocates overcoming such negative and traditionally feminine attributes as weakness and helplessness by replacing them with such positive characteristics as strength and defiance conventionally associated with masculinity.

Just as I did in this chapter, I will take up and expand upon select aspects of the analysis in an epilogue in order to end the monograph in a discursive mode of opening up rather than the more traditional one of narrowing down the argument in a conclusion. The epilogue will bring the discussion of the survivor figure full circle as it returns to Holocaust discourse in order to engage in an ethical critique of the survival lessons increasingly advocated in self-help literature that one can supposedly learn from the Holocaust in order to survive the apparently ubiquitous threats to one's life in present-day America.

References

Amato, J. (1990). *Victims and values: A history and theory of suffering*. New York: Praeger.

Arendt, H. (1963). *Eichmann in Jerusalem: A report on the banality of evil*. New York: Penguin.

Bauman, Z. (1998). The Holocaust's life as a ghost. *Tikkun, 13*(4), 33–38.

Bernstein, M. (1994). *Foregone conclusions: Against apocalyptic history*. Berkeley: University of California Press.

Binkley, S. (2000). Kitsch as a repetitive system: A Problem for the theory of taste hierarchy. *Journal of Material Culture, 5*(2), 131–152.

Boltanski, L. (1999). *Distant suffering: Morality, media, and politics*. Cambridge: Cambridge University Press.

Brooks, P. (1976). *The melodramatic imagination. Balzac, Henry James, melodrama, and the mode of excess*. New Haven: Yale University Press.

Caruth, C. (Ed.). (1995). *Trauma. Explorations in memory*. Baltimore: Johns Hopkins University Press.

Caruth, C. (1996). *Unclaimed experience. Trauma, narrative, and history*. Baltimore: Johns Hopkins University Press.

Chaumont, J.-M. (2001). *Die Konkurrenz der Opfer: Genozid, Identität und Anerkennung*. Lüneburg: Zu Klampen.

Cole, T. (1999). *Selling the holocaust. From Auschwitz to Schindler: How history is bought, packaged and sold*. New York: Routledge.

Cole, A. (2006). *The cult of true victimhood: From the war on welfare to the war on terror*. Stanford: Stanford University Press.

Dawidowicz, L. (1976). *A holocaust reader*. New York: Behrman House.

Fackenheim, E., Steiner, G., Popkin, R., & Wiesel, E. (1967). Jewish values in the post-holocaust future: A symposium. *Judaism, 3*, 266–299.

Felman, S., & Laub, D. (1992). *Testimony. Crises of witnessing in literature, psychoanalysis and history*. New York: Routledge.

Giddens, A. (1990). *The consequences of modernity*. Stanford: Stanford University Press.

Giesen, B. (2004). *Triumph and trauma*. Boulder, CO: Paradigm.

Greenberg, C. (1986). *The collected essays and criticism*. Chicago: University of Chicago Press.

Hacking, I. (1991). The making and molding of child abuse. *Critical Inquiry, 17*(2), 253–288.

Hacking, I. (1995). *Rewriting the soul. Multiple personality and the sciences of memory*. Princeton: Princeton University Press.

Hacking, I. (1996). Making up people. In T. C. Heller et al. (Eds.), *Reconstructing individualism: Autonomy, individuality and the self in western thought* (pp. 222–236). Stanford: Stanford University Press.

Horwitz, D. (2000). *Literary trauma: Sadism, memory, and sexual violence in American women's fiction*. Albany: SUNY Press.

Kansteiner, W. (2004). Genealogy of a category mistake. A critical intellectual history of the cultural trauma metaphor. *Rethinking History, 8*(2), 193–221.

Kansteiner, W. (2006). *In pursuit of German memory: History, television, and politics after Auschwitz*. Athens: Ohio University Press.

Kansteiner, W., & Weilnböck, H. (2008). Against the concept of cultural trauma. In A. Erll & A. Nünning (Eds.), *Cultural memory studies. An international and interdisciplinary handbook* (pp. 229–240). Berlin: de Gruyter.

Kaplan, E. A. (2005). *Trauma culture. The politics of terror and loss in media and literature*. New Brunswick: Rutgers University Press.

King, N. (2000). *Memory, narrative, identity: Remembering the self*. Edinburgh: Edinburgh University Press.

Kluger, R. (2003). *Still alive*. New York: Feminist Press.

Latour, B. (1987). *Science in action: How to follow scientists and engineers through society*. Cambridge: Harvard University Press.

Lennon, J., & Foley, M. (2000). *Dark tourism*. London: Continuum.

Leys, R. (2000). *Trauma. A genealogy*. Chicago: University of Chicago Press.

Luckhurst, R. (1998). The science-fictionalization of trauma: Remarks on narratives of alien abduction. *Science Fiction Studies, 15*(1), 29–52.

Luckhurst, R. (2008). *The trauma question*. New York: Routledge.

Margalit, A. (1988). The kitsch of Israel. In A. Margalit (Ed.), *Views in review: Politics and culture in the state of the Jews*. New York: Farar Straus Giroux.

Miller, N., & Tougaw, J. (2002). Introduction: Extremities. In N. Miller & J. Tougaw (Eds.), Extremities: Trauma, testimony and community (pp. 1–24). Urbana-Champaign: University of Illinois Press.

Minow, M. (1993). Surviving victim talk. *UCLA Law Review, 40*, 1411–1445.

Nadal, M., & Calvo, M. (Eds.). (2014). *Trauma in contemporary literature*. New York: Routledge.

Novick, P. (1999). *The holocaust in American life*. Boston: Houghton Mifflin.

Reich, T. (2007). *My holocaust*. New York: HarperCollins.

Robson, K. (2004). *Writing wounds. The inscription of trauma in post-1968 French women's life-writing*. Amsterdam: Rodopi.

Rothe, A. (2011). *Popular trauma culture: Selling the pain of others in the mass media*. New Brunswick: Rutgers University Press.

Ruthven, K. K. (2001). *Faking literature*. Cambridge: Cambridge University Press.

Sennett, R. (1977). *The fall of public man*. New York: Vintage Books.

Shandler, J. (2000). The man in the glass box: Watching the Eichmann trial on American television. In B. Zelizer (Ed.), *Visual culture and the holocaust* (pp. 91–110). New Brunswick: Rutgers University Press.

Sontag, S. (2004). *Regarding the pain of others*. New York: Picador.

Sturken, M. (2007). *Tourists of history: Memory, kitsch, and consumerism from Oklahoma City to Grund Zero*. Durham: Duke University Press.

von Plato, A. (2007). Geschichte ohne Zeitzeugen? Einige Fragen zur "Erfahrung" im Übergang von Zeitgeschichte zur Geschichte. In M. Elm & G. Kößler (Eds.), *Zeugenschaft des Holocaust. Zwischen Trauma, Tradierung und Ermittlung* (pp. 141–156). Frankfurt: Campus.

Weilnböck, H. (2008). The trauma must remain inaccessible to memory: Trauma melancholia and other (ab-) uses of trauma concepts in literary theory. Retrieved August 1, 2009 from.

Weissman, G. (2004). *Fantasies of witnessing. Postwar efforts to experience the holocaust*. Ithaca: Cornell University Press.

Whitehead, A. (2004). *Trauma fiction*. Edinburgh: Edinburgh University Press.

Wieviorka, A. (2006). *The era of the witness*. Ithaca: Cornell University Press.

Young, J. (1988). *Writing and rewriting the holocaust. Narrative and the consequences of interpretation*. Bloomington: University of Indiana Press.

Young, J. (1994). *The texture of memory: Holocaust memorials and meaning*. New Haven: Yale University Press.

Young, J. (1995). Parables of a survivor. *New Leader*, 17.

5 The Trauma of Modernism: Between Existential Indeterminacy and *Allegoresis*

Dennis Sobolev

5.1 Introduction

This essay has two goals; these goals are both opposed to one another and mutually complementary. First, it aims to underscore and analyze two general hermeneutic strategies of the cultural absorption and transformation of traumatic experiences, which seem to be highly significant for the understanding of the European and American literatures of the nineteenth and the twentieth centuries. These two hermeneutic strategies may be roughly defined as the search for an ultimate philosophical ground for the transcendence of the traumatic, on the one hand, and the acknowledgement of the insuperable semantic indeterminacy of human existence, on the other, which however does not render the human experience of suffering and trauma ontologically vacant. Therefore, when viewed from the perspective of the significance of the subjective, the former strategy elevates the human and the private into a figure for the universal, whereas the latter intensifies its materiality and refuses to empty them into the realm of the occasional and the contingent. Correspondingly, when viewed from the perspective of the cultural representations of the objective and the universal, the former strategy of dealing with the traumatic tends to deny the accessibility of the generally meaningful if the problem of the personal, the experiential, and the painful is ignored. In contrast, the latter hermeneutic strategy insists that the personal and the traumatic can be meaningfully articulated only if the temptation of their sublimation into the transpersonally meaningful and the figurative is thoroughly resisted.

Already this cursory description of the major interpretative strategies, whose poetic realization will be scrutinized in this essay, makes it clear that a significant element of philosophical and hermeneutic radicalism is implied by both of them. Moreover, this essay will focus on the cultural hermeneutics of the movement that is habitually represented as essentially and often radically posttraumatic: literary Modernism. Correspondingly, the philosophical radicalism of these strategies will be analyzed in their textual realizations *in extremis*—in the hope that this choice of a textual corpus will make both hermeneutic strategies more palpable and more easily comprehensible. At the same time, even though the representation of literary Modernism as posttraumatic is common among literary scholars and cultural historians, the exact modalities of the traumatic, as it is associated with Modernism, need further explanations. Moreover, as these explanations will differ from some of the major

D. Sobolev, Ph.D. (✉)
Department of Hebrew and Comparative Literature, University of Haifa, 199 Abba Khoushy Blvd., Mt. Carmel, Haifa 31905, Israel
e-mail: dennissobolev@hotmail.com

Y. Ataria et al. (eds.), *Interdisciplinary Handbook of Trauma and Culture*,
DOI 10.1007/978-3-319-29404-9_5

clichés that have been repeatedly used in the discussions of literary Modernism, and especially of its so-called "High Modernism" phase, the entire first section of this essay will address the question of the modalities of the traumatic behind the Modernist literary tradition. Without denying the traumatic nature of specific historical events—and, first and foremost, the horrors of the First World War—this section will argue that the historical framework of Modernism foregrounds its relation to another modality and probably a deeper layer of traumatic experience, which will be labeled as a "rupture in the episteme." It is partly because of these historical and somewhat polemical reasons that this essay will focus on the texts of the first Modernist in the English language—Gerard Manley Hopkins—whose poems were written a few decades before the First World War, even though they were published in its wake. Significantly, however, as will be shown throughout the analysis to follow, like much later "High Modernist" writings, Hopkins's poems are both explicitly posttraumatic and use the two above-mentioned radical hermeneutic strategies of the conceptualization of mental and physical suffering. Furthermore, if in the microcosm of a few sonnets these strategies can be analyzed in a relatively detailed and textually-oriented manner, a comparable analysis of their specific textual realizations in *Ulysses* or *The Trial* would require a full-length book. This "microcosmic" analysis, however, as will be stressed in the concluding section of this essay, is carried out in order to foreground the hermeneutic strategies that are common for literary Modernism, in general.

At the same time, as general as these goals may seem, this chapter does not aspire to propose any general theory of the hermeneutics of trauma in Modernism, let alone a general theory of the cultural hermeneutics of the traumatic. No such theory seems to be possible. On the contrary, as it seems, every period, every cultural movement and probably every writer have to deal with the traumatic anew, finding his or her own language, struggling to utter the ultimately ineffable, agonizing over the impossibility of transcending the ultimately intranscendable. And this is the second reason why this essay focuses on Hopkins's writings: even in comparison to writings that are as unrepeatable and often idiosyncratic as most major Modernist texts are, Hopkins's poems are usually considered to be among the most complex, the most inimitable, and the most idiosyncratic. By the same token, the analysis to follow will demonstrate the extreme singularity of the "counterpointed" relation between the two major poetic strategies of the traumatic in Hopkins. It is this textually-oriented clarification of the singularity of his hermeneutics of the traumatic—its complex and unrepeatable specificity, the singularity of the biographical circumstances that underlay it, its religious and philosophical assumptions, and its poetic articulations—that is the second major goal of this essay.

On a broader theoretical scale, it is this very duality—one may say, a paradox—that is at stake in this chapter. On the one hand, as will be shown below, Hopkins's representations and conceptualizations of the traumatic are strikingly personal and singular; as such, they stubbornly resist any attempts at their generalization in the form of a general theory of "poetry and trauma." On the other hand, as already said, in its complex, dialogical and dialectical form, Hopkins's poetry articulates the two major Modernist strategies of confronting the traumatic. Without a doubt, in Modernist literature the repertoire of such hermeneutic strategies of the traumatic is not limited to these two, nevertheless these strategies seem to be central both for Modernist literary practices and cultural self-consciousness. To use Althusser's well-known term in a slightly modified sense, such core hermeneutic strategies may be called "cultural dominants." It is from the repertoire of these cultural dominants of the hermeneutics of the traumatic, as they are accessible in a given period, that any writer—and probably any human being—is forced to construe, to construct, to write, to efface, and to rewrite anew, his or her own cultural hermeneutics of trauma. It is because of this reason that no general theory of the poetic hermeneutics of trauma is possible; nevertheless, what seems to be both possible and deeply necessary is the theoretical description of the historically specific repertoire of these dominant components of the hermeneutics of trauma. Correspondingly, it is with an eye on this difficult combination of analytical necessity and the impossibility of synthesis that this essay will have to proceed.

5.2 Modernism, Trauma, and a "Rupture in the Episteme"

Probably, the first thing most students of literature learn about Modernism is that the social and cultural changes that underlay its advent were of a deeply traumatic nature. When it comes to details, however, the First World War is usually discussed as the major traumatic event, and Modernism in literature—as being directly related to it. Probably, almost no one would doubt that there is a significant element of historical truth in this statement; nevertheless, under closer scrutiny the problem turns out to be much more complicated. As will be stressed below, literary Modernism emerged long before the First World War; correspondingly, the traumatic developments that underlay its emergence went far beyond the repeatedly discussed trauma of "the Great War," even though it is indeed the influence of this trauma that played a pivotal role in the recognition of the traumatic nature of a much broader range of human experience in the first half of the twentieth century. All this, however, seems to require much more detailed explanations.

Literary Modernism was much more than a change in style, in literary emphases or the modalities of cultural susceptibilities. However unforgettable, complex, and philosophically significant works it produced, as an artistic movement Modernism in literature and the visual arts was also what C. S. Peirce called an "index" (Peirce, 1932, pp. 143–144)—a visible cultural phenomenon and a sequence of cultural developments that possessed an intrinsic quality of a symptom, which pointed to much broader and far-reaching social, political, and cultural changes. Therefore, it is not occasional that in scholarly literature "modernism" is now being used in two essentially different senses: as a name for a loosely defined literary movement and as a designation for a social and cultural period—in other words, as the designations for the two components of a relation that, following C. S. Peirce, may be called "indexical." Yet, applying the term "index" to literary Modernism may also be misleading. In terms of Peirce's semiotics, "index" is supposed to be based on a relation between a cause and an effect; correspondingly, in different introductory books and courses on cultural theory, the notion of "index" is frequently explained through the example of smoke's relation to fire. In this sense, the Althusserian insistence on the "relative autonomy" of different "spheres" of culture may provide a necessary correction to this relation of causal determinism, as implied by the notion of "index" (Althusser, 1971, p. 130). At the same time, given this redefinition of the semiotic structure of the index by means of the notion of relative autonomy, the underscoring of the indexical nature of literary Modernism seems to be crucial for its understanding. It is in this sense of an intimate indexical relation to a very broad range of social, political, scientific, technological, and cultural developments that literary Modernism differs from more narrowly defined art trends such as Neo-Classicism, Symbolism, Futurism, or Hyperrealism. Certainly, each of these trends was also related to its social and cultural milieu through an elaborate texture of various and heterogeneous relations, and each of these trends had an indexical element to them. Yet, in literary Modernism this indexical element was essentially radicalized.

It is no less significant that Modernism articulated and attempted to come to terms with the social and cultural developments that were structured by rupture and essential discontinuity. Once again, a brief explanation seems to be necessary at this point. For a cultural historian, the perception of the social and cultural processes associated with early Modernism is somewhat paradoxical. At least until the First World War, those people who lived through these developments usually experienced them as being basically continuous with the past, even though it was widely recognized that the pace of change was steadily increasing. In contrast, from a retrospective viewpoint, in modernism a cultural rupture seems to be much more conspicuous than cultural continuity; moreover, in all probability, this was the most significant "rupture" within the history of European culture since the sixteenth century. A mention of the sixteenth century is not occasional in this context; since the early works of Foucault, the transition to "the Age of Reason" has been considered an archetype of a cultural rupture, as opposed to the belief in the basically continuous nature of cultural processes that was dominant at that time (Foucault, 1970, 1972). Although, since then, Foucault's work has frequently been criticized (yet even more frequently defended) from different perspectives, his model of the uneven development of culture, where periods of relative continuity are interrupted by the moments of discontinuity, is usually accepted. It is such moments, when the basic patterns of perception and the conceptualization of experience undergo a relatively rapid change that early Foucault referred to as a "rupture" in the "episteme."

Without a doubt, "modernism" in the broader socio-cultural sense indicates such a rupture in the episteme; and even in comparison to the sixteenth and seventeenth century this change happened very quickly. Within a few decades, an entire cultural world became partly non-existent, while another unknown world was rapidly emerging—whose promises and losses it was still difficult to foresee or estimate. In retrospect, it may well turn out that nowadays—with the advent of the "digital era," virtual communications, social networks, and the massive relocation of traditional industries to the space that only 20 years ago was habitually labeled as "the Third World"—we are living through another break in the episteme. Yet, it may equally turn out that these are only surface changes that do not affect the basic patterns of thought and experience. This is, however, one of those questions that the actual participants of historical events can rarely answer. At the same time, it seems that those who lived during the early modernist period did not know how deep and far-reaching the changes they were beginning to witness would actually be, and how traumatic this transition to a new social and cultural world would prove to be.

As regards the retrospective temporalization of this rupture in the episteme, different disciplines suggest slightly different temporal frameworks for the historical conceptualization of modernism (Armstrong, 2005; Bradshaw & Dettmar, 2005; Faulkner, 1977; Lewis, 2007). Sometimes a given event can be chosen as a symbolic beginning; among the earliest events marking the beginning of this "long modernism," the 1859 publication of Charles Darwin's *On the Origin of Species* is sometimes mentioned, as the 1865 exhibition of Edouard Manet's "Olympia" is mentioned as the symbolic beginning of modern art. There is a general consensus, however, that modernism as a broad cultural term applies to the period beginning somewhere around the 1870s. Correspondingly, it is to this period that literary Modernism as indexical to a radical change in the episteme, with all the traumatic implications of this rupture, may be reasonably applied. Significantly for the following discussion, the first of Hopkins's mature poems, *The Wreck of the Deutschland*, was written in 1875; his last sonnets were composed shortly before his death in 1889.

The attitudes towards this epistemic rupture were various and changing. As the usual historical narrative goes, although the horrors of rapid urbanization, mass poverty, the new forms of alienation and exploitation, as well as the increasing destruction of the natural environment, were often lamented, in most cases the scientific and technological advances of the time were enthusiastically welcomed and applauded. It was only the advent of the First World War that radically changed these dominant and usually optimistic attitudes towards the gradually emerging new social and cultural world. This positive emphasis was replaced by the stress placed on the destructive and traumatic character of these new developments, as well as the millions of dead, the trenches, the gas, and the tanks. Correspondingly, for many decades it was repeatedly suggested that a considerable part of literary Modernism—both in its broader sense and in the narrow sense of "High Modernism" in literature—was born out of these new types of postwar posttraumatic experience, its articulation and scrutiny. Indeed, the modalities of the traumatic, as they are identified and articulated in different Modernist texts, range from personal losses and suffering—through the poverty and alienation of growing urban spaces, the direct descriptions of the horrors of the First Word War and the partial collapse of European narcissistic cultural self-perceptions—to the general perception of human existence with its anxiety and finitude as intrinsically traumatic.

There are two main objections to this familiar representation. First, as has already been said, the beginning of cultural modernism, when it is conceptualized in the above sense of a rupture in the episteme, is usually identified by contemporary research at around the 1870s. Second, many of the central texts of literary Modernism, including those by Hopkins, Conrad, Joyce, Kafka, or Bely were written before the First World War. Little known before the war or even totally unknown, these writers seem to be those few whose cultural sensitivities to social and cultural changes, as well as the traumatic nature of these changes, went beyond the usual self-perceptions and self-representations of the pre-War European cultures. Correspondingly, from the historical point of view, it is not the emergence of Modernism, but rather its mass appeal, its perception as being able to speak directly about modern experiences, that is related to the First World War. What had earlier been perceived as a personal problem of this or that person, suddenly revealed itself as a common destiny, as the essentially tragic and traumatic nature of modern cultural and social experience. At the same time, an understanding of this traumatic core of modern experience was becoming increasingly difficult. As Joseph Wood Krutch stresses in *The Modern Temper* (1931, pp. 3–14), since the mid-nineteenth century the traditional strategies of interpreting human experience and the human place in the world, in general, appeared as less and less reliable. As a result, at the time of the emergence of Modernist literature, the growing need for a stable ground on which the hermeneutics of traumatic human experience could be based was paralleled by the cultural processes that created the situation when "mythology, religion, and philosophy" could no longer function as such grounds for "the interpretation of experience" (Krutch, 1931, p. 12).

The Modernist hermeneutics of dealing with this combination of traumatic experiences with the loss of a reliable hermeneutic ground is the main subject of this essay. As has already been said, in focusing on what may seem to be only a case study—the analysis of the two main hermeneutic strategies in the poetry of Gerard Manley Hopkins—I would like to explore the two main strategies of confronting the traumatic experiences that underlie the literature of Modernism: their radical allegorization, in the hope of arriving, to use Hopkins's own words, at a stable "ground of being," (*The Wreck of the Deutschland*, l. 254) and, conversely, the recognition of the essential and insurmountable semantic indeterminacy of human existence. What makes Hopkins's work especially significant from this point of view is not only its capacity for exemplifying these major hermeneutic strategies, nor even the fact that Hopkins seems to be the first poet to articulate both of them, while stressing their explicit relation to traumatic experiences. No less significant than this simultaneous articulation of the opposed interpretative strategies in their relation to suffering is the dialectical and dialogical relation between them, even though in Hopkins neither synthesis nor interpretative reconciliation are achieved through this dialectics. Nevertheless, this is not an example of Adorno's "negative dialectics" either (Adorno, 1973). Although this is indeed a dialectics without a synthesis, it is not a denial of a possibility of such synthesis. As will be shown below, while at the level of Hopkins's poetic practice the traumatic and painful experience is laid bare, the unresolved tension between the two major hermeneutic strategies opens itself to this experience without being able to heal, contain, rationalize, or efface it. Without a doubt, as a psychological condition this position is almost unbearable. Still, in contrast, as a poetic and philosophical stance it prefigures the entire history of Modernist literature in its repeated attempts to come to terms with this essential openness to the trauma of human existence. Let us see.

5.3 The First Modernist

Gerard Manley Hopkins was not only one of those writers whose work suddenly became famous following this change in cultural perceptions and sensitivities; it was discovered in the most literal sense of the word. Nowadays, Hopkins is usually considered as one of the greatest nineteenth-century poets, and he is one of the most often anthologized ones. For most readers, a mention of his writings—first of all poetic, but also philosophical, theological, and ars-poetic—immediately brings to mind their paradoxical combination of condensed visionary insights with some of the most tragic lines in modern poetry, philosophical meditations with a direct confessional mode. Over the course of the entire history of twentieth-century literary scholarship, a handful of his poetic works has proved to be one of the most difficult scholarly problems (Hartman, 1966, pp. 1–2). Hopkins's poems are known, often notoriously so, for their extreme complexity and semantic condensation, their revolutionary poetic language, rhetorical virtuosity, and the dislocation of familiar linguistic usage, as well as their intellectual tensions and unresolved questions. Given these difficulties of his poetic idiolect and his poetic forms, the difficulties that often seemed to be insurmountable for even his most close poet-friends, it is a most notable and somewhat paradoxical fact that his poetic standing outside the English-speaking world—from France and Italy to Japan and Korea—often seems to be even higher than within it.

In his lifetime, however, he was unable to publish a single work out of a relatively broad spectrum of his undoubtedly great texts. Even his friends tended to consider his poems as idiosyncrasies, whereas his colleagues and students in Dublin—at a provincial college which by that time had a reputation of being second-rate—were totally unaware of the fact that the person with whom they met on an everyday basis was probably the greatest poet of the generation. At least at this biographical level, a comparison to Kafka immediately comes to mind. In 1918, however—and the timing is significant given the role of the First World War in the change of literary sensibilities, preferences, and perceptions—Hopkins's friend Robert Bridges, now a poet-laureate, published a thin volume of the former's poems, accompanied by a preface that seemed more to apologize for their publication than to assert their literary value in any direct and unequivocal manner. At the same time, it is only the second 1930 edition that brought Hopkins his present fame, as well as the lasting and far-reaching influence on several generations of English-language writers. Examining the scholarly literature that focuses on his influence on both sides of the Atlantic, one gets the feeling that it is much easier to mention those poets who were not influenced by Hopkins than to list those who were; this list comprises such diverse and often opposed poets as W. H. Auden and Dylan Thomas, Elizabeth Bishop and Sylvia Plath, Robert Lowell and Ted Hughes, Theodore Roethke and Seamus Heaney, as well as many others, both religious and secular, philosophical and confessional. Put briefly, if in terms of a broader cultural history Hopkins's writings are indexical of that rupture in the episteme, which has been discussed above and whose meaning became comprehensible only much later, in more narrow terms of literary history his poems influenced and prefigured many of the most significant achievements in twentieth-century English-language poetry.

A brief detour through the biographical circumstances of Hopkins's life seems to be indispensable for understanding the hermeneutically-oriented discussion that follows. In his Oxford years, he was an outstanding student, brilliant in almost everything; he was awarded "double first" and called "the star of Balliol" (referring to Balliol College of Oxford University, where Hopkins studied) by Benjamin Jowett, who would later become the Master of the college. Hopkins could have chosen any path to success, be it social or academic, but he chose differently. In 1866, he converted to Roman Catholicism "just" because he thought that among different trends in Christianity and European philosophy, Catholicism was the closest to the truth; correspondingly, as an individual choice, this was the right thing to do. Notably, Hopkins did not make this decision in an act of blind passion; and he was well aware of the social consequences of his choice, even though he was probably incapable of assessing their entire range. His conversion caused a deep crisis in relations with his family—a crisis and alienation he was never able to overcome altogether. Given the social and cultural restrictions still imposed upon Catholics, this also meant an end to an academic career at a major institution, as well as blocking many other social paths. Shortly after the conversion, Hopkins would join the Jesuits and become a priest. He would go through long periods of training at Roehampton, Stonyhurst, and St. Beuno's and would also work as a priest at some of the poorest parishes in England, where he witnessed mass suffering, poverty. and human degradation. Despite the relatively rare moments of respite, like his "salad days" at St. Beuno's, Hopkins felt increasingly isolated from any intellectual milieu, where he could find understanding or appropriate interlocutors; he became increasingly depressed. As far as we know from his letters, diaries, and retreat notes, he never regretted his choice and never wavered in his allegiance; yet, there was also a gradual understanding that at the personal level this choice was essentially and irreparably destructive. In *The Wreck*, he describes his conversion as "I did say yes/O at lightning and lashed rod" (ll. 9–10).

The worst days, however, were yet to come. In 1884, Hopkins was transferred to Dublin, which in those days was in a state of dilapidation and mass poverty, and appointed the Professor of Greek at Catholic University, which was also going through difficult days. Here as a Catholic, Hopkins was alienated from other Englishmen; as an Englishman, he was alienated from the Irishmen. Formally, he received a substantial salary; yet, as he was a Jesuit, his salary reverted to the university as "a part of the much-needed funds for running the establishment" (Hopkins, 1956, p. 185; Martin, 1991, p. 363). If before he was often overburdened with work, now this burden became unbearable. In 1884, Hopkins wrote in one of his letters: "I have 557 papers on hand: let those who have been thro' the like say what this means" (Hopkins, 1955a, p. 123). In 1887, he checked 1795 exams, and in other years—between 1300 and 1800 (O'Flynn, 1987–1988, p. 176). The quantity was not the only problem. His notebook from the Dublin period indicates an almost unbridgeable gap between his standards and the actual level of these exams.[1] In addition, trying to be as scrupulous and attentive an examiner as he could, Hopkins spent much time calculating the exact grades and even divided the points he gave into fractions. "In the battered exercise-book called Hopkins's "Dublin Notebook" there are pages and pages containing thousands of examination ticks, marks, and occasional comments" (White, 1992, p. 372). This kind of work, alongside teaching, consumed practically all his time. In a letter to his mother, Hopkins writes: "I labour for what is worth little... And in doing this almost fruitless work I use up all opportunity of doing any other" (Hopkins, 1956, p. 185). Among others, this drudgery almost excluded any opportunity for writing poetry. He died from typhoid fever a few years later.

The brief biographical review presented above[2] is not meant to be a causal explanation of the traumatic experiences of Hopkins's life in Dublin, but only as a background to more easily understand these experiences, their major modalities, and poetic expression. In the final analysis, depending on one's background and specific circumstances, receiving professorship at the age of forty at a second-rate institution with loads of paperwork may be experienced as a significant success or a temporary obstacle, as a minor failure or as one's life tragedy. For Hopkins, however, it was closer to the latter. His letters written in Dublin testify that he suffered from constant fatigue, anemia, emotional exhaustion, intense

[1] Norman White writes: "Confronted with endless piles of examination scripts, he was shocked by the poor standard of answers, and by their grammar, expression, and spelling... Hopkins's bewildered and hopeless remarks reveal the fastidious distance between his standards and those of the students..." (White, 1992, pp. 371–372).

[2] For more detail, see Martin (1991), Mariani (2008), White (1992).

physical and mental suffering, incessant anxiety about the urgent work that needed to be completed, the long periods of insomnia, the recurrent feeling that he was gradually dying and, most importantly, deep depressions (White, 2002). However, the bouts of depression he feared most were those when he felt that madness might be approaching (Hopkins, 1955a, p. 139; Hopkins, 1955b, pp. 216, 222, 282; Hopkins, 1956, p. 256; Hopkins, 1959b, p. 262).

In sum, although Hopkins's did what he thought was philosophically, theologically and ethically right, this decision proved to be self-destructive. He found himself lonely and isolated, far from his family and his country, overburdened with relatively useless work, completely unknown as a poet, almost unable to pursue his literary writings, and doomed to unceasing suffering. It is only after the First World War that a comparable split between the world of thought and actual existence would become a much more commonly-shared cultural experience. Nevertheless, it is in Dublin that Hopkins wrote a series of sonnets that are variously referred to as "the terrible sonnets," "the dark sonnets" or "the sonnets of desolation." It is in these sonnets that he attempted to re-confront these experiences in the hopes of making sense out of them. As will be shown below, in these sonnets, while laying bare the various elements and causes of suffering, the hovering despair and the fear of approaching madness, Hopkins simultaneously followed both hermeneutic paths outlined above: the typological redemption of these experiences through the complex figure of *allegoresis* and its reversal, and the denial of their comprehensibility to the human mind. These sonnets proved to be an inexhaustible source of influence and inspiration for twentieth-century poetry.

5.4 Hopkins's Strategies of the Hermeneutics of the Existential

Translating suffering into meaning usually requires a relatively stable semantic foundation, on the basis of which human experience can be interpreted. However, it is this stable hermeneutic ground that gradually began to disappear in the second half of the nineteenth century, even though it was only in the twentieth century that European cultures faced and came to understand the entire range and consequences of this disappearance. At the same time, for a relatively long while, Hopkins felt that he was able to reestablish this hermeneutic ground for the interpretation of experience through the very radicalism of his act of conversion. At the beginning of the twenty-first century, Badiou would comment that truth as an "event" emerges through faithfulness to it (Badiou, 2001, pp. 40–56). In a letter to Canon Dixon, only a few years before his "dark sonnets," Hopkins writes:

> When a man has given himself to God's service, when he has denied himself and followed Christ, he has fitted himself to receive and does receive from God a special guidance, a more particular providence. This guidance is conveyed partly by the actions of other men, as his appointed superiors, and partly by direct light and inspiration. (Hopkins, 1955a, p. 93)

Thus, according to Hopkins, both external events and inner inspiration are more than just personal success or failure; they are the signs of divine will. A strange, almost puritan (or evangelical, to use a nineteenth century term), strain of thought surfaces in this letter. The results of Hopkins's incessant self-scrutiny were different at different times. "My heart," he writes in the autobiographical part of the 1875 *The Wreck of the Deutschland*, "but you were dovewinged, I can tell,/Carrier-witted, I am bold to boast,/To flash from the flame to flame then, tower from the grace to the grace" (ll. 22–24). Significantly, this was written in the period when Hopkins believed that he was making constant religious progress and when he even permitted himself to return to poetry, at a time when he still felt the "direct light and inspiration" to which he refers in the quotation above. However, as I have shown elsewhere, under closer scrutiny even this relatively early text is structured by an essential and insurmountable split between thought and existential experience (Sobolev, 2011, pp. 304–324).

The same is true on a broader scale. In Hopkins' poetry, hermeneutic certainties, which are based on clear theological declarations and doxological statements, were increasingly counterpointed with hermeneutic uncertainty and loss. In order to better understand this process, one may want to take a few steps backward and examine two poems that preceded the articulation of this double hermeneutics in the Dublin "dark" sonnets. "The Lantern out of Doors" focuses on a comparable alloy of human loneliness and divine concern. Hopkins describes a strange light in the night, and then, suspending the explanation of its origin, in the second quatrain turns to the existential realm: to the insuperable loneliness of the human being as the existential condition. Relating these apparently disparate subjects to one another, the sestet interprets the symbolic meaning of light in the first quatrain in terms of the human condition, as it is described in the second. Hopkins begins:

> Sometimes a lantern moves along the night.
> That interests our eyes. And who goes there?
> I think; where from and bound, I wonder, where,
> With, all down darkness wide, his wading light?
> (ll. 1–4)

As the poem opens with this vision of a glimmering light in the darkness, Hopkins stresses the contrast between the "wading" light that he sees and the surrounding night. The symbolic implications of this vision are quite clear: light is the central Biblical symbol of God, and light in darkness is a conventional image for divine concern. Moreover, as Gardner has pointed out, in Hopkins, in full accordance with the Biblical convention, fire and light are "divine symbols" (Gardner, 1948, 1: pp. 154–155). This symbolic answer, however, is to be withheld up to the end of the sonnet; at the beginning of the poem, Hopkins discusses the origin of the light in strictly realistic terms. The suspension of a symbolic meaning, which this reticence creates, enables him to introduce the second central theme of the sonnet: the theme of human loneliness. Moreover, this suspension makes it possible to foreground the experience of loneliness and its significance in strictly existential terms. Hopkins continues: "Men go by me…/…till death or distance buys them quite./Death or distance soon consumes them: wind,/What most I may eye after, be in at the end/I cannot, and out of sight is out of mind" (ll. 5–11) Thus, tacitly replacing the literal sense of the verb "to go" with its metaphorical meaning, Hopkins turns from an unnamed man with a lantern to the "men" he has encountered during his life. Significantly, these men are commodified: death "buys" and "consumes" them. In this final bargain with death, they turn into passive objects rather than human beings; they are represented as inanimate and incapable of returning one's affection. They come and go; little unifies them with other human beings; nothing remains of them in human memory. The human being is alone. As Joseph Brodsky would put this almost a 100 years later: "Man is alone, like a thought that is being forgotten" (Brodskii, 2014, v. 1, p. 688).

It is at this point in the articulation of human loneliness and reification that a radical hermeneutic turn takes place. After a seeming digression, Hopkins explains the symbolic meaning of the light he has seen in the first quatrain: divine love and concern. In contrast to the first quatrain, now that the vision of a passing unfamiliar man has been metaphorized and the theme of existential loneliness has been articulated, this translation of the vision of light in symbolic terms becomes especially meaningful. It is precisely because of this insuperable mundane loneliness that this translation of light as divine concern becomes significant not only in metaphysical, but also in existential terms. At the same time, anticipating much more direct expressions of hermeneutic disruptions, Hopkins refrains from explicit allegorization; he does not say, for example, that this wandering light in darkness is the sign of God's love and presence. Instead, he turns directly to divine concern, translating the figurative meaning of the first quatrain into the literal meaning of the sestet. In the second tercet, the interplay between the existential and the religious comes to the fore. Hopkins writes: "Christ minds: Christ's interest, what to avow or amend/There, eyes them, heart wants, care haunts, foot follows kind,/Their ransom, their rescue, and first, fast, last friend" (ll. 12–15). Thus, explicitly responding to the description of human loneliness in the first tercet and implicitly allegorizing the vision of light in the octave, Hopkins concludes that it is God who is both the Guide and the Friend. His choice of anthropomorphic diction, in turn, foregrounds the intersubjective dimension of his relationship with God, and thus stresses that divine concern, as Hopkins describes it, is not just transcendent supervision or the indifferent perfection of the world mechanism of the deists. This relationship belongs to the experiential, and not only to the theoretical plane. Miraculously, this triumphant revelation seems to resolve all the problems: his "first, fast, last friend" is certainly incomparable to any other kind of friendship. It is also noteworthy, however, that this happiness is extremely precarious: not only the speaker's happiness, but the very meaningfulness of his life hinges on the permanent feeling of divine concern through which the experience of ultimate human loneliness can be confronted, interpreted, and overcome.

This conclusion means that Hopkins's hermeneutics implies the possibility of the extremes of happiness and despair. On the one hand, in his "nature sonnets" of 1877–1878 complete detachment from the world, disinterestedness, and dispossession, make possible the intuition of divine presence in nature; Hopkins becomes able to transcend the limitations of his earthly existence and to partake in the eternal being of God (Sobolev, 2011, pp. 27–89). The God of Hopkins's poetry is a constant and sensitive listener to the human being, an interlocutor who answers through his natural manifestations. At the same time, if God ceases to answer, all these blessings inevitably turn into causes for suffering. The dazzling vision of nature becomes meaningless without the internal confidence in divine presence; as Hopkins says in the notes on Parmenides: "All things are upheld by instress and are meaningless without it" (Hopkins, 1959a, p. 127). Moreover, self-caused detachment, which once enabled the intuition of divine presence, has to prevent him from participating in the mundane life of the world, which could become a consolation. The dazzling world of poetic vision turns into a wasteland and plunges into darkness.

One of the first poems to register this transformation is the sonnet "The Candle Indoors." This poem is especially interesting for the current discussion since, as Hopkins himself says, it is "a companion to the Lantern" (Hopkins, 1955b, p. 84) discussed above. Moreover, both sonnets center on light, its sources, and symbolic potential. However, the differences are no less significant. If the former poem describes the relationship between the human being and divine presence in the world, the latter analyzes that between him and the divine presence within the human soul. And if the former celebrates the potential of happiness in *ultima solitudo*, the latter foregrounds its potential poignancy. As in the previous poem, "The Candle Indoors" begins with the same central image: that of a light in darkness; and, likewise, though the symbolic implication of this light is clear enough, it is to be withheld up to the sestet. The first quatrain describes, rather realistically, the picture of a lit candle, burning in the night; significantly, not all the elements of this picture can be potentially translated into symbolic terms: "yellowy moisture," for example, cannot. At the same time, the adjective "blear" already hints to the fact that the vision presented at the beginning of the poem is only a proleptic image of a clearer vision to be achieved; and the word "blissful" foreshadows the translation of light as grace. The second quatrain, which is also closely related to the existential realm, describes the presumed origin of this light; the candle helps unnamed hands to perform their daily drudgery ("fingers ply"). Going back to the autobiographical digression above, it is significant that this theme of drudgery is related to Hopkins's own presence as well. Describing his walk, he writes: "I plod wandering"; and since this phrase is the direct continuation of the previous one ("fingers ply/I plod"), it brings to the fore another sense of the verb "to plod": to drudge. This is still not drudgery in the sense of the thousands of exams Hopkins had to check in Dublin; yet it is noteworthy that in describing his thought, he introduces additional overtones of hard work. This parallelism implicitly makes his idle curiosity (his "a-wanting" to find out the source of light) closer to the hard work of "the eagerer a-wanting

Jessy or Jack/There God to aggrandise, God to glorify" (ll. 7–8); and thus it becomes a proleptic image of the sestet's allegorization of this "wondering" as a spiritual quest for grace.

At first sight, however, the phrase quoted above ("God to aggrandise, God to glorify") seems rather obscure; the only thing that becomes immediately clear is that "Jessy or Jack" refer to the archetypal common people. The question to be asked is why is their daily mundane work a sign of "eagerer" desire to praise and "glorify" God; and the answer to this question must be looked for in Hopkins's prose. In his notes on the *Principle of Foundation*, he writes:

> It is not only prayer that gives God glory but work. Smiting on an anvil, sawing a beam, whitewashing a wall, driving horses, sweeping, scouring, everything gives God some glory if being in his grace you do it as your duty. To go to communion worthily gives God great glory, but to take food in thankfulness and temperance gives him glory too. (Hopkins, 1959b, pp. 240–241)

Thus, like prayer, the exhausting earthly work of common men and their faithfulness to duty, glorify God. However, in order to be able to do this, they must perform their duties "in his grace." Correspondingly, if "Jessy or Jack" want to "aggrandise" God by means of their work, they have to make sure that their lives are open to grace; it is only this experience of grace that can turn the speaker's and his common people's "a-wanting" to praise God into a prayer. This understanding, in turn, helps to account for the transition from the octave to the sestet.

Although in this sestet Hopkins does not explicitly address the question of whether his common people receive grace, he turns directly to the meditation upon the relationship between grace and the unnamed "you." He begins with an imperative: "Come you indoors, come home; your fading fire/Mend first and vital candle in close heart's vault;/You there are master, do your own desire" (ll. 9–11). It is worth noting that in realistic terms this imperative applies neither to Hopkins nor to his common men: on the one hand, they are already inside; on the other hand, this house is not his. Breaking the symbolic continuity between the material world and the realm of spiritual truths, Hopkins uses some elements of the experience described in the octave in order to express an ethical imperative, pointing to a way from the darkness of external existence to the light of inner life: to the realm of grace, of divine presence. Within this allegorical space, already detached from the realistic plane, the sense of Hopkins's elliptical vocative "you" becomes extremely broad: potentially it may mean Hopkins himself, his archetypal working men and even the reader; it may apply to everybody from priest to peasant. The problem he addresses now is that of the relation between grace and humanity in general.

At the same time, the last line of the quotation above seems to pose a problem; it is not clear why the human being, rather than God, is called the "master" of the heart, of the realm of grace. In philosophical terms, an answer can be once again found in Hopkins's prose; according to him, the *arbitrium*, the elective will, which corresponds to the spiritual rather than empirical realm, is indeed unconditionally free (1959b, p. 149). In addition, Hopkins writes that it is only when man returns to grace ("candle") that he can become free: become the "master" of his inner life, of his "home"; otherwise, this home belongs to the devil. Nevertheless, even given this explanation, a disruptive undercurrent is still present in these lines. As already mentioned, in the first tercet neither the "candle" nor "home" is literal any more; the symbol has invisibly turned into an allegory: into the figure based on disruption (Benjamin, 1977; de Man, 1983). This seemingly minor shift foreshadows the development of the poem and mirrors a significant semantic difference between "The Candle Indoors" and its earlier "companion," "The Lantern out of Doors."

At first sight, up to this point the two poems conform to each other. However, there is also a conspicuous difference: if in the former poem light (divine presence) is "outdoors" in the external world, in nature, the latter indicates the only place of communication with God: the inwardness of the soul. However, nowhere—neither here nor his other poems or prose—does Hopkins say that the divine presence within the human soul is given to direct sensuous intuition (Sobolev,

2011, pp. 74–89). If in the earlier sonnet he refrained from discussing this split in the very center of the human soul, now the dark side of his conception of the human being comes to the fore. The inner life is referred to by means of the metaphor of the "vault" ("in close heart's vault"), which is hardly separable from its sense of a burial chamber. Death is smuggled into the very center of the soul; and this ambivance only prefigures the final statement of the poem, the statement which becomes especially palpable against the background of its companion poem. In the second tercet, Hopkins implicitly, yet unequivocally, states that grace is inaccessible to his unnamed interlocutor, to everyman: "What hinders? Are you beam-blind, yet to a fault/In a neighbour deft-handed? Are you that liar/And, cast by conscience out, spendsavour salt?" (ll. 12–14).

Whatever the explanation, it is clear enough that the human being cannot return to the divine presence within his or her soul. "What hinders" remains unexplained: this concluding tercet consists entirely of sentences with question marks. Hopkins propounds different hypotheses (hypocrisy, bad conscience), which might be able to explain this essential detachment of the human being from divine presence, but none are presented in the form of assertion. Significantly, in this tercet Hopkins draws upon the imagery from the Sermon on the Mount (Matthew 5–7; MacKenzie, 1990, p. 405). Referring to the pivotal point of evangelical history, he tries to account for the separation of the soul from God, but he cannot. At the same time, in the tercet the function of imagery is not restricted to this allusion to the Sermon on the Mount; it is interwoven within the sonnet's own tropological texture as well. When Hopkins writes "beam-blind," he evokes both the blindness to the beams of light, which are mentioned in the first quatrain, and the metaphorical beam that a hypocrite and sinner cannot see in his own eye (Matthew 7:3). The visible beam of light at the beginning of the poem turns at its end into the proverbial beam in the eye of the sinner, into an ultimate symbol of the latter's separation from grace. In contrast to "The Lantern out of Doors," the hermeneutics of light lays bare a split between it and existential experience, which defies explanation.

At the same time, this is not the denial of a possibility of the hermeneutics of human existence. In the sestet, Hopkins addresses an unnamed "you" rather than himself, and correspondingly manages to avoid the personal consequences of both the implicit separation of the human soul from divine presence in nature, which is seen against the background of "The Lantern out of Doors," and those of separation from the revitalizing divine presence within the soul, which is stated explicitly. In "The Candle Indoors," Hopkins both describes this experience and distances it. Yet, he distances himself from it only for a while, and it is only a little later that he will return to this experience in his dark sonnets. And if "The Candle Indoors" seems to retain a certain equilibrium between light and darkness—between divine imperative in the first tercet and the statement of the inaccessibility of grace in the second—in these sonnets the speaker is plunged deep into the experience of pain, loss, and darkness; the world of divine concern turns into a wilderness. Nevertheless, this change would not make Hopkins reject his existential hermeneutics as self-delusionary and stick to the assumption of the ultimate loss of meaning; paradoxically, it is this spiritual "wilderness" and darkness that will provide a number of partial typological answers to the unresolved questions of "The Candle Indoors."

5.5 In the Wilderness: Between Loss and Hope

A paralyzing experience of the wilderness had already been described by Hopkins in one of his early poems, which, though untitled, is traditionally published under the title "A Soliloquy of one of the spies left in the wilderness." The poem evokes an episode from Numbers (13–14), in which 12 spies, the vanguard of the Israelites, are sent by Moses to have a look at the Promised Land. The spies, frightened by the inhabitants of this land, though delighted by its beauty and richness, decide to bring back false news and try to dissuade the Jews from continuing their march. Hopkins's account of the story, however, significantly differs from the Biblical narration. His spy is frightened not by the inhabitants of this land, but rather by the wilderness itself and by surrounding death: "To-day/In hot sands perilous/He [Moses] hides our corpses dropping by the way/Wherein he makes us stray" (ll. 45–48). What was supposed to be the Promised Land, turns out to be a desert, a wasteland; and the spy cannot but yearn for a normal life, a normal attitude towards the world, for human happiness ("Egypt, the valley of our pleasance, there!... The comfortable gloom/After the sandfield and the unreined glare!" (ll. 13, 16–17). The spy ends his soliloquy in despair.

Hopkins's reasons for changing the Biblical narrative were never stated explicitly; yet one may arguably surmise that already at this early stage he was aware of the dark side of his philosophical and religious position with its radicalism, and already knew that its promised land of divine presence could easily turn into a spiritual wilderness. At the same time, he could not be unaware of the fact that the narrative of the spies is one of the traditional Christian examples of a failure of faith. And in this early poem, Hopkins who still feels God's immanent presence in the world, makes a clear-cut distinction between himself, as a poet, and this voice which fails to withstand the test of faith in the wilderness. Later on, however, the situation changes. By the end of the 1870s, Hopkins's poetry undergoes a radical change: the epiphany of divine presence in nature turns into inescapable loneliness, and Baroque exuberance makes way for harshness and seeming simplicity. During the almost 100 years of Hopkins studies, various hypotheses have been propounded in order to explain this change; most of them suggest that it resulted from Hopkins's constant exhaustion and feelings of loneliness, as well as the disappearance of God from his life. However, in human life (save, perhaps for that of the mystics) God neither appears nor disappears directly. Instead, certain events or psychological conditions, which in themselves may belong to completely mundane experience, can be interpreted as divine presence or absence; yet, as such, they can also be interpreted in entirely different directions. In other words, the feeling of God's immanence and that of his transcendence are contingent on an interpretative system. By the same token, what determines poetic expression is not only the experience itself, but rather its relation to a hermeneutic code and the latter's possible responses to the changes in one's existential situation. Correspondingly, one must analyze in a more detailed manner the hermeneutic strategies of Hopkins's presentation of existential experience, as well as the strategies by means of which he used to interpret the religious significance of his suffering and disappointments.

Hopkins's notes and diaries show that he repeatedly examined his life, again and again scrutinizing it as a text. As already mentioned, the justification of this hermeneutics was also at hand; Hopkins believed that after the self-sacrifices he had made, his experiences must have a divine meaning inscribed in them. The question to be asked now is what could be the meaning of suffering and loneliness, failure and loss, inner emptiness and the constant feeling of exhaustion, about which Hopkins repeatedly wrote during his Dublin years. On the one hand, they could be interpreted as divine signs of rejection, which, in all probability, foreshadow eternal damnation. In this case, one's sorrowful life is only a proleptic image of eternal pain. On the other hand, theologically, there exists another way to account for Hopkins's suffering, his sense of personal failure and even internal "darkness," as it is depicted in the dark sonnets and will be discussed below in more detail. They can be interpreted as a personal temptation, which is sent by God to the most upright and beloved. As such, they merge with Christ's temptation in the wilderness (Matthew 4:1–11; Luke 4:1–22) and his agony on the cross; pain becomes a sign of divine presence and redemption. Moreover, although in itself this interpretation is not necessarily related to mysticism, in Hopkins's poetic world, where divine presence and concern are constantly stressed, suffering and darkness as the signs of divine concern could easily be followed by a mystical echo (Sobolev, 2011, pp. 72–89). Hopkins's later poems show that it is the latter hermeneutic possibility that he often embraced, even though the interpretation of inner emptiness and pain as a proleptic image of damnation could not be discarded either. This possibility of the dual interpretation of suffering explains, to a considerable extent, the doubleness of Hopkins's late poetry with its paradoxical combination of the painful sense of detachment from God with the acute awareness of spiritual proximity to him. If the former is expressed in the famous invocation of the "dearest" "that lives alas! away" ("I wake and feel," l. 8); the latter surfaces in the self-identification with Biblical heroes, in *imitatio Christi*, and the direct invocations of God.

Let us take a closer look. Describing his life in Dublin, Hopkins repeatedly stressed his ostensible lack of inspiration and his inability to create. Paradoxically, these were the years when he wrote perhaps the most beautiful and, without doubt, the most tragic verses in the English poetry of the century; yet, an understanding of this was not what his incessant self-scrutiny yielded. In September 1885, he writes to Robert Bridges: "If I could but produce work I should not mind its being buried, silenced, and going no further; but it kills me to be time's eunuch and never to beget" (Hopkins, 1955b, p. 222). This is a simple indication, unredeemed by any consoling interpretation. Nevertheless, Hopkins's attitude towards his ostensible internal emptiness was not always like this; in January 1888, he writes to the same Bridges: "All impulse fails me: I can give myself no sufficient reason for going on. Nothing comes: I am a eunuch—but it is for the kingdom of heaven's sake" (Hopkins, 1955b, p. 270). In contrast to the previous description of inner emptiness and exhaustion, here Hopkins interprets them as necessary, perhaps even as a purgatory: as a way to heaven, as a sign of the highest hope. Both this self-representation as a "eunuch" and the intensity of faith, which is so conspicuous in this line, are reproduced in one of most his famous sonnets, "Thou art indeed just, Lord."

Apparent duality characterizes it. The sonnet voices internal pain, bitterness, and resentment; it centers on an outcry of pain. There is a broader picture as well; Hopkins portrays a world that is bereft of providence and divine justice. Like many others before and after him, he repeats Jeremiah's question, "why do sinners' ways prosper?" (l. 3) and then contrasts the prosperity of the sinners to his own ruined life ("Oh, the sots and thralls of lust/Do in spare hours more thrive that I that spend/Sir, life upon thy cause," "disappointment all I endeavor end[s]," "thou dost defeat, thwart me," (ll. 7–9, 4, 6–7). By the time of the sonnet's composition, Hopkins had already voiced the theme of personal failure in its relation to the incomprehensible divine will and the problem of divine justice in one of the dark sonnets, "To seem the stranger": "Only what word/Wisest my heart breeds dark heaven's baffling ban/Bars or hell's spell thwarts" (ll. 11–13). To understand the full significance of this insistence, one should recollect Hopkins's remark that he expects to receive special guidance from God; now this guidance seems only to point out his failures in contrast to the prosperity of sinners. In the second tercet of "Thou art indeed just, Lord," Hopkins adds that divine injustice does not apply only to external mundane failures; his internal life is permeated with the constant feeling of exhaustion and internal emptiness: "But not I build; no but strain,/Time's eunuch, and not breed one work that wakes" (ll. 12–13). This internal emptiness is even more poignant for, unlike earthly injustice, it cannot be ascribed to human vices; it must be the direct manifestation of divine will.

Nevertheless, the first line of the sonnet is a statement of faith, of the ability to withstand suffering and emptiness. Although Hopkins implies that he has forfeited the certainty of divine justice, he uses his soliloquy to restate it. He begins the sonnet with an invocation to God ("Thou art indeed just, Lord") and ends it with an even more direct address: "Mine, O thou lord of life" (l. 14). He stresses that, regardless of exhaustion and pain, God is still his God ("Mine"). Furthermore, in using the imagery of the battle and argument with God, the sonnet evokes both Jacob and Job. Implicitly comparing himself to Job ("Thou art indeed just, Lord… but, sir, so what I plead is just," ll. 1–2), he insists on both his uprightness and his right to speak to his creator. To compare himself to Jacob–Hopkins's "I contend/With

Thee" (ll. 1–2) explicitly echoes Jacob's struggle with God at Peniel in Genesis 32—means even more: Hopkins's confidence that eventually he will be blessed and will get a new life; "I have seen God face to face, and my life is preserved" (Genesis 32:30). Moreover, significantly, it is not only Hopkins's self-portrait, but also his description of ubiquitous mundane injustice, that are inseparable from Biblical overtones. The first two lines of the sonnet, as well as the climactic moment of the articulation of divine injustice ("Why do sinners' ways prosper?" l. 3), are the reiteration of the words of Jeremiah (12:1), and the epigraph brings this appropriation of the prophet's words to the fore. This, in turn, implies that even the most risky, seemingly heterodox, moments of questioning of the ways of God do not detach Hopkins from God; on the contrary, due to the condensed typological substructure of his questioning, it paradoxically shortens the distance between him and his creator. The word "contend" which Hopkins chooses for rendering Jeremiah's monologue adds an element of physical presence, however metaphorized, to this general description of Hopkins's dialogue with God.

5.6 Hopkins's Existential Hermeneutics: Between Despair and Allegoresis

A similar dialectics of suffering and divine presence, verging on almost physical contact, as well as a concordant typological structure, is present in the dark sonnets, and it becomes especially conspicuous in one of the darkest, "Carrion Comfort." Hopkins wrote that two of these sonnets were "written in blood" (1955b, p. 219), and it is usually assumed that one of them is "Carrion Comfort," whereas the other is either "I wake and feel" or "No worst, there is none" (Gardner, 1948, 2: p. 333; Mariani, 1970, pp. 197–248; MacKenzie, 1981, pp. 169–184). It is in these sonnets that the latent hermeneutic possibilities of Hopkins's hermeneutics of human experience are carried to extremes; these poems, as Rose puts it, seem "to teeter on the edge of blasphemy" (Rose, 1977, p. 207). "I wake and feel the fell of dark not day," writes Hopkins, "What hours, O what black hours we have spent/This night! What sights you, heart saw…//But where I say/Hours I mean years, mean life…" (ll. 1–3, 5–6). Human life and unceasing suffering become intrinsically and intimately linked to each other, whereas no explanation of this relation is suggested. In addition, as has been repeatedly noted by scholars, Hopkins's self-representation evokes the traditional images of the sufferings of the damned, including recurrent echoes from *Paradise Lost* (Sobolev, 2011). His representation of human existence almost merges with eternal suffering. And indeed Hopkins continues: "The lost are like this, and their scourge to be/As I am mine, their sweating selves; but worse" ("I wake and feel," ll. 13–14). As a result, the sonnet lays bare the experience of suffering, its pure irrationality and injustice, while refraining from any indication of a possibility of its explanation, understanding, or reversal. The only hermeneutic direction it indicates through the connotative and intertextual fields is even more disquieting in its linking of earthly to eternal suffering, and correspondingly, in a possibility it brings to the fore, without however voicing it, that the irrationality of earthly suffering may have no compensation in the world of eternity.

This theme, as well as the diction and tragic rhetoric of "I wake and feel," are further developed in another "dark sonnet": "No worst." Hopkins writes: "No worst, there is none. Pitched past pitch of grief,/More pangs will, schooled at forepangs, wilder wring" (ll. 1–2). Once again, the sonnet opens with the lines that articulate the experience of pain, both mental and physical, lasting and almost unbearable, irreversible, irrecuperable, while refusing to suggest any explanation for it, which can be comprehensible to the human mind. Instead, the text abounds with various expressions of anguish and grief: "grief," "pang," "cries," "chief-woe," "sorrow," "frightful," "wretch," among many others, all of them within the fourteen lines of the space of the sonnet. In the second part of the first octave, this description of pain is briefly interrupted by a question that invokes Christ and Mary. They are supposed to give relief, but apparently do not; "Comforter, where, where is your comforting?/ Mary, mother of us/where is your relief?" (ll. 3–4). Significantly, no such comfort is indicated in the poem; and after this question—which may be interpreted as either Jeremiah's requirement of justice or conversely as a rhetorical question voicing bitter resignation—Hopkins immediately returns to the description of suffering, both physical and mental: "O the mind, mind has mountains; cliffs of fall/Frightful, sheer, no man fathomed. Hold them cheap/May who ne'er hung here" (ll. 9–11).

Significantly, this depiction of the mind as a frightful and mortally dangerous landscape echoes those of Hopkins's letters that voice his fear of madness. In addition, as has been noted by several scholars, the sonnet's allusions to *King Lear*, culminating in "Here! creep,/Wretch, under a comfort serves in a whirlwind" (see, for example, White, 1986), add an intertextual dimension to this general expression of pain, loss, helplessness, and hopelessness, the feeling of mental collapse and inevitable death. Paradoxically, in the sonnet the only hope and consolation come from the very intensity of pain that may turn out to be overwhelming for the human mind and the body: "Nor does our small/Durance deal with that steep or deep," writes Hopkins (ll. 11–12). It is because of this human fragility that his "Fury had shrieked 'No ling-/Ering! Let me be fell: force I must be brief'" (No worst," ll. 7–8). Correspondingly, death as the final destruction of the human capacity for suffering, as well as sleep as its proleptic image, are the only explicit images of consolation, and their appearance concludes the sonnet: "Creep,/Wretch, under a comfort serves in a whirlwind: all/Life death does end and each day dies with sleep" (ll. 12–14). In a concordant fragment "The times are nightfall," composed around the same time, Hopkins writes that his life "makes welcome death, does dear forgetfulness."

At first sight, the world disclosed in "Carrion Comfort" is similar to its representation in "I wake and feel" and "No worst"; this is the world of darkness, violence, and overwhelming pain: both mental and physical. Once again Hopkins's representation of this world of darkness comprises a few explicit and implicit comparisons with hell; and the meditations of the speaker are characterized by dogmatic indeterminacy and metaphysical vertigo (Sobolev, 2011, pp. 246–252). Furthermore, like in "No worst," death seems to be the only hope and consolation such a world can give. However, to accept this consolation means to embrace the way of despair: to succumb to the temptation in the wilderness. And Hopkins begins his "Carrion Comfort," which was presumably written shortly after "No worst" (MacKenzie, 1990, pp. 449–450, 455), with the assertion that he can resist this temptation.

> Not, I'll not carrion comfort, Despair, not feast on thee;
> Not untwist—slack they may be—these last strands of man
> In me or, most weary, cry *I can no more*. I can;
> Can something, hope, wish day come, not choose not to be. (ll. 1–4)

Apostrophizing and capitalizing on despair, Hopkins transforms his resistance to its power into the medieval *psychomachia*: he dramatizes the psychological condition as a battle for the salvation of his soul, as a fight predetermined by God. As a result, his fight with despair, his resistance to the temptation of its "feast," becomes similar to the temptation of the spies, or even to that of Christ in the wilderness of the Judean desert. In September 1883, 2 years before the "dark sonnets," Hopkins wrote in his retreat notes: "In this evening's meditation on the Temptation I was with our Lord in the wilderness in spirit" (1959b, p. 253).

In the last line of the sonnet, Hopkins adds that this is not only a battle predetermined by God, but also a fight with God; he writes: "I wretch lay wrestling with (my God!) my God" ("Carrion Comfort," l. 14). This line is of paramount significance. It has often been argued by Hopkins scholars that in the dark sonnets God's immanence is replaced by his complete transcendence, that these sonnets, in James Olney's words, are the "tropes of absence" (Olney, 1993, p. 82). Yet, in "Carrion Comfort" Hopkins's explicit description of suffering as the "wrestling" with God makes this suggestion hardly tenable. On the contrary, this description of pain in itself becomes only a part of the battle which the sonnet dramatizes. Once again, typologically, it evokes Jacob's fight with God in Genesis 32. This is not the disappearance of God, but rather his most intense presence and such a proximity to him that one may easily interpret it as heterodoxy. Most significantly, however, the seeming repetition concluding the sonnet echoes the last words of Christ: "Eli, Eli, lama sabachthani?" (Matthew 27:46). Thus, although Hopkins presents his suffering as a purely irrational and irrecoverable experience, simultaneously, through the condensed reference to a number of Biblical paradigms, he re-presents it not only as deeply meaningful, but as a sign of the highest hope. A typological substructure transfigures personal anguish; and, conversely, it is the intensity of this anguish that makes possible participation in the Biblical history.

As in most typological representations in post-Reformation Christianity, a complex and bipartite rhetorical figure is involved here. A specific personal and existential experience is related to a Biblical episode, which it exemplifies and enacts, whereas episodes from the Hebrew Bible tend to be simultaneously interpreted as prefiguring even more basic "types" from the New Testament. All these types are perceived as being both literary ("historically") true, and simultaneously as embodying the most fundamental abstract theological and ethical meanings. In turn, these abstract meanings are projected upon the initial personal actions or experiences. In more technical terms, because of the double semantic detachment involved in this rhetorical operation, in such a representation the existential and the universal are related to each other not through the continuity of symbolic signification, but rather through the disruption of allegory. It is not by chance therefore that this typologically-oriented representation of painful and traumatic personal experiences concludes with the reiterations of the words of Christ, as both a central typological paradigm and the very basis for a possibility of any typological interpretation.

Thus, paradoxically enough, incessant suffering and the feeling of his life's collapse have only shortened the distance between Hopkins and his God. When Hopkins was able to perceive divine presence in nature, he wrote poems about nature; now, that this feeling has disappeared, he is forced to speak, to cry, directly to his only listener and his "first, fast, last friend" ("The Lantern out of Doors," l. 14) Moreover, whereas in the "nature sonnets" of 1877–1878 Hopkins was able to perceive divine presence only through detached, however attentive, vision, in the dark sonnets this presence is given to him in the immediate and unmediated experience, and it isexpressed in the metaphors of physical contact and aggression: in the bodily, almost erotic, proximity of "laying" and "wrestling." The invocation of God as a cosmic power, which in "Pied Beauty" "fathers forth" the world, in "Carrion Comfort" makes way for almost heretical intimacy. Here suffering and pain turn into the intimations—and I consciously pun upon this word here—of divine presence. This understanding, in turn, may shed light on the double meaning of diction in other dark sonnets. Thus, in "I wake and feel" Hopkins writes: "What hours, O what black hours we have spent/This night" (ll. 2–3). In the context of the poem, this "we" may mean "I, Hopkins, and my heart," even though this interpretation would make it a relatively awkward line, which is rarely found in Hopkins. Or, and this is much more plausible, this can be another echo of the same belief in presence and intimacy that was expressed in the line quoted above: "I was with our Lord in the wilderness in spirit" (Hopkins, 1959b, 253).

5.7 A Look Backwards: Poetics of Trauma Between the Collective and the Singular

It is high time now to return to a broader literary and cultural picture, at least for a short while. The two polar and radical literary strategies of confronting and understanding the traumatic experiences, with which Modernism was constantly engaged, were as follows. One could acknowledge existential pain, the loss of meaning, ontological disillusionment and the semantic indeterminacy of existence as the ultimate truth of being, the very truth of being human, and might even embrace them as the philosophical ground of a more authentic type of existence and behavior. Alternatively, one could aim to rewrite them in search of their figurative transfiguration within the relatively stable systems of religious or philosophical meaning. Correspondingly, if the latter strategy is frequently related to the articulation of philosophical nostalgia, the former is associated with its renouncement. However, most significant Modernist texts—including *The Castle*, *The Magic Mountain*, *Ulysses* and *To the Lighthouse*—are usually engaged in negotiating the gap between these two literary and philosophical strategies. In this sense, Hopkins is not only the first "Modernist" in English-language literature, his work is also a synecdoche for the major philosophical and hermeneutic concerns of literary Modernism.

At the same time, the case study carried out in this essay has demonstrated how the two major modernist approaches to the traumatic can be realized as more specific poetic perspectives and hermeneutic strategies. Moreover, this analysis has shown that this relatively common repertoire of the major strategies of the hermeneutics of the traumatic not only forms the basis of their individual specification, but also that of their reinterpretation in relation to one another. This is not only a hermeneutic space where the singularity of a poetic work can be realized, but also the space where the singularity of the human voice in its relation to the traumatic—and the existential in general—can become meaningful even against the background of the semantic bareness of human existence. Indeed, as has been shown above, on the one hand, Hopkins lays bare pain and suffering, loss and despair, death and the semantic indeterminacy of human existence. On the other hand, in direct opposition to the first strategy, his poetic representations of the traumatic draw upon the major typological paradigms of the Hebrew Bible and the New Testament. As a result, suffering reveals itself as essentially and initially allegorical, as the re-acting of the very paradigm of the meaningful—not a denial or a partial collapse of existential meaning, but its very revelation.

As has also been shown above, the relation between these basic hermeneutic strategies is no less important than the ways of their poetic realization and specification. The above analysis of the dark sonnets has not only illustrated these hermeneutic strategies, but has also demonstrated how their literary realization can call into question the very possibility of a compromise between them. Hopkins's major poetic and philosophical innovation, even in comparison to the much later writings of "High Modernism," is based on preventing these hermeneutic extremes from collapsing one into another, and moreover in refusing to negotiate the gap between them. On the one hand, finitude and pain, despair and madness, the loss of meaning are left in their complete barrenness, unredeemed by any sentimentality or self-irony. On the other, the possibility of meaning, the human need for meaning, and the hermeneutics of typological *allegoresis* are also left to stand in their totality and clarity, uncompromised by any incongruence with the existential or the historical. No compromise between them is either achieved or attempted; the tension between the bareness of the existential and the search for the meaning of suffering emerges in Hopkins's writings as central to human existence.

In order to foreground the figurative and philosophical specificity of this relation one may compare it to Joyce or Kafka, who have been mentioned above as concordant to Hopkins in many important senses. Nevertheless, the differences are no less significant. In *Ulysses*, the world of shops and cemeteries, pubs and brothels, and most importantly of existential emptiness, is not only permeated with symbols, but is also enveloped in a totalizing symbolic structure of the Odyssean myth, which it contradicts at every significant point. Yet this contradiction is not one of contrast, but rather that of discordance, ironic gap, and misplacement. In *The Castle*, the representation of the existential with its alienation and violence underscores its intrinsic requirement for figuration, its allegorical character; moreover, these representations both suggest a broad variety of allegorical meanings and deny a possibility of embracing these meanings (Sobolev, 2013).

There are two essentially different ways of looking at these three examples of Modernist writing: as it seems, paradoxically, both are accurate. One may underscore a concordant separation between the pain, the trauma, and the loneliness of the existential, on the one hand, and its transcendent figurative meanings, as they are both suggested and problematized by these texts, on the other. Conversely, in each of these cases one may underscore the meaningful singularity of the literary and philosophical stance that is taken by Hopkins, Joyce, or Kafka. To return to Hopkins, one should conclude that although his poetry can serve to better understand the major hermeneutic and literary strategies of confronting the traumatic in Modernist literature, it also provides a rare example of a philosophical stance that refuses any rhetorical, sentimental, or psychological solution to the problem of suffering, which it both articulates and confronts.

References

Adorno, T. W. (1973). *Negative dialectics*. New York: Seabury Press.

Althusser, L. (1971). *Lenin and philosophy and other essays*. London: New Left Books.

Armstrong, T. (2005). *Modernism: A cultural history*. Cambridge: Polity.

Badiou, A. (2001). *Ethics: An essay on the understanding of evil*. London, New York: Verso.

Benjamin, W (1977). *The origin of German tragic drama*. London: NLB.

Bradshaw, D., & Dettmar, K. J. H. (Eds.). (2005). *A companion to modernist literature and culture*. Oxford: Blackwell.

Brodskii, I. A. (2014). *Maloye sobranie sochinenii*. St. Petersburg: Azbuka.

De Man, P. (1983). The Rhetoric of Temporality. In P. de Man (Ed.), *Blindness and insight: Essays in the rhetoric of contemporary criticism* (2nd ed., pp. 187–228). Minneapolis: University of Minnesota Press.

Faulkner, P. (1977). *Modernism*. London: Methuen.

Foucault, M. (1970). *The order of things: An archaeology of the human sciences*. London: Tavistock Publications.

Foucault, M. (1972). *The archaeology of knowledge*. London: Tavistock Publications.

Gardner, W. H. (1948). *Gerard Manley Hopkins: A study of poetic idiosyncrasy in relation to poetic tradition*. London: Martin Secker & Warburg.

Hartman, G. (1966). Introduction: Poetry and justification. In G. Hartman (Ed.), *Hopkins: A collection of critical essays* (pp. 1–15). Englewood Cliffs, NJ: Prentice-Hall.

Hopkins, G. M. (1930). In R. Bridges & C. Williams (Eds.), *Poems of Gerard Manley Hopkins* (2nd ed.). London: Oxford University Press.

Hopkins, G. M. (1955a). In C. C. Abbott (Ed.), *The correspondence of Gerard Manley Hopkins and Richard Watson Dixon*. London: Oxford University Press, Geoffrey Cumberlenge.

Hopkins, G. M. (1955b). In C. C. Abbott (Ed.), *The letters of Gerard Manley Hopkins to Robert Bridges*. London: Oxford University Press, Geoffrey Cumberlege.

Hopkins, G. M. (1956). In C. C. Abbott (Ed.), *Further letters of Gerard Manley Hopkins, including his correspondence with Coventry Patmore*. London: Oxford University Press.

Hopkins, G. M. (1959a). In H. House & G. Storey (Eds.), *The journals and papers of Gerard Manley Hopkins*. Oxford: Oxford University Press.

Hopkins, G. M. (1959b). In C. Devlin (Ed.), *The sermons and devotional writings of Gerard Manley Hopkins*. London: Oxford University Press.

Krutch, J. W. (1931). *The modern temper: A study and confession*. New York: Harcourt, Brace.

Lewis, P. (2007). *The Cambridge introduction to modernism*. Cambridge: Cambridge University Press.

MacKenzie, N. H. (1981). *A reader's guide to Gerard Manley Hopkins*. Ithaca, NY: Cornell University Press.

MacKenzie, N. H. (1990). Commentary. In G. M. Hopkins (Ed.), *The poetical works of Gerard Manley Hopkins* (pp. 213–513). Oxford: Clarendon Press.

Mariani, P. (1970). *A commentary on the complete poems of Gerard Manley Hopkins*. Ithaca and London: Cornell University Press.

Mariani, P. (2008). *Gerard Manley Hopkins: A life*. New York: Viking.

Martin, R. B. (1991). *Gerard Manley Hopkins: A very private life*. London: Harper Collins: Flamingo.

O'Flynn, G. (1987–1988). Hopkins's teaching. *The Hopkins Quarterly*, 14.1–4:163–178.

Olney, J. (1993). *The language(s) of poetry: Walt Whitman, Emily Dickinson, Gerard Manley Hopkins*. Athens: University of Georgia Press.

Peirce, C. S. (1932). *Collected papers of Charles Sanders Peirce* (Vol. 2). Cambridge, MA: Harvard University Press and the Belknap Press.

Rose, A. M. (1977). Hopkins "Carrion Comfort": The artful disorder of prayer. *Victorian Poetry, 15*, 207–217.

Sobolev, D. (2011). *The split world of Gerard Manley Hopkins: An essay in semiotic phenomenology*. Washington, DC, Baltimore: The Catholic University of America Press.

Sobolev, D. (2013). Allegoria uMashmaut beYetsirat Kafka. In Z. Shamir, Y. Ataria, & H. Nagid (Eds.), *Kafka: Perspektivot hadashot* (pp. 24–67). Tel-Aviv: Safra (in Hebrew).

White, N. (1986). Hopkins' Sonnet "No worst, there is none" and the storm scenes in *King Lear. Victorian Poetry, 24*(1), 83–87.

White, N. (1992). *Hopkins: A literary biography*. Oxford: Clarendon.

White, N. (2002). *Hopkins in Ireland*. Dublin: University College Dublin Press.

6 Before Recognition: On the Aesthetics of Aftermath

Lisa Saltzman

6.1 Introduction

In strictly psychoanalytic terms, trauma describes a wound to the mind, an event so overwhelming that its understanding is necessarily deferred and perhaps only belatedly apprehended through its inadvertent repetition. Radically inassimilable, trauma tests the limits of representation. For much as the temporal economy of trauma is understood to be one of deferral, so too is the temporality of its representation. In other words, if there are certain events that we may only begin to assimilate long after their occurrence, then it is only in that process of belated encounter and understanding that we might begin to represent them, to shape them into aesthetic form (Caruth, 1996).

What do we do then, with a catastrophic event in which structures of deferral have been foreclosed, in which the divide between occurrence and representation collapses into the immediacy of live television coverage and urgent calls for commemoration? Furthermore, what do we do when repetition and representation are the defining characteristics of that catastrophic event, both in its occurrence and its transmission? Even before the relentless repetitions of televised instant replay began on September 11, 2001, repetition structured the event's very unfolding. It was only with the second plane's collision with the South Tower that the meaning of the first plane's collision with the North Tower became intelligible. With the second strike came the knowledge that what had happened to the first tower was not a freak accident but a deliberate act of terrorism. In repetition, meaning emerged. And a television audience participated in that movement from incomprehension to understanding and then witnessed it over and over again, a catastrophic event as visual spectacle, the visual field as a site of mediated yet immediate encounter.

In light of these events, a number of questions emerge: If the events of September 11th were indeed a traumatic event, how do we contemplate the question of their representation? Is their representation to be found in the media images, moving and still, through which the vast majority of spectators, even in New York, "witnessed" the events? Or is it to be found elsewhere, later, when artists and writers begin to reimagine and reconfigure those events into something that we might call art, or aesthetic representation? What constitutes that arena of representation? How and where do we begin to

L. Saltzman, Ph.D. (✉)
Professor and Chair of History of Art and the Andrew W. Mellon Foundation Chair in the Humanities, Bryn Mawr College, Bryn Mawr, PA 19010, USA
e-mail: lsaltzma@brynmawr.edu

Y. Ataria et al. (eds.), *Interdisciplinary Handbook of Trauma and Culture*,
DOI 10.1007/978-3-319-29404-9_6

think about aesthetics in the aftermath of September 11th? How do we understand the relation between trauma and representation? Did the unrelenting stream of media images overwhelm the psychic structures of deferral, forging and forcing a set of encounters in the time and place which might otherwise be held as the psychic space of refusal and refuge, but which here was already the site of representation? Or, might we instead conclude that for all the media images, video footage, memorial activity, and architectural planning, September 11th has yet to be encountered in any strict psychological sense, and in turn, has yet to be figured? In other words, did the visual economy of the events of September 11th trump the psychic economy of trauma, offering immediacy in place of belatedness, images in place of their impotence and impossibility? Or, might we conclude that for all its re-presentation, the events of September 11th have yet to be represented?

As a means of engaging these and other questions, the essay that follows will assemble and address a body of visual work that emerged in the aftermath of the events of September 11th. Turning first to Michael Arad's memorial proposal, *Reflecting Absence*, a piece that is at once a work of art and architecture, the essay will then survey and analyze a series of works that may be generally understood to have confronted these events in cultural form: Jonathan Borofksy's sculptural installation *Walking to the Sky*, Paul Chan's video installation *1st Light*, Pia Lindman's "portraits of grief," as well as her video projects *Viewing Platform* and *Waterline*, Art Spiegelman's graphic novel, *In the Shadow of No Towers* and Jonathan Safran Foer's photographically-illustrated work of literary fiction, *Extremely Loud and Incredibly Close*. Through a close reading of each project, indebted at once to the art historical project of exegesis and interpretation and the literature on trauma, the essay pursues the possibility that each work is not so much a post-traumatic representation of September 11th, but rather a cultural site in which the very impossibility of such representation is both theorized and figured.

6.2 Art, Architecture and Aftermath

What did we see in terms of visual representation? In addition to the stream of media images, iconic and particular, that captured the event or sequence of events of September 11th, and which taken together, form the visual archive of the event, work soon emerged that sought not to re-present that archive of images, but to engage the event from a position of aftermath and retrospection. Hans-Peter Feldman's *9/12 Front Page*, 2001, for example, undertook the fundamentally archival project of collecting the front pages of newspapers from cities around the world on the day after and arranging them for installation in a grid.[1]

Introducing a measure of belatedness to the insistent temporality of immediacy that characterized the representational economy of the event and its witnessing, much ensuing work typically took the form of the memorial. For example, if photographs of the missing posted around New York first served as signs of hope that the depicted might well be found, they all too quickly gave way to their funerary and memorial function, de facto shrines to those victims whose bodies were lost amidst the rubble. And such photographs, whether posted along the wall of St. Vincent's Hospital in Greenwich Village or, sometime later, printed, along with short biographies, as "Portraits of Grief" in the *New York Times*, came to function as a means of commemorating the victims of September 11th.

But if the assertion of human presence, through that memento that is the photograph, was an initial means of encountering, and countering, the individual losses of September 11th, it was not the only visual strategy in evidence. The successful proposals for the World Trade Center memorial competition, a competition announced as rubble and remains were still being cleared

[1] The piece was exhibited for the first time in Okwui Enwenzor's exhibition Archive Fever: Uses of the Document in Contemporary Art at the International Center for Photography in New York in the spring of 2008.

from the site, largely avoided such claims to presence, forgoing the power and poignancy of figurative images for visual instantiations of their impossibility and inadequacy, putting forth in its place absence as aesthetic form. In the winning proposal, for example, Michael Arad demarcated the bases of Yamasaki's Twin Towers with two massive reflecting pools. Their walled edges etch onto the landscape the reconstituted architectural footprints of each lost object, the twin towers, already uncanny doubles even at the moment of their creation and construction. Negative space concretized as memorial form, Arad's proposal attempts to address loss, to express loss, through its monumentalizing of and insistence upon absence.

Arad's memorial proposal countered and inverted the almost redemptive forms of *Tribute of Light*, which on March 11, 2002, repeating the form of Yamasaki's Twin Towers in two intense, ascending beams, temporarily restored the skyline of Lower Manhattan by making visible again, even if only as spectral trace, the irredeemably absent architecture. In contradistinction, Arad's memorial is recessed in the earth, two depressed voids that continue the vector of downward motion that was the collapse of the Twin Towers, the desperate plunge that was the descent of the "falling man." A gravitational movement whose trajectory and force is echoed in the waterfalls that cascade down the surfaces of the recessed bounding walls, the perpetual cycle of water also repeats something of the logic of the video loop that first imaged, but in its repetition then supplanted or simply became our memory of the event, representation replacing anything like an experience of the real.

In formal terms, it may be said that Arad's memorial proposal reprised or echoed certain crucial aspects of Daniel Libeskind's initial architectural plan for the World Trade Center. Though now much modified, Libeskind's plan captured the imaginations of its judges and a broader public in part for the symbolism of its soaring architectural form, the 1776 foot Freedom Tower, a building conceived to condense and restore to the skyline of Lower Manhattan something of the monumental presence of the Twin Towers, while also echoing and emblematizing all that is signified by the torch held aloft by the Statue of Liberty. Its appeal lay as well in its insistence on maintaining and foregrounding the exposed subterranean structure of the World Trade Center, the retaining wall that had held back the waters of the Hudson. Its surface marked and scarred by the traces of the site and its destruction, an architectural remainder and reminder, at once survivor and witness, Libeskind's exposed slurry wall managed also to repeat, or at least recall in its minimalist form and recessional relation to its site, something of the visual language and symbolism of Maya Lin's Vietnam Veterans memorial, that monumental form whose departure from traditional figurative practices has come to define a mode of memorial architecture in the present (Abramson, 1996).

Unlike Libeskind's proposed inclusion of a literal survivor, the slurry wall, Arad's design provides not so much a trace of the lost object, or in this case, objects, namely the Twin Towers and all they represented, but rather, the illusion of their tracing. Unlike Libeskind's slurry wall, in Arad's design there is no relation, beyond the symbolic, to the lost towers. Even as Arad's walls of water take and map as their site the former footprints of the Twin Towers, demarcating as massive voids the areas from which the towers rose, the walls are not, of course, actual architectural footprints. They are, instead, something like an architectural site plan grafted belatedly onto the landscape of death and destruction. Collapsed and cleared away, the towers left no footprints, no markers, and no imprint. In the memorial landscape that is now the new World Trade Center, save the slurry wall, there is little trace of what once was. Unlike an actual footprint, an imprint or outline that bears the trace of what stood above it, of the massive buildings that once pressed their weight upon the surface of the earth, of the looming towers that once rose above the streets of Lower Manhattan, Arad's memorial footprints, his walls of water, his monumental silhouettes, are not an actual trace of what once rose above that now hallowed ground. Their imprint is only imagined, a means of belatedly marking, memorializing that which remains irredeemably lost.

Individual and collective, private and public, such explicitly memorial work established something of the aesthetic terms for visual representation in the aftermath of September 11th. Whether offering up a photograph of a missing victim or demarcating the architectural footprint of an absent skyscraper, such work insisted on asserting the material trace of that which once was, staking a claim to presence even as it acknowledged an irredeemable absence. This work did not repeat the images of destruction. This work did not show death or suffering. Instead, this work marked out spaces, photographic and topographic, that might hold the place of what was lost, that might open onto a time for memory. Of course, the temporary shrines have long-since disappeared and Arad's project, as well as the vestige of Libeskind's, has now been realized. But perhaps it is in that interval between those two moments, past and present, then and now, an interval that we might understand to be that psychic space of deferral, the very province of trauma, that we might glimpse something of what aesthetics look like in the aftermath of September 11th. And it is thus that I turn more fully to the arena of contemporary art.

6.3 Art and Aftermath

One such glimpse of aesthetic possibility could be found in Jonathan Borofsky's sculptural installation *Walking to the Sky*. Organized by the Public Art Fund and temporarily installed at Rockefeller Center in September and October of 2004, the sculpture was certainly among the most monumental of artistic projects to emerge in the aftermath of September 11th, comprised as it was of a 100-foot-tall stainless steel pole, rising from the earth at a precipitous angle. Despite its daunting slope, the pole serves as a pathway for a group of figures, ranging from young children to briefcase-toting professionals, seven of whom stride up the steep incline while three more watch from its base. Of course, Borofsky had already exhibited two precursors to this piece in the 1990s—*Man Walking to the Sky* at Documenta IX in Kassel, Germany in 1992 and *Woman Walking to the Sky* in Strasbourg, France in 1994, so it is not as if the kernel of the work was explicitly conceived for, or even necessarily alludes to the events of September 11th. Nevertheless, in its monumental re-conception and aggregation of the ascending figures for its installation at Rockefeller Center, the image of ascension was mobilized as if to counter and reverse, if not also redeem, both the loss of the towers and all those who plunged to their deaths. And it is precisely the embodiment of aspiration in the individual figures—the eager step of a girl setting off for school, the purposeful strides of a businessman and woman heading to another day of work—that gives the piece its poignancy. With each iteration of that vigorous step, these gravity-defying figures reach forward with a confidence that can only be seen as naïve, and in turn, tragic in the aftermath of the events the sculpture does not and yet, by virtue of its location, temporally and spatially, unavoidably commemorates.

If Borofsky's sculptural figures seem to strive for an unattainable place beyond their present, that no-place that we call utopia, they also reach, as sculptural figures, for a kind of universalism, each an assiduously generic version of a set of types. Emptied of the specificity of actual portraits, Borofsky's sculptural figures come to function as something closer to abstractions, each offering up the idea of individuals in place of actual individuals. As such, even if the seeds of the piece long predate the events of September 11th, Borofsky's return to the generic climbers provides him, and us, with a sculptural language with which to gesture toward, even if not directly represent the victims. Perhaps, in offering us an aesthetic environment, an aesthetic experience, that so plainly reverses the logic and images of the events of September 11th, we are made to produce for ourselves, to recall, the images that issued forth from the event. Against Borofsky's utopian vision of brightly-clad professionals ascending toward their promising futures, against Borofsky's mythic vision of eager children climbing a sculptural beanstalk, we may think of an all-too-real vision, the monochromatic palette of survivors covered head-to-toe in ash, the horrifying spectacle of bodies falling from such an unfathomable height, the idea, if not the image, of those victims incinerated or asphyxiated in the World Trade Center. This is to say, standing before Borofsky's piece, we may call to mind, remember, something of that day, those events, indeed, those victims. But we just as well may not. We may see the piece differently for its installation in New York after September 11th. But for all the ways in which Borofsky's conception comes to mean in the aftermath of September 11th, nothing of its aesthetic project can be understood as an explicit response to that day or those events.

Something quite different is at work in a piece conceived fully in the aftermath of September 11th, Paul Chan's cycle *The 7 Lights*. Deriving its structure from the biblical story of creation and taking its aesthetic cues and philosophical inspiration from, among other sources, Pliny and Plato, Chan's cycle is comprised of six silent digital video projections and a set of drawings on blank musical scores. In its orchestration of light and shadow, stillness and movement, the cycle is by no means simply a response to the events of September 11th. Indeed, Chan's piece shares much with the work of a number of contemporary artists—Kara Walker and William Kentridge foremost among them—who, since the early 1990s, have mobilized the structure and idea of a shadow as a means of figuring obliquely moments of historical trauma that test the limits of representation. Yet, at the same time, Chan's piece *is* a response to September 11th, as its iconographic elements and narrative programs, for all their obscurity, make insistently clear.

1st Light, a piece that since 2005, has been exhibited more widely on its own than it has within the context of the entire cycle—in addition to its inclusion in the complete cycle at the New Museum's exhibition of Chan's work in the spring of 2008, *1st Light* has been installed, among other locations, at the Whitney Biennial in the spring of 2006, at the Fabric Workshop in Philadelphia in the fall of 2006, and at the Hirshhorn Museum and Sculpture Garden in Washington, DC in the summer of 2008, as part of the exhibition *The Cinema Effect: Illusion, Reality, and the Moving Image*—and elicits inevitable associations with the visual experience, the visual archive, of September 11th. Suffused at the outset with warm reds and yellows, the colors of dawn, the piece gradually gives way to daylight and the emergence of silhouettes, the visual illusion, through visual occlusion, of form. If at first we see, as if through a window, the establishing shot of a wire, a telephone pole, and then a flock of birds, a number of objects soon emerge, among them eyeglasses, a cell phone, folding chairs. Following the birds in flight, these objects rise slowly from the base of the projected light-field to the top; often breaking apart as they do so. They are then joined by larger objects, though not to scale, among them, bicycles and police cars. The ascent of these objects is then interrupted by a rapidly falling body, only to be followed by more bodies, falling singly or in pairs or groups, a meteor shower of human forms. Finally, color seeps back into the scene, washes of dark blue and violet. Night falls. The apocalyptic vision gives way to darkness. And then we begin again.

Projected onto the floor, the piece does not insist upon a grounding edge. Even as we come to understand its orientation, given the structuring illusion of the silhouetted telephone pole, we can just as easily walk to the top of the visual field and watch the scene in reverse, objects falling gracefully to the ground, bodies ascending. The same counter-factual logic that propels Borofsky's figures skyward operates here as well. But here the evocation is less of an alternate reality, even if it does allow us the possibility of reorienting the world and rewriting its script, than a prior reality, the fugitive images conjuring up in their visual effects something of an earlier moment of image-making and viewing. Chan's video projections, for all their digital production, invoke not only that philosophical space of Plato's cave, but also that visual space that was the theater of the magic lantern. His choreography of light and shadow, his orchestration of silhouetted objects in motion, returns us to these earlier moments of visual spectacle, of phenakisticscopes and stroboscopes, of zoetropes and praxinoscopes, when to see the image of the world was to witness something fleeting and wondrous. These pre-cinematic technologies gave their viewers images as if they had been magically reconstituted by light and shadow alone. And Chan's cycle restores something of that visual magic to the contemporary arena of the gallery.

To see Chan's work, then, is to experience something of an art historical anachronism (Didi-Huberman, 2000). It is to be both in and out of time, at once illuminated by the glow of the digital present, yet somehow also bathed in the darkness of the pre-cinematic theater of illusion, whose origins may be found in the chamber that was the camera obscura. In witnessing Chan's work, we are situated in a temporal arena of dislocation, of return and repetition, the logic of the video loop by which the work is structured instantiating the temporal economy of historical return staged within. In other words, in experiencing Chan's work, we are situated in the temporal dimension of repetition and return, seeing images that repeat something of the visual archive of a recent past, September 11th, through a visual technology that digitally simulates the visual spectacles of an earlier epoch. In this doubled position of repetition and return, we experience something of the temporal economy of belatedness. Moreover, if Chan's work produces a kind of temporal suspension, in and out of time, it also induces a further dislocation, this time a spatial one. For to see Chan's work, is also to stand before a visual schema that embraces the notion of inversion. As in the camera obscura, in the darkened gallery, Chan's image is always, in some sense, upside down. And we cannot right it. Just as we know, with even the most rudimentary or intuitive grasp of the laws of physics, that these sorts of objects should not rise from the ground, we also know, with a certainty that is borne of ethics, that bodies should not fall from the sky.

6.4 Grief and Witness

If, in their different ways, Borofsky's *Walking to the Sky* and Chan's *The 7 Lights* stand as examples, even if by no means exemplars, of artistic responses to the traumatic events of September 11th, neither should they be called upon to bear the burden of that psychological challenge or that aesthetic and ethical responsibility. For even as each may be seen to allude to the events of September 11th, neither makes explicit claims to treating those events or that subject. As installed in the sculpture garden of the Nasher Sculpture Center in Dallas, Texas, where it was subsequently acquired, Borofsky's *Walking to the Sky* has far less specificity in its allusive possibilities than it did when installed in New York. If anything, we see it in relation to his other work, his sculptures of figures walking to the sky as another means of figuring the impossibility of counting to infinity. And Chan's *1st Light*, for all the potency of its iconography of falling bodies and of objects and detritus blown toward the sky, is but one element in a cycle of works that engage questions of creation and destruction in the context of epic, rather than historical time, and do so in a shifting set of institutional contexts. If there is a historical specificity in Chan's work, it is more often expressed quite directly, as it has been in his animated Iraq pieces or in his site-specific staging of Beckett's *Waiting for Godot* in the Ninth Ward, in New Orleans, a city that is still waiting for all the help that it deserves in the aftermath of the destruction wrought by Hurricane Katrina.

Certainly, there are works of contemporary art that more explicitly take on the events and impact of September 11th as their point of departure. The work of Pia Lindman, for example, engaged the responses that emerged in the aftermath of September 11th, making gestures of grief or the very act of witness its subject. Her ongoing *New York Times Project*, begun in 2002, collected images of mourners from the *New York Times* for one year. From these media images of mourners, were they New Yorkers in the aftermath of the attack on the World Trade Center or those grieving in the aftermath of terrorist attacks elsewhere around the world, Lindman made drawings, what could be called her own "portraits of grief." Re-enacting these poses in a set of performances from 2003 to 2005, Lindman also re-enacted them in front of a video camera, for the piece *Lakonikon*, also printing the poses as stills and tracing them in charcoal on vellum. The vellum drawings, now at multiple removes from the photographs of mourners they took as their subject, were collected in the book *Black Square*. These pieces, which move in and between the media of performance, video, and drawing continue something of Lindman's abiding interest in the body as a kind of affective archive, a repository of gestures that contain within them the registers of emotion, even as her work seems to dislocate emotion from embodiment. In such contemporaneous work as *Fascia*, which employed a mechanical device to shape and stretch her face into expressions, or *Domo and its Double*, a piece in which she filmed herself mimicking the gestures of a robot and in a process similar to *Lakonikon*, traced the stills as drawings, Lindman emerges as a kind of anti-Greuze, physiognomy giving way to technology, the face no longer a semiotic template of feeling, but instead a manipulable and programmable machine. But it is her video projects, *Viewing Platform*, and *Waterline*, both from 2002, that inaugurate a specific concern with sites of historical trauma and its challenge to representational dynamics.

Both pieces take the World Trade Center as their subject, but fully from a position of aftermath and belated witness. *Viewing Platform* depicts the viewing stand erected before the cavernous pit of ruins at the site of the World Trade Center. Created from sixty minutes of footage shot from a fixed perspective, cut into one-minute transparent segments and layered into a video loop, the resulting piece is an evanescent palimpsest of spectral figures, ghostly witnesses looking onto a scene of aftermath. Its companion piece, *Waterline*, puts that camera in motion, suspended on a fishing pole and bobbing through the waters of the Hudson. Against the fixed stare of the mounted camera, which records the actions of the belated witnesses, here the camera is the witness, its literally fluid movements capturing everything from the waves in the Hudson and the traffic on the West Side Highway to the skyline of Lower Manhattan, now missing its most defining architecture. Fixed or felicitous, the camera in Lindman's work depicts the site of the World Trade Center, but already at a remove, both spatial and temporal. If one piece captures the belated act of witnessing, only to erase that very act from the record, transforming spectator into apparitional blur, the other renders vision itself unstable, dislocated from the structuring armature of a tripod or a body and given over to tides and currents.

Perhaps what is most crucial about Lindman's World Trade Center pieces in relation to the questions posed here is that at the same time that they approach their subject, they move away from it. They do so not only in structural terms, building in to their realization a degree of temporal and topographic remove. They do so in historical terms, shifting their gaze from the landscape and geography of Lower Manhattan toward a topography of destruction that predates the events of September 11th. For after making these pieces, Lindman traveled east, first to Berlin and then to Warsaw, where she reprised some of the visual strategies of these site-specific pieces as she took on the legacy of fascism and the Second World War. And it is that extension, that historical opening onto earlier moments of catastrophe that makes her work so significant, not only in the site-specific contexts of its creation, but in the context of aesthetics in the aftermath of atrocity. To represent the events and aftermath of September 11th is less to enter into a new aesthetic era than to return to an aesthetic arena that precedes that moment in 2001, whether we understand art after Auschwitz to follow from a moment of aesthetic rupture or not. It is to understand that aesthetics have already been shaped by catastrophes that may be said to both demand and defy representation. Artists work as much in the aftermath of that aesthetic legacy, as they do in the aftermath of the particular events they may choose to engage (Saltzman, 1999).

6.5 Images in Spite of All: The Graphic Novel

All that said, rather than continue to discuss works of contemporary art, I want to turn in conclusion to two books, Art Spiegelman's, 2004 *In the Shadow of No Towers* and Jonathan Safran Foer's, 2006 *Extremely Loud and Incredibly*

Close, both of which help to further a discussion of questions of aesthetics, and aesthetic representation, in the aftermath of the traumatic events of September 11th. What distinguishes these two literary works from all those that emerged in the aftermath of September 11, as, for example, Don DeLillo's 2007 *Falling Man* and Joseph O'Neill's 2008 *Netherland*, is that while each takes the form of the book, and involves textual narratives, each is also, to varying degrees, composed of and concerned with images. Perhaps most significant about these works, at least in terms of the discussion underway here, is that even as each strives to represent something of the events and legacy of September 11th, whether in word or image, each also engages the aesthetic challenge, if not impossibility, of taking on such a subject. In the end, each work is as much the offering up of a set of ethical questions in textual form as it is the putting forth of a set of aesthetic responses, be they visual or literary.

Art Spiegelman's *In the Shadow of No Towers*, which narrates, among other things, the experience of eyewitness to the events of September 11th in Lower Manhattan, may be said to have taken shape in their immediate aftermath, even if the book did not appear until 2004. Its cover, an Ad Reinhardt-inspired black-on-black image of the towers, repeats, as its ground, the image Spiegelman created for the cover of the post-September 11th issue of *The New Yorker*, published just 6 days after the attack. The book's contents emerged in the weeks and months that followed. With an open invitation from Michael Naumann, the editor and publisher of *Die Zeit*, Spiegelman was given the opportunity to create a set of ten large-scale broadsheet pages, a template for his signature "comix," a form and a forum in which to work through his experience of the events and their aftermath. The book gathers and reproduces as sequential narrative the color broadsheets. It also reproduces a set of historic cartoons, selected by Spiegelman and reflecting his own research into his medium during the days and months that followed September 11th, that present something of a history of newspaper comics and illustrate the degree to which newspaper comics could to be seen to have engaged historic events. The book is introduced by a preface by Spiegelman that explains the book's conception and realization.

As the title, and title image, of Spiegelman's book make clear, the shadow, that quintessential index of bodily presence and proximity, of physical continuity and contiguity, is here a means of expressing an irredeemable absence and irrevocable break. Already an utterly immaterial form, the semblance of a sign that is nothing more than a disturbance in the visual field, an occlusion of light, the shadow, for Spiegelman, is a shadow in the absence of a body, which is to say, a shadow that is only ideational, that is, in other words, fully spectral. For, of course, there is no shadow without the towers. And there are, of course, after the events of the morning of September 11, 2001, no towers. That said, even as Spiegelman's shadow fully gives way to its essential non-essence, even as it is de-materialized into the void that it always already was, it also emerges a symbolic form, a metaphoric means of conjuring the experience of living and working in Lower Manhattan in the aftermath of witnessing the collapse of the Twin Towers, of seeing that spectacle both as an eyewitness and as a viewer of media images. For even if there is no longer an actual shadow, even if the towers leave no material, visible trace, for Spiegelman, the events of September 11th cast an enormous shadow. His book is a means of addressing, if not re-dressing, that shadow, that is at once a void and an ideational presence, that shadow that is the space of aftermath.

Thus, even as he structures his project around that void and asserts it as an irredeemable absence, he also fills that space left by the event and its aftermath with a story, a story that is at once memoir, meditation, and political critique. He fills that space with images, among them the repeated evocation of an image that was neither photographed nor filmed on that morning but that, as Spiegelman writes in the preface to his work, "remains burned onto the inside of my eyelids several years later… the image of the looming north tower's glowing bones just before it vaporized" (Spiegelman, 2004, n.p). Against the archive of images that we have all seen,

Spiegelman introduces, as an image that he cannot quite capture but that he comes to depict, grainy and pixilated, over and over again, an image that conveys, in its very etiolation and evanescence, the asymptotic task of representing the traumatic. It is and is not what Spiegelman saw, what Spiegelman remembers. And even if he were able to reproduce the image that is seared into his visual memory, it would never fully represent his experience of witness, let alone the experience of witness of those who did not survive (Agamben, 1999).

What emerges in the broadsheets is a depiction of Spiegelman's growing awareness that, with the events of September 11th, he had entered into the historical time of trauma. As he remarks in the preface, *In the Shadow of No Towers* was written from "that fault-line where World History and Personal History collide" (Spiegelman, 2004, n.p.). If, with the events of September 11, Spiegelman steps into that grey zone of witnessing in which we both see and fail to see the catastrophe unfolding before us, standing on a fault-line that opens onto an abyss, Spiegelman also straddles that generational fault-line that both connects him to and divides him from his parents' generation, victims and survivors of the Holocaust whose story forms the kernel of his earlier project, the graphic novel *Maus*. It would seem, one fault-line opens into or onto another. As Spiegelman writes in the third installment of broadsheets, the author appearing in an inset of small black-and-white frames that reprise his visual style and his persona as mouse, in *Maus*: "I remember my father trying to describe what the smoke in Auschwitz smelled like.... The closest he got was telling me it was "indescribable"... That's exactly what the air in Lower Manhattan smelled like after Sept. 11" (Spiegelman, 2004, p. 3). Here, his experience of trying to describe something about New York in the aftermath of September 11 brings Artie closer to his father trying to describe the smoke in Auschwitz. And yet, it by no means equips him with the representational tools to describe that which cannot be put into language, even as it sets the two in relation. The equivalency he establishes turns on a description of an experience that remains "indescribable." And what does it mean to compare the indescribable?

Kaleidoscopic in its fracturing of both stylistic and narrative content—Spiegelman mobilizes a history of cartoon styles and characters that are both his own and those of his predecessors in the genre, the broadsheets move in and out of historical time, into what, as I have already suggested in the case of Paul Chan's work, may well be the space of traumatic time. In Spiegelman's *In the Shadow of No Towers*, we have stepped into the chasm that is the fault-line that cleaves traumatic experience from that of the everyday. In the juxtapositions that define the visual structure of *In the Shadow of No Towers*, it would seem that traumatic time defies historical time. Even as Spiegelman narrates and depicts something of the situation in the present, it is interrupted and inflected by the past. Quotations of visual styles and characters, both his own and those of other cartoonists, animate the broadsheets. If September 11th names the event that structures and motivates the story that is told, in word and image, it also names the event, the traumatic experience, that undoes the telling of the story, that unmoors the characters from their historical location, that opens the fault-line into and out of which a set of representations both emerge and return.

6.6 Images in Spite of All II: The (Illustrated) Novel

Such unmooring is central to Jonathan Safran Foer's *Extremely Loud and Incredibly Close*, a novel, conceived in word and image, that is perhaps the fullest aesthetic response to the traumatic events of September 11th yet to emerge, partly for its attention to the very problems trauma poses to memory, and, in turn, to works of memorial and acts of representation. Punctuated, if not in any strict sense illustrated, by images throughout, Safran Foer's novel closes with 29 pages of images, grainy black-and-white photographs, a sequence of images that reverse the very real trajectory of the falling man, even if this counter-factual reversal is also a means of acknowledging, once and for all, the horrible truth of that day; namely, destruction, death, and national vulnerability. Narrated by the precocious, imaginative, grief-stricken 9-year-old New Yorker, Oskar Schell, whose father was killed in the World Trade Center, and interspersed, at regular intervals, by the voices of two others—Oskar's absent grandfather, writing letters to Oskar's father that he never receives, and Oskar's doting grandmother, writing words to Oskar that he never sees, the novel is also interspersed with images, images that form the entirety of another book, whose existence and relevance will only belatedly be revealed, namely, Oskar's own creation, a scrapbook of images entitled *Stuff That Happened to Me*.

If the novel's central protagonist, Oskar Schell, is something of a repetition and reimagining of another literary Oskar, namely, Oscar Matzerath, the traumatized child at the center of Günther Grass's post-Holocaust novel, *The Tin Drum* (1959), with the distinction that the tambourine, not the tin drum, is the instrument of Safran Foer's self-proclaimed "percussionist," the novel's form bears more relation to Grass's émigré compatriot, W.G. Sebald, whose hybrid use of fact and fiction, word and image in such works as *The Emigrants*, 1992, and *Austerlitz*, 2001, allowed him to engage with particular acuity the historical legacy of the Holocaust. Oskar's story is propelled by his efforts to come to terms with the traumatic event of his father's death on September 11th, a project largely displaced into his quest to solve what he understands to be a mystery, the ownership and function of a key, stashed in a vase in Oskar's father's closet. But that paternal death, and the larger context of its occurrence, is not the only trauma structuring the novel. It is a novel limned by trauma. Two generations ago, the man and woman who would become Oskar's paternal grandparents survived the bombings of Dresden. Their postwar reunion in New York both creates and in some ways destroys the family into which Oskar is born, a family that was already destroyed, even before it had begun. For the man once loved the woman's beloved only sister, killed in the war while carrying their unborn child. Oskar's grandparents are thus linked, and ultimately separated, by their shared, yet utterly individual losses. That Oskar loses his father in the collapse of the World Trade Tower, is, then, already something of a repetition, yet another chapter in a familial history structured by devastating losses, losses that began in the fire-bombings of Dresden but that were compounded by the emotional consequences of living, or, in some sense, not living, in the aftermath of trauma.

The novel is particularly attentive to the spaces of memory that trauma both demands and defies. At the very outset of the novel, a novel that moves back and forth in time, both within the present and the past, just as we are getting to know something of Oskar's emotional and imaginative life, he proposes the following:

> So what about skyscrapers for dead people that were built down? They could be underneath the skyscrapers for living people that are built up. You could bury people 100 floors down, and a whole dead world could be underneath the living one. Sometimes I think it would be weird if there were a skyscraper that moved up and down while its elevator stayed in place. So if you wanted to go to the 95th floor, you'd just press the 95 button and the 95th floor would come to you. Also, that could be extremely useful, because if you're on the 95th floor, and a plane hits below you, the building could take you to the ground, and everyone could be safe, even if you left your birdseed shirt at home that day. (Foer, 2006, p. 3)

As Oskar, who has only just witnessed the burial of his father's empty coffin, imagines both a proper place of burial and a proper, if preposterous, plan for urban security: he moves back and forth between the unreal fact of his father's death and the bizarre logic of his symbolic burial, all the while imagining a world, a set of architectural spaces, and safety garments, in which such deaths would be impossible. An attempt less to assimilate than to counter the utterly inassimilable fact of his father's death and absent body, Oskar echoes the fiction of closure in which he is forced to participate at his father's funeral by proposing a set of fictions of his own, retractable towers and birdseed shirts, imaginative inventions to foreclose the loss he cannot yet bear to make his own.

The struggle to live in the aftermath of loss permeates the novel, even when we encounter its secondary characters. One is Mr. Black, who will serve as a surrogate grandfather for Oskar, until he unwittingly encounters his own, the mysterious "renter," who, in the aftermath of September 11th, takes up residence in his grandmother's guestroom, and transforms his bed into a sculptural monument to his deceased wife. As he explains to Oskar, he has hammered a nail into the bed frame every morning since she died. There are now 8629 nails; Mr. Black has been a widower for nearly 25 years. The bed is a magnetic force-field of grief, a monument to a marriage that ended all too soon.

With an eye to the kinds of material traces that would seem to bear witness to a life, but, in the end, do not—the repeated signature of Oskar's father, testing pens, in an art supply store on 93rd Street, is revealed, 225 pages later, to be the signature of his supposedly absent grandfather—Safran Foer produces a novel that is filled with images and evocations of the impossible spaces, the absent places, where memory of loss can and cannot take place, where lives can and cannot be lived, where traumatic events can and cannot be represented. That Oskar's grandparents, whose lives in exile are structured by the silences and absences of presumed muteness and blindness, construct a mode of living in which their apartment is increasingly filled with "nothing places," spaces in which they can cease to exist for each other, even before one will literally leave the other while she is pregnant with the son he will then never see, is but one narrative space of impossibility. There is also the achingly sad fact of the empty novel of the grandmother's life, written with a typewriter with no ribbon, 2000 blank pages testifying not to the historical narrative of the life lived, but to the emotional economy of the present, in which blindness is put forth as one more "nothing place" of safety, even if it is a self-destructive fiction. While Oskar's mute grandfather is consumed with guilt that he has given his blind wife a typewriter with no ribbon, and in turn pretends to read words that do not exist, his wife, by no means as blind as she pretends to be, goes into the guest room in which she types and pretends to write, hitting the space bar again and again and again, refusing to transform her life into narrative form, offering only blankness. As she writes, to Oskar, in a letter that he never sees, but that expresses both her knowledge of the fiction and futility of her autobiographical project and the ways in which irredeemable losses have ruptured her biography with the fissures that describe a psychic topography of trauma, "My life story was spaces" (Foer, 2006, p. 176).

In a novel of "nothing places" and empty spaces, there is also, given the grandfather's postwar muteness, a conversational arena structured as much by silence as by speech. The grandfather's muteness compromises the ability of the couple to communicate from the very moment they meet. Gestures, signs, and the written word replace the reciprocity of speech. That the grandmother's sight is failing certainly complicates the visual dimension of their communication. When communication depends on the visual, sight is required. And when, years after their separation, Oskar's grandfather returns to New York to grieve with his wife for their lost son and telephones from the airport, a futile conversation ensues, the grandfather treating the keypad of the payphone as if it were a mechanism for text messages and the grandmother hearing only electronic beeps. Standing in the airport, despite his wife's obvious inability to understand his call, Oskar's grandfather persists in typing his words, for hours, producing a cryptic two and a half page text of all that has happened since he last saw his wife, from the motivation for his departure to the reason for his return, a string of numbers, a stream of noise.

A phone call that is received but fails to communicate, that cannot be heard because it has never been spoken, the grandfather's call repeats something of the set of phone calls that structure the novel, the calls that Oskar's father places to the apartment in the minutes before his death that are never answered. The first five attempts at communication, at contact, are recorded on their answering machine, at 8:52, 9:12, 9:31, 9:46, and 10:04 am. Oskar plays back these calls upon entering his apartment, sent home from school once the city begins to understand what has happened. The final call comes in once Oskar has listened to the others, at 10:22 am. Oskar sees that it is his father's caller ID. But he does not pick up. He only listens. And then, in an act that he imagines will protect his mother, who, unbeknownst to Oskar, has spoken to her husband on her cell phone, Oskar runs out to Radio Shack to buy an identical phone, onto which he copies their recorded greeting and then stashes the old phone, with the record of his father's final calls, in his closet. It is at Radio Shack that Oskar sees, on a television, that one of the towers had fallen. Over the course of the novel, Oskar will listen to these recordings, save the final call. But it is only in the presence of his grandfather, that sympathetic stranger, that he will play all of the messages, even the last one, a broken set of words attempting to make contact with his son as his fate becomes clear.

Oskar's unwitting encounter with his grandfather, and all that ensues, is recounted in a final letter the grandfather writes to his deceased son that completes the collection of letters, from grandfather to father, that have been stored, unsent, in a suitcase that the grandfather brings back from Dresden, his second emigration from that city, and that will be buried, by Oskar and the grandfather, in a final escapade, in the empty paternal/filial coffin. Printed in an increasingly dense type, line atop line, word atop word, the grandfather's final unread letter is literally unreadable. Unlike the cryptogram of telephone keypad numbers that we might well attempt to decode, the grandfather's final epistle concludes in three pages of such dense typography that it is indecipherable. Like a painting by Glenn Ligon, the words devolve from clarity to obscurity, words interred upon the very surface of their inscription, instantiating and anticipating their final burial, their literal encryption.

That the novel ends, to return to the set of images with which I began my discussion of Safran Foer, with an illusion of ascension, is by no means the utopian gesture it could well be in other hands. It was the work of Oskar, whose collection of images punctuates the novel, an attempt to tell (himself) a different story, to hold at bay the grim reality of his father's death. Oskar's picture book, much like Oskar's journey through the city, in search of the owner of the mysterious key, is an attempt to create a space in which to contain, if not contend with, the traumatic event of his father's death, perhaps even in a desperate jump from the towers. Much like the spaces and non-spaces, the unconventional memorial gestures that structure the novel, Oskar's book, Oskar's imagistic story, is a place in which the work of memory might take place, even if it is held at bay. Taken together, the multiple narratives, epistolary, autobiographical, and more conventionally novelistic, produce something of a memorial landscape, a narrative environment that offers up an aesthetic topography of remembrance, but also, importantly, of forgetting.

Were a novel to stand as a work of memorial, or, more to the point, as set of propositions, or a proposal, for what representation might look like in the aftermath of the traumatic events of September 11th, indeed, simply in the aftermath of trauma, Safran Foer's *Extremely Loud and Incredibly Close* is certainly a good candidate. All too aware, as its title suggests, of its proximity to the event whose consequences it takes as its subject, Safran Foer nevertheless pursues the limits and limitations of aesthetic forms. And in so doing, Safran Foer's hybrid novel emerges as a site of aesthetic possibility. Set against the architectural and memorial plans for the World Trade Center, juxtaposed with the visual work that took September 11th as their subject, if only at times obliquely, Safran Foer's novel is a work not just of literary and historical imagination, but of visual imagination. Catalyzed by events that, in the simultaneity of their media capture and transmission, collapsed the very distinction between trauma and its representation, Safran Foer's novel provides a narrative context, an emotional framework, a space, indeed, of deferral, in which to begin to make sense of those events in narrative and visual form, even as they continue to defy and test the limits of our understanding. As such, Safran Foer's work stands as emblematic of the relation between trauma and representation, his richly imagined and vividly illustrated novel, functioning as a vexed but vital site of encounter. Indeed, his work, like each of the work's discussed here, is ultimately yet one more asymptotic approach to a set of traumatic experiences that remain stubbornly, necessarily, just beyond the reach of representation, even as they continue to demand voice and form. So it is that we tarry with trauma in cultural terms.

References

Abramson, D. (1996). Maya Lin and the 1960s: Monuments, time-lines and minimalism. *Critical Inquiry, 22*(4), 679–709.

Agamben, G. (1999). *Remnants of Auschwitz: The witness and the archive. Trans. Daniel Heller-Roazen* (pp. 15–39). New York: Zone Books.

Caruth, C. (1996). *Unclaimed experience: Trauma, narrative and history*. Baltimore: Johns Hopkins University Press.

Didi-Huberman, G. (2000). *Devant le temps: Histoire de l'art et anachronisme des images*. Paris: Minuit.

Safran Foer, J. (2006). *Extremely loud and incredibly close*. Boston: Houghton Mifflin.

Saltzman, L. (1999). *Anselm Kiefer and art after Auschwitz*. New York: Cambridge University Press.

Spiegelman, A. (2004). *In the shadow of no towers*. New York: Pantheon.

From Hiroshima to Fukushima: Comics and Animation as Subversive Agents of Memory in Japan

7

Ory Bartal

7.1 Introduction

In the Second World War, the atrocities of humanity reached new heights with the Jewish Holocaust in Europe and the nuclear holocaust in Japan. These traumas, which took place under the auspices of the nations that were considered the most civilized in human history (Germany and America), and that were led by a totalitarian regime and a liberal democratic regime, respectively, have driven mankind to grow weary of grand ideologies, whichever they may be. The modernist faith in progress and evolution, rooted in notions of enlightenment and optimism that view the world as progressing toward a better future and man as a rational creature that strives for freedom and enlightened form of government, suffered a harsh blow in light of these devastating events. This process, which would later be given the moniker "the end of ideology," spawned a new perception which no longer put much stock in the state and the establishment, and instead centered on the individual's internal struggle. This new reality, which allows for pluralism, was one of the constitutive psychological motives of postmodern thought, which broke down traditional and dichotomous modernist divisions between margins and center and between high and low culture. One of the signs of the postmodern era is the rise in prominence of the products of popular culture and mass media, including comic books and animation films, that took the postmodern blurring of borders to the extreme by depicting traumatic historical events from the modern era, namely the Jewish Holocaust and the nuclear holocaust, in a format perceived as popular, low, and mainly comical. Despite the rise in eminence of popular culture and the cancellation of the high-low dichotomy, this crossing of lines created a stir and public debate surrounding the legitimacy of a format of this kind to portray these fraught events (Weinbaum, 1991).

While European and American comic books depicting the Jewish Holocaust, like Art Spiegelman's *Maus*, for example, caused a public uproar (Blich, 2013), publications of this kind are still marginal compared to the official publications of the education system, books, museums, documentary movies, and documentation of private memories of survivors. In contrast with this type of memory, Japan offers an interesting case study for the way graphic novels and animation serve as a key agent that shapes the collective memory of the nuclear holocaust. The Japanese case evokes several questions, namely: why did the Japanese choose to present the atrocities of war in this medium? How did it allow the

O. Bartal, Ph.D. (✉)
Department of History and Theory, Bezalel Academy of Arts and Design, Jerusalem Mount Scopus, P.O. Box 24046, Jerusalem 91240, Israel
e-mail: ory_bartal@yahoo.com

Y. Ataria et al. (eds.), *Interdisciplinary Handbook of Trauma and Culture*,
DOI 10.1007/978-3-319-29404-9_7

presentation of a new historiography and the processing and construction of new memory? What is the subversive role graphic novels and animation play in Japan in relation to the official channels that deal with the representation of the nuclear holocaust?

In the attempt to answer these questions, this article will argue that the products of popular culture, such as comic books and animation, serve as a powerful tool for processing a traumatic historical event. The article will open with a theoretical discussion of the difference between methodological historical research and personal memories portrayed in popular culture, and the way that in the postmodern era, personal memories complement, and at times replace, the state-official historical narrative. The discussion will then move to the way that the comic book format, which is essentially different from a history book, facilitates a different type of processing of traumatic memories. As a case study of these ideas, this article will present the treatment of Japanese manga and anime of the memory of the nuclear holocaust, the way that they allowed the survivors of the atomic bomb to be heard, and how the Japanese reader/viewer processed a national memory underplayed in the history books. This process was made possible due to the general traits of this medium, the place it holds in Japanese culture, and the historical context of the conflictual memory.

7.2 History and Memory

History and memory are the bricks that bind together a group of people and build their culture. Every culture has institutions entrusted with the role of recounting its history—the education system, pedagogic programs, national museums, television programs, and documentary films. These official agents construct the collective subconscious and formulate a common experience the nucleus of which is events that took place within the history of that group. However, these official narratives do not always coincide with private memories of individuals who experienced the events first-hand. Traditionally, history and memory were considered contradictory terms, since memory is personal and has no place in the research of traditional history, which presents historical facts as self-evident (Lipsitz, 1990).

In her book *Hiroshima Traces* Lisa Yoneyama discusses the scholarly attitude toward the question of "memory," perceived as incongruent with "history," claiming that "memory is often associated with myth or fiction and is opposed to history as it is written by historians" (Napier, 2005). The subject of myth versus history is particularly poignant in the discussion of the Jewish Holocaust and the nuclear holocaust in Japan, which are singular historical events that represent nothing other than themselves. Auschwitz and Hiroshima have become metametaphors and prototypes of human suffering of a surreal and mythical nature, which sometimes cover over private memories and stories, as they were experienced by the people who lived through them.

In the past, historians who dealt with subjective-collective interpretation were inclined to be skeptical toward personal memories as research materials, due to their subjective, retrospective, changing, and consequently unreliable nature (Watchel, 1990). However, in the wake of the poststructuralist and deconstructivist movements that perceived collective consciousness as oppressive, there has been a shift in the attitude toward history and memory. Some philosophers rejected the conservative perception of history and offered a new paradigm of history devoid of a chronological sequence of events. Derrida, for instance, offers a perception of temporality as "repetition with a change" (Lipsitz, 1990). Events, according to him, do not simply take place, but rather reoccur as they attach and reattach in ways that illuminate, and do not repress, the many differences encompassed in the event (Lipsitz, 1990). Foucault, on the other hand, sees historical narrative as tainted by the discourse of power. In his view, the traditional historical story does not wish to present meaning but rather bolster the establishment that writes it, through the notion that there is a common human history, an idea that expands the establishment's hold over its people to the level of human existence (Lipsitz, 1990). While these perspectives tend to reject linear history,

George Lipsitz (1990) maintains that there is justification for history, since it unfolds many possibilities for understanding the present. In his book *Time Passages: Collective Memory and American Popular Culture*, Lipsitz introduces the revolutionary idea that "history became one of the disciplines of memory" (1990, p. 6). And indeed, in the postmodern age when central narratives have lost their validity and traditional dichotomies are blurred, personal memories began to permeate the historical narrative. Kerwin Klein explains that the new approach allowed historians to process personal recollections, perceived as individual mental events, into collective memories that form the collective consciousness. Thus, personal and collective memories have turned into a reservoir of research subjects, and memory was given the status of a historical agent (Kerwin, 2000). The discourse of memory was a "natural fit" with postmodernism, and its allusive, fragmentary, and changing nature no longer poses a threat to the credibility of the research, but rather adds more depth and substance to it and to a large degree makes it more accessible (Selzer, 2009).

How are these theories being adapted in the research of the holocaust? In her discussion of the nuclear holocaust, Yoneyama maintains that the dichotomy of myth/history is problematic since the production of knowledge about the past always entails the assertion of power and is accompanied by elements of oppression and repression. She suggests that her readers will do well to keep in mind that they are embarking on research into the past with the knowledge that "historical truth" is only available through the mediation of a given category and of representation and a process of labeling (Napier, 2005). For instance, the term "received history," coined by James Young (2000), refers to the historical story constructed by the second generation of the Holocaust as a memory mediated through family memories, photographs, movies, books, and historical testaments 50 years after the events. Marian Hirsch (1997) ventures further on the subject of mediated memory, with the expression "postmemory," which describes memory differentiated from regular memory, since it is formed not by remembering a historical event, but by formulating a new memory from the imagination and experiences of traumatic narratives that preceded the birth of those who remember and shaped their life story. Postmemory is not a black hole or a lacuna in memory. On the contrary, it is an obsessive memory, relentless and structured like memory itself and therefore it also constructs a historical memory (Hirsch, 1997). And so, memory and history have turned into concepts that act together in the construction of the historical story while maintaining equilibrium.

7.3 Memory and Popular Culture

This article addresses popular culture and its products as a new agent of memory. Popular culture products, which gained prominence in the postmodern era, are agents founded on materials that are not dictated by the official institutions, but are built from the ground up without a guiding hand and recount the stories and memories of private individuals. The new technology that has engendered a plethora of media channels—the Internet that provides access to infinite knowledge and social media platforms like Facebook—is a powerful agent in the processes of dissolution and formation of a new collective memory and often prescribes a new construction of memory (Stiegler, 2010).

In the age of new media channels such as these, a new semiotic order has been created, canceling the difference between presented and representing, while between reality and its representation emerged the simulacrum in which the image, according to Baudrillard, is found in the realm that lies beyond the difference between real and the imaginary; this is not always a reflection of reality/history, but rather becomes the only reality that exists in the mind of the viewer (Baudrillard, 1995). This new reality also generates new "memories" that over time produce a new outlook on history.

At the same time, the popular culture industries manufacture different products—such as memorabilia or meaningful objects—that hold memories that compensate for the absence of a "real" memory. The dialogue between object and memory formulates a living connection with the past as it gives presence to the memory, which is vital to the foundation and shaping of a sense of identity of individuals and groups. Memory objects such as these often construct—for an individual, a group, or a nation—"memories" that are not always associated with reality (Weitz & Strauss, 2009). In Japan, we may think of the graphic novel and animation as the products of popular culture that in the 1980s became a subversive agent of memory facilitating the processing of traumatic events such as the nuclear holocaust. However, before I approach the subject of why such cultural products became the carriers of the memory of Japan's nuclear holocaust and the type of memory they present, I will turn to the unique traits of the medium of animation and comics.

7.4 Comics as a Memory Agent

The first comic books appeared in Japan in the nineteenth century, when Katsushika Hokusai coined the name *Manga*, literally "whimsical drawings," and produced notebooks packed with such paintings.[1] The enthusiastic reception they received is reminiscent of the reception of the illustrated scrolls of the Heian period in Japan (AD 794–1185) or the woodprints in medieval Europe; they provided a world of gestures and dramatic displays that are inevitably absent from the written word or painting.[2] Like prints, modern comics provide very little information, forcing the viewer to complete the scarce hints provided by the few lines of text with his own interpretation. For our discussion here, it is also significant that there is a difference in the memory of what had been transmitted by pictures and what had been transmitted verbally. Friedlander maintains that recounting the history of the Holocaust creates a distance from historical facts due to the use of a rational language, which protects us from the inconceivable past (Lentin, 2002). Just as rationality distances us from the memory of the past, documentary photographs can create a similar distance. Hirsch claims (after Kristeva) that photographs of the Holocaust are shorthand for the representation of the terrible atrocity: when we see an emaciated figure behind a barbwire fence we "see" the Holocaust. However, she also claims that the multiplication of such pictures and photographs, while powerful, is also paralyzing, debilitating, and diminishes our capacity to process the apocalyptic events of the twentieth century (Hirsch, 1997). She explains (after Barthes) that the photographs of the Holocaust are like "relics," or "fragmentary sources" that do not recall the past and do not allow a processing of grief, but rather block the past and become counter-memory. The photographs are often an affirmation of death and facilitate repression and oblivion as a result of the viewer's preexisting knowledge that the people in the photograph died a horrible death.

In contrast with the photographs or historical story, the medium of animation offers an integration of image and text that facilitates the processing of memory. The continuity of comics, as opposed to photographs, creates a sequence of images that portray not just death or agony, but life as a whole. In addition, comics have the structure of a collage, they are fast-paced, contain some specific information, many "comic reliefs," and are accompanied by gibberish such as "Byou" (to signify wind) and onomatopoeia such as "woof-woof." Even if the comics address every possible subject matter, these are imbued with the naiveté of initial formulation, which has not yet learned of complexity (Reinhart, 2000, p. 123). McLuhan referred to comics as cold low-resolution media means that forces the reader to be highly involved as a creator of meaning and as a participant who imagines what has not been said. He calls this form of creation of meaning

[1] Katsushika Hokusai painted 15 comic books entitled *Hokusai Manga*, which featured ironic paintings of people, landscape, and supernatural elements. They were published in 1814. On the reception of woodprints in medieval Europe, see: McLuhan (2003).

[2] In this context it is worth mentioning early works executed in this form like the Scrolls of Frolicking Animals (*Chōjū-jinbutsu-giga*) in twelfth century Japan, or the Bayeux Tapestry of the eleventh century, commemorating the triumph of William the Conqueror in the Battle of Hastings. It is interesting to note that the tapestry portrays not just the triumph but also the terrors of war and suffering.

"Do It Yourself" and that it allows the viewer to be an active participant in the construction of the historical story (McLuhan, 1964, p. 190). Therefore, McLuhan claimed that the "medium is the message," which is to say, the comics medium presents the historical story in a very different way to other media. Due to the association of image and text, the nature of the image, and affiliation with the world of games and entertainment, one could see comics, the graphic novel, *manga*, and animation as media that invite the viewer/reader to a new form of observation and *a different viewing category* compared with watching a documentary, a film, or indeed, observing reality. The comics, graphic novel, manga, and animation are iconic signs, meaning (after Baudrillard) signs that hold a relation of similarity with reality, but are not reality itself and therefore supposedly present fiction. In contrast, documentary photography is an indexical sign—a sign that stems from a causal relation with the object in reality and therefore supposedly presents the "photographic truth." The viewers of a documentary films and photography have a sensory filter that allows them to look at things from a distance and without experiencing pain—like the employment of a particular cognitive dissonance that allows them to continue functioning despite the sights. The iconic nature of the media of comics and animation allows the presentation of traumatic past events that are difficult to watch in the medium of documentary photography. Comics and animation, which traditionally portrayed fairytales, fictional narratives, and superheroes, are perceived by the reader/viewer as fiction, and therefore allow for the depiction of an event that resembles the catastrophic event, but is not the actual event. Thus, the medium creates a distance that does not engender resistance and renders the traumatic memory accessible (Raz, 2008). Even when the medium presents realistic images, the eye and consciousness can deal with them without triggering the cognitive dissonance mechanism, thanks to the iconic nature of comics. This medium, which according to Marshall McLuhan offers a cool and ridiculous repeat of the different forms of warm media means, provides an opportunity for cultural therapy in which the reader/viewer is given an opportunity to visit a repressed place, which is difficult to access via other media, in a safe mode (McLuhan, 1964). Consequently, the use of popular culture materials, including the comic format, which developed as a subversive genre, has become a new agent of memory that constructs a "low memory," which undermines the official high memory and assists in shattering myths and metanarratives constructed in the institutional culture.[3] The remainder of the article will focus on the Japanese as a case study.

7.5 The Memory of the Nuclear Holocaust

An exhibition featuring contemporary Japanese culture was held in New York in 2005. The exhibition's title, "Little Boy," was on the one hand a play on the Western image of the Japanese as comics-reading little children, and on the other hand also referred to the nickname of the atomic bomb that was dropped on Hiroshima.[4] The exhibition, which was given the subtitle, "The Arts of Japan's Exploding Sub-Culture," displayed popular cultural products, from toys to computer games, that in some related way to the atomic bomb. The exhibition linked together popular culture with the atomic bomb and presented, among other things, the processing of the memory of the nuclear holocaust as it is expressed in popular culture, *manga*, and *anime*. The exhibition's curator, the artist

[3]Comics, which developed as a subversive genre, have been often perceived as a threat to the institutional contents. In the 1950s, the American "comics code" was formed, determining the sanctioned contents in comics, since it was perceived as a format containing violent contents endangering youth's morals. In Japan, in the 1990s, after the murder of young girls by a comic's reader, the police raided comics shops, outlawed hundreds of titles, summoned makers for questioning, and started monitoring the contents of comics.

[4]The two atomic bombs (one using uranium and the other plutonium) that were dropped on Hiroshima and Nagasaki were nicknamed after their shape. The plutonium bomb had a stubby rounded shape and was thus named Fat Man. The uranium bomb was long and slim in comparison and gained the moniker Little Boy. Giving nicknames to atomic bombs was probably a way to cope with the aggressive bombardment on the side of the aggressors.

Takashi Murakami, wanted to showcase the fact that the memory of the war, the defeat, and the nuclear holocaust are nowadays commemorated in Japan through popular culture: more so in computer games, toys, or apocalyptic animation films than through the official channels of history books, memorial services, or museums.[5]

Indeed, it would seem that the processing of the memory of the bombing of Hiroshima and Nagasaki has been conducted in Japan via popular media, namely comics or science fiction (sci-fi) movies. Most of these do not address the historical story but rather divert the issue and tackle the horrors of a nuclear holocaust through science fiction. Specifically, from the 1950s onward, the commemoration of the nuclear holocaust in Japan has been redirected to fiction through King Kong-type horror movies. In 1954, 9 years after the atomic bomb was dropped on Hiroshima, the Americans conducted a hydrogen bomb experiment in the Bikini Islands in the Pacific Ocean. The experiment impacted the Japanese fishing boat "Lucky Dragon #5" (*Daigo Fukuryū Maru*), which had some survivors of the Hiroshima nuclear holocaust on board. This event enflamed the raw nerves of Japanese sensitivity to the use of nuclear weapons. That same year, in the wake of that incident, the first film in what would be the most successful series in Japanese cinematic history was released—*Godzilla* (*gojira*). The movie opens with the disappearance of the boat *eiko-maru* near Odo Island. A specialist by the name of Yamane arrives at the island to investigate the event and finds giant footsteps contaminated by radioactivity (Strontium-90). Yamane discovers a giant dinosaur in the sea that has been awakened from its slumber and mutated as a result of a nuclear experiment. He returns to Tokyo and presents his findings before the Japanese parliament. One of the parliament members declares that it would be imprudent to publicize that Godzilla is the outcome of the atomic bomb, seeing as information of this kind might carry adverse repercussions in the international arena, due to the delicate relationship with the US—a statement that generates protest and heated discussion in the assembly. However, the truth is made public when Godzilla attacks Tokyo and with bursts of atomic fire it issues from its mouth causing numerous casualties, injuries, and widespread devastation. The government wishes to have Godzilla killed, but Yamane claims that it would be unwise since it survived the atomic bomb and should be studied in order to learn how to survive the next bomb. In the meantime, it turns out that a Japanese scientist by the name of Dr. Daisuke Serizawa has a new weapon (Oxygen Destroyer), which is even more powerful than the atomic bomb. However, he refuses to use it, saying that if it would be used even once, politicians all over the world would try to use it as a new weapon. Finally, he uses the weapon to kill Godzilla, but then destroys all his research, as he realizes that the weapon is as deadly as the monster and that demolishing the weapon is for the good of mankind.

The movie portrays a prehistoric creature awakened from its slumber and mutated due to a hydrogen bomb experiment in the Pacific Ocean. The prehistoric monster arrives in Japan, where it demolishes entire cities. The American nuclear experiment, which took place in the Pacific Ocean, similarly brought about mass devastation in Japan—this time in the indirect way of a monster and cinematic fiction. The film, in the guise of popular culture, implicitly speaks of the terrors of the bomb—an issue which was still under-processed in 1954. The movie indirectly addresses the enemy and the American conqueror through the genre of a monster movie (*kaiju eiga*), since the government did not wish to trigger anti-American sentiments while the Americans were helping restore Japan from its wreckage. The movie raises issues that were legitimate in terms of public agenda, yet were supposed to be left unspoken—could the Americans

[5]Murakami Takashi, the most influential contemporary pop-artist, sees himself as an artist, entrepreneur, curator, and art theoretician. He views art as something that encompasses creativity, production, theory, distribution, and marketing. Murakami studied the visual languages of popular culture and consumer culture and used it to create works of art that present consumer culture and its products as a reflection of thought patterns and cultural structures. His works present *kawaii* culture, the processing of nuclear holocaust memories, and subconscious fantasies that often appear in popular Japanese culture.

be blamed for the nuclear holocaust? Is it right to create a weapon more powerful than the atomic bomb? The popularity of the film stems from the fact that the Japanese saw it as a mirror and a reflection of the trauma of a society that collapsed in the past and can collapse again in the present, as well as of their anti-American sentiments which at the time remained unspoken (Sawaragi, 2005).

In 1973, the movie *Japan Sinks* (*nihon chinbotsu*) directed by Shiro Moritani was released. Based on a bestselling novel of that year by the author Sankyo Komatsu, the movie dealt with the subject of total destruction. Both the book and the movie recount the Japanese archipelagoes' sink into the abyss in the aftermath of an earthquake, volcanic eruptions, and giant tsunamis, as the surviving Japanese refugees are forced to flee to all corners of the earth (Sawaragi, 2005). The successful book was adapted into a 15 volume *manga* series, and a 2006 film by Shinki Higuchi in which the ending was changed. This film opens with an earthquake and the volcanic eruption of Mount Fuji, after which the geologist Tadokoro discovers that the Japanese archipelago is about to sink due to a geological fracture that destroys the bottommost stratum of the land. In the film, natural catastrophes demolish extensive areas of Japan, and some 80 million people perish. A state of emergency is declared and Tokodoro has a plan to rescue Japan: nuclear warheads are to be positioned around Japan, in order to detach it from the geological stratum that pulls it down. Tokodoro accomplishes his plan and a major explosion that looks like a succession of atomic mushrooms saves Japan. The 1970s book and movie shocked Japanese readers and viewers and while it was published during the Japanese economic boom which promised a bright future, the book became the most popular bestseller in Japanese history up to that point (4 million copies sold), and was adapted into a film and a television series (1975). The book's popularity probably stemmed from the fact that the Japanese saw it as a reflection of the big bang that took place in the past and could take place in the present, with the shift from a nuclear holocaust to a natural disaster, which Japan had known on a smaller scale (Sawaragi, 2005). However, the film introduces a new perspective—the atomic warheads are what saves Japan. The film gives an expression to the thoughts that lurk beneath the surface in Japan and remain unspoken: the atomic bomb and the ensuing holocaust have stopped the war and thus saved what was left of Japan after the war and prevented its total collapse. The bomb also allowed the Americans to conquer and build Japan after the war. In 2007, the Japanese Minster of Defense Kyūma Fumio was forced to resign after he said that the American use of atomic bomb against the terrors performed by his country at the time was necessary. His words, perceived outside Japan as extreme rightwing sentiments, constitute an acceptable, albeit unexpressed, way of thinking in Japan. The Minster of Defense, who is supposed to adhere to the official line, had to pay the cost of tarnishing the national conviction. But the movie, as a subversive agent of popular culture, facilitated the processing of the bomb in a new way—as a weapon that stopped the collapse of Japan into total oblivion.

1974 Saw the release of one of the first and most significant animation series: *Space Battleship Yamato* (*uchū senkan yamato*) by the creator Leiji Matsumoto and director Yoshinobu Nishizaki.[6] The story begins in the year 2199, when the Earth is devastated by nuclear bombs and most of the population move underground. It is estimated that within a year radioactive contamination will reach the survivors' subterranean dwelling. Just when it looks like mankind is on the brink of extinction, two Earth space pilots, Susumo Kodai and Daisuke Shima, discover a message from the planet Iscandar, which has possession of the technology that can rehabilitate

[6]The series was a cult phenomenon in Japan, comparable to "Star Trek" and "Star Wars" in the West, and its success led to the production of a film entitled *Arrivederci Yamato*, in which the Yamato crew is facing a new enemy called "Comet Empire." The film was a hit and led to a second series of the television show. Later two other movies were made: *Yamato: The New Voyage* and *Be Forever Yamato*. Following the success of these movies, a third season of the series was produced, in which the Earth is at the center of a battle between Deslar (leader of the Gamilon aliens) and the Bolar Federation. The events of the series were concluded in the film *End of Yamato*. The original series aired on Israeli Television in the early 1980s with the title *Space Pioneers*.

planet Earth. A special team led by captain Okita goes out to space on the state-of-the-art spaceship Yamato, an illustrated upgrade of the real Japanese battleship that was sunk in World War II. The team has a very limited time frame in which to find Iscandar and return to Earth, yet during their journey, time after time they are forced to fight the aliens of Gamilon, who are trying to prevent them from reaching their destination.

Animation artist Leiji Matsumoto, the son of a fighter pilot in the Japanese Royal Air Force during World War II, imbued the series with a strong militant nationalistic tone. The opening scene takes place during World War II, when American fighter jets sink the Yamato. This scene is accompanied by a soundtrack identified with the Gamilon aliens, thus the American enemy becomes an alien of no cultural affiliation, so that they can be portrayed without directly generating anti-American sentiments and the series was even distributed in the US. The fact that the Earth is obliterated by nuclear bombings is of course an analogy to the atomic bombs dropped on Japan during the Second World War; however, it is displaced from the US–Japan war to the war between the aliens and Earth. Susan Napier explains how the series *Space Battleship Yamato* goes beyond memory and oblivion and helps process history anew. Through the medium of animation and the genre (futuristic sci-fi), the series revisits the experience of war and allows the viewer a new processing of the trauma of defeat by presenting countless repetitions of attack and devastation from World War II. The processing of the trauma culminates in the eventual success of Yamato's mission to save human civilization. The animation offers the viewers the opportunity to indirectly access the moment the battleship Yamato was destroyed and then successfully escape what seemed like total devastation. The ship that plummets to peril and is immediately rescued can also be understood as a plunge into the collective subconscious of postwar Japanese civilians. Thus, in the vein of the films discussed above, this *anime* series constitute a form of cultural therapy in which the viewers are confronted over and over again with loss and defeat, but which offer a soothing and comforting end.[7] However, this series—unlike *Godzilla* or *Japan Sinks*—touches on historical materials that are directly linked with the war, and are therefore presented in the medium of animation in order to sidestep the direct gaze of the viewer (Napier, 2005). The fantasy animation that portray historical events transform real events to symbols that are easier to deal with. In this case, the ship becomes a symbol, not only of the final battle of the Second World War, but also of Japan. More than the atom bombs, which Marilyn Ivy sees as emblematic to the loss of Japan (Ivy, 1995)—the ship Yamato (the original as well as the animated ship) is metaphorical for Japanese identity, both because Yamato is Japan's original ancient name, and because the ship Yamato that was sunk in 1945 was the flagship of the Japanese Navy and became a symbol of destruction and loss. This symbol gains new meaning when it becomes a metaphor for resurrection and hope through the medium of animation. The ship is transformed from an emblem of prewar Japanese militarism to a global spaceship of peace and love. In the film, the Japanese people and warship Yamato gain a new signifier and new meaning—they are the saviors of the world.

This series and its sequels were the beginning of an entire genre of apocalyptic manga series and animation films that indirectly reference the memory of defeat and the war and nuclear holocaust through the portrayal of life on planet Earth after a third world war. The movie *Akira* (1988), for instance, opens with a scene of an atom bomb which is dropped on Tokyo in 1988 and starts a third world war. Neo-Tokyo, which is built on the ruins of Tokyo, is ruled by violent gangs and antigovernment terrorism. The movie begins with an accident that awakens super powers in the movie's hero Tetsuo, who decides to free Akira—a boy with strong telekinetic powers whose abilities and the explosion he caused led to

[7]For more on the term "Cultural Therapy" in the context of Japanese animation film see: Napier, Susan, "World War II Trauma, Memory and Fantasy in Japanese Animation," in *The Asia-Pacific Journal: Japan focus* (online article).

the eruption of the third world war. Akira is a small, plump boy (a visual paraphrase on the nickname of the atomic bomb) whose powers took over his personality, leaving a character that is unable to speak or express emotions. After the war, he is kept in cryonic storage under the Olympic stadium site, but Tetsuo awakens him and his powers bring about the devastation of Neo-Tokyo once again. The film presents the human destructive impulse and portrays an unfamiliar destructive force, stronger than any known to date. This is a reference to the atomic bomb whose full force and the devastation it harbored were still unknown, until it was dropped on Japan. The movie goes on to raise questions concerning the future and development of weapons of mass destruction by the scientific community.

Other films offer a subtler message, like *Nausicaä of the Valley of the Wind* (*kaze no tani no naushika*) (1984) that portrayed the legend of a princess who lives in a postapocalyptic kingdom that has its own bioengineered ecological system. The story takes place in the aftermath of a global war, in which industrialized civilization has self-destructed. Although mankind survives, the surface of the earth and the seas are still extremely polluted, reminiscent of the devastation and radioactive contamination in the wake of the atomic bomb. In the movie, most of the earth is covered by the Sea of Corruption, a bioengineered toxic forest of fungal life and plants that is gradually expanding, taking over what little open land is left. Mankind is trying to survive in the polluted lands beyond the forest, a survival that entails fierce battles over the scant resources that remain. On the backdrop of the wars for survival raging between people and between humanity and nature, the princess fights to bring about a peaceful coexistence among the people of her world, as well as between humanity and nature. Set in a postapocalyptic future, the movie addresses some big questions concerning the nature of civilization, violence, and the destructiveness of mankind, as well as desperation in the face of cycles of violence that have plagued the world again and again throughout history. Yet at the same time it offers hope for a peaceful coexistence. Without mentioning the Second World War, the film creates a "model reader," to use Eco's term, who is capable of actualizing the meaning and decoding the narrative (Bondanella, 1997). In this case, of a narrative of civilians who experienced total destruction and radioactive contamination.

This popular genre of movies based in a third world war, apocalypse, and total devastation enjoyed immense popularity. The question is: why did the fantasy of an apocalyptic world and stories of total destruction emerge in Japan at the height of its economic prosperity? And why were these movies so successful and why did they strike such a chord with the Japanese audience?

The success of the sci-fi genre in cinema and animation in Japan revealed that below the surface of its economic success, the collective Japanese consciousness is teeming with monsters (Godzillas), created by the atomic bomb and defeat in WWII. They inhabit the subconscious as a deep-rooted fear of total devastation. Since these existential anxieties did not have a proper place in official social consciousness, they found their way into popular culture. As I have already mentioned, the memory of the Jewish Holocaust has also been processed in comic books; however, in Israel the memory and trauma were managed primarily through the education system, museums, documentary films, and television programs on memorial days that recount and present testaments of survivors. Comics that discuss the Holocaust mainly address the second generation and its attempt to fathom the horrors of the Holocaust in a personal context (Blich, 2013). In Japan, on the other hand, the memory of the actual nuclear holocaust has been processed through the genre of animation, purportedly a medium devoid of depth, that engages in fantasy and belongs to the popular entertainment industry that is usually divorced from historical perspective and expression, which begs the question—why? The answer to this question lies in what the flatness of the medium allows, as I explained at the beginning of this article. However, in order to understand the success of this genre in Japan we should examine the historical context of Japan alongside the place of *manga* and *anime* in Japanese culture.

7.6 Japan and the Memory of the Atomic Bomb

Japan was the victim of a nuclear holocaust, but that memory could not have been presented outside the context of Japan's war crimes against the people of Asia as a tyrannical oppressor and an ally of the Nazi and Fascist regimes (memory that the Japanese strive to repress). In its relationship with the US, which helped rebuild Japan after the war and still holds close financial ties with it, the government refrained from bringing up the American responsibility for the nuclear holocaust, so as to not trigger anti-American sentiments in Japan. The processing of the memory that includes both shame and guilt is therefore conflictual, since the Japanese were both the aggressor and the victim, a fact that diminishes the psychological space for processing the memory. Consequently, until the 1990s, the memory of the war and the nuclear holocaust had undergone only partial and fragmentary processing. History teachers in Japan could choose from a variety of history books sanctioned by the Ministry of Education, including books that whitewash the war crimes and rearrange Japanese history, or justify Japan's aggression by presenting Japan's declaration of war as an act of liberating Asia from Western powers.[8] In the 1990s, in the wake of Japan's return to the international Asian arena, South Korea and China raised subjects such as Japan's accountability for the war and the inadequate apology to its victims. This accusation was not conducive to an international discussion of Japan's casualties in the war, and is one of the reasons that the memory of the bomb is not mentioned in Japan, even in the national memorial services, apart from the modest ceremony in the Hiroshima Peace Memorial Park, on the anniversary of the atomic bombing.

The younger generation in Japan, which was raised after the war under the umbrella of the American military protection, detached itself from the wars in which America was involved (Korea, Vietnam, and the Cold War), focusing on peace and the developing economy in Japan. At the same time, they watched as the world armed itself with nuclear weapons as part of the Cold War, pursued nuclear experiments that exceeded the bomb dropped on Hiroshima, and the unfolding of nuclear disasters like Chernobyl—all these touched the raw nerves of the Japanese people, particularly sensitive to nuclear power, since they are the only ones who understood what it really meant. Furthermore, since the Japanese constitution does not allow the maintenance of armed forces, there was nothing they could do to prevent it. They started to feel powerless, even worse—that their protection depended on the Americans, former enemies who continued conducting nuclear experiments (Sawaragi, 2005). All these complex fears and memories never made their way from the subconscious to the consciousness in a legitimate way and remained an unvoiced anxiety. Yet, the desire to revisit the traumatic experience of the war and understand it did not disappear. Yoshikuni Igarashi believes that since the economic success and cultural prosperity of today's Japan is entirely based on the infrastructure built in Japan during the 1950s and 1960s, after the defeat, the return to the defeat is a natural process of a society that feels a need to examine its origins in order to comprehend its present. Nevertheless, according to Igarashi, due to the conflictual memory, the desire to express the experience of war can only take place in the form of repeating the experience of defeat, caught up in the contradictory need to remember and at the same time forget (Napier, 2005).

Since Japan has been denied the use of weapons by its constitution, war was relocated to computer games based on animation and *manga*, and the management of the anxiety or the desire to experience the war have found their way to watching animated war movies. *Manga* and *anime*, which blossomed in Japan in the 1970s and 1980s, exceeding the popularity of cinema, allowed a space in which the fear could be channeled in an

[8]The processing of the memory of war in Japan, which was very limited, focused on Japan's victimhood, while its war crimes in Asia were covered up or described as attempts to free Asia from colonialism, see: Orr (2001). However, we should also mention that there were literary artworks, films, documentaries, and activists (like the China-Japan Friendship Association) that addressed the uneasy subject of Japan's blame and war crimes during the war.

indirect way. In these media, it is possible to approach the subject in a playful manner that oscillates between fiction and reality without an explicit connection to political and historical reality. Computer games and films that present a narrative of a third world war, nuclear holocaust, and apocalypse, were in fact a displacement of the repressed fears to a fictional world—which for the Japanese is not fictional at all. They encrypted the fear in a medium that belongs to the world of fantasy and thus permitted the discourse about this anxiety. These media engage with total devastation and apocalypse and present the ruin alongside the recovery of postwar Japanese society; allowing the younger audience born after the war to comprehend the backstory of the rise of modern Japan as well as disconnect it from traditional Japan.

In the 1980s, these fictional movies were joined by another genre of animation films portraying war and nuclear holocaust: docu-animation films of Second World War survivors who felt a need to tell their stories and the horrors they experienced.[9] Animation films of this kind portray the transformation in the attitude toward the atomic bomb and the shift in its symbolic meaning after the end of the Second World War. In the late 1960s, even during student riots, the radical left movements that protested the ailments of Japanese society stayed away from volatile issues such as the emperor's culpability for the war. Although the emperor was a symbol of the devastating war, there was never a wide public debate surrounding his responsibility during his lifetime. However, in the late 1980s, with the end of Emperor Hirohito's reign, there was a change in the attitude toward the war and the bomb in Japanese society. These docu-animation films serve as the trailblazers for this discourse. One such docu-animation is the 1988 film *Grave of the Fireflies* (*hotaru no haka*), based on the autobiography by Nosaka Akiyuki that relates the hardships of Japanese civilians during the Second World War in the city of Kobe. The autobiography relates an untold story related to the American bombardments before Hiroshima and Nagasaki, which were among the most devastating known prior to Hiroshima and Nagasaki. The story is told from the perspective of a brother and sister who are trying to survive after their parents are killed by the American bombings. Through the personal story, the viewer manages to connect to the difficult memories of civilians who lived through the war and do not speak about it, since Japan does not dare talk about the suffering of its civilians in light of the war crimes and suffering it inflicted on the people of Asia; and of course, when the victims are mentioned, they are naturally identified as the victims of the atomic bomb and the suffering of other civilians is forgotten.

Another docu-animation film is the autobiographical story of Keiji Nakazawa who experienced in person the bomb dropped on Hiroshima. *Barefoot Gen* (*hadashi no gen*) was first published in 1973 as a series in the comic book "Weekly Shonen Jump" (*Shukan Shonen Jampu*). The series was later (1975) bound into a book with a preface written by Art Spigelman, which was translated to many languages and adapted as an animation film (1983). The film portrays Gen's family and life in Hiroshima during the war, prior to the bombing. The day of the Hiroshima bombing is depicted in great detail, including the horrors that ensued in its wake. Gen runs home to discover that he had lost his entire family except for his mother who gave birth that day to a baby sister. He then describes the days following the bombing: the hospitals crowded with casualties, the search for food, and the troops who come to help and contract different diseases caused by radiation. In contrast with the shift of war films to sci-fi films depicting a third world war, *Barefoot Gen* deals explicitly with the bomb and presents the atrocities of the nuclear holocaust to the general public for the first time. To quote Nakawaza himself: "They wanted to know what the war and the atomic bombing was really like. It was the first time people had heard the truth. That's what they told me everywhere I went.... The government probably doesn't want to risk encouraging anti-American sentiment. But the facts are the facts" (The Comics Journal 2003).

[9]Although these films are in animation format, they constitute living testimonies of survivors, much like testimonies of Holocaust survivors in documentary films.

In this sentence, Nakawaza highlights the possibility for trauma survivors to testify and thereby undermine the oppressive official memory. He presents the power of a personal memory as a part of the historical story. In an interview with Asai Motofumi, head of the Hiroshima Peace Institute, Nakawaza condemns the inhumanity of the American enemy that used unconventional weapons on civilians, and particularly the use of war as an excuse for experimenting with different atomic bombs (uranium and plutonium) (Asai, 2007). He also does not spare the imperial system that allowed such a crime to take place in its country and did not prevent while it could have acceded to the Potsdam Declaration and the demand for the Japanese to surrender. He goes on to criticize the conduct of the Japanese government during the war and its combativeness that brought the bomb on Japan, as well as its responsibility for the repression of the trauma after the war when it did not agree to publicize photographs from Hiroshima in order to avoid generating anti-American sentiments in Japan. Nakazawa raises the question: why did the government not demand of the US to assume responsibility for the crime and apologize to the victims? Why was it so scared of generating anti-American sentiments and telling the story? He claims that the Atomic Bomb Casualty Commission nominated by the government has done nothing for the survivors" (The Comics Journal 2003).[10] He also criticizes Japanese society that discriminated against the survivors and did not help them rehabilitate or find employment, pushing survivors to lose hope and even commit suicide despite having survived the bombing. These severe allegations and the anger over the fact that the atomic bomb survivors were not given the chance to be heard and the Japanese people the chance to process the memory, are presented in a *manga* format. Nakazawa recalls that when the *manga* was published he received many letters from Japanese who asked "Is it real?" "Tell us more," "We never thought that the war and the atomic bombing were so terrible." Today *Barefoot Gen* is a mandatory book in elementary and middle school libraries, despite its antiwar and anti-imperial nature. It replaces the missing information in the elementary and middle school history books and gives the pupils an opportunity to engage with history via familiar media. Nakazawa was a pioneer in speaking openly about the atomic bomb and from his *manga* the young generation in Japanese learned about what took place in the war. And thus, the cloak of popular culture—*manga* and animation—permitted the subversive criticism to bypasses the unofficial censorship of a government that did not make public the photographs and history of the nuclear holocaust. As blockbusters, these movies became a part of the collective memory of the younger generation in Japan.[11]

7.7 The Nuclear Holocaust and the Jewish Holocaust

I will illustrate my contentions about the importance of the medium, its subversive nature, and its role in processing the memory, through the graphic novel *Message to Adolf* (*adolf ni tsugu*) by Osamu Tezuka. This graphic novel (published as a serial in 1983–1985) has a unique way of processing the memory and is perhaps the most significant in this genre. *Message to Adolf* is a novel that interweaves fiction and reality through the story of three Adolfs: Adolf Kaufman (a German-Japanese boy), Adolf Kamil (a Jewish boy) and Adolf Hitler. The plot follows the three Adolfs on the background of the Second World War in the Far East and in Europe, when Adolf Kaufman is sent to Germany and joins the Nazi army, and Adolf Kamil becomes a Zionist who arrives in Israel after the war. The graphic novel, which presents an antinationalistic and pacifist position, is unique in Japan, as it portrays historical materials (including a timeline of the war)

[10] Keiji Nakazawa claims that the commission has done nothing for the survivors except conduct research on behalf of the government, like comparing children who were not impacted by the bomb with children who were impacted by it.

[11] In the 2000s more films dealing with the subject were released, like *Town of Evening Calm* and *Country of Cherry Blossoms* by Konyo Fumiyo.

that are not featured in Japanese textbooks, like the war crimes the Japanese army committed against the people of Asia. In the *manga* format, Osamu not only presents historical materials but also targets the conduct of the Japanese government during the war and reveals the materials repressed in the memory of the Japanese people. The historical materials can be read easier due to the medium and due to the blurring between the fictional narrative and historical facts. This graphic novel provides Japanese readers, who are the second generation after the Second World War, with the opportunity to look at the terrible acts committed by the Japanese army through the story of an individual's memory. This complex issue of processing the historical memory of the aggressor also came up in the German education system in 2007, when history teachers presented to children aged 9–13 (third generation) the events of Nazi Germany and the Holocaust through two graphic novels. These novels, published in Amsterdam by the illustrators Eric Heuvel and Ruud van der Rol, were entitled *The Search* (*Die Suche*) and the sequel *The Revelation* (*Die Entdeckung*). These comics became an important part of a case study in Germany, after one of the most extensive studies conducted by the University of Oldenburg revealed that almost 20 % of school pupils in Germany know very little or nothing at all about the Holocaust (Lautenschläger, 2008).

However, the graphic novel *Message to Adolf* helped the processing of this complex memory in a surprising and indirect way through a literary device that allows the reader to process the memory in an unconscious manner. Osamu creates two leading protagonists named Adolf: the first is the German-Japanese boy (who represents the Japan–Germany axis during the war), and the second is the Jewish boy (who represents the victim and then the fighter). Both are represented as the two sides of Adolf Hitler, since Hitler is described in the story as an Aryan-Jew (in the story his mother conceived after she was raped by a Jewish employer). In the story, the divided Adolf becomes a symbol of Japan during the war—an extremely cruel country but also the victim of a nuclear holocaust. The reader identifies with both sides through the coming of age experiences of the two Adolfs—on the one hand the process of brainwashing that can turn a relatively normal person to absolute evil, and on the other hand the experience of victimhood. The reader can empathize with the incredibly complex memory of Japan as it was both an aggressor and a victim.

Today too, in an age of information freedom where there is no need to circumvent censorship, comics are still used as a channel for processing trauma in Japan. After the tsunami and nuclear reactor disaster in the Tokohu area in March 2011, several *manga* depicting the catastrophe were published. The reportage comic *The Day Japan and I Shook* written by Suzuki Miso, covers the aftermath of the earthquake and tsunami. Suzuki describes his decision to write the *manga* in the first chapter, explaining that: "Scenes of the tsunami swallowing up cars and houses crisscross my mind. With so many people having lost their homes, their families, their land, living in refugee camps and in fear of radiation, what kind of *manga* should one draw? Is it the time to even be drawing *manga*?" (Holmberg, 2011). He thus decided to write about his personal experiences through the story of his daughter who was stuck in Disneyland after the earthquake until the following morning, when the trains and buses resumed operation. Another *manga* that was published in a personal blog and became very popular was *Field of Cole* by Mihoko Ishizawa, which described personal stories of the victims of the tsunami. It was read online by many people who contacted Ishizawa to convey how helpful and comforting they found the *manga* (Ishizawa, 2012). Neither *manga* addresses issues of repressed memory processing or reveal information that was suppressed by the government, but were a channel that helped the public deal with the traumas. Unsurprisingly, a *manga* called *Phaethon* by Yamagishi Ryōko that gained a great deal of popularity was again an indirect story about the nuclear disaster that took place in Chernobyl from 1988, republished online after the Fukushima event (Thornber, 2013).

7.8 Conclusion

The graphic novels and animation films presented in this article manifest the Japanese need to return to a trauma that merges guilt and shame, acknowledge it, and give it a place in contemporary life. The portrayal of events through comics performs a twofold action. First, in the guise of popular culture as action and sci-fi films, the memories and stories are transformed into myth and fantasy, creating a new experience that sheds light on obscured memory layers considered illegitimate in the official culture, and allow the processing of repressed and unbearable memories. For instance, Japanese animation films address questions that were viewed as subversive and were silenced by the government, such as: Why did the nuclear holocaust take place? Who is responsible for it? And why was there discrimination against survivors? Secondly, the paradoxical union of the format of comics and horror story allows the reader to associate the historical story (which the first generation had experienced) with the story of the second generation's contemporary life and create a new memory, this time not a historical memory, but rather private history and memory that merge the two narratives into one coherent story. Films in the genre of docu-animation such as *The Grave of Fireflies* and *Barefoot Gen* are not merely the autobiographical stories of the protagonists, but also the story of an entire generation who wish to process the memory in order to survive and live their lives normally in contemporary Japan; a generation that understand the traumatic events not as a historical story but as the "return of the repressed," which helps them comprehend the formative story of their lives, its foundation through the traumas that influenced them before they were even born. The integration of personal memories with postmemory memories helped the second generation reader fathom the story of the nuclear holocaust, which seemed distant and inconceivable in the current reality of wealth, globalization, and ostentatious consumer culture, as an integral part of life. The protagonists of films such as *Barefoot Gen* explain that not forgetting promotes forgiveness. The reconstruction work generates a change in the traumatic memory and allows it to be transformed from a common memory to a deep personal memory, uniting the two narratives on the individual level and reminding young people in Japan that the Hiroshima experience (this time not as a metaphor) is not a story of the past but a central part in the story of their contemporary lives (Friedländer, 1992; Langer, 1991). After the private memory found its context in the narrative of collective memory, the reader can revisit the deciphered past and formulate a coherent historical story through feedback, based on historical facts alongside private memories. Thus, the media of *manga* and animation that expand the historical story, by blurring the lines between history and memory and between objectivity and subjectivity, help the second generation to construct a complete and coherent identity that allows them to live at peace with themselves in the present. As such, in Japan, comics, the graphic novel, and animation have become agents of memory that undermine the institutional culture, the informal censorship of the government, and the censorship of the individual's consciousness through repression.

References

Asai, M. (2007). Barefoot Gen, the atomic bomb and I: The Hiroshima legacy. *Hiroshima Research News, 10*(2), 4–5.

Baudrillard, J. (1995). *Simulacra and simulation*. Ann Arbor: University of Michigan Press.

Blich, B. (2013). *Can we learn from pictures?* California: David Publishing Company.

Bondanella, P. (1997). *Umberto Eco and the open text: Semiotics, fiction, popular culture* (p. 90). New York: Cambridge University Press.

Friedländer, S. (1992). Introduction. In Saul Friedländer (Ed.), *Probing the limits of representation: Nazism and the "Final Solution"*. (p. 42) Cambridge, MA: Harvard University Press.

Hirsch, M. (1997). *Family frames: Photography, narrative and postmemory*. Cambridge, MA: Harvard University Press.

Holmberg, R. (2011). Manga 3.11: The tsunami, the Japanese publishing industry, Suzuki Miso's Reportage, and the One Piece lifeboat in *The Comics Journal*.

Ishizawa, M. (2012). Interview of Ishizawa by Chris Cooper on March 15 2012 in Tokyo. Bloomberg Business. Retrieved April 15, 2015 from https://www.youtube.com/watch?v=_CgaHibz7F8.

Ivy, M. (1995). *Discourses of the vanishing: Modernity, Phantasm, Japan* (p. 14). Chicago: The University of Chicago Press.

Kerwin, L. K. (2000). On the emergence of memory in historical discourse. *Representations, 69*, 136. Special Issue: Grounds for Remembering.

Langer, L. L. (1991). *Holocaust testimonies: The Ruins of memory*. New Haven: Yale University Press.

Lautenschläger, R. (2008). *Much discussed: Comic about the Holocaust given try-out in history lessons*, Online-Redaktion, Goethe-Institute, Helsinki, Finland. Retrieved April 15, 2015 from http://mucz-lbv-002.goethe.de/ges/pok/dun/en3955257.htm.

Lentin, R. (2002). Postmemory, received history and the return of the Auschwitz code in Eurozine. *On-Line Journal*. Retrieved April 15, 2015 from http://www.eurozine.com/articles/2002-09-06-lentin-en.html.

Lipsitz, G. (1990). *Time passages: Collective memory and American popular culture*. Minneapolis: University of Minnesota Press.

McLuhan, M. (1964, 2003). *Understanding media*. Tel-Aviv: Bavel Publishing. [Hebrew].

Nakazawa, K. (2003). An interview in *The Comics Journal* # 256.

Napier, S. J. (2005). World War II as trauma, memory and fantasy in Japanese animation. *The Asia-Pacific Journal: Japan Focus*. Retrieved April 15, 2015 from http://www.japanfocus.org/-Susan_J_-Napier/1972.

Orr, J. (2001). *Victim as Hero: Ideologies of peace and national identity in postwar Japan*. Honolulu: University of Hawai'i Press.

Raz, Y. (2008). Visual evidences: History and memory in Israeli cinema. *The Journal of Israeli History: Politics, Society, Culture, 14*, 6. Hebrew.

Reinhart, T. (2000). *From Cubism to Madonna. Subject & representation in 20th century art*. Tel-Aviv: Hakibbutz Hameuhad Publishing. Hebrew.

Sawaragi, N. (2005). On the Battlefield of "Superflat". In Takashi, Murakami (Ed.), Little boy: The art of Japan's exploding sub-culture (pp. 187–205). New Haven: Yale University Press.

Selzer, A. (2009). Freedom *"Still my soul demands"—growing up in a Jewish family in Inter-War Poland*, Unpublished dissertation, Bar-Ilan University. [Hebrew].

Stiegler, B. (2010). Memory. In W. J. T. Mitchell & M. B. N. Hansen (Eds.), *Critical terms for media studies* (pp. 64–87). Chicago: University Of Chicago Press.

Thornber, K. (2013). *Ecoambiguity: Environmental crises and East Asian literatures* (p. 487). Ann Arbor: University of Michigan Press.

Watchel, N. (1990). Introduction. In Marie-Noëlle Bourguet, Lucette Valensi, Nathan Wachtel (Eds.), *Between memory and history* (p. 4). New York: Harwood Academic.

Weinbaum, L. (1991). Holocaust as comics series—Maus/Art Spigelman. *Nativ—Journal of Politics and the Arts, 1*(18), 69–71, [Hebrew].

Weitz, Y., & Strauss, S. (2009). Memorabilia: A case study of women migrant workers in Israel. In Bar-On Yaarah & Tarazi Ezri (Eds.), *In our Backyards* (p. 185). Jerusalem: Bezalel Academy of Arts and Design.

Young, J. (2000). *At memory's edge: After-images of the holocaust in contemporary art and architecture*. New Haven: Yale University Press.

8 Performative Recollection: Koizumi Meiro Representations of *Kamikaze* Pilots and the Trauma of the Asia-Pacific War in Japan

Ayelet Zohar

8.1 Preamble

A young man dressed in a *kamikaze* pilot outfit, bandages covering his wounds, his face whitened as a ghost, crawls and limps though the streets and shopping districts of Tokyo. The passers-by stare at him with awe, stopping momentarily or completely ignore the youngster as they turn around and rush away. The aviator calls out "Chieko!" before he falls again to the ground… .

Koizumi Meiro's (b. 1976, Gunma, Japan) video project, *Voice of a Dead Hero* (Koizumi, 2009) (Fig. 8.1),[1] is a documentation of the performance described above as it takes place throughout the streets of Tokyo and ends with the passage into Yasukuni Shrine at the center of the city.[2] Koizumi, a young Japanese artist who has appropriated the image of the *kamikaze* pilot as a metonymy of war, specifically, the memory of the Asia-Pacific War, uses this icon to express his criticism toward the controversial acts, and to bring forward some aspects of the trauma.

This chapter explores the links between trauma and image within the framework of Koizumi's work, the concept of *performativity* and the practice of *performance*, the notion of the trauma of the Third Generation in Japan after the Asia-Pacific War, and the ways in which the younger generation of artists makes use of documentary, as well as staged and performed photography strategies, to form their critique. My argument is that despite the intensive attempts of Japanese authorities and governmental agencies (such as the Ministry of Education, and the activities of Historical Revisionism that flourish within Japan's academic system) to delete the discussion of the war and its traumas, the memory of the Asia-Pacific War is not pushed into oblivion, but rather is being presented and perpetuated, especially by film makers, as well as contemporary artists, in their attempt to understand the ailments of the past, the problems of the present, and possible solutions for the future. Photography and video-art, in this context, become tools for self-expression, methods for reshaping and questioning the harsh realities of the past through the possibility to perform and reenact the events that were denied and concealed by their parents and grandparents generation.

[1] To view Koizumi's video, go to: http://www.meirokoizumi.com/.

[2] Yasukuni Jinja (Shrine) is a controversial shrine at central Tokyo. It is notorious for storing the ashes of Asia-Pacific War criminals, and thus draws much public criticism whenever a Japanese politician chooses to visit the place. For extensive discussion of the site and its significance, see Jiji News Agency (2015). "It's 'natural' for leaders to visit Yasukuni, Abe says," *Japan Times*, Feb 18th 2015, http://www.japantimes.co.jp/news/2015/02/18/national/politics-diplomacy/its-natural-for-leaders-to-visit-yasukuni-abe-says/#.VbyGrvmqqko [Accessed Aug. 1st, 2015].

A. Zohar, Ph.D. (✉)
Art History Department, Tel Aviv University, Tel Aviv, Israel
e-mail: azohar@post.tau.ac.il

Y. Ataria et al. (eds.), *Interdisciplinary Handbook of Trauma and Culture*, DOI 10.1007/978-3-319-29404-9_8

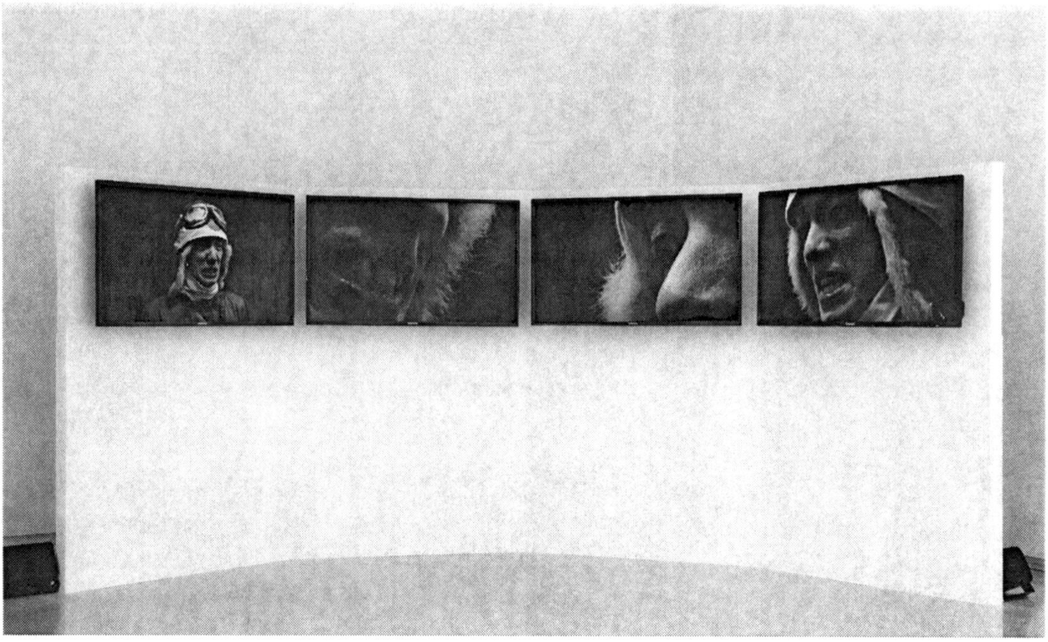

Fig. 8.1 Koizumi Meiro, *Voice of a Dead Hero*, 2009 four-channel video installation at the The Genia Schreiber Tel Aviv University Art Gallery, 2015

The use of photography to reconstruct and show the images of the past is a central concept in this chapter. Moreover, this practice is deeply linked to the experience of the Third Generation (to the war trauma, and the distance of time experienced from the actual events that created the trauma). Borrowing from the expression of the field of Trauma Studies (LaCapra, 1999, p. 43–85), the idea of a Third Generation is often used in the context of Holocaust Studies and other contexts of psychological and sociological trauma (Caruth, 1996). Researchers in the field have coined it to suggest that traumas can be inherited or culturally transmitted. Third Generation members have a very remote experience of the trauma itself, yet in contrast to First Generation members who experienced the events, and the Second Generation who lived with collective memories of the trauma, the Third Generation is in a position where the past does not dominate the present, and the future holds much more promise. Hence, their attitude toward past memory is complex and interesting, and does not necessarily follow common expectations of remembrance (Klein, 2007).

In the context of the Jewish Holocaust of World War II, Third Generation members were born into an atmosphere of "Remember, Don't Forget." The idea of remembrance seems like a common command, but Third Generation members sometimes find it difficult to follow this order. In her text on testimonial videos and the encounter of Third Generation members with these documentary materials, Amelia Klein notes the desire to formulate their own perspective on war-remembrance, which involves individual memory-work, or "working through" the material in a personal manner (Klein, 2007, pp. 137–138). Agata Kula sees Third Generation interviewers "reveal common tension between perpetuating memory […] and their desire to move forward and celebrate more positive aspects" (Klein, 2007 p. 137). Klein adds that Third Generation members working out their attitudes toward (Holocaust) remembrance is a complex issue, one that may take a lifetime to resolve. On the other hand, according to Dominique LaCapra, people may resist this process of "fidelity to trauma, a feeling that one must somehow keep faith with it," as shaping one's own memory may feel like betrayal of the dead. Therefore, some would prefer to remain within the trauma (LaCapra, 1999, pp. 22, 70). Michael Roth, on the other hand, considers issues of memory and trauma, and the challenges these pose to historiography, through his work on the value of the archive for the visual arts. He also states the importance of representation as part of the processing of traumatic events, and the fragmenting capacity of photography as a means to deconstruct time and trauma (Roth, 2012, pp. 77, 178). David Stahl, on the other hand, refers to the possibilities of literature and art to serve as modes for assimilating and coping with the traumatic events of wartime Japan, their extreme violence, and their ideological reconstruction of the individual. In his view, in order to be able to assimilate traumatic experience, it is a necessity to constitute the (visual) presence of that trauma, without which, it will never be resolved or assimilated (Stahl, 2010, pp. 1–4).

In this chapter, through the analysis of Koizumi's video-art, I arrive at an understanding of situations that reflect on memories and traumas associated with the Asia-Pacific War, giving special attention to issues concerning *performance* and *performativity* in relation to war memory, expanding on the discussion of past trauma and its embodiment and reenactment in the present. In *The Performative Force of Photography*, Laura Levine suggests a bridge over the gap between the concept of "performance" and that of "photography": performance is a concept (and an art form) that relates to the ephemeral and to a living form of change and movement, while photography is conceived as a medium of visual immobility, which makes it a perfect medium for archiving and stabilizing categories and meaning—especially those related to trauma (Levine, 2009, pp. 328–329). This idea is built on Roland Barthes' suggestion that photographic stability is designed by posing, which has a theatrical quality to it and is designed for the camera's gaze (Barthes, 1980, p. 78). Levine continues by offering a reconsideration of Barthes concept in relation to J. L. Austin's concept of "speech acts": suggesting that photographs serve as "speech acts," emphasizing the inter-subjective relations that initiate the photograph's performative force and meaning (Kaye, 2006). Ariela Azoulay, on the other hand, insists that the performative reconstruction of the photograph as "performative force" is created by its spectator, who contextualizes the image and gives it meaning (Azoulay, 2008, p. 14).

In light of the previous ideas that situate the photographic image under the performative lens, my discussion of Koizumi's work suggests that the format of performance (in front of the camera) is a powerful tool of remembrance and memory, that helps to bring back the controversial memories of the war in a tangible/visual manner, that enables a fruitful discussion of trauma in general, and in the current example is situated specifically within Japanese society. Koizumi's different video projects are at the core of this discourse and practice, his work permits a direct encounter with images pushed into oblivion, and allows viewers to take a first step on the long journey of Japan's reengagement with war memory and its responsibility for war and postwar issues. In Koizumi's videos, performance is a means of cultural visualization of the forgotten and repressed, and the return of the trauma in a mode that enables remembrance and the working through of issues of memory and *postmemory* (Hirsch, 2012), as means of working through the traumatic experience.

8.2 War Trauma in Japan

In his quintessential text *Imagined Communities* (Anderson, 1983), Benedict Anderson identifies that the core of Nationalism lies at the need to create a collective, Master Narrative that most members of the community can identify with. Anderson's argument proceeds to identify these Master Narratives at moments the community commemorates and lionizes, such as the establishment of the nation, or moments of glory and success, that most members of the community (nation) can strongly identify with. For most countries building such Master Narrative is part of a dominant discourse that explains the nation's history and becomes a central element in its collective memory. This Master Narrative contains collective memories of glorious accomplishments, usually linked to the foundation of the nation, victory in wars, and successful achievements that became a keystone of national solidarity (Gellner, 2006). However, in recent decades, there is tendency to incorporate guilt-inducing historical events—exposing narratives of horror and misery as part of a nation's unifying Master Narratives—that challenge the Master Narratives of heroism. Good examples are the collective experience of the Jewish Holocaust, or the memory of slavery and extreme forms of racism in the collective memory of American citizens of African heritage (Barkan, 2000). As these historical events tend to breed more guilt and shame rather than honor and pride, the dark memories are no longer safely hidden away from foreign eyes. In the current reality, after long years of silence and shame, those who were victimized during the war became empowered and demanded justice from perpetrators. In many cases, perpetration of horrific acts is committed by a small minority but they still tint the nation sense of the majority, because the atrocities were committed in the name of the nation. Hence, trauma becomes more complex, and is not only associated with the victims, but indeed, is becoming increasingly associated with the perpetrators as well. Perpetrators face the judgment of history as empowered victims mobilize to bring them to justice (Tsutsui, 2009, p. 1391).

Literature on collective trauma has noted several aspects that reoccur in societies marked by perpetrators of the trauma: first there is forgetting/repression, followed by phases of distortion, displacement, and justification (Giesen, 2004a). Other responses after the perpetuation of a trauma may include denial (common in Japan and in Germany), reversal, projection, and depersonalization as the modes of coping with perpetuation of trauma. Although not quite common in social terminology, where we identify the trauma with the victim, Giesen has brought forward the problem regarding the trauma of the perpetrators, especially in the years following the crime, and the generations born after the aggressive events become part of their collective history. Hence, the trauma as discussed in this context is broader than the common division between perpetrator and victim, and concerns issues related to Third Generation of both sides (Giesen, 2004b). Giesen traces the trajectory of this pattern in Germany, and lists phases of: denial, silence, demonization, criminalization, withdrawal, collective guilt, objectification, and metaphysical guilt (Jaspers, 1961). Since Japan has suffered from the trauma of the atomic bombs at the end of the war, the main strategy has been to focus on the victims of trauma and ignore the trauma perpetrated by Japan's aggressiveness during the war (Tsutsui, p. 1393). In post-1945 Japan, main critics of perpetrations have been linked to opposition parties, generally of progressive or leftist political orientation, while defenders of perpetrations generally tend to be conservative or right leaning (Gluck, 1993, pp. 64–95).

The past two decades mark a dramatic change in the cultural atmosphere of Japan. During this period, following the collapse of Japanese financial markets in 1989 and the continuing recession, deep social change, and continuing public discussion of the past were brought to the forefront. After long decades of denial and ignoring the Japanese responsibility for military aggression in Asia, the last two decades, since 1995, mark a time of significant change in public attitude in Japan—one that has been more open discourse and reflected an ability to consider issues of guilt and responsibility (Tsutsui, 2009, pp. 1413–1414). Nonetheless, conservative discourses that have presented the war using nostalgic imagery have also been present and to a certain degree, dominate areas of film, visual, and popular culture (Sakamoto, 2015, pp. 158–184).

After decades when public discourses in Japan concentrated on the trauma of Hiroshima and Nagasaki, and the victimization of Japan, the process of rethinking wartime trauma has seen the return and expansion of public discussions of Japan's aggression during the war, and its continued approach to refrain from public engagement with discourses of war responsibility, affect, and memory (Tsurumi, 2015). Yet, specters of the wartime era continue to haunt the present through tensions in Japan's relations with its neighbors in

East Asia.[3] Attitudes toward war memory in Japan range from the silence of the First Generation, to the practical rehabilitation of the Second Generation, to the youth of the Third Generation (born after the1970s), who argue for facing the dilemmas, pain, and suffering of the past by accepting the idea of Japan's responsibility in a more direct and honest manner. This chapter concentrates on the work of a young artist who belongs to the Third Generation group in Japan, aspiring to represent the contemporary spectrum of visual interpretation that reconsiders and re-represents these dilemmas; that refuse to let the subject sink into oblivion.[4]

8.3 The *Kamikaze*: Guilt and Nostalgia

Since the events of the war and their particular images are generally being eradicated from the Japanese landscape and cultural memory, backed by government policies that have made a huge effort to avoid having the subject brought up in the public sphere (Nishio & Fujioka, 1996; Nozaki & Inokuchi, 2002), many artists have chosen modes of reconstruction and repetition of images and memories associated with the Asia-Pacific War and times gone by,[5] while others have searched the historical arena for evidence and testimonies of the lost past, in an archeological manner.[6] Hence, strategies of representation in the field of contemporary Japanese photography and video-art are diverse. Some consist of performance and its documentation, while others concentrate on evidence and testimony, or collecting documentation in a manner that allows for the reconstruction of the past through its fragmentation, including snap-shots, photojournalism, documentation, performance, projection, and multiplication (of channels) in video art (Cotton, 2004).

One image that carries controversial aspects of war memory is that of the *kamikaze* pilot. For Western audiences, the image of the *kamikaze* is often associated with pictures of airplanes crashing into US vessels in the Pacific Ocean, evoking images of suicide-bombers fanatically flying to their cruel death in the name of the Emperor, with brutality and inhumane feeling (Ohnuki-Tierney, 2002, pp. 157–163). Contrary to these images that flourish in Western culture, Japanese views of the practice are quite different: first, the word *kamikaze* is associated with wartime propaganda language, and thus is not in use today. Instead, the honorific term *tokkōtai*—special attack unit—is used in Japanese.[7] Secondly, in Japan, the memory of the young men flying to their death is a personal matter—these are the sons, the relatives, friends, classmates, neighbors of people still living today, and so their image is very human, connected to stories and events, and they are often portrayed as the victims of the unfortunate circumstances of the end of the Asia-Pacific War in the Pacific Theatre. Their images often evoke a romantic memory of exceptional young men, university students, and

[3] Professor Carol Gluck, George Sansom Professor of History and Professor of East Asian Language and Cultures, Department of History and Department of East Asian Languages and Cultures, in a presentation entitled, "Past Obsessions: World War II in History and Memory" considered this issue extensively (Boston College, March 20, Gluck 2013). A similar discussion was also presented in Jerusalem under the title, "Modern Japan and the Work of History" (The Historical Society of Israel, Jerusalem, May, Gluck 2014).

[4] The 2014 Yokohama Triennale, curated by the photographer Morimura Yasuama, one of the participants in the current show, was titled "ART Fahrenheit 451: Sailing into the Sea of Oblivion." Although not a direct reference to the war and its remembrance, the title indicates the problem of oblivion and forgetting the past.

[5] Some of the artists using performance strategies to reconstruct war memory include Morimura Yasumasa, Shimada Yoshiko, Tsukada Mamoru, and Yamashiro Chikako. See Zohar (2015).

[6] Among artists using documentary strategies are: Ishiuchi Miyako, Shitamichi Motoyuki, Suzuki Norio, as well as certain aspects in Yamashiro Chikako's work. See Zohar (2015).

[7] References to the image of the *kamikaze* as fanatical, cruel, and inhumane can be found in many American historical and fiction films describing the war in the Pacific. See, for example, *The World at War*: episode 22: "Japan: 1941–1945" (Browne, Raggett, & Isaacs, 1974); episode 23: "Pacific: February 1942–July 1945," (Pett, Wheeler & Isaacs, 1974), ITV Channel, UK, 1973-4. Kevin Watson and Ed Topor, dirs. *Kamikaze: Death From the Sky* MPI Home Video, 1989.

well-trained officers who served as pilots in the Imperial Navy and were sent off to their cruel death with no choice in the matter.

Since the end of the Asia-Pacific War, *kamikaze* pilots have been the subjects of numerous cultural products, including the publication of their personal diaries (Ohnuki-Tierney, 2006; Yamanouchi & Joseph, 2000), and the creation of films and novels, where the portrayal of the young men is nostalgic and romantic (Sakamoto, 2008). Notable in this context are several recent films, such as *Ā kessen kōkūtai Ah* (*Battle Air Unit*, 2005), featuring right-wing activist Toshio Kodama; the film *Ore wa kimi no tameni koso shini ni iku* (*For Those We Love*, 2007), by the ex-governor of Tokyo, Ishihara Shintaro (2007), which tells the story of Torihama Tome, *Mother of the Tokkotai*, and her personal view of the young men on the eve of their departures; or *Eien no zero* (*Eternal Zero*), Hyakuta Naoki's 2009 best seller, made into a movie in 2013 (Yamazaki, 2013).[8] The gap between the government's denial of war responsibility in discourse, forgetfulness on war-related matters, and the romantic images of the *tokkōtai* pilots that flourish in popular Japanese culture, represent the open ground into which Koizumi's work intervenes in an attempt to generate a performance related to memory and remembrance, rather than oblivion or over-romanticized nostalgia of the past.

Most of the novels and films about *tokkōtai* pilots present a fundamental dilemma: were the young men volunteering to go on their last mission, readily dedicated to sacrifice their lives for the emperor? Or were they pushed into their mission by the authorities that left no other recourse for the men, and forced them to proceed on their one-way mission? (Ohnuki-Tierney 2002, pp. 169–176). The dilemma is presented in various ways—some showing pilots expressing discomfort and mild objections about performing their last mission, contemplating their families (The Eternal Zero), while others express their hesitation (*Boku wa kimi no tame shini ni iku*), or even show them shot dead in their cockpit, before sinking onto the US vessels in an unwilling act (August Moon Sonata).

[8] See bibliography for further details.

Therefore, I would like to discuss an alternative model of considering the trauma of *kamikaze* within Japanese society, and show how performative methods may be a fruitful approach to bringing the image back and re-evaluating the trauma of the perpetrator in a more direct manner.

8.4 Photography, Video-Art, and Third Generation Trauma

The use of photographic work as an approach to war memory appeared in Japan as early as 1948. The first series of photographs by Kimura Ihei (Kajiya, 2014; Kimura et al., 1949), Domon Ken, and Tōmatsu Shōmei (Feltens, 2011, 2012) were followed by multiple projects that looked into the remains of the atomic bombs and their killing power. In his chapter on "The Intolerable Image," Jacque Rancière discusses the options suggested by photographs with unbearable visual content, so that they cause restraint—a restraint that fundamentally represents the spectator's anxiety, rising through the intensity and magnitude of the trauma, that their intolerability touches upon the spectator's (human) condition beyond comprehension, as they cannot bare the truth relayed through the photograph (Rancière, 2009, p. 88).

Yet, the value of "truth" and "testimony" attached to photographic practice resulted in many images produced during the war and post-war era being put in locked military or national archives, where they were categorized as "documents" and "evidence." Recent trends in contemporary art opened the visual experience embraced in these images under the broadening span of the art world. Many genres of photography, previously considered "nonartistic," have been analyzed and discussed under new methodologies and theoretical tools, while artists began using documentary practices to create their work.

After the financial collapse of 1989, followed by *the two lost decades* of economic recession, the overassured Japan of the 1980s went through a watershed crisis to be reflected in social and cultural experience. Young men and women, especially artists, film makers, and novelists started to raise questions concerning the suppressed memories of the Asia-Pacific War responsibility in Japan, Japan's current position in and toward Asia,[9] with Koizumi Meiro being one of the most important players in this field. My suggestion to consider his projects within this framework, and under the notion of Third Generation is grounded in the idea that the silence around war memory in Japan was replaced with a new approach of rethinking the disputed past and Koizumi was able to create several projects that expanded recognition of this perpetration of trauma, as well as the trauma of the perpetator.

With the above ideas in mind, Koizumi Meiro's *kamikaze* pilots' play a central role in the reconstruction of the images of war trauma. The image of the *kamikaze* as a quintessential icon of the perpetrator resurfaces in Koizumi's video-art, questioning the history of the parents and grandparents generations, daring to delve into the memory of events of the war years. This inquiry is in opposition to contemporary nostalgia of wartime bravery and ability (Seaton, 2010), or the collective perplexity after the long recession in Japan. Although there are many valuable documentary-based projects in the contemporary Japanese photography and video-art scene, I chose to discuss Koizumi's projects that follow the performative act and its value in the reactivation of trauma and memory (Zohar, 2015).

8.5 Performative Recollection: Four Aspects

To be able to discuss the relationship of Trauma and the Performative, I present some aspects concerning the relations of Third Generation artists to the First Generation who "witnessed massive traumatic events connected so deeply to the previous generation's remembrances of the past that they identify that connection as a form of *memory*, and that, in certain extreme circumstances, memory *can* be transferred to those who were not actually there to live an event" (Hirsch, 2012, p. 3). Hence, one of the powerful and effective methods for facing a trauma by those who have not experienced it directly, is through the practice of performance. The *performative recollection*, as I have coined this practice, is based on the possibility of construing an event, and repeating it in a dislocated manner, enabling an experience beyond the immediate and the daily.

8.5.1 Performative Presence in Photography

First, *Performative Recollection* employs theories of the *performative* in photography, for which David Green and Joanna Lowry's writings are helpful in understanding the performance that lies at the core of the works discussed (Green & Lowry, 2003). Green and Lowry suggest that the *performative* act of picture-taking overcomes the transparency of the image as a "window" to reality (Walton, 1984, p. 246–247). While the rupture between "image" and "representation of reality" was identified early on by several art historians as the core of conceptual photography and its processual consciousness, Green and Lowry open a possibility for photography to become a platform onto which memory, emotions, and desires can perform. Rather than expecting photography to become a documentary mechanism of "real" things it becomes a performance of presence, or a manifestation of the absent, and, in this sense, it can be a crucial tool in the performance of memory and recollection. This concept underlines the photographic language of the projects presented in this text.

8.5.2 The Performative Body

The second idea of the *performative* comes from Judith Butler's employment of this rupture as it occurs in relation to the performance of the body in terms of gender, sexuality, melancholy, and trauma (Butler, 1990, pp. 31–32). In the context of Butler's discourse, the performance is perceived as a reactivation of the imagined trauma

[9] See, for example, Murakami Haruki, *The Wind-Up Bird Chronicle* (1994), Aida Makoto's *The War Picture Returns* series (1996), and Murakami Takashi's *Little Boy* project (2004).

and as a mode of materialization and embodiment of the traumatic image that occupies cultural and social memory. In the Japanese experience, the specific connection between war, trauma, and performance is presented in unpredictable ways as reenactment of moments of extreme violence and sexuality and their way of repeating the trauma retained in the body—as presented in the many bodily actions Koizumi brings forward—from limping to masturbation, from becoming a ghost to playing dead on the ground.

8.5.3 The Parafictional

The third concept employed is a reading of how Koizumi's project relates to Carrie Lambert-Beatty's idea of the *parafictional* (Lambert-Beatty, 2009). *Parafictional* is a term referring to an occurrence that inhabits the space between the *fictional* and the *real*. Lambert-Beatty's notion is helpful in understanding the underlying format of the performances presented in this text (Currie & Ichino, 2013), and "the way performance plays with viewers' belief in representations of the real in art and art's separateness from life" (Lambert-Beatty, 2009, pp. 54–56). Lambert-Beattie has taken her term from the idea of "Speech Acts" discussed by J. L. Austin—the idea that the speech itself is a performance of the act in itself, not a replacement or a representation, but a performance of meaning and affect (Austin, 1962). Differing from the *performative*, which I relate to the repetition of specific images well preserved in cultural memory (like the image of the Emperor or General MacArthur), the *parafictional* refers to repetition of generic images, as common categories—such as "comfort woman" or "imperial soldier" or "*kamikaze* pilot." By restaging a generic image of "soldier" or "*kamikaze*" within the contemporary settings of postwar Japan, the tensions between past and present, empire and democracy, war and peace, all become highly charged and quite effective in terms of their impact on the viewer. By staging a scene and reviving a moment of the past inserted into the present, Koizumi is able to perform the memory and reconstruct a historical instance in a critical and reflective manner that allows future experiences to reshape, restage, and reform the experience of the past.

8.5.4 Performative Engagement: Political and Aesthetic

The fourth source of the theoretical analysis of *performative recollection* relates to Jacques Rancière's association of *the political* with the *aesthetic*, reflecting on the nature of artists' engagement with social and communal circumstances, and how these are an activated opportunity of *performative recollections in the plural form* (Rancière, 2004, pp. 42–45, 2010, pp. 105–111). Rancière's concept is augmented through projects that employ a relationship, a dialog, or some sort of plural interaction between an individual (artist) and a chorus (collective/society).

The following sections consider different performances and their respective characteristics in relation to the various iterations of performative recollection described above.

8.6 Koizumi Meiro: The *kamikaze* Projects

Koizumi Meiro created a series of seven projects that challenge the concept of the *kamikaze* pilot, conflating the images of the *tokkōtai* pilot and the myths around these men with the environment of everyday life in contemporary Japan. While keeping in mind the ideas developed above, I analyze Koizumi's project in relation to the different aspects of the perpetrator's trauma, and dedicate special attention to Koizumi's embodiment of power and subjective obedience, as his mode of representing aspects of responsibility, obedience, will, and conformity. I indicate how each and every scene staged or documented by Koizumi holds a potential critique toward conservative attitudes of nationalism, patriotism, and self-sacrifice.

Below I closely analyze two of Koizumi's projects, one of a fictional nature, the other (made

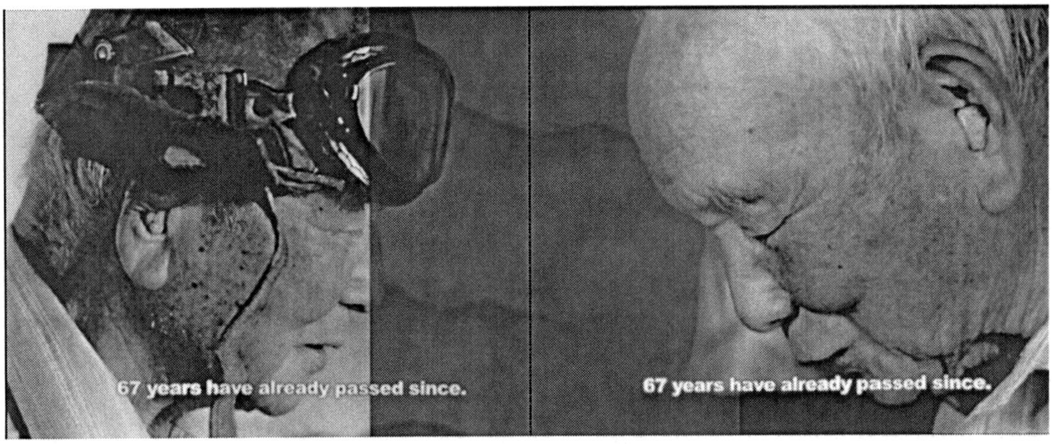

Fig. 8.2 Koizumi Meiro, *Double Projection #1: Where Silence Fails*, 2012 two channels video projection, 14 min

of two parallel installations) based on documentary footage, showing how Koizumi utilizes the medium of video-art as a mechanism of remembrance, and confrontation with the trauma of the perpetrator, as well as the social and cultural critique of contemporary conservative trends. Notable among his videos are the theatrical projects, including a *kamikaze* pilot who gives his departure speech, confronted with the voice of the director and his crying mother's voice who calls for his refusal to depart, begging him to stay behind; a performance of the infamous Ōnishi Takijiro, the man who conceived the idea and commanded the *kamikaze* pilot units at the end of the Asia-Pacific War plans his *harakiri*, while playing with a chunk of clay between his legs, a scene turned into a farce by mixing images of suicide and masturbation together in *Melodrama for Men no. 1* (2008); a couple, a blind man and a blind woman are having their last supper together before the departure of the man in *Defect in Vision* (2013); in this group of fictional narratives, I analyze what seems to me as the most important *parafictional* piece—*Voice of a Dead hero*.

There are two documented interviews with an ex-*tokkōtai* pilot, Itazu Tadasu, who survived due to coincidence (*Double Projection #1: Where Silence Fails* (2013)) (Fig. 8.2), and a second interview with a *kamikaze* pilot's girlfriend, Nagura Kazuko, and the vivid memories she still holds to this day (*Double Projection #2: When Her Prayer is Heard* (2013)) (Fig. 8.4). The two projects present a mode of intervention interfering with the documentary process as a comment on reality in a way that raises two central questions: is there such big difference between fictional and documentary practices, given that both are based on reenactments of memories, and the ways reality is being presented? The second question asks, what is the role of the director as the person in charge of constructing and retelling the stories told in the images, and how much influence does he have on the actors? In other words, how do we obey or accept orders without questioning their logic or aim?

8.7 The Fictional Projects

8.7.1 Voice of a Dead Hero (2009)

In the first part of Koizumi's video *Voice of a Dead Hero* (Fig. 8.3), he quotes parts of Anazawa Toshio's letter to his girlfriend Sonoda Chieko, a romantic text of an immature and unattainable love between two young people (Ohnuki-Tierney, 2006; Sasaki, 1996). The text contains numerous references to his love and his hope to come back, as well as his understanding of himself as a victim, "fallen cherry blossom," but does not contain any references to the Emperor.

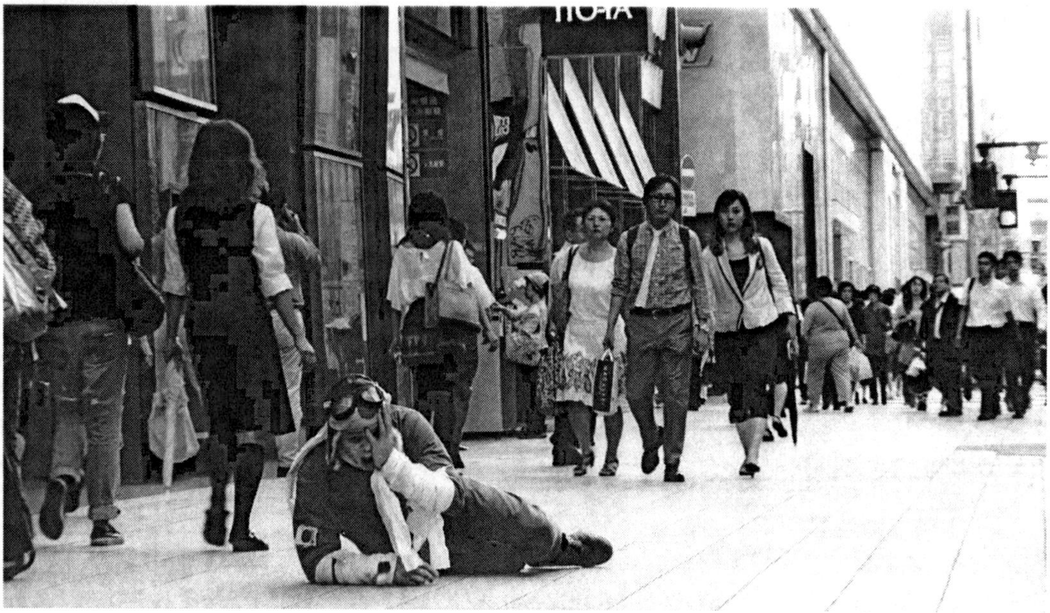

Fig. 8.3 Koizumi Meiro, *Voice of a Dead Hero*, 2009 14:14 min. Still from video

The text is a famous piece in Japan's collective memory, and Anazawa's romantic letter to Chieko is known to many, therefore, Koizumi's choice of the image of a particular pilot, gives this piece the personal touch of a historical drama. The original text of the letter, incorporated in a fictional scene, is a play between memory and presence, past and present, and makes the long forgotten text a tool to make the past present.

In the second part, the wounded Anazawa (Koizumi himself, his face whitened like a ghost) limps, stumbles, falls, and crawls his way through different parts of Tokyo—including elegant Ginza, some subway stations, open streets, and neighborhoods—while crowds turn around, ignore him, and rush away. Some curious young men take a closer look, and someone even asks if he is okay. But the general atmosphere reflects the loneliness and solitude of the wounded aviator who calls out Chieko's name. In the third part, the limping pilot arrives at the long path leading into Yasukuni Shrine.[10] The camera is stable at this point; from afar we see the Torii[11] just before the entrance, while Koizumi/Anazawa gradually disappears from the viewer's eyes. In this scene, he completes what for many had been a wartime promise: all souls gather at Yasukuni after the battle, thus Yasukuni as a final destination became a metonymy for wartime Japan.

Koizumi's choice to bring the image of the *kamikaze* back into the central arena reflects a point of view that criticizes the romantic, tear-jerking narratives described above. His video projections challenge the double meaning attached to the term *kamikaze*/*tokkōtai*, confronting and tackling the painful memory not by glorifying and retelling sad stories of death and agony, but instead by taking an active step to insert the images of the pilots into the texture of contemporary Japanese society. The piece questions the norms and attitudes in mainstream Japanese society by using the *parafictional* method of intervention—a fictional image implanted into daily reality, taking a critical point of view to oppose the nationalistic, romantic, and emotional images suggested in Japanese cinema. In this piece, Koizumi's strategy is *parafictional* because it

[10] For extensive discussion of the site and its significance, see Akiko Takenaka (2015).

[11] Torii is square-shape gate, made of two beams and two columns in front of a Shinto shrine.

brings the past into the present and reexamines its effect here and now, not just as a distant memory of the romanticized times-gone-by, located within a highly space of the film studio. By inserting the pilot into the present, Koizumi examines the actual effect of such an act, posing an inquiry, making the passers-by face the question: what would *you* do, if you had to confront a *kamikaze* pilot today, on the street, or if this were your brother, lover or friend, or even if you had to become one? In this sense, the presence of Koizumi, disguised as Anazawa, acting like a *kamikaze* pilot in the midst of modern Tokyo recalls the events that transpired upon Onoda Hiroo's return, and the negative reaction of the general public in modern, democratized Japan to the presence of a fossilized imperial, military past reemerging in its midst (Zohar, 2017). By drawing a route that winds between prominent points in Tokyo—symbolically ending at the controversial Yasukuni Shrine—Koizumi embodies the traumas of the past as a trajectory that leads into the present.

On one hand, the *kamikaze* pilot is an embodiment of obedience, although several researchers have taken on the task of exposing traces of disobedience and disagreement. When Koizumi himself, dressed as a *kamikaze* pilot, crawls like a wounded soldier through train stations, shopping districts, and elegant parts of Tokyo, he conflates past and present, wartime discourses and contemporary views. In *Voice of a Dead Hero* we learn from the quoted text and the wounded *kamikaze* pilot that he is not just a generic image of a *kamikaze*, but actually a specific person and a particular memory. Koizumi's *kamikaze* act is fundamentally different from the *kamikaze*'s flight: his is a documented performance, the action of an artist experienced in the neutral space of the art gallery or the museum, aimed to arouse the attention of the audience, to evoke their response to questions long ignored and deliberately forced into oblivion—because they point to some very painful, and possibly unanswerable, issues. Koizumi's *kamikaze*'s wounded walk marks a trajectory that crosses the areas of contemporary Tokyo, but it ends in Kudanshita, in the shrine that lies at the heart of the city and at the heart of some its politicians and leaders, and the recent changes to Article 9 of the Japanese Constitution (The Peace Article), to allow the reestablishment of a Japanese military. The presence of the dislocated *kamikaze* pilot on the contemporary scene serves as a reminder, a metonymy of times of war, and a big question mark concerning the desire to see these scenes return. The young, courageous artist brings back an image in order to show that implemented changes to Article 9 of the Japanese constitution[12] are not just mere talk or a textual deed, but indeed, have a profound effect on the lives of young men and women, civilians and paramilitary, urban dwellers and rural farmers. In a nomadic act, the artist embodies memories and long-forgotten images in order to remind ministers and governors that the horrors of war, and the trauma of loss and injury, are only a few steps away, and that one should tread with great care so as not to fall back into nconflict and hostilities.

8.8 The Documentary Projects

8.8.1 Double Projection #1: Where Silence Fails (2013); Double Projection #2: When Her Prayer Is Heard (2014)

While a documented interview is an event quite different from the staged act of professional actor, the manipulations entailed in editing and screening can be quite similar, making the end product not as different as would be expected.

[12] Article 9 of the Japanese Constitution refers to the pacifist aspect of postwar Japan, and reads: "Aspiring sincerely to an international peace based on justice and order, the Japanese people forever renounce war as a sovereign right of the nation and the threat or use of force as means of settling international disputes. To accomplish the aim of the preceding paragraph, land, sea, and air forces, as well as other war potential, will never be maintained. The right of belligerency of the state will not be recognized." In Aug. 2014, Japanese government suggested to reinterpret Article 9 so that it will allow Japan to exercise the right of "collective self defense" and perform military action if one of its allies were to be attacked. The reinterpretation is considered a breach of Japan's post-1945 pacifistic policies.

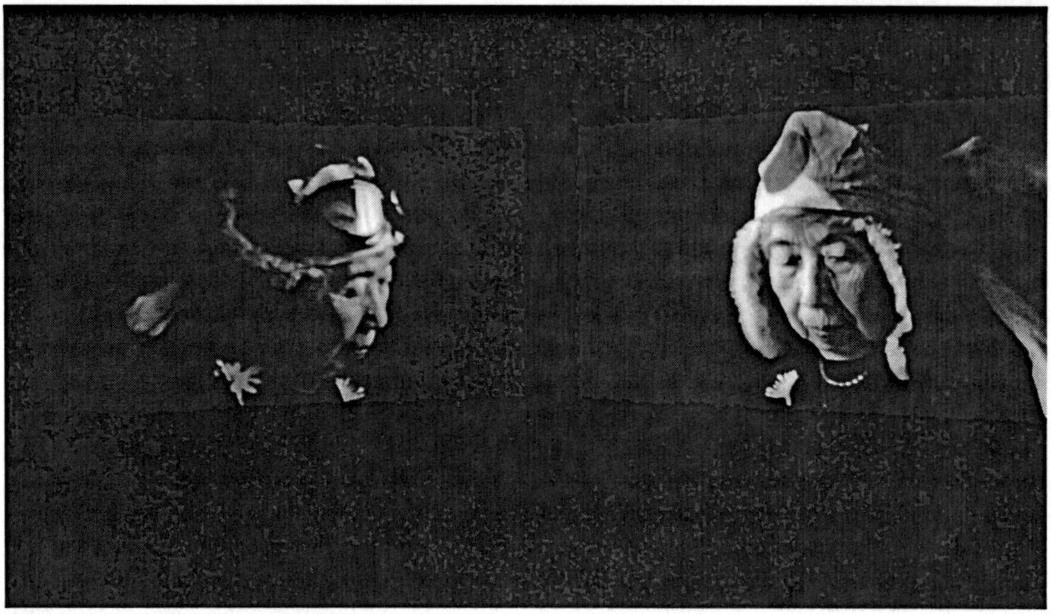

Fig. 8.4 Koizumi Meiro, *Double Projection #2: When Her Prayer is Heard*, 2014 Two-channel video projection, 20 min

The two pieces included under the title *Double Projection* were produced as a process relating to the genre of documentary film making: the starting point of these works is the footage taken during interview with the persona presented, and only on the latter part of the project is a fictional element brought in, making the central figure confront its own memory and fantasy. The tradition of testimony, a personal account of the events at the core of the *memory video*, is a familiar practice since the interviews conducted by Claude Lanzmann with Holocaust survivors in his 1985 *Shoah* mega-project (Felman & Laub, 1991). Koizumi brings the interviews of the surviving *kamikaze* pilot, and the girlfriend of a pilot who lost his life in a manner that at first seems to echo a testimonial video, yet it gradually develops into something quite different—at certain intervals, we identify Koizumi's interference in the scene in a manner quite similar to the way he interrupts and enforces his idea on the actor in *Portrait of a Young Samurai* (2009). Due to this presence and the sound of instructions given to the main characters, the video somehow moves from the territory of pure testimony, in a singular voice, into the arena of a dialog. Nonetheless, it is not a dialog of equal voices negotiating questions and answers, but rather, it becomes a manifestation of power relations, of dominance and obedience, as it becomes clearer that Koizumi performs the role of an order-giving director and the person in front of the camera is complying with his ideas and his orders. Nagura is better in adapting into the situations suggested by Koizumi, while Itazu finds it hard to obey and collaborate, and sticks to his singular lines.[13]

While Koizumi does not attempt to present historical authenticity or display a factual past, he is successful in embodying past trauma within the present tense, while flirting with history. This is brought about through the (distorting) use of memory and personal conviction, where the reminiscences of the past in the ex-*kamikaze* pilot and the *kamikaze*'s girlfriend story, their recollections

[13] I have interviewed Koizumi on the event of the "Third Generation: Wartime Memory in Photography and Video Art" conference at Tel Aviv University, 9 June 2015; I was also present in Koizumi's vivid discussion with Tokyo University Students concerning their reactions to his video-works at the Graduate School of Education, University of Tokyo, Hongo Campus, class of Professor Yūki Megumi, 3 July 2015. See also: Sumitomo Fumihiko (2015), "How Do We Find Ourselves in Koizumi Meiro's Work," *Koizumi Meirō: Trapped Voice Would Dream of Silence* (exh. cat. Arts Maebashi, Mar–June 2015) 54–61.

of the trauma of departure, separation and loss lived through the past seven decades, dictates the rhythm, and contents of the piece. Historical fact is played down in favor of a more emotional memory; images presented in memory (the last day's stroll together in the park, the last flight and the broken engine, etc.) evoke remembrance are at the center of the performance. Rather than historical accuracy, Koizumi's appearance and revealing of the directing orders and presence of guiding instructions draws the trajectory that runs between the past and present. At a certain point Koizumi leads his presenters to perform the images of their lost beloved partners—Nagura enters the persona of her lost Ken-chan, while Itazu is leading a conversation with his lost partner Ashida-kun. A strong sense of intimacy and closeness is projected from these fictional conversations, and the audience reacts with emotional identification with the person in front and the suffering they went through, despite the fact that the film is looking into a memory reconstruction of *kamikaze* pilots, war perpetuators, people whose images of fanatic aggression dominate Western media. In these videos Koizumi successfully works against two dominant trends—that of Western interpretation of the inhuman, fanatical *kamikaze* pilot, while simultaneously he is also able to deconstruct the nostalgic, over-romanticized image of the *kamikaze* pilot in recent conservative Japanese circles. The social, political, and even psychological discourses prompted by these "testimonial" videos represents an opportunity for the Japanese and international audience to face their worst fears and the images of wartime perpetrators, and see that the story contains multiple angles of personal experience.

8.9 Conclusion

In this chapter, I have developed the idea of perpetrator's trauma, and how it has been experienced in Japan over the past 70 years. This reflects a process where young people who are of the Third Generation after the war trauma, are involved in the discussion of memory and testimony, as an opposition to denial and oblivion. I have presented the *kamikaze* videos of Koizumi as an example that facilitates a discussion on how performative strategies serve the process of embodiments and manifestation of trauma—a process which I have coined *performative recollection*—aiming to show that the performance practiced, through theatrically staged acts and documented testimonials, plays a crucial role in the ability to face the dilemmas of that trauma. I suggested four separate interpretations that relate to the *performative* act and to its meaning in the process of remembrance and handling of trauma: the performative presence in photography, the performative body, the *parafictional*, and the performative engagement with the political and aesthetic. With these concepts in mind, I have shown how Koizumi's video works engages with the problematic image of the *kamikaze* pilot and its multilayered meaning in Japanese society, as a platform through which to reinvoke the traumatic issues related to war responsibility within Japanese culture and society. While many in Japan are engaged in long and multiple discussions on the identity and characteristics of their society, its relations with Asia and its place in the West, its past, and its future—it seems that the true and responsible discussion of the war and its atrocities, especially from the point of view of Japan's responsibility for its aggressions during the war are still lacking in many ways. The specific discussion brought about in this chapter was concerned with these debates, how their attention needs a shift toward remembrance of the past. And more than anything else, Koizumi works perform how the trauma of the war remains affective at the present, and therefore, in order to reexamine, reevaluate, and understand the present there is a need to engage with the past.

References

Anderson, B. (1983). *Imagined communities: Reflections on the origins and spread of nationalism*. London: Verso.
Austin, J. L. (1962). *How to do things with words*. London: Oxford University Press.
Azoulay, A. (2008). *The civil contract of photography*. Cambridge, MA: MIT Press.
Barkan, E. (2000). *The guilt of nations: Restitution and negotiating historical injustices*. Baltimore, MD: Johns Hopkins University Press.

Barthes, R. (1980). *Camera lucida*. New York: Hill and Wang.

Browne, C., Raggett, H., & Isaacs, J. (1973). Episode 22: Japan: 1941-1945, *The world at war* (TV series), UK: Thames TV.

Butler, J. (1990). *Gender trouble*. London: Routledge.

Caruth, C. (1996). *Unclaimed experience: Trauma, narrative and history*. Baltimore, MD: Johns Hopkins University Press.

Cotton, C. (2004). *The photograph as contemporary art*. London: Thames & Hudson.

Currie, G., & Ichino, A. (2013). Imagination and make-believe. In B. Gaut & D. McIver Lopes (Eds.), *The Routledge companion to aesthetics* (pp. 320–339). London: Routledge.

Felman, S., & Laub, D. (Eds.). (1991). *The return of the voice: Claude Lanzmann's Shoah, Ch. 7 in testimony: Crises of witnessing in literature, psychoanalysis, and history* (pp. 204–283). New York and London: Routledge.

Feltens, F. (2011). Realist betweenness and collective victims: Domon Ken's *Hiroshima*, Unpublished paper.

Feltens, F. (2012). Constructing collective victims, Domon Ken and Tōmatsu Shomei, two Japanese photographers, Modern Art Asia, Selected Research Papers, Issues 1–8, London: Enzo Art Publishing.

Gellner, E. (2006). *Nations and nationalism*. Malden, MA: Blackwell Publication.

Giesen, B. (2004a). *Triumph and trauma*. Boulder, CO: Paradigm Publishers.

Giesen, B. (2004b). The trauma of the perpetrators: The Holocaust as the traumatic reference of German national identity. In J. C. Alexander, R. Eyerman, B. Giesen, N. J. Smelser, P. Sztompka, et al. (Eds.), *Cultural trauma and collective identity* (pp. 112–154). Berkeley, CA: University of California Press.

Gluck, C. (1993). The past in the present. In A. Gordon (Ed.), *Postwar Japan as history* (pp. 64–95). Berkeley, CA: University of California Press.

Gluck, C. (2013). Past obsessions: World war II in history and memory (lecture), Boston College.

Gluck, C. (2014). *Modern Japan and the work of history (lecture series)*. Jerusalem: The Historical Society of Israel.

Green, D., & Lowry, J. (2003). From presence to the performative: Rethinking photographic indexicality. In D. G. Maidstone (Ed.), *Where is the photograph?* (pp. 47–60). Brighton: Photoforum. Photoworks.

Hirsch, M. (2012). *The generation of postmemory: Writing and visual culture after the Holocaust*. New York: Columbia University Press.

Jaspers, K. (2001, 1961). The question of German guilt. New York: Fordham University Press.

Jiji News Agency (2015). It's "natural" for leaders to visit Yasukuni, Abe says. *Japan Times*, February 18, 2015. Retrieved August 1, 2015 from http://www.japantimes.co.jp/news/2015/02/18/national/politics-diplomacy/its-natural-for-leaders-to-visit-yasukuni-abe-says/#.VbyGrvmqqko.

Kajiya, K. (2014). Kami no ue no kankō—(Living Hiroshima) to kokusai kankōchika (a tour on paper: "Living Hiroshima" and the making of international tourist ground), bakushinchi 1945-1952 (*Photographs of the Centre of Explosion 1945-1952 issue*), Photographers' Gallery Press No. 12, Tokyo: Photographers' Gallery.

Kaye, N. (2006). Displaced events: Photographic memory and performance art. In A. Kuhn & K. E. McAllister (Eds.), *Locating memory: Photographic acts* (pp. 173–197). New York and Oxford: Berghahn Books.

Kimura, I., Kikuchi, S., Ōki, M., Asano, T., Hara, H., Tagawa, S., et al. (1949). *Living Hiroshima*. Hiroshima: Tourist Association Press.

Klein, A. (2007). Memory-work: Video-testimony, Holocaust remembrance and the third generation. *Holocaust Studies: A Journal of Culture and History, 13*(2–3), 129–150.

Koizumi, M. (2009). *Voice of a Dead Hero* (video art), single-channel video projection, 21 min.

Koizumi, M. (2009). *Portrait of a Young Samurai* (video art), four-channel video projection, 9:37 min.

Koizumi, M. (2013). *Double projection #1: Where silence fails* (video art), two-channels video projection, 15:48 min.

Koizumi M. (2013). *Double projection #2: When her prayer is heard* (video art), two-channels video projection, 15:48 min.

LaCapra, D. (1999). *Writing history, writing trauma*. Baltimore, MD: Johns Hopkins University Press.

Lambert-Beatty, C. (2009). Make-believe: Parafiction and plausibility. *October 129* (Summer 2009), 51–84.

Levine, L. (2009). The performative force of photography. *Photography & Culture, 2*(3), 327–336.

Nishio, K., & Fujioka, N. (1996). *Kokumin no Yudan—Rekishi Kyokasho ga Abunai! (The Negligence of the Nation—History Textbooks Are in Danger!)*. Tokyo: PHP Kenkyujo.

Nozaki, Y., & Inokuchi, H. (2002). Japanese education, nationalism, and Ienaga Saburo's textbook lawsuits. In L. Hein & M. Selden (Eds.), *Censoring history: Citizenship and memory in Japan, Germany and the United States* (pp. 96–126). Armonk, NY: M.E. Sharpe.

Ohnuki-Tierney, E. (2002). *Kamikaze, cherry blossoms and nationalisms: The militarization of aesthetics in Japanese history*. Chicago and London: The University of Chicago Press.

Ohnuki-Tierney, E. (2006). *Kamikaze diaries: Reflections of Japanese student soldiers*. Chicago and London: The University of Chicago Press.

Rancière, J. (2004). *The aesthetics of politics (Trans. G. Rockhill)*. London and New York: Continuum.

Rancière, J. (2009). *The emancipated spectator (Trans. G. Elliot)*. London and New York: Verso.

Rancière, J. (2010). *Dissensus: On politics and aesthetics (Ed. and Trans. S. Corcoran)*. London and New York: Continuum.

Roth, M. S. (2012). *Memory, trauma, and history: Essays on living with the past*. New York: Columbia University Press.

Sakamoto, R. (2008). Will you go to war? Or will you stop being Japanese? Nationalism and history in Kobayashi

Yoshinori's Sensoron. *Asia Pacific Journal Japan Focus* 2632, Retrieved August 1, 2015 from http://japanfocus.org/-Rumi-Sakamoto/2632/article.html.

Sakamoto, R. (2015). Mobilizing affect for collective war memory: *Kamikaze* images in Yūshūkan. *Cultural Studies, 29*(2), 158–184.

Sasaki, M. (1996). Who became *Kamikaze* pilots, and how did they feel about their mission? *The Concord Review, 7*(1), 187–190.

Seaton, P. A. (2010). *Japan's contested war memories: The "memory rifts" in historical consciousness of world war II*. London: Routledge.

Stahl, D. (2010). *Brill's Japanese studies library 34: Imag(in)ing the war in Japan: Representing and responding to trauma in post-war literature and film*. Leiden: Brill.

Sumitomo Fumihiko. (2015). How do we find ourselves in Koizumi Meiro's work. In *Koizumi Meirō: Trapped voice would dream of silence* (pp. 54–61) exh. cat. Arts Maebashi.

Takenaka, A. (2015). *Yasukuni Shrine: History, memory and Japan's unending postwar*. Honolulu: University of Hawai'i Press.

Taku, S., & Ishihara S. (2007). *For those we love* (俺は君のためにこそ死ににいく) (motion picture). Nippon Television Company. Toei films.

Tsurumi, K. (2015). *Social change and the individual: Japan before and after defeat in world war II*. Princeton, NJ: Princeton University Press.

Tsutsui, K. (2009). The trajectory of perpetrators trauma. *Social Forces, 87*(3), 1389–1422.

Walton, K. L. (1984). Transparent pictures: On the nature of photographic realism. *Critical Inquiry, 11*(2), 246–277.

Watson, K., & Topor, E. (1989). *Kamikaze: Death from the sky* (motion picture). MPI home video.

Wheeler, D., Pett, J., & Isaacs, J. (1973). Episode 23: Pacific: February 1942–July 1945, *The world at war* (TV series), UK: Thames TV.

Yamanouchi, M., & Joseph L. Q. (2000). *Listen to the voices from the sea*. Scranton: The University of Scranton Press. English translation of: nihon senbotsu gakusei no shuki (日本戦歿学生の手記) (1993 [1949]). *kike wadatsumi no koe*(きけ、わだつみの声) Tokyo: Kobusha.

Yamazaki, T. (2013). *The eternal zero* (永遠の0) (motion picture). Toho films.

Zohar, A. (2015). Introduction. In: Beyond Hiroshima: The return of the Repressed—Wartime memory, peformativity and the documentary in contemporary Japanese Photography and video art, exh. cat (pp. 7–18). Tel Aviv: The Genia Schreiber Tel Aviv University Art Gallery.

Zohar, A. (2017). Performativity and invisibility: Asia-Pacific war memory in Japanese photography in Tsukada Mamoru's *Identical Twins* series (2003) and Suzuki Norio's photos of Onoda Hiroo (1974), *positions: asia critique* (forthcoming, Vol. 25 issue 2).

9 Architecture and Trauma

Teresa Stoppani

9.1 Introduction

"Trauma" and "architecture" are terms characterized by an intrinsic ambiguity in relation to their historical and cultural contexts. Both, in different ways, indicate cultural constructs that change through time (the definition of "trauma," indeed, has a recent history), and continue to adjust to the needs, events, body of knowledge, and disciplinary positions of their times.

Spanning and embracing the ambiguities of "trauma" and "architecture," this chapter defines and explores the "trauma of architecture," that is, the effects of traumatic events on architecture. What trauma do we need to consider here, though? Physical or psychological? And is it always possible to trace a clear distinction between the two? Psychological trauma is fundamentally a disorder of memory, and what crucially defines it is its relation to time and to "normal" consciousness. Frozen in time, the traumatic experience is relived in a traumatic present and escapes efforts to represent it *as* past.

Is it then legitimate to suggest that architecture can be "psychologically" traumatized, beyond the evident effects of violent destructions and physical damages: That is, can architecture be traumatized as a discipline? How is the architectural discipline wounded and shocked, and how does it react to the shock? And how does architecture respond to trauma, using its own languages, histories, and forms of representation, in an attempt to incorporate it? This text discusses the different modes of these responses within the discipline of architecture.

In the background of these considerations lies the historically established foundational relation between architecture and the human organism: a relation that, beyond anthropomorphism, has always been grounded on ideas of proportion and connectivity, function and growth, evolution and change in time, linking the workings of architecture to the physiology of the body. According to these definitions architecture lives, and in living it can be traumatized. This genealogy of architecture also allows for a transposition of the idea of trauma from the body of architecture as an object to the complex system of social, functional, and temporal relations that are embedded in the process of architectural making.

What this text explores is not the relation between the traumatic event and the physical body of architecture (its buildings), but the more complex and temporally dilated workings of the effects of the traumatic event through architecture as a practice and a discipline. Trauma is therefore considered as a temporal becoming, much as is the process of architecture, and their

T. Stoppani, M.Arch., Ph.D. (✉)
School of Art Architecture and Design,
Leeds Beckett University, Broadcasting Place,
Leeds, LS2 9EN, UK
e-mail: T.Stoppani@leedsbeckett.ac.uk

Y. Ataria et al. (eds.), *Interdisciplinary Handbook of Trauma and Culture*,
DOI 10.1007/978-3-319-29404-9_9

relationship is examined as a complex process of interactions which affect the body of architecture as well as its pasts, its memories, its narratives, and its languages.

Sigmund Freud's fundamental idea of *Nachträglichkeit* or "deferred action" of the trauma is important in an architectural discourse on trauma, as it distinguishes between the traumatic event or experience and its delayed revival as a memory. Transposed onto architecture, the idea of "deferred action" can be applied to the time of the project, to study how a traumatized discipline responds in time: the different ways in which architecture elaborates the trauma to produce not only spatially and temporally situated physical responses, but also transformations of the discipline at large, with a further deferred effect in both time and space.

Through a series of examples, this chapter explores those practices which, operating in architecture and around it, process the issues that traumatic events raise for the discipline of architecture. Different responses emerge that attempt to appropriate the work of trauma within architecture: from the (re)design of the traumatic event within the conventions of architectural representation, to political strategies for its urban diffusion and social redistribution; from the reinvention of a cartography of urban memory, to design strategies that imitate the forms of destruction, to an understanding of the violence of architecture that reveals the intrinsic and originary traumatized nature of architecture.

In the aftermath of the events of 9/11 in New York, theoretical architectural projects proposed different ways to process the trauma that the terrorist attack had inflicted not only upon buildings, but also on the role and the status of architecture in society. Lieven De Boeck's ex-post drawings of the event in *Fireworks II. Le Blue du Ciel* remain specifically architectural, offering a visual graphic representation of the traumatic event that appropriates it to architecture, in a meticulous attempt to understand and process facts and data through the conventions of architectural representation (plan, section, and elevation drawings).

Michael Sorkin's socially and politically engaged architectural criticism and design proposals offer a different strategy of appropriation of the trauma, through a diffusion and redistribution in the social.

In the case of the *Urbicide Sarajevo* project, the architectural response to prolonged urban warfare comes in the form of a reinvented cartography of the city that visually documents, categorizes, and systematically maps the instances of physical damage and destruction of buildings. War introduces an alternative logic that induces a re-categorization of architecture, foreign to the criteria of its aesthetics and production; and the *Urbicide* project, while painstakingly detailed, remains unable to find a synthesis and declares the impossibility of articulating a linear narrative of the traumatic event and its consequences.

Produced as an architectural response to the effects of the war in Sarajevo, Lebbeus Woods's *Wararchitecture* projects offer a very prolific catalogue of design solutions resolved and expressed in a highly personal architectural style. Yet, they too remain incapable of constructing a response other than by embracing, as the title of the series suggests, the language and the aesthetic of the trauma, ultimately showing the failure of a mimetic approach.

The theoretical background of these questions and approaches is the critical position developed by Bernard Tschumi in the 1970s with his work on architecture and violence, which questions the nature of architecture through writings, drawings, and theoretical design projects. On the grounds of Tschumi's work it is possible to develop the relationship between architecture and trauma even further. Architecture can be traumatized, and the traumatic effects are recorded and expressed on its body, while they are also reflected in its project; traumas affect changes in the discipline and its forms of representation both visual and social. What are the changes that trauma produces on architecture as a discipline then, and how does trauma affect architectural discourse and forms of expression? In his early writings and projects Tschumi explored the violence exerted on architecture and exposed the nature of the violence of architecture (that violence on space and bodies can be performed *by* architecture). Here the idea of architecture's intrinsic violence is developed further, to suggest that architecture is always already traumatized as it defines itself through a subject–object relation. The possibility is thus opened up to use architecture's intrinsic trauma (traumatized nature) as a critical tool for architecture's auto-analysis and self-development.

9.2 Analogies to Transitions: Architecture as a Body

In her book *Trauma: A Genealogy* (2000), Ruth Leys points out that post-traumatic stress disorder (PTSD) was first officially recognized and defined by the American Psychiatric Association only in 1980. But the history of trauma and its consequences on the psyche are much older, and Leys sets out to document the different and often contradictory positions and theories that, in time, have contributed to the development of the definition of trauma.[1] Ley's genealogy of trauma shows that the definition of the term oscillates even within the work of the same psychiatrist, and that the ambiguity of the term, and of the approaches to it, persists today.[2]

> Post-traumatic stress disorder is fundamentally a disorder of memory. The idea is that, owing to the emotions of terror and surprise caused by certain events, the mind is split or dissociated: it is unable to register the wound to the psyche because the ordinary mechanisms of awareness and cognition are destroyed. As a result, the victim is unable to recollect and integrate the hurtful experience in normal consciousness; instead, she is haunted or possessed by intrusive traumatic memories. The experience of the trauma, fixed or frozen in time, refuses to be represented *as* past, but is perpetually re-experienced in a painful, dissociated, traumatic present. (Leys, 2000, p. 2)

This preamble can offer some clues to the notes on architecture and trauma that follow here, as some of the terms it introduces can be applied significantly to architecture.

What does one speak of when one speaks of trauma and architecture? Can architecture be traumatized, and what is the trauma of architecture? If trauma occurs when terror and surprise or, in transposing trauma to architecture, violence and suddenness destroy "ordinary mechanisms of awareness and cognition," what is it that is destroyed of architecture when architecture is traumatized? I suggest here that it is not only the body of architecture, its physical edifice, that is traumatized. The whole discipline of architecture, its history, assumptions, knowledge, and practices are affected, as architecture is always already invested by social, political, economic, ideological, and symbolic values. The dual nature of trauma, physical and psychological, also lies at the origin and definition of the medical term, suspended between the body and the mind, the medico-surgical and the psychological-psychiatric.

Leys invokes "Morton Prince, Josef Breuer, Sigmund Freud, and other turn of the century figures to describe the wounding of the *mind* brought about by sudden, unexpected, emotional shock" (Leys, 2000, p. 4). If we accept these early definitions, how is the "mind" of architecture shocked and wounded, and how does architecture react to the shock? What allows this transfer of feelings, altered perceptions, and memories from an individual and a society to their built environment, and to architecture as the key discipline that defines it?

If architecture can be traumatized it is because of its ongoing relation with human beings, not only in its definition, but also in its making and changing. We can argue that architecture lives because it lives with man, rather than saying that human beings simply inhabit architecture. This relationship is in fact much more complex: architecture is not only the habitat of human life, but

[1] "[F]ar from being a timeless entity with an intrinsic unity [...] PTSD is a historical construct that has been 'glued together by the practices, technologies, and narratives with which it is diagnosed, studied, treated, and represented and by the various interests, institutions, and moral arguments that mobilized these efforts and resources.'" (Leys, 2000, p. 6). Leys quotes Young, Allan (1995). *The Harmony of Illusions: Inventing Post-Traumatic Stress Disorder*. Princeton, NJ: Princeton University Press, 5.

[2] "[...] the oscillation between mimesis and antimimesis that has structured the history of trauma all along (Leys, 2000, p. 14). 'The history of trauma itself is marked by an alternation between episodes of forgetting and remembering'" (Leys, 2000, p. 15).

also the product of such inhabitation, as well as the result of the application of a knowledge that developed in time. But there is more at stake. Architecture is not only a container, a supporter, but a product of life; architecture is also a cultural and symbolic production, always invested with political and ideological meanings that reflect those of the society it hosts and represents. Architecture changes with life and culture; in this sense, it lives.

The association of architecture with the human body and human life is not relevant only when discussing trauma, traumatic effects on architecture, and architecture's response to these effects. Both the form and the function of architecture, as a dynamic relational system, have always been associated with those of an organism, particularly the human organism. Western architecture was defined, from its very origins, in relation to the forms and the proportions of the human body. While the relation to nature at large was always mediated by a material and structural intervention, both culturally and technologically influenced (think for instance of the myth of the primitive hut as the origin of architecture, which does not imitate the tree structure but uses and combines trees to produce its own structure), the relation to the human body has always been direct, and a certain anthropomorphism has always informed architecture. The forms and proportions of the Greek orders imitated those of masculine or feminine human bodies, and Renaissance architecture organized its spaces according to harmonic proportions that were intended to elevate them to the divine by imitating the terrestrial "perfection" of the human body. We are all familiar with the figure of Leonardo's (1452–1519) Vitruvian Man, inscribed in a circle and taken as rule and measure for an umbilically centered universe, and with Leon Battista Alberti's (1404–1472) suggestive image of the city as a well-functioning body, whose head, heart, intestines, and other parts are ideally informed in their distribution, relation, and function by the different components of a human body (Alberti, 1755, 1988). Passages of Francesco di Giorgio Martini's (1439–1501/2) treatise on architecture further develop this relation, also adding illustrations that may seem naïve but are self-explanatory, and well express the widely shared assumption that the human body, the body of architecture, and the body of the city are connected by correspondences that go beyond formal similitude and also structure their function (di Giorgio Martini, 1967).

Less well-known passages of Antonio Averlino il Filarete's (c.1400–1469) treatise on architecture[3] further focus on the physiology of the body (human and architectural), concentrating on the issue of the production of architecture and its analogy to human reproduction (Filarete, 1972). Here, in an apparently bemusing narrative, the architect, as author of the project of architecture, is presented not as the father but as the mother of architecture, the father being instead the client, who both initiates the project and makes its realization possible. As mother of architecture, the architect makes, revises, and develops his (her?) project, in a design process that is explicitly referred to as "gestation." The architect then delivers the architectural "baby" in the form of an architectural model and with the support of the client then nurses it to completion with the construction of the building. While obsolete in its representation of authorship and the relationship between architectural design and construction, Filarete's text remains crucial today—beyond the transgender twist of his narrative—as it performs a double shift in the definition of architecture (Agrest, 1988). The making of architecture is defined here as a dynamic, negotiated, and collaborative process: before, around, and beyond the production of the object-building acts a complex network of voices, forces, desires, specialisms, intentions, and possibilities. More importantly, architecture is defined as a temporal entity that evolves in time, in the process of its making, as well as in the alterations of its inhabitation. According to this narrative, as early as its embryonic state, architecture possesses a story of change, of variation, of adjustments in time. Even in the Renaissance, dominated by images of harmonic proportion, the analogy of architecture with the body pushed beyond the figure of

[3] Filarete (1972). For the English translation, see: Filarete (1965).

an idealized, well-proportioned body, and took on the body's time, physiology, and occasional messy malfunctionings.

Can architecture be traumatized then? Can architecture, as psychology did, perform a transposition of the idea of trauma from the body of architecture to the complex system of social, functional, temporal relations that are embedded in the making of architecture and embodied in its object? And if so, what is a traumatized architecture? In other words, how does trauma work on architecture as a body and on architecture as a practice and a discipline?

Trauma, Ruth Leys explains, "was originally the term for a surgical wound, conceived on the model of a rupture of the skin or protective envelope of the body resulting in a catastrophic global reaction in the entire organism" (Leys, 2000, p. 19). The idea of trauma as the rupture of a protective envelope easily suggests the possibility that the idea of "from the body to the mind" can indeed be extended to architecture, thus returning trauma, in a sense, to the body—the body of architecture and inhabitant of architecture. It is important to understand that these transpositions are not merely formal analogies, but need to be considered as processes in time when they refer to architecture. The "transposition" of the medico-surgical notion of trauma into psychology and psychiatry is well described by Jean Laplanche (1924–2012). Laplanche explains that in physical trauma there are "a series of gradations linking major impairments of tissue to decreasingly perceptible degrees of damage, but that would nevertheless be of the same nature" and produce "histological damage and, ultimately, intracellular damage. The trauma would proceed, as it were, to a kind of self-extenuation, but without losing its nature, until it reached a certain limit, that limit being precisely what we call 'psychical trauma'" (Laplanche, 1976, pp. 129–130).

There are here a few points that offer a key to better understanding the relation of trauma to architecture. Trauma is not a sudden event, violently triggered and enacted (the rupture of the protective envelope), but rather the series of reactions that the event triggers and that spread out, in time-space, in the body. Trauma is therefore a temporal becoming. The transition from the body to the psyche, then, is not marked by a discontinuity. This is not an analogy but a continuum of becoming of the organism, be it a body or the body of architecture. Architecture too, then, can be seen, not as a wounded body, but as an organism that progressively reacts to a triggering rupture. The relationship between trauma and architecture is thus a complex process of interactions, and, as in psychology, the body of architecture—its pasts, memories, and languages—is affected.

The very ambiguity of the notion of trauma, once it is applied to architecture, exposes the equally complex and ambiguous nature of architecture. That architecture is not only an affected and then reacting body, but an active and changing repository of memories, as well as a form of expression and communication, can be further clarified if another aspect of psychological trauma is considered as well. Leys observes that the temporality of the continuity between physical and psychological trauma suggested by Laplanche needs to be further complicated and that "an entirely different direction was taken by Freud [...] [as he] stressed the role of a post-traumatic 'incubation' or latency period of psychic elaboration, in ways that made the traumatic experience irreducible to the idea of a purely physiological causal sequence" (Leys, 2000, p. 19). Sigmund Freud's (1856–1939) fundamental contribution to the debate is important for an architectural discourse on trauma, as it distinguishes between the traumatic event or experience and its delayed revival as a memory. Freud's *Nachträglichkeit*, or "deferred action," suggests a "temporal delay or latency through which the past was available only by a deferred act of understanding and interpretation" (Leys, 2000, p. 20; Freud, 2001).[4] This becomes crucial when we consider architecture as a project, whether in response to a traumatic event or not, as it brings into the discourse the temporality that characterizes its process. Beyond and before the more evident time of the building and its inhabitation, there exists in architecture, essential to it, the time of the project, what Filarete in

[4] Leys, 2000, p. 20. Leys refers here to Freud's *The Psychopathology of Everyday Life* (1901) (Freud, 2001).

the 1400s had referred to as the gestation of the architectural idea ("Before the architect gives birth, he should dream about his conception, think about it, and turn it over in his mind in many ways for 7–9 months, just as a woman carries her child in her body for 7–9 months" (Filarete, 1965, pp. 15–16). But how is this project altered when it is assaulted from the outside, and how does it perform these alterations?

The following notes do not aim to offer a survey of cases where trauma and architecture intersected in the history of humanity. The task would be both endless and always insufficient, not only in its dimensions, but also for its intrinsic Borgesian impossibility.[5] Architecture that is, is always traumatized—by life, by history, by ideas, and by events that are outside architecture but affect it. On the other hand, architecture always traumatizes its immediate context, its inhabitants, its environment, and ultimately the planet. The study of this aspect of the relationship between architecture and trauma is therefore an issue of gradation, scale, velocity, and pace. What is important instead is to understand the possible articulations that the relation of trauma and architecture can take. These notes offer a very small selection of cases that are paradigmatic in defining the possible articulation of such relations.[6]

9.3 Under Attack: Violence on Architecture

On the 11th of September 2001, violence hit architecture in a sudden and unexpected way, with a speed that is unconceivable in architecture, and in a carefully choreographed manner. The terrorist attack on the towers of the World Trade Center in New York City was not only swift and swiftly doubled, but also magnified in its scale, dimension, conflict, political significance, and human tragedy. The Boeing Airliners that were flown into the symbols of American global economical power destroyed buildings and lives while also attacking values, meanings, political and economic systems, and beliefs. Architecture was muted as a discipline, physically pulverized, and stunned as a discourse. Beyond the human tragedy that resulted from the attacks, architecture too had to cope. Beyond the immediate impact and destruction of the buildings, the trauma of the attack slowly worked its effects through architecture, triggering a questioning of the roles, the meanings, the weaknesses, and the responsibilities of the discipline, from its vertical ambitions to the moral issues of representation that are imbedded within it.

While the general architectural debate following 9/11 concerned itself with the meaning and the legitimacy of wanting to build higher and higher, the problem of the aestheticization of the ruin, the issues of memory and monumentalization, and the effect of land value and speculation,[7] Belgian architect Lieven De Boeck (1971–) produced a critical architectural response to the events. His project *Fireworks II, Le Bleu du Ciel*—the title an obvious homage to Tschumi's homonymous project and to his references to the

[5]In two short fictions Jorge Luis Borges tells stories of excess of information and of identity with the represented or narrated object. In "On Exactitude in Science," Borges (1975) tells of a map that becomes gradually so accurate that it coincides with the territory which it represents, and is therefore useless. Similarly, in "Funes the Memorious" of Borges (2000) the protagonist Ireneo Funes remembers everything, and therefore cannot live.

[6]A series of recent publications have specifically addressed the effects of war, violence, and trauma on the urban environment. This is not the purpose of this chapter, which focuses instead on the relationship between architecture and traumatic events by looking at how the latter produce critical responses and transformations of architecture as a discipline. On war, violence, and trauma and the city see, for instance, and to cite just a few recent publications: Graham (2004), Koolhaas, Bouman, and Wigley (2007), Lahoud, Rice, and Burke (2010), Forensic Architecture (2014).

[7]I have discussed these, as well as the other New York cases examined here, in relation to the idea of "disaster" in Stoppani (2012). The essay considers the irruption of the artificial disaster, as "designed destructive event," in the order of the project of architecture. It explores a series of architectural modes of practice which work on and with the energy released by the disastrous event, suggesting that silence, or the project of the silence of architecture, is an act of design too.

writings of Georges Bataille[8] (both discussed below)—focused on the planning and the unfolding of the traumatic event, redefining it and reliving it as a choreographed architectural act. In *Fireworks II,* the planning and the execution of the attack are turned into architectural drawings, diagrams, legends, and data sheets. Architecture reappropriates, incorporates, and graphically reenacts the violent attack as a strategy to cope with it, in an attempt to reorder, categorize, and normalize what is not normal within architectural knowledge and the media.

After the traumatic events, De Boeck's project condensed the planning, the unfolding, and the consequences of the attack in a series of architectural documents, reconstructing and reinterpreting the facts *in* architecture. The figurative (the drawings of the explosions), the descriptive (architectural drawings of the buildings and the airplanes), the diagrammatic (the reconstruction of flight paths and timelines), and the quantitative (the calculations and display of times, distances, geographical coordinates, speeds, weights) are combined in a synthesis that employs varied architectural media. The project focuses on the details and the measurements of the event itself rather than its aftermath, and the explosions become part of the architectural project that is represented. De Boeck reads the repeated attack on the Twin Towers as an architectural performance. He even reminds us that the pilot who flew the first plane into the North Tower was an architect who had graduated in Cairo and specialized in urban planning and preservation at Hamburg TU.

Here, as if in a process of healing that does not propose a reconstruction but instead offers a reframing and a reinterpretation, the architectural project mimics the project of the attack. Thus appropriated into architecture, the attack will continue to affect (disturb?) the discipline, ultimately forcing it to elaborate a response, at least in the form of an exorcizing representation performed through its habitual conventional media. This project strips architecture to its bare essentials, outside humanitarian concerns, political and ideological connotations, and corporate real estate values, and in doing so, paradoxically, it exposes the trauma suffered by architecture and its internal linguistic response. De Boeck analyzes the event "as an architectural enterprise, as an act that gains significance from an architectural point of view" (Davidts, 2005, p. 242).

The site plan, flight positioning and data, coordinates and times, together with conventional architectural drawings—plans, sections, and elevations—are used here to represent the traumatic event and the architectural understanding of it.

Immediately after 9/11, various sponsored exhibitions, publications, and design competitions called for architectural proposals for the reconstruction of the World Trade Center site and for monumental commemorations of the event. The installment at Ground Zero would not only indicate the tabula rasa caused by the terrorist attack, but also suggest the possibility of an optimistic and amnesiac new beginning, for both the site and its architecture. Prompted by urgency, by the vitalistic reaction of the city, and by the enormous political and financial interests invested in the site, the reconstruction proposals, and in particular Daniel Libeskind's winning project, all displayed a will to forget and carry on, building higher and higher in optimistic commemoration of the event. What was lacking in these mostly conventional and then successfully realized proposals was the critical distance that was demanded of architecture after 9/11. De Boeck's theoretical exercise with the *Fireworks II* project proposed instead an analytical understanding and critical denunciation of the events, and as such remains controversially and uncomfortably active within the discipline. It shows why and how architecture should have engaged with the events of 9/11, responding not with an amnesiac (re)construction, but with a critical reconsideration of the role of architecture in society.

What does this mean in terms of the specifics of architecture? The extreme event exposes the complexities, limitations, and conflicts that inhabit architecture, invested as it is by "other" systems of signification. Beyond the symbolism of a late modern international building complex

[8]Georges Bataille's novella *Le Bleu du Ciel*, set in the civil war of Franco's Spain, was written in 1935, but published only in 1957. See Bataille (2001).

that had come to represent a center of global economic influence, the Twin Towers were also the icon of a myth of renewed birth and indomitable progress that is exquisitely "New York." Superimposed on these ideas, De Boeck's attempt is specifically architectural; it reappropriates the event to architecture, incorporating it in the project: he creates trauma *as* architecture.

De Boeck's work concentrates on 9/11 as a traumatic event, proposing an architectural aftermath of formal and linguistic re-elaboration. The writings and theoretical projects proposed by Michael Sorkin (1948–) in the period that immediately followed 9/11 develop, instead, a slow reaction in time that moves away from the idea of the traumatic moment, and evolve a strategy of change and reconstruction (therapy?) that gradually spreads in time and space (Sorkin, 2003). Sorkin suggests that "the process of recovery would involve repeated mapping of the meanings not just of the site but of the very idea of site" (Sorkin, 2003, pp. 8–9),[9] and his proposal suggests a series of social and political interventions that would not concentrate exclusively on the physical site of the 9/11 attack, but would combine the redevelopment of the Lower Manhattan site with a comprehensive redistribution plan throughout the city (November 2001). Mirroring this strategy, Sorkin's projects for the World Trade Center site, initially similar to other conventional architectural responses (a reconstruction of twinned towers), gradually dissolved the architectural form, moving from the idea of the tower to the proposal of a protective berm around the explosion craters, to a huge geodesic dome, to its opening up into a group of smaller torqued towers, and to their eventual disappearance, as in the blossoming, opening up, and ultimate undoing of a flower. Sorkin's critical responses remained firmly based on design, but they became increasingly focused on devising strategies for the wider city rather than on the definition of closed forms for the Ground Zero site. In the end, his *Back to Zero* project (April 2003) returns the site to the city as an open public park that maintains the gigantic footprints of the World Trade Center towers but covers everything in grass, because "Nothing need be built there" (Sorkin, 2003, p. 137).

Responding to an architecture that rushed a reaction of reconstruction and verticalism and left many questions unanswered, Sorkin proposes an architecture that can be formally silent but socially relevant. "Build nothing" is not "do nothing," and it addresses the political agency of an architecture that aims to be globally and internationally effective beyond its formal resolution. "Perhaps this is a scar that should simply be left. Perhaps the billions should be spent improving transportation and building in neglected parts of the city [and] of the world" (Sorkin, 2003, p. 23). Sorkin's *Back to Zero* project called for an architectural silence capable of reappropriating the terrorists' symbolic appropriation of architectural space. Proposing architecture as a practice of social collective engagement, and speaking up against the US imperialism that had indirectly enabled that symbolic appropriation, Sorkin's "silent" project for Ground Zero proposed a constant reminder of the ghost presence of the traumatic event—not as a celebration of the ruin, but as a form of reactivation for collective public reuse.

Beyond the devastating dimension of the human tragedy, the attacks of 9/11 also raised questions about architecture. In different ways, Lieven De Boeck's and Michael Sorkin's projects attempted to "speak of the unspeakable" (Lewis Herman, 1992; Leys, 2000, p. 109) in architecture, in response to the trauma that had hit architecture too. From the personal and yet universal to the socially engaged and yet dislocated, they aimed to find the architectural truth of 9/11, "because telling that truth has not merely a personal therapeutic but a public or collective value as well" (Leys, 2000, p. 109). "Remembering and telling the truth about terrible events are prerequisites both for the restoration of the social order and for the healing of individual victims" (Lewis Herman, 1992, p. 1).

[9] More morbidly, for Daniel Libeskind, the architect of the reconstruction, these measurements could include the mapping of all the bodies and body parts found on the site. See Libeskind (2004), p. 50.

9.4 Traces and Scars: Urbicide and Wararchitecture

On the 16th of March 1994, during the war in former Yugoslavia, while Sarajevo was still under siege, five members of the Architects Association Das-Sabih escaped from Sarajevo with documentary materials that were recordings of the systematic destruction of the city with photographs, maps, video footage, audio, and written accounts. The materials would become *Wararchitecture-Sarajevo: a Wounded City*, a travelling multimedia exhibition that showed the world the destruction of the architecture of Sarajevo. (The exhibition was first presented at the Arc en Rêve Centre d'Architecture in Bordeaux in 1994, then at the Centre Georges Pompidou in Paris, and subsequently travelled to numerous museum and galleries around the world as an itinerant architectural witness of the destruction.) *Urbicide Sarajevo, A Wararchitecture Dossier* (1994), which accompanied the exhibition and circulated even more widely, documents the systematic destruction of the city's monuments and buildings. The dossier offers a systematic survey of the damages to buildings and structures, organized in a chronological/stylistic order according to four architectural periods.[10] The scale of the disaster is measured in details of destruction such as hit by hit, fire by fire, and grenade by grenade. Each piece of damage is photographically documented, described in lists that read like inverted architectural specification documents, and recorded on cadastral maps and city maps. Yet, as both the war and the documents were still being made at the time the city was being destroyed, the documents were presented in an unordered *open archive* of loose sheets that could be rearranged, reworked, and complemented with new ones, in an ongoing survey that was offered without commentary, as a silent witness.

Painfully and painstakingly precise, photos, mappings, and words documented a siege perpetrated in *time*. War, here, becomes as slow as architecture and its making. The destruction proceeds systematically but slowly, piecemeal, in a time so extended that, as in the long exposure of early photographs, human presence is erased and its traces only remain in the objects that are left behind. Documenting buildings according to the chronological order of their making rather than by the time of their destruction, this systematic account of damages does not count deaths. There are no people in this documentation, no information on human lives lost, and no blood. The photos are published in black and white, and their emphasis thus falls onto the incompleteness and the unraveling of the built forms. Mute, scarred, and burnt, the buildings, or what remains of them, carry the loss and bear witness to the traumatic event. Weak and vulnerable, structurally damaged, and collapsed, they become both precarious records and symbols. But both the precarious and the symbolic are so diffuse in this Sarajevo that they become part of the urban tissue, beyond a single architectural object, in a new disquieting continuity. The photographic documentation then becomes insufficient and unstructured, and the visual record of the damaged fragment, or the lost detail, works only when it is considered in the plural, as a series. The photographic reportage is complemented by the mapping of the damages. Detailed and annotated with accuracy, the maps are even more powerful than the photographs, as they enter both public buildings and private lives with the precision of a surgical knife. Like the archive that they accompany, these maps are unfinished, only provisionally wrought; and while most of the wounds of the physical city will heal, bear scars but grow new tissue in them, these maps (and photographs) remain charged with the role of defining (and remembering) the moment of the traumatic event. And yet even the event here is multiple, fractured, and repeated again and again and again, and yet never identical to itself.

The *Urbicide Sarajevo* dossier, characterized by the precision of its data and the systematic organization of its details against the historical

[10] "Oriental period, Oriental influences until 1878," "Austro-Hungarian period, European influences until 1918," "Period between the two wars, Modern period until 1941," "Post war period, contemporary architecture, until 1992."

and architectural background of the city, becomes a critical project. The survey of the damages could have been structured in a moment-by-moment chronological account of the instances of destruction, or in a neighborhood-by-neighborhood spatial description. Instead, the dossier is placed within the discipline of architecture, providing a historical background to what has been erased from the body of the city. It also chooses to operate in space-time, using the conventional tools of architectural and urban representation (the photo, the plan, the text) to produce an archive in progress that remains open to future strategies of intervention. The materials are thus presented in a loose-leaf folio that avoids any linear narrative, and their sequence remains re-combinable.

The maps represent the synthetic moment of this process, but they too are renegotiable. While photos can be added to photos, and words to the list of damages, the map remains subject to constant reworking. Encoded, synoptic, and dynamic, the map represents at once the pre-existing context and the formal effect of the damage. It also records the production of the photographic documentation; open and instrumental, it offers basic information for potential reconstruction projects. The map also becomes the representation of the work of war on architecture, as it records buildings that have become relevant or representative for their damages rather than for their historical or architectural qualities. Here the war produces, and the map records, an alternative logic that establishes new categories, blind to aesthetic and stylistic criteria as well as to the utilitarian and infrastructural reason of architecture. The survey, ranging from the city scale to the microdetail of damage to a single building, produces a reading of the city as an organic, wounded, and traumatized but still living body. The pain of the wounds seems even bigger because it is so diffuse, so extensive, and yet so precisely and clinically articulated by the dossier's legends: "direct hit, direct hit in the roof, direct hit in the façade, roof damage, partly burnt, completely burnt down, completely destroyed" (Association of Architects DAS-SABIH Sarajevo, 1994) produce a new glossary of spatial and architectural classification whose entries and definitions are determined by absence and defined by what is materially missing.

The *Urbicide Sarajevo* dossier is a precise survey, an archive, a tour guide, a plan for reconstruction; but, as an unstructured catalogue, it is also a monument, a witness, a mute book, a nonlinear account, openly structured to be as heterogeneous and as pluralistic as the culture of Sarajevo itself. A memory that can be selectively and differently reactivated, *Urbicide Sarajevo* is also a project that chooses not to design. It does not offer sets of building instructions and it does not devise spatial arrangements. On the one hand, the project declares the impossibility of articulating a linear narrative of the traumatic event, and of producing an exhaustive account of it. Not only will this document (the map or the archive) be always in the making (incomplete); but it will also be always insufficient to the object of its representation. On the other hand, the recording of the urban trauma takes place in and on the city itself: the buildings and their remains become the inscription (the tracing) of the war, a three-dimensional rendering of the horror. But above all, *Urbicide Sarajevo* is a project about the distance that it produces, about its "editing out," about what it does not say and what it does not show.

While the *Urbicide Sarajevo* dossier was presented around the world, American architect Lebbeus Woods (1940–2012) produced his own *War and Architecture* project, which addresses the conditions of Sarajevo after the siege of 1992–1996, proposing that cities devastated by war should not restore their buildings in a way that erases the evidence of the destruction, but should express the traces of their wounds by incorporating them into the architectural projects of reconstruction (Woods, 1993). For Woods, building is "an aggressive, even warlike act" (Woods, 1995, p. 50) and therefore the traumatic effects of war on architecture are not external to it, but bring to paradoxical extremes the violence that is intrinsic to architecture. Indeed, the violence released by war questions architecture's own performances and rituals, ultimately exposing violence as an integral part of the architectural project and organism. For Woods, the reconstruction of the city should acknowledge the damages of war and build around them a "new tissue" of "scabs," "scars," and "insertions" (these are the titles of Woods's projects for Sarajevo) to be grafted on its wounded fabric and buildings (Woods, 1993).

While the architects of Das-Sabih had documented the traumatic events of Sarajevo by recording the physical damages, Woods accepts the damages and works with them, assimilating the workings (destructions) of war and incorporating them in his architectural project (their undoings are turned into makings). Here, architecture and war are no longer mutually exclusive but coexist in the same cityscape where destruction and a process of rebuilding by grafts and insertions can happen simultaneously. Yet, what remains excluded from Woods's project is the idea of the city as a functioning organism, as a system of interconnected spaces, and as a network of energy. The piecemeal repairs performed by Woods's projects propose a new aesthetic of reconstruction, but do not address the city as such, apparently ignoring the fact that the damage may spread beyond the eye and beyond isolated damaged structures, into an invisible realm that ranges from hidden building structures and urban networks to the environmental and psychological comfort of the inhabitants.

For Woods, architecture's possibility of survival in a context of random destruction lies in its fluidity and adaptability. He propounds an architecture that operates by moves rather than rules: quick, shifty, adaptable, and able to make do with given precarious conditions and makeshift materials; an architecture characterized not by the forms it produces, but by the moves that generate it. Different formal outcomes, regimes of ownership, and occupations are determined by the specificity of the situation. The architectural forms produced are always unpredictable, constantly changing, and always incorporating different times and durations: the sudden time of the explosion, the quick time of collapse, and the slow or broken time of a makeshift construction. This is a design strategy that claims to assimilate contemporary strategies of war: the urban raid and the guerrilla, rather than the frontal array and confrontation of regular armies. Woods suggests that the project is not only formal and proposes, in fact, a political and social strategy of survival through occupation tactics and a new regime of ownership. The design projects, however, remain trapped in a mimetic response to the traumatic event, materializing the effects of the trauma into an architectural translation (transposition) of its effects. Instead of producing a distance and a response, architecture here becomes the formal language for the concretion of the trauma, thus reducing any tension and stifling any possibility of change.

Too quickly and too literally, Woods's projects "transpose" the trauma into architecture without constructing any distance from it. Frozen in the time and in the forms of a building (or building repair), the matter and the forces of architecture are composed according to the rules of a project of destruction whose finality was other than form making. Woods's *wararchitecture* literally traces the forms produced by war, constructing the craters, using as a mold the urban gaps produced by the explosions, thereby embracing a rhetoric of destruction that is not indifferent to the formal appeals of the architecture of deconstruction. What remains unresolved here is the possibility (and the responsibility) for architecture to go beyond a formal strategy of given forms and to propose instead a strategy of *making* form that affects and organizes space.

Woods's projects for Sarajevo perform a mimesis of trauma, a sort of architectural "hypnotic imitation or identification" (Leys, 2000, p. 8) that "preclude[s] the kind of spectacular distance necessary for cognitive knowledge of what had happened" (Leys, 2000, pp. 8–9). Like the "altered" traumatized subject, his proposals are reduced to "nothing more than a series of heterogeneous and dissociated roles," and the trauma remains, defined by "multiple borrowing" (Roustang cited in Leys 200, p. 9). Traumatized, Woods's projects remain imprisoned in a rhetorical imitation and repetition of the forms of war, unable to suggest a way forward.

9.5 Languages and Ruptures: The Violence of Architecture

> 1. There is no architecture without action, no architecture without events, no architecture without program.
> 2. *By extension, there is no architecture without violence.*
>
> -Bernard Tschumi (1994b)

Architecture can be subjected to trauma, and this remains recorded and expressed on its body and is reflected in its project. But what are the changes that trauma produces on architecture as a discipline, and how does it affect its discourse? And what if the trauma that affects and changes architecture is self-generated, a rupture internal to the discipline? The idea that architecture and violence may intersect in ways that are different from that of an extreme attack on a predefined, static, and passive architectural edifice is long established and deeply encoded in the architectural discourse (Wigley, 1993; Fernandez-Galiano, 2000; Kenzari & Fierro, 2008; Piquard & Swenarton, 2011).

Recent positions in trauma studies "hold that the traumatic event is encoded in the brain in a different way from ordinary memory" (Leys, 2000, p. 6).

> Bessel A. van der Kolk suggests that traumatic memory may be less like what some theorists have called "declarative" or "narrative" memory, involving the ability to be consciously aware of and verbally narrate events that have happened to the individual, than like the "implicit" or "nondeclarative" memory, involving bodily memories of skills, habits, reflex actions, and classically conditioned responses that lie outside verbal-semantic-linguistic representation (Leys, 2000, p. 7).

The architectural discourse has similarly shifted in the last half a century from the verbal-semantic-linguistic approach to concerns with the physical, the material, and the bodily. Yet, it is important here to consider the relationship between architecture and trauma within the frame of the crucial questions that originated in the 1960s and 1970s in the work on architecture as a semiotic system of, among others, philosopher Jacques Derrida, semiologist Umberto Eco, and architect Bernard Tschumi.

It is particularly the work of Bernard Tschumi (1944–) that directly and explicitly addresses the idea of the violence of architecture, as performed by architecture on space, on its environment, on its inhabitants, as well as on its own structures, rules, and conventions of representation. Tschumi drew from the work of French philosopher and polemical intellectual Georges Bataille (1897–1962), whose writings exposed architecture's compromised relationship with society as a subservient form of expression of hierarchical power systems that celebrates and perpetuates authority (Hollier, 1989). Bataille performed an irreverent critique of all forms of authority, and his writings challenged all established forms of knowledge and expressions of power, architecture included (Martin, 1990, pp. 23–25). For instance, Bataille reads the pyramid as an expression of a static hierarchical social structure and as a form representative of a structured system of knowledge, while the labyrinth represents, for him, the never fully knowable and representable image of a world of human relations that are always in the making, produced by fluid associations, and always threatened by sudden reconfiguration.

Tschumi embraces the idea of architecture as dynamic and relational, and sets out to challenge its forms of conventional representation. In order to question the stability of architecture and to represent it as a structure that is subject to ongoing transformations beyond and behind the appearances of its firmness, Tschumi's architectural projects experiment with languages and media borrowed from other disciplines. His early works propose architecture as political demonstrations, as social and political manifestoes, as advertisements that show improper uses of architectural spaces or their decay and ruination in time (Tschumi, 1979), and as performances that dissolve the solidity and permanence of architecture altogether. Tschumi's project of explosive *Fireworks* (1974; performed again in 1992 in the Tschumi-designed Parc de la Villette in Paris, and then in 2009 at the Architectural Association in London) proposes a staged and timed fireworks performance where architecture becomes an explosive event: immaterial, ephemeral, sudden, and violent and yet designed, measured, instructed, and built (if only for only a few minutes). Dissolved in an ephemeral choreography for a designed violent release of energy, architecture is intentionally reduced to some of its paroxysmal moments in order to reveal and release energies that are always present, dormant, or hidden and usually very slow, in any architecture. Architecture is no longer a restrictive container or a constrictive frame for the event, but the designed event itself, and the energy released by it is translated in a system of spatiotemporal organizations (the explosion of the fireworks) that are anticipated (designed and represented) by a script and a set of drawings and notations.[11]

Working from "inside" architecture but appropriating themes developed in philosophy, film, and semiotics, Tschumi theorizes the intrinsic violence of architecture to emphasize its dynamic aspect. Action, explosion, destruction, and violence become in his work both goals and mediums for the expression of an architectural project that refuses to privilege space and includes the time of the event. Architecture is presented as a tensioned ground of confrontation between objects and man, each operating according to a different logic. Each intrusion of the human body in the established order of architecture violates and at the same time animates a construct that would otherwise remain inert, and as such would not be true architecture but only its image. The violence on architecture that brings about its physical destruction is therefore reframed as the paroxysmal manifestation of "the intensity of a relationship between individuals and their surrounding spaces" (Tschumi, 1994b, p. 122) that exists also in calm conditions of apparent stability. But this relationship is not so straightforward. The presence and the movement of bodies in space constitute already an architectural act, in which "bodies carve all sorts of new and unexpected spaces, through fluid or erratic motions" (Tschumi, 1994b, p. 123). And while bodies produce disturbances in the architectural order, architecture inflicts control and restriction onto the body in motion, and is in itself "violence ritualized" (Tschumi, 1994b, p. 125) that freezes and repeatedly restages the relationships between action and space. Codified architecture solidifies this relationship in a procedural prescription of iterated acts.

In parallel with his writings, Tschumi's architectural projects aim to operate between the violence that is already embedded and codified in architecture, and the violence of the body that disrupts the order of architecture. By deprogramming, by introducing the unexpected, and by breaking away from the rituals that architecture solidifies, Tschumi's interventions question the relation of architecture to life, inhabitation, and movement. The deliberate introduction of unusual or misplaced actions in architecture releases the energy that is frozen in this relationship, and challenges the codification of architecture and its representations, revealing the transgression that is already at play in architecture. What Tschumi defines as "programmatic violence" (Tschumi, 1994b, p. 134), far from being metaphoric, intervenes not only in the architectural representation but also on the material structures of architecture, and indeed on human bodies. This violence "encompasses those uses, actions, events, and programs which, by accident or by design, are specifically evil and destructive. Among them are killing, internment and torture, which become slaughterhouses, concentration camps or torture chambers" (Tschumi, 1994b, p. 134). Tschumi does not seem to distinguish between accidental and designed violent acts, and yet he concentrates mainly on actions that require not only an intentionality but also a project, a detailed strategy of implementation in space and time, and often, in group acts, a choreography of movement.

In the same years when he was theorizing the violence of architecture and designing pyrotechnic explosions, Tschumi produced the *Manhattan Transcripts* (1976–1981), a series of theoretical projects that propose a system to represent not only the structure and the form of architecture,

[11] The explosive and instantaneous theoretical provocation of the *Fireworks* was enacted again in 1992, with their display in the Tschumi-designed Parc de la Villette in Paris, and in 2009 at the Architectural Association in London.

but also its time and the dynamic release of its energy in relation with inhabitation. Architecture is critically reconsidered in the context of the city, as it is primarily in the city that architecture has to deal with phenomena that are out of its control, and these are often violent. In the *Manhattan Transcripts* "the idea of order is constantly questioned, challenged, pushed to the edge" (Tschumi, 1989, pp. 174–183), and conventional representations of architecture (plan, section, elevation, axonometric or perspectival view) are reinvented, and the projects are represented by the triad of "space-event-movement," transcribed, respectively, by the drawing, the photograph, and the diagram, always presented together. Extreme programs and violent actions that exceed the common notion of "function" are introduced to separate the project from both architectural form and social conventions. Presented as stages for and participants in a murder, a chase, a suicide, and an explosion of institutional structures, the four projects of the series—*The Park*, *The Street (Border Crossing)*, *The Tower (The Fall)*, and *The Block*[12]—dissect and disrupt the architectural discipline and the given orders of the city, in a crescendo that focuses on its in-between spaces, borders, and limits. In the last of the Transcripts, *The Block* (1976–1981), groups of acrobats, skaters, soldiers, dancers, and football players progressively transgress their routines and break loose from their choreographed movements, attacking, gradually deconstructing, and eventually exploding block courtyards that contain them. The observer's point of view becomes itself dynamic and involved in the action, no longer able to measure and control space, but only to experience it through a disoriented exploring eye. Space, movement, and event progress towards dynamic articulations that undermine the integrity and the boundaries of the image (frame). Addition, repetition, and disjunction are the tools that Tschumi uses to represent these broken spaces and their activities. The project "play[s] with the fragments of a given reality" and uses them as materials of architecture (Tschumi, 1994a, p. 8), but remains incapable of reconstructing the broken whole, or finding an alternative synthetic medium to represent it. The *Transcripts*, Tschumi explains, "never attempt to transcend the contradictions between object, man and event in order to bring them to a new synthesis: on the contrary, they aim to maintain these contradictions in a dynamic manner, in a new relation of indifference, reciprocity or conflict" (Tschumi, 1994a, xxi).

The *Transcripts* questions the discipline from within while proposing transdisciplinary openings for a redefinition of architecture. Tschumi's theoretical works from the 1970s seem to move away from explicit political and social concerns to concentrate on the investigation of the forms and the languages of architecture. Yet, architectural

[12]The first of *The Manhattan Transcripts*, *The Park*, illustrates in a series of plates the dynamics of a homicide in New York's Central Park. The narration by images of the event (photographs), the recording of the movements performed (diagrams), and the documentation of the architectural settings (plans) are juxtaposed, and only together they define the space-event of the park. The extreme activities of the homicide-investigation-chase-capture provide the narrative with a free movement that involves and transgresses the built structures. The second transcript, *The Street (Border Crossing)*, illustrates the east-west crossing of Manhattan along Forty-second Street, tracing the movements of a chase that carves new in-between spaces in the street facades by penetrating the buildings' fronts. The dynamic "transcription" of the project disrupts the continuity of the façades and detaches them from the volume of the buildings behind, redesigning street and block interiors as a continuous sequence of movements, spaces, and actions. In the third transcript, *The Tower (The Fall)*, the fatal fall (voluntary or induced?) of the prisoner of a Manhattan skyscraper produces an unconventional vertical reading of the space of the tower, as the falling body moves from floor to floor. Breaking through the horizontal layers of the building the falling body produces an altered perception of the spaces, defying any distinction determined by use and reading them as a vertical filmic sequence. The fourth transcript, *The Block*, sets in motion five inner courtyards of a Manhattan block with a series of "programmatic impossibilities" of contradictory events and spaces. Choreographed group movements by acrobats, skaters, soldiers, dancers, and football players progressively break loose and transgress their routines, attacking, gradually deconstructing, and eventually exploding the architectural spaces that contain them. This last project represents spaces through perspective views that are gradually multiplied and exploded, as the observer's point of view becomes itself dynamic and involved in the action.

manifestos, firework displays, urban narratives, and their graphic representations in the form of "transcripts" are projects that combine architecture's formal concerns with a social and political critique of the hierarchies of space and power. Tschumi theorizes the effect of a traumatic event *on* architecture as a release of the violence *of* architecture itself that breaks not only the architectural object but also its conventional forms of representation. Photograph, notation diagram, and drawing are used together to "transcribe" the traumatic event that ultimately releases the violence embedded in architecture. Architecture thus appropriates the event, and the violence that invests it conflagrates, in one moment, all the roles—shelter, representation, symbolism, and power—that architecture normally plays in day-to-day experience. Architectural representation, *what* architecture represents and *how* it represents, is also transformed.

9.6 Intrinsically Traumatized: Architecture as a Relational System

Architectural responses to traumatic events that affect architecture are significant when, beyond instances of immediate physical reconstruction, they engage in investigations that aim to expose the internal and diffuse ruptures of the discipline that the traumatic event both triggers and uncovers. The examples discussed in this chapter show how in this process a series of disciplinary assumptions are questioned: the integrity and the solidity of the architectural edifice (9/11 and the critical responses by De Boeck and by Sorkin; Tschumi's 1970s' projects); the static and lasting nature of the building (Woods's *Wararchitecture*); the proper and functional use of the building (Tschumi and Woods); the power of the symbolic role of architecture in society (9/11 and Sarajevo's *Urbicide* dossier); and architecture's different forms of representation, through both images and the built environment (De Boeck, *Urbicide* dossier, Tschumi). Architectural investigations that engage with traumatic events, those which refrain from an amnesiac reconstruction hubris, ultimately expose the very nature of architecture as dynamic, changing, fragile, exposed, as well as slow, restrictive, and both controlling and controlled. What emerges from these architectural auto-analyses is a fractured discipline, both violent and traumatized from its onset, in its antagonistic and duplicitous relationships with its environment, its context, its sites, and its inhabitants, and ambiguously performing in different guises, throughout its history, between the natural and the artificial, the static and the dynamic, the solid and the ephemeral, and the oppressive and the empowering. Architecture is thus posited as intrinsically traumatized in its foundational act, where the trauma resides in the very relational nature of architecture (Stoppani, 2015).

It was Freudian psychoanalyst Sandor Ferenczi (1873–1933) who "posited *two different models* of traumatic splitting and of the imitative mechanisms connected with them" (Leys, 2000, p. 124). In Ferenczi's first model of trauma, which Ruth Leys calls the *originary* model, "splitting was imagined as producing the separation of the ego from the object," while the second model, which Leys calls the *postoriginary* model, splitting was imagined "as taking place on the basis of an already existing ego" (Leys, 2000, p. 124). "Trauma and splitting on the postoriginary model were pathological and exceptional processes that happened to the already constituted subject—the human being in the postoriginary condition" (Leys, 2000, p. 125; Dupont, 1988) but the "originary" trauma is intrinsic to the making of the subject, as it "was the very process which constituted the subject *as* a subject by the splitting apart of the ego from the objective world. Trauma and splitting on this model were absolutely originary for the subject–object opposition and hence were normal and inescapable" (Leys, 2000, p. 125; Dupont, 1988). Ferenczi's subject–object opposition is different from Freud's subject-subject opposition,[13]

[13]"Like Freud, Ferenczi in his *Clinical Diary* posited an original state of infantile psychic repose whose disturbance by excitation starts the process of reality judgment. But unlike Freud, Ferenczi tended to focus less on the disturbing force of the infant's unmet internal needs (the role of desire) than on the disrupting power of external objects, especially the will of another human being" (Leys, 2000, p. 127).

and allows us to see the "original" trauma of the subject–object opposition as "normal" to the definition of the subject. For Ferenczi, trauma and splitting occur in the individual for "the mere existence of *objects as such*" (Leys, 2000, p. 130); they originate the subject and the psychic development that follows. Trauma and splitting are both intrinsic to and necessary for the self-definition of the subject. Leys writes of a *traumatogenesis* of normality (Leys, 2000, p. 130).[14]

This latter point becomes relevant when considering architectural discourse and production as a cultural construct that contributes to the creation of the subject–object opposition. If we consider it as an object, as a given, architecture is one of those objects (a complex and composite one) that, opposing the (human) subject, contributes to the definition of the subject itself. But considered as a subject (that is, in its becoming), architecture defines itself by differentiating and constructing the ambiguous foundational oppositions that I have referred to above. As a discourse and as a discipline, architecture needs to construct itself as a subject.

When considering architecture in relation to trauma, a few distinctions must be made. Architecture as a discipline is a constantly changing body of knowledge and a critical cultural construct that is always already embedded in and defined by its sociopolitical contexts. Beyond the material destruction of buildings and its effects on the body of architecture's edifices, architecture as a discipline can be traumatized by external events. The traumatic process that ensues after and beyond the sudden violence of the traumatic event affects the architectural discipline, triggering reconsideration and transformation. The relationship between architecture and trauma is not restricted to the time of the violent event and to its physical destructive effect, but develops in time through the "body" of the discipline, reconfiguring its relationship to its own past and affecting its processes of space and form making. The examples considered above show that such processes are both intrinsic to and necessary for architecture to perform a sort of disciplinary auto-analysis, critical to its ability to transform itself in relation to changing contexts. Indeed, the traumatic process affects architecture not only when it is triggered by a planned or accidental external event, but also when it is intrinsic to the relational nature of architecture itself, and can be introduced (or designed) in a process of critical (self)definition. The violence that architecture both performs and is affected by (and that Tschumi has released, represented, and harnessed in his projects and argumentations) shows that architecture is a relational system, intrinsically (originarily) traumatized. Like the subject, and as a subject, architecture needs, as it were, to define itself through an originary traumatic process of differentiation and opposition.

[14] It is the originary traumatic relation with objects that "brings the ego into being by separating it off from the world of objects. Indeed, the more Ferenczi extends his analysis of trauma back in time to the very origins of subjectivity, the more trauma and splitting are held to occur prior to any properly intersubjective encounter. From this point of view, it is not the accidental imposition of an alien *human will* that traumatizes the individual but the mere existence of *objects as such*. We might describe this as a normalization of the idea of trauma, or better, as a *traumatogenesis* of normality, as traumatic splitting emerges on Ferenczi's first or originary model as a normal and necessary stage in psychic development" (Leys, 2000, p. 130).

References

Agrest, D. I. (1988). Architecture from without: Body, logic, and sex. *Assemblage, 7*(10), 28–41.

Alberti, L. B. (1755). *Ten books of architecture. (De Re Aedificatoria).* Translated from Latin by James Leoni (1986). New York, NY: Dover.

Alberti, L. B. (1988). *On the art of building in ten books* (Translated by Joseph Rykwert, Neil Leach, and Robert Tavernor). Cambridge, MA: MIT Press.

American Psychiatric Association. (1980). *Diagnostic and statistical manual of mental disorders.* Washington, DC: American Psychiatric Press Inc.

Association of Architects DAS-SABIH Sarajevo. (1994). *Urbicide Sarajevo, A Wararchitecture Dossier.* Paris, France: Ministere de l'Equipement, des Transports et du Tourisme, Direction de l'Architecture et de l'Urbanisme. A selection of images from the catalogue is available at: http://imaginarymuseum.org/MHV/PZImhv/UrbicideSarajevo.html.

Bataille, G. (2001). *Blue of noon.* London: Penguin.

Borges, J. L. (1975). *A universal history of infamy* (Trans. Norman Thomas de Giovanni). London: Penguin Books.

Borges, J. L. (2000). *Labyrinths* (Trans. James E. Irby). London: Penguin Classics.

Davidts, W. (2005). Home call: A case in architectural storytelling. Reflections on the work of Lieven De Boeck. *dlk (de loeiende koe), 9*(2), 236–251.

di Giorgio Martini, F. (1967). In C. Maltese (Ed.), *Trattati di architettura ingegneria e arte militare*. Transcription by Livia Maltese Degrassi. Milan: Il Polifilo.

Dupont, J. (Ed.). (1988). *The clinical diary of Sándor Ferenczi*. Cambridge, MA: Harvard University Press.

Fernandez-Galiano, L. (2000). *Fire and memory. On architecture and energy*. Cambridge, MA and London: MIT Press.

Filarete, A. (1965). *Treatise on architecture; being the treatise by Antonio di Piero Averlino, known as Filarete*. Translated with an introd. and notes by John R. Spencer. Yale Publications in the History of Art, 16. New Haven, CT: Yale University Press.

Filarete, A. (1972). In A. Maria Finoli & L. Grassi (Eds.), *Trattato di architettura*. Translation and notes by Liliana Grassi. Classici italiani di scienze, techniche e arti. Milan: Il Polifilo.

Filarete, A. (Antonio Averlino). (1965). *Trattato d'architettura (1461-63); Treatise on architecture*. Translated, with an introduction and notes, by John R. Spencer (Vol. 2). New Haven: Yale University Press.

Forensic Architecture (Ed.). (2014). *Forensis: The architecture of public truth*. Berlin: Sternberg Press.

Freud, S. (2001). *The psychopathology of everyday life. Complete psychological works of Sigmund Freud* (Vol. 6). London: Vintage Classics.

Graham, S. (Ed.). (2004). *Cities, war, and terrorism*. Oxford: Blackwell.

Hollier, D. (1989). *Against architecture. The writings of Georges Bataille*. Cambridge MA and London: MIT Press.

Lahoud, A., Rice, C., & Burke, A. (Eds.). (2010). Post-traumatic urbanism. *AD Architectural Design, 80*(5).

van der Kolk B. A. et al. (Eds.). (1996). *Traumatic stress: The effects of overwhelming experience on mind, body and society*. New York, NY: Guilford Press.

Piquard, B., & Swenarton, M. (Eds.). (2011). Architecture and conflict. *The Journal of Architecture, 16*(1).

Wigley, M. (Ed.). (1993). *Assemblage, 20*(4) (violence, space).

Koolhaas, R., Bouman, O., & M. Wigley, M. (Eds.). (2007). *Cities unbuilt. Volume, 11*(1). Archis.

Kenzari, B., & Fierro, A. (Eds.). (2008). *Architecture and violence*. Barcelona: Actar.

Laplanche, J. (1976). *Life and death in psychoanalysis*. Baltimore, MD: The Johns Hopkins University Press.

Lewis Herman, J. (1992). *Trauma and recovery*. New York: Basic Books.

Leys, R. (2000). *Trauma: A genealogy*. Chicago, IL and London: The University of Chicago Press.

Libeskind, D. (2004). *Breaking ground. Adventures in life and architecture* (p. 50). London: John Murray.

Martin, L. (1990). Transpositions: On the intellectual origins of Tschumi's architectural theory. *Assemblage, 11*(4), 23–35.

Roustang, F. (1988). Foreword. In M. Borch-Jacobsen (Ed.), *The Freudian subject*. Stanford, CA: Palgrave Macmillan.

Sorkin, M. (2003). *Starting from zero. Reconstructing downtown New York*. New York, NY: Routledge.

Stoppani, T. (2012). The architecture of the disaster. *Space & Culture, 15*(2). In D. Wills, C. Moore & J. McKim (Eds.), *Spaces of terror and risk* (pp. 138–153).

Stoppani, T. (2015). Relational architecture: Dense voids and violent laughters. *Field: A Free Journal for Architecture, 2*(1), 97–111. Sheffield: University of Sheffield, www.field-journal.org.

Tschumi, B. (1979). *Architectural manifestos*. London: Architectural Association.

Tschumi, B. (1989). Parc de la Villette, Paris. In A. Papadakis, C. Cooke, & A. Benjamin (Eds.), *Deconstruction* (pp. 174–183). London: Academy Editions.

Tschumi, B. (1994a). *The Manhattan transcripts*. London: Academy Editions.

Tschumi, B. (1994b). Violence of architecture. In B. Tschumi (Ed.), *Architecture and disjunction* (pp. 121–137). Cambridge, MA: MIT Press.

Woods, L. (1993). *War and architecture* (Pamphlet architecture, Vol. 15). New York, NY: Princeton Architectural Press.

Woods, L. (1995). Everyday war. In P. Lang (Ed.), *Mortal City* (pp. 47–53). New York, NY: Princeton Architectural Press.

Young, A. (1995). *The harmony of illusions: Inventing post-traumatic stress disorder*. Princeton, NJ: Princeton University Press.

10 Art as the Transport-Station of Trauma

Bracha Lichtenberg Ettinger

The place of art is for me the transport-station of trauma: a transport-station that, more than a place, is rather a space that allows for certain occasions of occurrence and of encounter, which will become the realization of what I call *borderlinking and borderspacing in a matrixial trans-subjective space*, by way of experiencing with an object or process of creation. The transport is expected in this station, and it is possible, but the transport-station does not promise that passage of remnants of trauma will actually take place in it; it only supplies the space for this occasion. The passage is expected but uncertain; the transport does not happen in each encounter and for every gazing subject. The matrixial trans-subjective field is a field in whose scope there is no point to speak neither of such certainty nor of absolute hazard. Likewise, it is pointless to evoke there the whole subject, a definite hindrance of encounter, a neat split between subject and object, a total evacuating of the subject, or its shattering into endless particles. In this psychic field, a gathering of several of its potential intended correspondents is possible—of several, and not of all of them, and not at just any moment—in their actualization as partial-objects and partial-subjects, between presence and absence.

B.L. Ettinger, Ph.D. (✉)
Marcel Duchamp Chair and Professor of Psychoanalysis and Art at The European Graduate School/EGS, Saas-Fee, Switzerland
e-mail: brachastudio@gmail.com

Beauty that I find in contemporary artworks that interest me, whose source is the trauma to which it also returns and appeals, is not the beauty as "private" or as that upon which a consensus of taste can be reached, but is a kind of encounter that perhaps we are trying to avoid much more than aspiring to arrive at, because the beautiful, as Rilke says, is but the beginning of the horrible in which—in this dawning—we can hardly stand.

We can hardly stand at the threshold of that horrible, at that threshold which maybe is but, as Lacan puts it in his 7th seminar, the limit, the frontier of death—or should we say of self-death?—in life, where life glimpses death as if from its inside (Lacan, 1992). Could such a limit be experienced, via artworking, as a threshold and a passage to the Other? And if so, is it only the death frontier that is traversed here? Is death the only domain of the beyond?

The beauty that Rilke evokes refers to the individual that, isolated in its interior, relates to an object contracting toward itself; that is, Rilke refers to a distinct and pivotal individual. And in Lacan's view, beauty refers to the individual on the edges of the border that must incise it. Such a concept of beauty, that refers to a Beyond, is immediately associated for us with the Sublime, if a transgression to the Beyond is working through it. We can meditate on its meaning as a ready, a *between Beauty and Sublime,* if the limit loses its function of a frontier. The limit frontier

Y. Ataria et al. (eds.), *Interdisciplinary Handbook of Trauma and Culture*,
DOI 10.1007/978-3-319-29404-9_10

described by Lacan that separates the subject from the death drive cuts the subject also from feminine sexuality, and constructs the "woman" as absent, and her "rapport" as "impossible," and her self as out-of-existence and significance.

Against the option of a separating limit frontier as the carrier of beauty's palpitations, I would like to speak of a limit transmuted into a threshold that allows the passage between beauty and the Sublime. Here we can conceive of an occasion for realization of an unavoidable encounter with remnants of trauma, in the mental stratum of trans-subjectivity, in a certain jointness that becomes possible only *with-in differentiation,* in a co-emergence with-one-another that is not assimilation and fusion, in a psychic dimension where a web of connections inside and outside the individual's limits, and a self-mutual but nonsymmetrical transgression of these limits, does not favor the total separation of the distinct individual either from the death drive or from the feminine. This web, which is not only a feminine "beyond-the-phallus" web, but also an originary matrixial web, is tragic in many senses, but is not melancholic, hysterical, or psychotic, despite its psychotic potentiality that stems from this non-separation itself and from this transgression itself. Such realization of encounter via the artwork penetrates into, impregnates, and creates further encounters between the artist and the world, the artist and the object, the artist and the Other, and artists and viewers. The realization of such an encounter transforms the *tableau* and is transformed by it into a transport-station of trauma. Beauty, for Lacan, concerns the individual that trembles on the limit of the border that splits it—and this limit is in fact the barrier of "castration anxiety" as shaped by the discourse concerning sexuality from the viewpoint of male development: a limit that tears the individual subject—male or female—apart, both from feminine sexuality, always still intermingled with closeness and attraction toward the archaic mother, and from revelations of death drive. In other words, it tears the individual subject away from the regression into psychosis, or rather into the womb-as-symbiotic-autism-and-psychosis. Theory, that produces the subject thus split, where negation of the feminine is constructed as a defense against insanity, also produces by the same move some unequivocal consanguinity between femininity and psychosis, the feminine and art object, the feminine and loss, and the feminine and sacrifice. It resonates all through Western culture, for example in the classical structuring of the figure of the artist as a creative subject that shapes its object and as the loss of the woman or the mother, or the structuring of the woman as an object sacrificed to creation and replaced by it—the list is long, from the myth of Orpheus to Duchamp's "Bride" (Ettinger, 2000; Huhn, 1993).

The foreclosure of the feminine is vital for the phallic subject because it stands for the split from the death drive in many intricate ways. The idea of death is closely connected to the feminine in Western culture and is very strongly embedded inside Freudian psychoanalysis in general and in the Lacanian theory in particular, where the feminine is closely assimilated to fusion, undifferentiation, autism, and psychosis, all manifestations of deep regression and of the activity of the death drive. The matter of the split from the death drive, which is in fact the split from the feminine, moves us to analyze further the matter of the relation between the beautiful and the tragic as Lacan knit them: the effect of beauty results from the rapport of the subject with the "horizon" of life, from the artist's traversing, via the elected figure through which he/she speaks (and we add: through which he/she sees), to what he calls "the second death." For Antigone, life "can only be lived or thought about, from the place of that limit where her life is already lost, where she is already on the other side. But from that place she can see it and live it in the form of something already lost" (Lacan, 1992, p. 280) his place, behind this limit, that during life usually can't be traversed because it is well carved and kept—it protects the subject and the subject preserves it—this place, detached from historical time, is for Lacan the source from which artistic creation emerges toward a surface that yearns for its unique value—the unique value of the place beyond the limit of life—in a world of solid partitions of separation of the Real both from language, in the sense that the Symbolic produces the Real as what it lacks, and from the social context, in the sense that "castration" is the barrier of the total prohibition of the mother-child early "incest" that duplicates the total break-off from the archaic mother. That is, this place is the limit of the law that is also offered as its origin, upon which the replacement of any event with a symbol and the replacement of every object by another object, while keeping their value intact, become possible. While the kept "same" value of what is forever absent is the phallus itself, its embodied price is the woman as archaic-m/Other or as a body-psyche Thing. But the beautiful in artwork is the result of the capture of a *unique value* of the Thing, which is out of that chain of objects, of the event that is outside the chain of events, of an unplaceable place and of time out of historical time, which glitters from the other side behind this invisible and untraversable limit—of their capture by the surface of passion in its turning into an image, bypassing the phallic value that took their place.

I propose to add the idea of *non-life,* and of *feminine borderswerving, borderlinking, and borderspacing,* to the heart of the thinking about the creative moment and its "soul" by means of a different kind of woman-archaic-m/Other-Thing. This would mean, to paraphrase Lacan's expression, a life that can be lived or thought about, from the place of that limit where life is yet to come, where she is already on the other side, but seeing it and living it in the form of something not already here in time or place. In other words, not only *death* and the *foreclosed femininity,* but also the *archaic trauma and jouissance*—to begin with those that any potential subject experiences *with* its becoming-archaic-m/Other, and later on any trauma and jouissance produced in a similar sphere of *jointness* and mounted upon similar nonconscious lanes—are those unique values behind the phallic limit that the artist tries to capture and the artwork treasures. Their inscription in the domain of feminine sexuality or in the domain of death drive inside an *only phallic* paradigm is what imprisons the affected traces of these events in a circular way, in psychoanalytic tradition, in a frame of an experience outside any symbolization, and which each symbolization is supposed to reject, in a circular way again, onto the domains of feminine sexuality and death drive *as* the foreclosed and the abject. I suggest that a certain hybridization of the margins of these two domains—non-life and the feminine—can become a source of a feminine difference whose sense can be accessed and can engender a configuration of symbologenic liberty, born from this particular *occasion for occurrence and encounter. This feminine difference is neither a configuration of dependency derived from disguising oneself in a phallic masque (from* femininity *as masquerade* as for Joan Rivière, on to parody and irony in Judith Butler's terms) nor is it a revolt or a struggle with the phallic texture *(the feminine as the moment of rupture and negativity* as for Julia Kristeva, or as the *total Otherness and the contrary,* as for the early Lévinas). It is not a total Other either (as for Lévinas and Lacan). We can advance along this route of thinking if we free ourselves, not only from the compulsion to disqualify whatever is glimpsed from beyond the border of the One-subject life as mystical or psychotic, but also from perceiving the borderline itself as a split and a frontier limit and if we distinguish between subjectivity and the individual, between full presence and pres*ab*sence, and between total absence and disabsence.[1]

But for a moment, let's continue to reflect upon Lacan's ideas. If the surface of passion captures such a "unique value" while making an image out of it, this image creates a barrier and is created as a barrier that blocks the fluidity or the passage of the subject to the other side, be it death or now also more explicitly the feminine, and therefore the effect of beauty is a "blindness effect" (Lacan, 1992, p. 281). The beautiful blinds from the other side when blindness is structured as the arrest of impulsive passion,

[1] The expression *presabsence* came up during the long conversations between Ghislaine Szpeker-Benat and myself around the translation of some of my concepts into French and the difficulty of finding proper words to describe the almost-presence of the matrixial object and the almost-absence of the matrixial *objet a,* as well as the between-presence-and-absence status of the matrixial partial-subject.

which engenders desire. (It was Freud who structured blindness as "castration" in his article "The 'Uncanny'" that deals with the aesthetic experience (Freud, 1919).) The function of the beautiful is precisely "to reveal to us the site of man's relationship to his own death, and to reveal it to us in a blinding flash only" (Lacan, 1992, p. 295 *translation modified*). The beautiful is a limit of a sphere that we can approach only from the outside, a phenomenological limit which allows us to reflect on what is behind the untraversable borderline. "Outrage" is the term that carries, according to Lacan, the crossing of this invisible borderline, a crossing which allows us to join beauty with desire. The meaning of "outrage" is "to go 'out' or beyond" ("aller outre, outre-passer," Lacan, 1992, p. 281), to transgress, and this transgression is the tragic esthetic effect, like that of Antigone, this "most strange and most profound of effects" (Lacan, 1992, p. 248) that arises in the limit zone between life and death, where a fate notches its verdict and a death is lived by anticipation, being a death that crosses over into the sphere of life and interlaces within the texture of a life that moves into the realm of death. Thus, "the glow of beauty coincides with the moment of transgression" (Lacan, 1992, p. 281) and of the desecration of the limit.

The esthetic question engages both death and the beauty-ideal. For Lacan, the beauty-ideal operates at a limit materialized and represented in art by the human body that envelops "all possible phantasies" of human desire and creates a barrier which transports the "relationships of the human being to its own death." (Lacan, 1992, p. 260). "Outrage" is, first of all, wrath and fury about the unbelievable and the inhuman. It is not just any transgression toward death; it is the scandal and the disgrace; it is the transgression to the inhuman and the horrible. Thus, the beautiful, as for Rilke, is the beginning of the horrible, captured in an image or an object, or it is its limit to which we still have some access, which keeps us distant from transgression in reality but allows us to glimpse our own death. While the body carries the rapport of the human being to its death, as an image it also obstructs the passage to the experience of that horrible; the "effect of beauty derives from the relationship of the hero to the limit" (Lacan, 1992, p. 286). I suggest that not only death and the feminine, as defined by a phallic framework, but also the archaic trauma and jouissance, experienced in jointness-in-differentiating with the archaic-m/Other-to-be, are those inaccessible unique values behind the limit. Would they not be appropriately intuited by this zone "between life and death" (Lacan, 1992, p. 280) that attracts Antigone? But we need to consider, now, going further and beyond the idea of death as that only limit; there is another kind of unique value. The archaic trauma and jouissance, experienced in jointness-in-differentiating with the archaic m/Other, are interwoven inside the limit itself, and transform the limit itself into a threshold.

In the elucidation of the scopic drive and the desire to see, for Lacan in his *Seminar XI*, the unique value is articulated by the gaze structured as a lacking object, as an *objet (a)* (Lacan, 1964). The painter lays down his armed gaze, he surrenders in order to meet the *objet (a)* of the gaze that approaches him as if from the outside. The painter's gesture concludes an interior internal stroke that resembles the one that participates in the process of regression that intends to satisfy fixated partial impulses, but instead it creates—as in a backward movement, as in a reversal of the course of mental time—a stimulus toward which the stroke appears already as a response.

The gaze as a lack is behind the borderline of this move and emerges from behind the horizon, from a place or time where or when it touched the Thing from an intimate exterior captured in the interior of its psyche. Now it is that gaze, that absence, that seduces the painter's caressing attack; it horrifies her touch or fascinates it, and it enchants it—and her—on the borderline of the Irreal.

Face to face with the astounding and horrible force of the gaze arising on the horizon, still impregnated with residues of archaic pain or pleasure of jouissance, the artist yields its consciousness, and consciousness can only come in the aftermath to arrest the artist's stroke or conclude it by assigning images and symbols for what was up till then the unnamed, the immemorial, the invisible, and the unintelligible.

The archaic jouissance, saturated with pain or pleasure, is the traumatic wound, beyond the border. The traumatic jouissance is considered inaccessible to the subject, and if it appears by way of the *objet (a)* only then the evasive flickering of its momentary disclosure in the picture, whatever presentifies its absence, can be understood in Lacan's theory as "a phallic ghost." The phallic ghost seals its imprints in the plans of the Symbolic, the Imaginary, and the Real. It also gives their relations with each other, around each event, their own twisting signature. In the plan of the Real, the link of the phallus to the male body is most tightly kept, but this linkage is duplicated, even if by way of lack and loss, in the other two plans as well, in the correlation between the male sexual organ, the potentiality related to its action, the phantasms associated with it, the image, and the concept that corresponds to it, even though the concept itself already appears as neutral, and Lacan shows us how, as a concept, the phallus is at the service of both male and female individuals and if not in the same way, then at least on the same level. The phallic viewpoint with its concepts of subject and object is not free from the imprints of the body, be it even by consideration of the plan of the Real only. But since this body is male, the artist—male or female—that encounters this gaze can only turn into a man-artist.

The archaic jouissance saturated with pain or pleasure, that is the traumatic wound beyond the border, is indeed inaccessible to the subject in as much as it is phallic. But the One-and-Only phallic difference is not the only one, because there are other figures of loss. The archaic Woman-m/Other should not be understood only, as Lacan suggests, as absence—as "in the field of the Thing" and as the "other-Thing that lies beyond" (Lacan, 1992, p. 214, 298) where she can only be sacrificed, eliminated, and evaporated—but also, as I view it, in the field of Event and Encounter, where she is an almost-other-Event-Encounter that is border-linked to the I, and is therefore in presabsence. In the matrixial borderspace, another artist appears. Here, where I and non-I co-emerge and co-fade, composite partial subjectivity produces, shares, and transmits assembled, impure, and diffracted objects and absorbs their loss and their dispersion via a conductible borderlink, so that absence is des-absented, and presence diminuated but not extinguished.

The sphere where the woman-m/Other is not an other-Thing-as-absence is the matrixial sphere. Here, the subject lives in a borderspace between not-yet-life and the feminine, where the encounter-Thing and the Thing-event have some border-accessivity. This sphere is modeled upon the feminine/pre-birth intimate sharing in jouissance, trauma, and phantasy. Elaborating such a sphere between non-life and life in the feminine upon the rapport between the subject-to-be and the becoming-m/Other-to-be—and, on the level of the Real, between the fetus and the female body-and-psyche—should not lead us mistakenly to look for the sense of the matrixial encounter-Thing and Thing-event in nature. Female sexual bodily specificity allows for thinking primary co-affectivity. It supplies an apparatus of a sense-making. Her sexual difference, like his sexual difference, is a thinking apparatus. A sexual difference has always served to explore the intimate and the public and to articulate the conscious and the unconscious, and it has always supplied the archetypes and the ideals for the soul, and shaped the ideas of beauty. It has always been a thinking machine. The womb, which is a female bodily specificity, stands here for a sensing-and-thinking apparatus as well as for a psychic capacity for shareability that is based upon borderlinking to a female body. This borderlinking permits differentiation-in-co-emergence and separation-in-jointness, which take their sense from a continuous reattuning of distance-in-proximity between partial-subjects and partial-subjects. I and non-I interweave their borderlinks in a process I have named "metramorphosis," activating relations-without-relating on the borders of presence and absence.

The matrixial affect, which creates the metramorphosis and is created by it, is the affect of the Thing that marks together an I with a non-I in co-emergence and co-fading. The matrixial affect diffracts a difference on the level of the Thing when it signals that some-Thing happens, and that a transition from Thing to object takes place without a total separation from the Thing. A minimal sense of differentiation-in-togetherness is tracing itself beyond the signal, between signal and significance, testifying that partial subjectivity is already involved in this move, that someones are there to be affected, and that these someones are not just objects: they are wit(h)nessing. A web of movements of borderlinking, between subjects and partial-subjects and between partial-subjects and partial objects, becomes a psychic space of trans-subjectivity when matrixial affects signal that a passage from Thing to object-and-subject takes place in jointness. This passage is in itself a minimal sense, and it works for more meaning through the work of art.

Borderlinking is thus enabled by a minimal difference of affect or by affective minimal differentiation, in the passage from Thing-Event and Thing-Encounter into partial-subject and partial-object. The metramorphosis is a passageway through which matrixial affects, events, materials, and modes of becoming infiltrate just into the nonconscious margins of the Symbolic to enable the transformation, to transgress the borders of the individual subject, and to establish inter-psychic designified communication. Metramorphosis does not remain on the level of the Real, forever designifying into absence. It is a joint awakening of unthoughtful-knowledge on the borderline, and an inscription of the encounter in traces within it, traces that open a space in and along the borderline itself. The metramorphosis is thus a co-affectivity and coactivity that opens the borderline between subjects and between subject and object into a space, that occasion a linking and a mutation into a threshold, so that the absolute separation between subjects upon the pattern of cut/split/castration from the Other-Thing—a separation which in fact is the pattern of elimination of the archaic m/Other-Event-Encounter—becomes impossible. This is because the borderline loses its frontier quality momentarily and surrenders to the transitive movement.

Metramorphosis is a poietic process of affective-emotive borderswerving: a process of differentiating during borderspacing and border blinking by affective differentiating, which is from the outset transgressive. It is a process of inscriptive exchange between/within several matrixial entities. Border swerving dissolves the individual borderlines so that they become thresholds that allow a passage, which, for each participant, captivates what I call a surplus of fragility. The knowledge of being-born-together—co-naissance—in a matrixial alliance insinuates a crossed transcription of a transcryption. It hurts. We are hurt in the sub-knowledge of which we receive a sense in visual arts by inventing or joining a screen where an originary matrixial repression—a process of repression by fading-in-transformation—is inverted, because it allows the originary matrixial transitive trauma some veiled visibility via a touching gaze that approaches it, from within-outside, and makes us fragile via wit(h)nessing the trauma of the Other and of the world. We are hurt, but we are also solaced.

The matrixial impossibility of not-sharing with the Other and with the world is profoundly fragilizing. We are sharing in, beyond our intention or will, and this sharing within requires its price and initiates its beauty. Where the other-Thing is not eliminated and the object is not entirely lost, and where the object approaches the subject without a schism, the link to the archaic m/Other-Encounter-Event is always maintained in some aspects and on a certain level, moving us closer to the archaic space in between no-thing and some-thing. In the matrixial sphere it is possible to describe the emanation of the gaze in artwork not as a phallic ghost, and to describe the "uncanny" experience without castration anxiety. Since metramorphic swerving is a sexual differentiating based on webbing of links and not on essence or negation, I have called "woman" this interlaced trans-subjectivity that is not confined to the contours of the one-body in which inside and outside converge without fusion and disabsence can't reach full presence or total absence. The artist, who is working through traces coming from the immemorial, not only of herself but of others to whom she is borderlinked—which opens lanes to deepen a singular metramorphosis in the matrixial field—is a woman-artist even when she is a man. She wanders with her spirit's eyes, mounted upon her erotic antennae, and she channels anew trauma(s) and jouissance(s) coming from non-I(s) that are linked to her in the matrixial borderspace. Her art works through to bifurcate, disperse and rejoin anew, but in difference, the traces that whoever was there had lost during its wandering, and she is acting on/from the borderline, transcribing it while sketching it and displaying it and opening it wide, to turn it into a threshold and transform it into yet another borderspace.

The matrixial swerving and differentiating are affective gestures that implicate the borderlines between psychic elements that "belong" to several individuals, to different persons. Subjectivity here becomes both diffracted and assembled, both dispersed, partial, and in alliance. Here, the borderline does not function as a frontier-barrier any more. Here come to pass and turn expressive a *lightning of passage*, if to use Foucault's expression together with what Lyotard calls a *spasm* that becomes a joint spasm. Each borderline is, then, also a breadth, a space where affect and trace join in a kind of sense of the individual-in-jointness and become a transitive sense. The matrixial difference, as transgressive swerving and differentiating, implicates a borderline and acts along its length, condensing and opening it into a space, while also diffracting it into few nonconscious lanes. The matrixial borderline interweaves a nonconscious trans-subjectivity, composed of trauma and jouissance. In itself it is the composite of psychic events of encounter, wrapped with affects and memory traces, which shapes and exposes its sense. If transgression, after Foucault, traverses and re-traverses a line that closes itself from behind again and again in a short flickering of a wave, a borderline that retreats anew straight to the horizon of the untraversable, it seems to me that its action receives an unconscious meaning that concerns the human condition only in the partial and shared matrixial borderspace, in the trans-subjective expanse of the individual-in-jointness. Here, in this sphere, the Foucauldian transgression is, indeed, not motivated by negativity or subversion and does not cause the alterity beyond the invisible and untraversable limit to appear as mirror image or mimetic image, because it does not act as a phallic being in expanses conditioned by structures of castration, right from the start. Maybe the matrixial transgression is this desecration that is neither violence in a partitioned world (in the ethical world) nor a victory on barriers that it effaces (in a dialectical, revolutionary world (Foucault, 1994, p. 238). This desecration is a measure of swerving, digression and deviation, reception, and transportation and transmission of the spaces[1] opened at the heart of the borderline itself, which is both the laying out of the marks that create this difference and the traces that this layout leaves around, if and when it occasions the dispersion of the marks and the traces between someone and someother.

The feminine-matrixial difference, which is an impregnation of a borderline—that is not a frontier-barrier of disconnection and separation that hides effacement and displacement behind its action—is originary. This difference is a passage into a sense, not grasped until this moment, which is not dependent upon the schism between signifier and signified, between subject and object, and even between the masculine and the feminine as gender-identities. The matrixial difference is a subjective dimension not derived from the exchange of signifiers that does not refer to the phallic field and to the rift of castration, except on a secondary level of dialectics. This difference is a swerve, intertwined in borderlinking, in plaiting and interweaving of borderlines, and in the opening of a borderspace that the interwoven plaits create. Such a feminine difference is not the effect of social structuring (gender), neither is it the effect of essentialistic raw data that encodes biological difference. This difference is woven in the *relationship to* the female body that is different when you have and when you don't have a female body. This relationship, that creates the difference of the alike and not of the same or of the opposite, is human already at the level of the Real and therefore it is captured already in some human language—be it, to begin with, only the designified language of bodily signs, and the language of affective channeling, and the language of transference that "speaks" with its sensations and affections, and the esthetic language.

The archaic pain or jouissance, that is the-traumatic wound beyond the limit, is inaccessible to the subject wherever it is phallic. The limit, in the phallus, corresponds to the *Ketz* as described in the "Book of Zohar"; the Ketz as a limit is an end, and the end is *the place of no memory.* If the immemorial, the no-memory par excellence, the total Otherness, is the woman-as-archaic m/Other, then her place of no-memory is the final station, from which no transmission is possible.

But where the subject is also matrixial, such no-transmission is impossible. It is impossible for the subject not to be accessible to the traumatic shared-in-difference wound; it is impossible for the subject to tear itself away from the archaic pain or jouissance, and not only of oneself, but also of several others borderlinked to the self upon the pattern of this borderlinking to the archaic-becoming-m/Other. And if in the phallic field, *not to be disconnected* from the immemorial between life and non-life means psychosis, in the matrixial sphere a total disconnection from it is in itself a madness, because in the feminine there is a memory-of-oblivion of and in the borderline a memory of oblivion, different from no-memory in its transgressive affectability, that transmits onward the immemorial. The *Ketz*—a frontier and an end, turns into a *Katze*—a borderline as an open limit, an edge (both words derive from the same root in Hebrew), because where the limit is fluid, crumbled, joined together, and bordersverved in the Real or by artworking to become an edge, the borderline becomes a space and the *Katze* is then *a transport-station of trauma.* Back to Lacan. Beauty, in the form and image of the human body, is the last barrier from the Otherness "beyond" which the artist experiences the "second death." But it can now also be understood, bending toward the Sublime, as a special reactivating of this supplementary femininity, because the same border which serves both as the barrier from the second death and as the barrier from direct apprehension of "sexual rapport," from these relationships which are, according to Lacan, both feminine and "impossible" (Ettinger, 1998a; Lacan, 1972–1973), can become a threshold. In the domain of esthetics, the borderline that separates the human being from experiencing the second death—from the articulation of death in life—converges with the frontier that separates the human being from articulation of the feminine. In the phallic structure, the figure-of-art that transgress this borderline, whether like Oedipus or like Tiresias, is sacrificed to blindness or death. There, for Lacan, even though transgression is feminine, it is not accessible, not to men and not to women either. I am suggesting that from a matrixial angle we can't speak of such a total inaccessibility, rejection, or abjection of the transgressive femininity, but rather of separation-in-jointness with it, whose risks and wonders are beyond the phallic scope. If transgression operates here from the start in a joint borderspace, the inscriptions of the human body within a feminine sphere and their move as what I have named transcryptum toward the visible by art (Ettinger, 1999) are not the last barrier from the Otherness-beyond, but are the creation of a transport-station that enables the passage to partial matrixial almost-otherness. For that reason the poietic-aesthetic feminine transgression vibrates between the beautiful and the Sublime but leads, at the same time, to the domain of ethics, by the operation of wit(h)nessing (Ettinger, 1998b).

Different aspects of trauma and jouissance are dispersed by and with affects, and their traces circulate between I and non-I. Events that profoundly concern my soul and psyche, and that I can't contain and elaborate entirely, are transformed and they fade away and get dispersed in others that thus become wit(h)nesses of/to my own trauma. We can think of events whose traumatic weight is so heavy that I would not be able to contain its memory traces at all. In the matrixial borderspace "my" traces will transgress my limits and will be inscribed in another so that the other crossed in/by me will mentally elaborate them for me. Thus, the "uterine" transgression, in which partial sharing in/of jouissance and trauma takes place, is a model for a particular human transgression, for a wit(h)nessing within the other, that gives birth to phantasms and produces its own trauma and desire. And beauty-affected-by-the-Sublime that is folded in such an occasion disables the obstruction of access to the pain of the Other. Thus, the desire to join-in-difference and differentiate-in-joining with the Other doesn't promise any peace and harmony, because joining is first of all joining within/by the trauma that weakens and bifurcates me, and creates a danger of regression and dispersal in the process of receiving, passing on, and transmitting.

A loss by definitive cut to a point of no trace and no memory is, in the matrixial space, a horror beyond its scope and an implored missing of the occasion of/for encounter. Here, the experience of anticipated future-death in the actual present is not entirely divorced from experiencing life in non-life or in, before and with no-more giving life and yet, co-birth and co-emergence that are no refuge or hideaway from the anxiety of fading and death. Death drive that arises at the horizon of visibility in the tableau is linked to the experience of co-emergence. The effect of beauty-inclined-toward-the-Sublime indicates not only the place of relationships to one's own anticipated death, but also the feminine zone of me "without me" (Lévinas & Ettinger, 1993), the site of the rapport with the death of the other (as the "feminine" for Lévinas), and also the site of the rapport with the non-life in me and in the other—this matrixial feminine with-in-out place which is a before-as-beside time. The effect of this Sublime-beauty is the effect of borderlinking with what had caused the trauma of the other, for whom and in whose place I channel an affective memory, I process the immemorial and transform the memory traces of oblivion, of the other and of the world, and inscribe them fa painting for fa first time.

The matrixial sphere with its processes of metramorphosis forms a difference that is feminine in the sense that it is abstracted from borderlinking to female body. It is also a feminine difference in the sense of the transgression beyond the phallic subjectivizing scope. But it is, before any considerations of this axis, an originary difference. For the matrixial subject, the archaic m/Other is not evacuated or eliminated, she is abpresenced; the subject is still and always somehow borderlinked to the archaic m/Other, and the almost-lost object is still and always partial and trans-subjective. In disabsence, the encounter-Thing and the Thing-event are still offering witness of her abpresence, to any subject that surrenders to trans-subjectivity. The subjective-object, like the fetus between living and not-living-yet, carrying the in-between possibility of future-living and of not-living-any-more, is a trans-subjective-object for another subject who relates to it. The subject, borderlinked to the other as the archaic m/Other while borderlinking to the trans-subjective-object, becomes partial by this same move. It also becomes fragile because it trembles on the borders and transgresses into a zone where in life the non-life is accessed affectedly. The "woman"-artist transgressively accesses the dimension of non-living in life, and experiences the other-*qua*-partial-trans-subjective-object as a desperate part of her own not-One-self that is calling upon her self.

With the affective experience of living non-life in life I would like now to emphasize the profound difference that the idea of the matrix allows us to meditate upon, in relation to the esthetic experience, between death on the one hand and non-life on the other hand, or even between not-yet life, no-more life, non-life, killing, and death. When Antigone, according to Lacan, lives in a "zone between life and death," although she is not yet dead, she is "eliminated from the world of the living" (Lacan, 1992, p. 280). I will paraphrase this idea to say: in the feminine, the artist between life and non-life is not eliminated from the world of living but suffers from the no-memory or the immemorial of the other and of the world, and labors to transport traces of/from the crypted phantoms of the Other and of the world, into the light of partial visibility.

If the esthetic question then engages both the relations between death and the beautiful, and the relations between co-emergence and co-fading that resonate the linkage between life and non-life, then the artist desires to transform death, non-life, not-yet-life, and no-more-life of itself and of the world into art as the theater of the not-One soul, with its jouissance and its trauma. An artist-as-"woman," engaged in co-emerging, co-fading, transcryption, and cross-inscription of traces, is not a celibate subject-hero relating to a limit, but a fragmented and partial interlaced trans-subjectivity, rendered fragile by her wit(h) nessing and transforming, time after time, the limit into a threshold.

The artist-woman wit(h)nesses trauma not necessarily with a direct experience of the event that caused it—trauma of Other, and of the m/Other's others, and of the world—and engraves its unforgettable memory of oblivion in the painting. Affective matrixial trail skirts on sensations' edges and trembles at the limits of the visible when a passion—created by the erotic antenna of the psyche, which is not an isolated drive but an impulse-toward-the-other—immersed in relations of sharing-in-differentiating, becomes a transgressive desire that does receive a human sense, between sign and signification, and does not remain inhuman. When a world, internal and external, from which the artist-woman transfers, through which she traverses and from which she transmits onward, becomes shared with-in-difference via artwork, this world is being presenced; it flickers with lights and spasms and with this lightning of passage in which the painting awakes its strange beauty, pain, and languishing. This beauty is both emergence and fading in the process of making a difference and is the opening of a space at the heart of the border.

No content, no form, and no image can guarantee that such beauty-inclined-toward-the-Sublime will arise, but an occasion for it is opened. A potentiality to infiltrate into and deface the borderspace together with others becomes such a beauty when the painting vibrates, and the spectator attracts to itself and transmits, back to it and onward to others, in the trajectories of the impulse of the wit(h) nessing touching gaze, an affected openness to borderlinking. The *impossibility of not transgressing* demands its own price and sprouts its own sublime-beauty. And the working through of an artwork that also supplies with moments of *Hesed,* of grace and solace, is but *the deepening and widening of the threshold of fragility* at the transport-station of trauma.

This chapter was printed in *Bracha Lichtenberg Ettinger: Artworking 1985–1999.* Brussels: Palais des Beaux-arts, Ghent: Ludion, 2000.

References

Ludion & Brussels: BOZAR – Palais des Beaux Arts, 2000), 91–115.

Ettinger, B. L. (1998a). Supplementary Jouissance. In *The almanac of psychoanalysis* (Vol. 1) Tel Aviv: GIEP.

Ettinger, B. L. (1998b). Wit(h)nessing trauma and the Gaze. In *The fascinating face of Flanders.* Stad Antwerpen.

Ettinger, B. L. (1999). Transcryptum: Memory tracing in/for/with the other. In *La Ville, le Jardin, la Mémoire.* Rome: Villa Medici Publication.

Ettinger, B. L. (2000). Weaving a woman artist within the matrixial encounter-event. In *Regard et éspace-de-bords matrixiels,* Brussels: La Lettre Volée.

Foucault, M. (1994). Préface à la transgression (en hommage à George Bataille). In *Dits et écrits 1954–1988* (Vol. 1). Paris: NRF/Gallimard.

Freud, S. (1919). The "Uncanny." In *Standard edition of the works of Sigmund Freud,* XVIL (pp. 217–252). London: Hogarth, 1955.

Huhn, R. (1993). Moving omissions and hollow spots into the field of vision. In *Catalogue: matrix—borderlines.* Oxford: MoMA.

Lacan, J. [1959–1960] (1992). In J. -A. Miller (Ed.), *Le Séminaire de Jacques Lacan. Livre VII. L'éthique de la psychanalyse.* Paris: Seuil. 1986. Trans, as the ethics of psycho-analysis Denis Porter. London: Routledge.

Lacan, J. (1964). In J. -A. Miller (Ed.), *Le Séminaire de Jacques Lacan. Livre XI. Les quatre concepts fondamentaux de la psychanalyse.* Paris: Seuil, 1973. Trans. Alan Sheridan as the four fundamental concepts of psycho-analysis. New York: Norton, 1981.

Lacan, J. (1972–1973). In J. -A. Miller (Ed.), *Le Séminaire de Jacques Lacan. Livre XX. Encore.* Paris: Seuil, 1975.

Lévinas, E., & Ettinger, B. L. (1993). *Time is the breath of the spirit.* Oxford: MOMA.

Part II

Theory of Trauma

The Trauma of Philosophy

11

Frank Seeburger

To think the disaster (if this is possible, and it is not possible inasmuch as we suspect that the disaster is thought)

Maurice Blanchot (1986, p. 1)

We can only hope in what is without remedy.

Giorgio Agamben (1993, p. 102)

11.1 Introduction

What is philosophically interesting about trauma, whether personal or cultural? What sorts of philosophical questions does it raise? What impact does it have upon such traditional philosophical concepts as truth, time, identity, subjectivity, power, and being itself—and even upon philosophy's own understanding of itself?

The story of the emergence of the modern concept of trauma, as well as sustained inquiry into trauma and its effects down to and including contemporary trauma studies, not only parallels but also often intersects with the story of the development of philosophy during the same period, especially though not exclusively in what is often called "continental European" philosophy. Philosophers themselves write relatively rarely about trauma as such, at least using that term.[1] Nevertheless, when we in effect put philosophy in dialogue with trauma, in the modern sense of the latter term, then we can begin to discern what I take to be a noteworthy convergence between certain key movements of thought in contemporary philosophy, on the one hand, and the evolution of the concept and study of trauma, on the other. For me in my own work as a philosopher at least, that convergence became so increasingly evident, when I did put philosophy in dialogue with trauma in my own thought, that the term *trauma* eventually suggested itself to me as a crucial trope for philosophy itself, not only in its contemporary form but also all the way back to its beginning among the ancient Greeks. In this chapter, I will attempt to share with readers what I have learned about both trauma and philosophy in my own process of responding to that suggestion.

In the first section of this chapter, "Defining Trauma," I will begin with the ancient Greeks, and the birth of philosophy among them. I will start by suggesting a sense in which trauma might plausibly be seen as defining philosophy itself in its very birth, and to have been in that sense a "defining" trauma. That points to *one* way of taking my intentionally ambiguous title for my first section: "defining trauma" in the sense that it was the trauma that did the defining—with philosophy being what that trauma defined. Because philosophy has itself, since its beginnings among the Greeks, been centrally concerned with what has

[1] For one notable exception, see Brison (2002). In addition, philosophers have often expressed themselves after certain traumatic events affecting entire communities have occurred. After September 11, 2001, for example, a number of philosophers offered thoughtful and thought-provoking analyses. Important examples are: Habermas and Derrida in Borradori (2003), Butler (2004, 2009), Derrida (2005), and Žižek (2002).

F. Seeburger, Ph.D. (✉)
Department of Philosophy, University of Denver,
1941 Diamond Dr., Longmont, CO 80504, USA
e-mail: frank.seeburger@gmail.com

Y. Ataria et al. (eds.), *Interdisciplinary Handbook of Trauma and Culture*,
DOI 10.1007/978-3-319-29404-9_11

often been called the very search for "definitions," I will then shift attention to the question of how trauma itself is to be defined—the philosophical task of "defining" trauma in turn, which is the second way of taking the section title, such that it would now be philosophy that is doing the defining, and trauma that is getting defined.

After that opening section, I will then take up, in Sects. 11.2–11.5 of this chapter, four of what I have come to think of as codefinitive aspects of trauma: its "belatedness" (Sect. 11.2), its "excessiveness" (Sect. 11.3), its "importunity" (Sect. 11.4), and its "irremediability" (Sect. 11.5). In each of these four characteristics, trauma presents significant challenges to traditional philosophical conceptions. Accordingly, in each Sects. 11.2–11.5, I will briefly address how the feature of trauma at issue becomes traumatic, as it were, for traditional philosophy and its self-understanding. To put that a bit differently: in the pertinent second parts of each of those four sections, I will suggest just a few ways in which "the trauma of philosophy" in the sense of trauma as it comes to be philosophically defined, becomes "the trauma of philosophy" in the sense of the trauma that philosophy itself undergoes, when it tries to think trauma.

As the remark I just made about the twofold structure of Sects. 11.2–11.5 suggests, it is not only my title for the first section of this chapter (Defining Trauma) that is intentionally ambiguous. So, too, is my title for the whole chapter, "The Trauma of Philosophy"—which I have used again as the title for the sixth and final section of this chapter, in which I turn directly to the correspondences that are there between developments of the modern concept and study of trauma, on the one hand, and developments in modern philosophy as such, on the other.

There are at least *three* senses that can be given to "the trauma of philosophy." I have already touched on two. The first is the sense whereby the expression "the trauma of philosophy" is taken to mean what I would call "philosophically purified" trauma. That is, the expression means something such as "trauma, insofar as it might engage the philosopher's interest," or "trauma insofar as one's attention to it is confined to what is philosophically interesting about it." "The trauma of philosophy" would thus be trauma insofar as it interests philosophy. The second sense, in contrast, takes "the trauma of philosophy" to mean "trauma, insofar as philosophy itself undergoes trauma"—the trauma that happens *to* philosophy itself. It would be trauma, not insofar as it *interests* philosophy, but insofar as it *befalls* philosophy. Finally, the *third* sense of "the trauma of philosophy" is one in which "the trauma of philosophy" would mean neither trauma insofar as it interests philosophy nor trauma insofar as it befalls philosophy. Instead, it would mean the trauma that philosophy itself *is*.

All three senses of "the trauma of philosophy" are actually at issue in each of the sections of this chapter. However, in Sects. 11.1–11.5 the interplay of the first two senses is dominant. That is especially so by virtue of the twofold structure I have given Sects. 11.2–11.5, since in each of those sections I first consider one of what I take to be the four most philosophically interesting features of trauma (the first sense of "the trauma of philosophy") and then turn to some remarks about the challenge trauma issues to philosophy in that feature (the trauma with which taking an interest in trauma ends up, as it were, traumatizing philosophy in turn: the second sense of "the trauma of philosophy"). In contrast, in my sixth and final section I will, as it were, tell the traumatic tale of philosophy itself—or, more precisely, retell that tale as other philosophers, as I read them, have already told it, using their own terms. Thus, it is in the final section that the third sense of "the trauma of philosophy" comes to sound more clearly: the trauma that philosophy itself is.

11.2 Defining Trauma

In more than one way, philosophy itself can be at least plausibly viewed as arising from trauma, or at least amidst trauma. To begin merely with the external circumstances surrounding its historical emergence, what came to be called "philosophy" itself began not in Greece proper, in the bosom of Greek culture at home with itself, but at the peripheries of "Greater Greece," in the Greek colonies of Asia Minor and Italy, places where a multiplicity of diverse cultural influences came together unexpectedly. Encounters with other cultures—as is true of all encounters with what the influential philosopher Emanuel Levinas called "the Other" (Levinas, 1969)—always carry at least some degree of traumatic impact; and it under just such conditions that the way of thinking that came—two centuries later in the works of Plato—to be called "philosophy" was born.

With regard to considerations internal to philosophy as such, rather than just the historical setting within which it emerged, Aristotle, Plato's most famous student, characterized philosophy as having its true beginning—in Greek, its *arche*, a word from which derive various modern English words, including "archaic," "archeology," as well as the suffix "-archy" in such terms as "anarchy" and "oligarchy"—in "wonder;" that condition of coming suddenly to be "dumb-struck," as we say, before the majesty or mystery or simply magnitude of what captures our attention. Being struck dumb in wonder gets thought going. Such a stroke brings one up short and takes one's breath away, to use two other common ways of speaking. They cast one out of the familiar and everyday, and disorient one. In all these ways, being struck with wonder can plausibly be said to be *traumatic*, even though the experience of wonder does not normally carry the strongly negative, painful affect we ordinarily associate with trauma.

Thus—and, in fact, in more senses than the two just mentioned: the external circumstances of philosophy's origin, and the internal nature of that origin itself—trauma can plausibly be seen as defining philosophy ever since its Greek beginnings. In turn, however, once traumatically triggered and eventually come round at last to wonder in the face of trauma itself, it is not at all against its nature for philosophy to set about trying to define trauma in turn.

Indeed, at least since Plato, what has counted as *the* definitive philosophical question has been, "What *is* … such and such?" So, for example, in Plato's *Republic* Socrates asks, "What is *justice*?" In the *Meno*, it is, "What is *virtue*?" It is *courage* in the *Laches*, *piety* in the *Euthyphro*, and so on—in all the Platonic–Socratic dialogues in search of a "definition." It would not be inappropriate, therefore, to begin a philosophical inquiry into trauma with the question of just what trauma itself *is*.

Trauma, of course, is simply the Greek word for "wound." "Hurt" and "defeat" are also possible synonyms for the Greek term. Etymology tells us that *trauma* derives from the presumed Proto-Indo-European root **trau-*, which itself comes from **tere-*, meaning "to rub, turn, rub by turning, or bore"—as even just a trickle of water sustained over a long enough time can bore a hole in rock, for example—and with derivatives referring to twisting, piercing, and the like. From **tere-*, it is relevant to note, the English word *throw* also ultimately derives. That latter word in turn, the modern English *throw*, comes more immediately from the Old English *þrawan*, meaning "to twist, turn, writhe, or curl," and related to Welsh *taraw*, "to strike." In Old English itself, however, *þrawan* was not the usual word for "to throw." Rather, that was *weorpan*, from which, in turn, the modern English *warp* derives, which is related to German *wurf*, derived from the verb *werfen*, meaning "to throw, cast, or hurl."

All of which is just what trauma does. Trauma throws, casts, hurls, twists, and turns those it strikes, rubbing them raw as it bores into them, making them writhe and curl. Clearly, then, the verbal definition of *trauma* as "wound" is appropriate.

There are wounds, however, and then there are wounds.

Accordingly, any philosophical endeavor to define trauma would need to consider just what differentiates a wound that is genuinely *traumatic*, in the full modern sense of that term, from one that is not. After all, not every wound—every "trauma" in the original Greek sense that included any physical cuts, scrapes, burns, gashes, breaks, and smashes such as are still treated today in hospital "trauma wards"—is traumatic in the sense at issue for Freud and others who stamped the term with its full modern sense during the turn from the nineteenth to the twentieth century. Only some of a hospital trauma-ward's traumas are traumatic in that full modern sense. Furthermore, sometimes wounds in the more limited sense turn out to be traumatic only to some of those they strike, not to all. For some, for example, the breaking of a leg may have no more properly traumatic impact than a much lesser physical wound might have on others; but for the next person, that same break may be deeply traumatizing. It all depends on the circumstances.

What are the "circumstances" at issue, those that make a wound "traumatic" in the full modern sense that might be of interest to philosophy? In philosophy itself that question might traditionally be worded as one about the definitive characteristics of trauma—or, in its classic Aristotelian formulation, a question about the *specific difference* between wounds properly called traumatic and wounds *in general*.

Addressing *that* question would then yield something like a philosophical definition of trauma, a sketch of just what trauma "is," philosophically considered. However, that alone would still not fully explain why trauma should be of any such special *philosophical* interest that philosophers would even bother with trying to define it in the first place. Given what trauma is, philosophically defined, what difference does trauma make to philosophy?

As I read it, the history of the emergence of the modern concept of trauma (see Fassin & Rechtman, 2009 for a good general account of that history) suggests that trauma is characterized by the inextricable interconnection of what I will group under the four following features: (1) *belatedness*, (2) *excessiveness*, (3) *importunity*, and (4) *irremediability*. The conjunction of those four characteristics reveals, in my judgment, the full face of trauma—wherein, as is common to faces and proper to characteristics, character expresses itself. I will consider each characteristic in turn, and indicate some of the challenges that each one issues to philosophy, disrupting traditional philosophical conceptions.

My indications are meant to be suggestive only. As befits the very excessiveness of trauma itself as I will address it below, I make no claim to being exhaustive.

11.3 Belatedness

There is evidence that the word *trauma* first entered common English usage in the 1690s and was first used then in the relatively simple medical sense of a physical wound, some blow stuck against and into the body. However, in the 1890s, 200 years after it first entered common English, the term started to be used regularly in the sense of a "psychic" wound as well; a wound to the "mind" or "spirit"—both of which are possible translations of the Greek term *psyche* (*Online Etymology Dictionary*). Specifically, the term came to be extended to cover psychic wounds made by an experiential throw, strike, or turn that may well have caused little or no visible, physical wound at all.

Some of what is especially of philosophical interest about trauma begins to emerge in considering just what sorts of situations occasioned that linguistic shift, whereby in the 1890s the term *trauma* came suddenly, as such shifts are reckoned, to be extended to cover not only physical but also purely psychic wounds. What motivated that shift was the coming of the railroad—and what came along down the rails with it. As railroad tracks and train transportation of goods and persons became more and more common, so too did railroad accidents. In turn, as the number of the victims of such accidents grew, so did the number of lawsuits brought on behalf of those victims, against those who owned, operated, and profited from the railroads and their traffic. Among such suits, an increasingly significant number started to come from those who had been involved in train wrecks and walked away apparently unscathed, but who at shorter or greater durations *after* the accident began to show emotional and behavioral disorders for which no underlying, theretofore hidden *physical* damage could be found. It was adjudication of the issue of the legal liability, if any, for such supposedly *belated* manifestations of such accidents that drove the extension of the term *trauma* to cover cases of that sort, where no physical, bodily trauma ever became visible, but yet significant "wounding" had apparently occurred.

Freud was among the most important of those who helped forge for the new, extended usage of the word *trauma*; the dominant role it has had ever since. Today, someone who says that some event was "traumatic" is ordinarily just understood to be using the term in that more or less Freudian way, rather than in the original, restricted medical sense. Central to Freud's own thinking about trauma is precisely the *belatedness* at issue.

What I am calling "belatedness" is in Freud's German *Nachträglichkeit*, a substantive form derived from the adjective/adverb *nachträglich*. Original translations of Freud's works into English used "deferred action" and "delayed action" to try to capture the sense of the German term. In French, what has become the most common translation is *après-coup*, from *après*, "after," and *coup*, "strike" or "blow." Ordinarily, in French usage *après-coup* simply means "afterwards." However, used not only in the general context of Freud and psychoanalysis but also and especially with reference to trauma, *après-coup* might best be translated, with closer attention to its literal meaning, as "after-shock." So translated, the term is well suited indeed to capture something important about trauma, since traumatic shock definitively sets up waves upon waves of aftershocks.

More is at stake in the belatedness of trauma, however, than the fact that trauma sets off aftershocks. So do earthquakes. What sets trauma apart might be captured by saying that trauma is like an earthquake that does not "register" at all when it first strikes, even on the most sensitive equipment, but that it registers only later. Trauma is just such a shock that manages to register only *belatedly*, in its aftershocks.

How does this first of my four features of trauma, its belatedness, challenge philosophy?

Above all, the belatedness of traumatic shock disruptively challenges the traditional philosophical conception of time and temporality. Trauma time is not the time that ticks off in obedience to the clock. The time that trauma itself "temporalizes," to borrow a key term from Heidegger (1962)—that is, time as trauma concretely spreads or opens it up into the three dimensions of "past," "present," and "future"—is not time in the sense given paradigmatic formulation long ago by Aristotle, who defined it in Book IV of his *Physics* as the "number" of motion, its measure with respect to "before" and "after," as counted out by the succession of "nows" as they tick by.

In Aristotelian time, time as measured by clocks, the past is defined as what already happened and is now over and done with: what once *was* but *is* no longer. Similarly, the future is defined as what has not happened yet and is still to come: what *will be* but *is* not yet. That leaves only the present to truly *be* now. By the traditional concept, the "motion" (as Aristotle calls it) that the instants of time measure out is the very process of "becoming" itself, of "generation and corruption"—arising or coming to be, only then to pass on by again, ceasing any longer to be, giving way to whatever comes next, only for that also to pass by and yield in turn to whatever comes after that, over and over again without end.

Time, so conceived in terms of what passes by "in" time, as it were, was always traditionally juxtaposed to "eternity," itself conceived as what remains untouched by time, "outside" and "beyond" it: the "*supra*-temporal," which always *is* and never *becomes*. Nietzsche, about the same time that the modern concept of trauma was first beginning to develop, insightfully noted that in this traditional conception of time, with its radical opposition of time to eternity, it is really the *past* that takes priority over the other two temporal dimensions, the future and the present. Thus, in *Thus Spoke Zarathustra* (1954, p. 252) he writes simply of "time, and its 'it was!'" Time is, in effect, a machine for generating ever more of the past.

In the temporality proper to trauma, however, the time of the clock—time as traditionally conceived—gets split asunder. In trauma time, as we might call it, the past of trauma is not, in fact, already over and done with. To borrow a famous line from William Faulkner (1950, p. 80), when it comes to the traumatic: "The past is never dead. It's not even past." Indeed, and even more radically, in trauma time it is not just that the past is not past—that is, not just not already passed by and over and done with. It is *still to come*. In trauma time, the past is the future.

Yet it is also the present, insofar as traumatic experience keeps on repeating itself. That is at the heart of Faulkner's insight that the traumatic past never dies, but continues to be all too alive in the present. The time of the clock is a time that will not stay, but always passes on. In contrast, the time of trauma is a stuck time that never passes, no matter how much those stuck within it may wish it would or how hard they may try to make pass.

How are we to think such time, the time of trauma, a time that disrupts the traditional philosophical concept of time and time's passing? That, in short, is the challenge that the "belatedness" characteristic of trauma puts to philosophy.

To address that challenge requires rethinking the entire concept of time—or, rather, just how we go about *conceptualizing* time. For example, "time" is commonly taken to be a highly "abstract" matter, and certainly the traditional conceptualization of time that goes back to Aristotle treats it as a pure abstraction. After all, what could be more "abstract" than *number* and *motion*, those key elements of the Aristotelian definition of time, as recounted above? *Clock*-time is as abstract as can be. In contrast, however, there is nothing more *concrete* than trauma time. The time of trauma, the time trauma "takes," is in fact so *excessively* concrete that it *overwhelms* all endeavors to "comprehend" it in mental "abstractions"—a point with which I will begin my discussion of the second feature of trauma, its "excessiveness."

11.4 Excessiveness

Trauma exceeds the capacity of those it strikes to "process" it. That is the "excessiveness" that co-constitutes trauma, along with "belatedness" and the other two characteristics I am considering. Indeed, it is largely due to its *excessiveness* that trauma always registers only *belatedly*, "after" its initial strike or shock, in its "aftershocks"—in a sort of continuing, continual attempt to catch up with itself. To that degree, the belatedness of trauma is rooted in its excessiveness.

The excessiveness of trauma is its incomprehensible comprehensiveness.

In *The Language of Psychoanalysis* (1973), which became a classic of psychoanalytic literature after its initial publication in France in 1967, Jean Laplanche and J. B. Pontalis provide an exhaustive dictionary of key psychoanalytic terms in the concrete history of their usage within the definitive texts of Freud and subsequent psychoanalysts. Under the entry for "Deferred Action; Deferred" in the English translation of their work, Laplanche and Pontalis remark that in Freud's own definitive conception of *Nachträglichkeit* "[i] t is not lived experience in general that undergoes a deferred revision, but, specifically, whatever it has been impossible in the first instance to incorporate fully into a meaningful context." They immediately go on to add: "The traumatic event is the epitome of such unassimilated experience" (Laplanche & Pontalis, 1973, p. 112).

A sympathetic "deferred revision" of those very remarks today, a revision consistent with Laplanche's and Pontalis's own later works, might well drop the qualifier "in the first instance" in the first line just quoted, and change "unassimilat-*ed*" into "inassimil-*able*" in the second. Such revision would help to bring out that what makes an event traumatic in the first place, in the fullest and richest sense of that term at issue for Freud and psychoanalysis in general, is that the event altogether exceeds the capacities of those to whom it happens to "assimilate" it by somehow giving it "meaning" in the ongoing context of their lives. Instead, all they can do in the face of it, when it initially strikes, is to swoon, one way or another.

When first struck by trauma, those so struck may swoon by entirely losing consciousness. More often, however, the swooning takes the form of a modification of awareness whereby those struck by trauma manage somehow to anesthetize themselves sufficiently against its impact that they can survive it—literally, "overlive" it: live on through and beyond it. Either way, the swoon, the numbing, bears witness that the traumatic blow overflows and overwhelms the capacity of those it strikes to *comprehend* what has befallen them. The traumatized cannot "get their minds around" what has happened to them, as we say colloquially.

That colloquial way of speaking actually captures the literal sense of the word *comprehend*, from Latin *com-*, which here carries the sense of "completely," and *prehendere*, "to catch hold of, seize." To comprehend is to encompass in thought. The excessiveness of trauma is its *incomprehensibility*, in that literal sense.

In turn, that incomprehensibility of traumatic experience is linked, paradoxical as it may sound to say it this way, with the *comprehensiveness* of that same experience. A remark heard frequently from trauma survivors is that after the traumatic event "nothing will ever be the same again." That common remark points to the connection between the incomprehensibly of trauma and its comprehensiveness. What makes an event traumatic in the first place—what makes it so excessive and, therewith, beyond all possibility of comprehension and timely response—is precisely the way in which the event changes not just one thing or one limited range of things, but "*everything*." (In that way, traumatic experience resembles mystical experience, as it also resembles, to give an example from the literature of twentieth century, "existential" philosophy, what Albert Camus called the experience of "the absurd." The connections between all three—the traumatic, the mystical, and the absurd of Camus are well worth philosophical reflection, but to pursue them here would take me too far afield.)

If it is the traditional understanding of *time* that the *belatedness* of trauma disrupts and challenges most directly, in its *excessiveness* trauma begins to disrupt and challenge the traditional philosophical understanding even of *being* as such—and all that goes with it, such as the very idea of "definition," pointedly including the endeavor to give a philosophical definition of trauma itself. Since Plato and, especially, Aristotle, the very notion of definition—the very definition of definition itself, as it were—has been yoked with that of being, and both together with the idea of "limits," which itself has been inseparable from the idea of comprehension, for that matter.

Define comes from Latin *definire*, "to limit, determine, explain," itself from *de-*, in this case used in its intensive or completive sense of "down to the bottom, totally" and hence "completely," and *finire* "to bound, limit," from *finis* "boundary, end." To de-fine is to de-limit, in the sense of drawing the boundaries or borders around something, confining it within its own proper outline or "form"—a favorite term for both Plato and Aristotle, it is worth noting.

But "by definition," as we can rightly say, trauma is that which de-fines or de-limits itself in a very different sense of the prefix *de-*, the purely *privative* sense that is its most common usage in modern English, whereby it functions to undo, cancel, or negate the verb to which it is prefixed, as in the words *defrost*, *de-ice*, *defuse*, and *de-escalate*. "By definition"—which means here: by virtue of the very tendency, sense, direction, or aim of the word, sign, hint, or mark—trauma *exceeds* all limits and undoes all efforts to con-fine it within any boundaries by giving it a clear "definition" in the sense traditionally understood in philosophy. By definition, trauma cannot be defined (including, by the way and for clarity's sake, being defined as "something undefined or even un-definable" since, for one thing, not everything undefined or even un-definable is traumatic).

By thus disrupting the traditional philosophical understanding of what it means to define something, trauma also disrupts, as some of my ways of speaking in the preceding paragraph already suggest, the understanding of such notions as that of marks, hints, signs, or words, that is, of *language* and *signification* themselves. Indeed, by disrupting our way of thinking of definitions and delimitations, trauma also disrupts a whole series of other philosophical concepts connected with that of definition, which is itself, to return to where I began this foray into undoing definition, inseparable from the very concept of being.

In the first place, the very concept of "concept" itself is another concept that the excessiveness of trauma disrupts: the concept of "concept," from Latin *con-* plus *capere*, "to take," from the presumed Indo-European root **kap-*, "to grasp," and used since the fourteenth century with the meaning "take into the mind." Yet, as I began this section by observing, that is precisely what trauma exceeds: the traumatized mind's capacity to "take it in." To rethink the concept of concept in dialogue with trauma, philosophy is thus challenged to rethink just what it is to "think" something in the first place.

In twentieth century philosophy, Heidegger attempted to rethink thinking itself in just such a way. For Heidegger (1968), thinking ceases to be "conceptual" in the standard sense and gets recast as a *recalling* or *recollection* of what calls thinking itself forth and, as such, is always prior to, and inexhaustible by, the thought that *responds* to that original and originating call. What is more, the call of that which calls thinking forth in calling for thinking is what, according to Heidegger (1971), resounds throughout *language*, which thus comes to be thought no longer as a mere means of conveying information, but as what first of all *lets* whatever is *be*—what in one essay (1998) he calls the very "house of Being." These and other elements of Heidegger's thought are rich with suggestions of just what a thinking that tries, in dialogue with trauma, to rethink the nature of thinking itself, and along with it the nature of speaking and language, might look like.

At any rate, trauma's challenge to philosophy to rethink thinking itself cuts to the very heart of the whole philosophical enterprise. As American philosophy Matthew Lipman, whose influential "Philosophy for Children Program" grew out of Lipman's own attempts to address the trauma with which the student movement of the 1960s and 1970s faced American university education (Lipman, Sharp, & Oscanyan, 1980), once defined it, philosophy is "thinking devoted to the improvement of thinking" (Lipman, 1984, p. 51). Accordingly, in challenging philosophy to rethink the whole nature of thinking itself, trauma strikes at the very center of the philosophical enterprise.

11.5 Importunity

By its belatedly excessive, swoon-inducing, incomprehensible comprehensiveness, trauma not only challenges *philosophy* at is very center, but also sets itself up at the very center of any *life* that survives it—that is, any life that literally "over-lives" trauma, "lives through" it. Trauma, once it strikes, continues thereafter to constitute the very dead center of the ongoing lives of those it has struck.

That expression, "*dead center*," is particularly apt—doubly so, in fact. First, the numbness, the deadening, that allows trauma survivors *to* survive, does indeed come to constitute a continuing deadness in the ongoing survivors' lives. Second, that very deadness or numbness in turn takes up a position dead center, as we say, in those subsequent lives, as is manifest in what Freud called the "repetition compulsion": the compulsion to keep on repeating in one's life, in one form or another, the trauma-inducing situation.

Indeed, Freud himself saw clearly that numbness in the face of trauma and the compulsion to repeat the traumatic situation—which is to say the *deadness* and the *centrality* of trauma—go inseparably together. He held that they are really just two sides of one and the same overall effect of traumatic experience. In effect, a traumatic blow raises a question that importunes a response from those whom it addresses, yet at the same time it addresses them with such force as to render them senseless, and therefore incapable even of hearing the question, let alone giving it any adequate answer.

Once posed, however, the question that trauma puts to those it strikes continues to demand an answer. The clamor for an answer grows louder and louder, in fact, the longer it is delayed. That is true in large part because of the very nature of the question being posed. Another, equally frequent remark from trauma survivors, besides the one about nothing ever being the same for them again after they have been traumatized, is that they can "never forget" what happened to them, either. (See, for example: Brison, 2002; Caruth, 1995, 1996; Felman & Laub, 1992; Glassner & Krell, 2006; Herman, 1992; Lifton, 1979.) In fact, the two remarks can easily be taken to be just two different ways of saying the same thing: Because trauma changes everything, whatever we do to try to forget it ends up just confirming yet again that nothing will ever be the same again.

Thus, the importunity of trauma is tied to the excessiveness of trauma through the comprehensiveness of the traumatic impact. What is more, the ineluctable importunity of trauma also links into the incomprehensibility that, together with its comprehensiveness, constitutes trauma's excessiveness.

Something Heraclitus said at the very dawn of philosophy seems prescient today in its obvious relevance to traumatic importunity. "How could one escape the notice of what never sets?" asked Heraclitus two and one-half millennia ago (1964, p. 69). To what Heraclitus thus gives us from so long ago, back at the very beginning of philosophy's long history, can fruitfully be coupled an insight from the contemporary French phenomenological philosopher Jean-Louis Chrétien today, at the very end of that same long road. In *The Unforgettable and the Unhoped For*, Chrétien (2002) notes that it is only what can never be remembered that is truly unforgettable.

In that sense the call "never to forget" a trauma—for example, the oft-heard call never to forget the Holocaust, or more recently the attacks on the Twin Towers in New York in September 2001, or more recently yet the Boston Marathon bombings in April 2013—is always redundant. Trauma cannot be held in memory, not because it is so easy to forget, but because it can never be put there, in memory, in the first place, such that it ever *could* be forgotten. (Within trauma studies themselves, there is wide debate about the related issue of what has been called "the crisis of witnessing.") (See, for example: Felman & Laub, 1992; Laub & Auerhahn, 1995.) In philosophy, perhaps the most important relevant reflection is to be found in Agamben (1999). When Nietzsche underwent his own final mental collapse in the streets of Turin, Italy, in January of 1889, one of the missives of madness he fired off to his friends back in Basel said that the problem was not so much finding him in the first place, but forgetting him once he was found. That message applies to all traumas, not just the trauma that Nietzsche himself was—which brings me to the fourth of the features intertwining in trauma to make it philosophically interesting, trauma's irremediability.

First, however, I want once again to suggest a few more of the disruptive challenges trauma puts to philosophy by way of this third feature, its importunity.

Trauma importunes those it touches to rethink the meaning of their lives, and their ever-impending deaths. No less does it importune philosophy to rethink the basic concepts of life, death, and the relation between them—as the Holocaust, and especially the living-dead "*Muselmänner*" (Muslims), as they were called in the Nazi death camps, gives Italian philosopher Giorgio Agamben (1998, 1999) impetus to rethink them, for example. In *Beyond the Pleasure Principle*, one of the key texts for his formulation and development of his own concept of trauma, Freud linked the compulsion to keep on repeating traumatic experiences to what he introduced in that text as "the death drive," a drive he placed in perpetual conflict with the "pleasure drive" that he references in the book's title (Freud, 1950).

As it emerges in his thought, there is actually a sort of double deadliness about the "repetition compulsion" triggered by trauma. First, as discussed already above, Freud taught that the compulsion to repeat was but one side of the two-sided psychic effect of trauma, that compulsion always being coupled with, and indeed arising from, the numbing or deadening of the state of "shock" trauma triggers by virtue of its incomprehensible excessiveness. Added to that, in its very compulsiveness the repetition compulsion is more suggestive of the mechanism in an automaton than of an adaptive response-pattern in a living being. The compulsion to repeat that arises from trauma has a machine-like deadening deadness of its own.

Freud sets up the relationship between his two "drives" as a dualistic opposition, casting their contest in ancient Greek terms as that between *Eros* and *Thanatos*, Love and Death. However, the details of his account, as well as his repeated returns to re-account for the relation in his later thought until his death, suggest that the two are locked in an embrace that is itself difficult to sort out with regard to its being a love-lock or a death-hold, as it were. The importunate demands trauma placed upon his thought seem to have driven Freud himself to point to an intimate lacing together of the two drives, such that in the heart of life one cannot escape death, nor can death, buried in its grave, escape a certain animation, a literal liveliness.

This compulsively, repetitively importunate deadness at the very heart of life itself defies any effort to avoid or remove it, either through expulsion and defense against its return or through any sort of final, up-lifting, Hegelian synthesis wherein the opposition between death and life—Freud's two "drives"—would somehow be overcome in some higher unity.

Thus, at the very core of what I have been calling the importunity of trauma lies a conflict that can neither be expelled nor, more crucially for modern philosophy, "sublimated" (in Hegel's German: "*aufgehoben*") into some higher concept wherein the conflict gets resolved. By the irresolvable yet abidingly importunate nature of that conflict at its center, trauma disrupts and challenges not only traditional philosophical conceptions of life and death, but also the even broader and deeper philosophical categories—including some that have been fundamental for philosophy ever since Plato. Above all, serious dialogue with trauma challenges philosophy to rethink what Plato in the *Sophist* presents as among the most fundamental of all philosophical categories: the categories of "identity" and "difference"—"sameness" and "otherness"—themselves.

Some endeavors to begin doing just the sort of rethinking trauma requires emerge in some recent philosophical work, especially that of Heidegger (1969) and Heidegger's onetime pupil Emanuel Levinas (1969). Furthermore, as Heidegger suggests, the roots for such rethinking of how it stands between identity and difference, sameness and otherness, can already be discerned in German Idealism—especially in the later Schelling, but also even in Hegel himself.

Ever since Aristotle, Heidegger observes, the standard formula for identity has been "A = A." It then took more than two millennia, by Heidegger's account, before the German Idealists were able to realize that such identity, the equality of the self with itself, was no simple given. It had to be *established*, as we might put it—no less than the universal human "equality" proclaimed, along with "liberty" and "fraternity," in the great French Revolution of 1789, had to be (as it still remains to be) established. The German Idealists thus introduced—to go back to Heidegger's own account, which itself hearkens back especially to Hegel and his terminology—*mediation* into the very heart of identity. Heidegger's own thought in turn—drawing closer at this point to antecedents in the later Schelling rather than to Hegel—endeavors to clear the way for *difference* to install itself at the center of *identity*, as an "a-byss" (*Ab-grund*) out of which identity, as the very "ground" or "basis" (*Grund*) of whatever is, must first arise.

Insofar as trauma breaks the connection of simple equality of oneself with oneself, it calls for such philosophical endeavors as Heidegger's. Trauma introduces just such an irreducible disparity into selfhood, an original difference into identity itself, as Heidegger explores in his thinking. To borrow the title of one of twentieth century French philosopher Paul Ricoeur's final books (1992), in trauma one no longer encounters oneself, but instead encounters *Oneself as Another*. From a Levinasian perspective—and Ricoeur's book is in part an attempt to incorporate Levinasian themes into his own thought—we might say that trauma breaks open the "totality" within which "the ego" seeks to secure itself by excluding from that totality whatever is not "the Same" as itself. Trauma shatters that totality, and opens "the Same" to "the Other"—an "Other" that the self, according to Ricoeur's eventual response, finally discovers always already to have been there at the very center of itself.

Thus, as manifest in trauma, the relationship not only between life and death, but also, and even more fundamentally, between identity and difference, sameness and otherness, as such can be grasped neither as mutually exclusive opposition nor as dialectically inclusive synthesis. Facing trauma puts philosophy in the position of having to rethink all those basic concepts. The rupture of relations, even if only relations of simple opposition, between the two anchors of such fundamental binaries of thought, proves to be beyond fixing by traditional philosophical means. That is itself traumatic for philosophy, confronting it with the task of leaning how still to think of, and in terms of, ruptures that remain beyond remedy—which brings me to my fourth and final characteristic of trauma: its irremediability.

11.6 Irremediability

By virtue of the belatedness that always attaches not accidentally but definitively to it, one can never catch up, as it were, with remembering trauma. The traumatic experience is always already beyond recall just as soon as it happens. In *that* sense, in fact, traumatic experience could be said to never really be "experienced" at all: made to be an event *within* experience. Rather, it is one that *defines the very parameters of subsequent experience*. Traumatic experience is the encounter with the unsurpassable bounds of experience itself, the experience of an ultimate limit to what can be experienced, but which as such belongs *to* experience itself, de-fining and de-limiting it as such—a center of deadness that henceforth sits dead in the very center of experience itself, centering it.

To say, as I just did in the preceding paragraph, that there is a sense in which "traumatic experience could be said never really to be 'experienced' at all," is not to say that no one is ever traumatized. It is not to deny that trauma occurs. In fact, to make my point I could say that it is only those who *have* been struck by traumatic blows—only, that is, trauma *survivors*—who "could be said never really to 'experience' trauma" in the sense I mean. Accordingly, if trauma survivors themselves can be said in that sense "never to have experienced trauma," that is not at all in the sense that they have never been struck by traumatic blows, as someone who was said "never to have experienced divorce" would typically be taken to be someone who has never been divorced. Paradoxically put, it would only be those who *have* experienced trauma who have never *experienced* it, in the sense at issue. It is precisely as what remains not only un-experienc*ed* but also un-experience-*able* that, once it *is* "experienced" (that is, once the traumatic blow has been struck), trauma ever after remains the doubly dead center around which survivors' lives must subsequently revolve.

Insofar as that is the case, there is no resolution to that perpetual revolution. In that sense, trauma cannot be "fixed." That is, the traumatic event can never be canceled out, in effect, and the traumatized individual returned to an original trauma-free condition. In an important way, the traumatic wound always remains open (Seeburger, 2013).

Not only can trauma in that sense not be "fixed," but also all endeavors to "recover" from it always come too late, at least if by *recovery* one means the same as *cure*, in the sense of complete elimination. Caught up in traumatic belatedness, endeavors to find such eliminative recovery always fall short. Overwhelmed by the excessiveness of trauma's incomprehensible comprehensiveness, they are always still subject to its importunate demands.

In the sense at issue, there is therefore no "remedy" to trauma, which is to say, to repeat, no means of counteracting it in such a way as to eliminate it. There is no "curing" of it, in that sense—just as, according to AA's "Big Book," *Alcoholics Anonymous*, there is no "cure" for alcoholism (Alcoholics Anonymous, 2001). There is no "getting over" it, at least if one thinks of that the same way we think of getting over a cold, or getting over a hurdle on our way to achieving some goal. The harder and more compulsively we keep on repeating the attempt to get over trauma in that sense—as the very un-stilled, un-still-able importunity of trauma itself dictates that we indeed *will*, until and unless we can finally find and learn another way of understanding and approaching "getting over" it—the more trauma clings to us, like our own shadow does when we try to outrun it.

If by "recovery" from trauma we mean any return to a presumed pre-traumatic or non-traumatized condition, a condition in which the traumatic event is somehow canceled out and everything is made "as good as new," as the saying goes, then I would say that there is *no* recovery from trauma. If that is the sort of thing we mean by "getting over" trauma, then I would say that the only way of ever genuinely getting over trauma is by letting go of the very effort to "get over" it.

Recovery from trauma cannot be a matter of finally succeeding in closing the wound. It must instead be a matter of learning to let the wound stay open—of learning how to stay open *to it*, rather than stiffening to defend oneself against it and against any further wounding. In *Genesis*, the Biblical Jacob comes away with the mark of a permanent limp from his night-long wrestling match with the angel—which is to say the manifestation—of God. Just so is it characteristic of trauma, once it strikes, permanently thereafter to hobble those it has struck.

In the case of this fourth and final characteristic of trauma that I am considering, its "irremediability," there is good evidence that philosophy has already gone a long way toward responding in advance to the challenge that trauma, through that feature, addresses to it. That challenge is, above all, to rethink the nature of such interconnected categories as health, vitality, recovery, disease, and healing. I will give what for me is a prime example of how such rethinking has already been well underway for some time.

Late in the nineteenth century, Nietzsche suggested that our whole way of thinking about health and vitality needs to be radically revised. Instead of thinking of health and vitality in terms of the *absence* of sickness or disease, he said, we need to start thinking of the former in terms of the capacity to *tolerate* the latter. Thus, the more disease and disorder the organism can digest and actively incorporate into itself without succumbing, the more alive and healthy the organism.

Nietzsche pointedly extended that idea to cover not only single individuals but also communities and peoples as a whole. Thus, he maintained, the healthiest, most vital and vibrant societies are not those from which crime and social disorder has been most completely eliminated, but those that are able to tolerate the very highest degree of criminality and deviation and still keep buzzing right along.

That counter-intuitive projection of life and health need not be confined within the philosophical borders within which Nietzsche himself formulated it, the borders of his metaphysics—or, as he would have it, given his own usage of such traditional philosophical terms, his anti-metaphysics—of the "Will to Power." Rather, the new understanding that he outlines is itself vital and healthy enough easily to tolerate being torn from the philosophical womb wherein it was born, and cast loose to fend for itself. It is certainly the sort of disruptive, disrupted reinterpretation of what it means to be fully alive and glowing with health that *trauma* challenges thought to offer.

By such an interpretation, to "recover" from trauma—just as, not at all accidentally, to recover from alcoholism or other addictions—is not to be "cured" of the effects of trauma, and most certainly not to manage at last to ensconce oneself in some sort of bubble of complete security against future traumatization. Indeed, all efforts at such cure and elimination can ultimately only strengthen the importunity of trauma, turning up the volume of trauma's compulsively repeated insistence on being faced and no longer avoided. The greater the effort to close the traumatic wound and insure oneself against any further such wounding, the more compulsively the trauma repeats itself, demanding proper attention. Such attempts, either individually or collectively, to secure oneself against trauma thus only worsen the devastation. In that way—to borrow again from Nietzsche—the wasteland can only grow.

Thus, especially with regard to this fourth feature of trauma, what I am calling its irremediability, philosophy has already more than begun to meet the challenge that trauma issues to thinking. Furthermore, from later modern philosophy beginning with Nietzsche, both trauma studies and, far more importantly, individuals and societies struck by trauma can perhaps begin to learn new, genuinely healing ways to face trauma and the irreparable changes it brings.

That the philosophy of the last century and a half contains such resources for trauma studies and above all for trauma survivors themselves, may well be because during that time philosophy at last ceased—or at least began to cease—to avoid the trauma at its own center and began instead to face it. At any rate, having opened this chapter by remarking that in multiple senses philosophy itself can plausibly be said to have been born in trauma, I will end it with a reflection on how the entire trajectory of philosophy across its history from the ancient Greeks to the present day can itself be read as a story of trauma and, even more importantly, of the possibility of genuine recovery from it.

That very tale of the whole history of philosophy as a story of trauma is, in fact, nothing I am making up on my own. It is a tale already told by various, important, recent philosophers themselves. In the sixth and final part of this chapter, I will briefly retell the story that some of those philosophers themselves have already told. I will thereby also try to show the very convergence of recent philosophy and the recently emergent study of trauma to which I also pointed when I began.

11.7 The Trauma of Philosophy

Nietzsche, with whom I ended the preceding section, is also good for beginning this one. Nietzsche himself treats the whole history of philosophy as a story of the long recovery from an initial trauma, though he does not use that specific term. He provides perhaps his own best summary of the story in *Twilight of the Idols*, one of his final works, written not long before he suffered mental collapse early in 1889, never to return to full lucidity before his death in 1900. In that late work, in a single brief passage of only a little over a page in length (1954, pp. 485–486), he recounts, as he puts it himself in the title to the piece, "How the 'True World' Finally Became a Fable: The History of an Error." The history—that is, the (presumably) "true" story—at issue is that of the emergence, spread, and eventually final, total victory of what Nietzsche labels "nihilism," which he describes and defines in turn as "the de-valuation of all values." It is the emptying of everything of all "value," casting humanity adrift in eternally recurring meaninglessness.

Although, as I have said, Nietzsche does not highlight the term *trauma* in his account of nihilism, his "history of an error," surely nothing could be more traumatic than what he describes! The triumph of nihilism, conceived as the stripping of all meaning from human life, is a traumatic blow to the very heart of humanity itself. That trauma does not just strike certain individual human beings or certain human communities. Rather, as Nietzsche conceives nihilism, the blow that it delivers strikes at the very core of the *humanity* of humankind as such.

As he recounts the history of philosophy, Nietzsche gives a nice ironic twist to the standard, traditional depiction of Plato by identifying the latter as the one to have taken the first definitive step along the road of nihilism itself. Nietzsche maintains that it is from the very emergence of the notion of a "true" world—the world as it truly is, according to Plato, when at last we rise to the level of the purely intellectual vision of what he calls Ideas or Forms—in distinction from the world of mere sensory appearance or semblance, that nihilism actually takes birth. Christianity, by another wonderfully ironic twist, then takes the next major step along the nihilistic road, followed by Kant and German Idealism, then by nineteenth century positivism, and finally culminating in Nietzsche himself—or at least in what he heralds.

The same nihilism the history of which he thus recounts in *Twilight of the Idols* is the black snake that, in a parable from his earlier *Thus Spoke Zarathustra*, has crawled into the throat of humanity, figured in the parable as a sleeping shepherd, and bitten itself fast there, to the horror of Zarathustra, who has chanced upon the scene in a dream. Filled with dread, hatred, and nausea, along with a sickening pity, Zarathustra (1954, p. 271) finds welling up from everything within him the cry, "Bite! Bite its head off! Bite!"

Thus, as though it were not bad enough already that an ugly, revolting black snake has bitten itself fast inside humanity's own throat, that same humanity is now called upon to stop struggling and trying to pull the awful thing out, and instead to bite *into* it! Bite into it—and let all the pus and blood and ooze of it fill one's mouth till it runs out the corners, and trickles down the throat into the stomach? One is tempted to ape Herman Melville's character "Bartleby, the Scrivener," and reply that one would prefer not to.

What more wonderful image of trauma itself could be asked for? That is most especially true for the depiction of the road of "recovery" from trauma, the "overcoming" of it, that Nietzsche's image contains: recovery consisting precisely in *abandoning* the effort to eradicate the trauma and get back to one's business as usual, instead turning *into* the trauma, *opening to it*, and to all the horror and loathing it brings with it. Furthermore, conjoining the parable in *Zarathustra* with the history from the later *Twilight of the Idols* lets one see the entire arc of philosophy from its beginnings with the ancient Greeks down to the present day—and beyond, into the future that opens out only in the completion of that arc in the turn whereby everything "reverses" itself, and a paradoxical "recovery" occurs—as but a single tale. That tale is one of traumatic numbing and compulsive repetition until, at last, the importunity of the trauma grows so great that it can no longer be avoided or expelled, and must instead be ingested and digested, to transform the deadness at its center into the very gate through which one enters into life.

It is actually that very same gate through which another German philosopher also bade his readers enter, in a work he began during World War I, while he was a soldier on the Eastern Front, and finished shortly after the war, in 1919, 30 years after Nietzsche's breakdown in Turin. Franz Rosenzweig was a friend and collaborator with Martin Buber and one of the most vital agents of the resurgence of Judaism and the Jewish community in Germany between the two World Wars, before the Nazis and their death camps. Rosenzweig ends *The Star of Redemption*, his major work, with just that gate, even using that very term to name the closing section of the entire, three-part book. The gate at issue leads, to use Rosenzweig's own last two words in the book: "Into life" (1985, p. 424).

As for that *from or out of which* that final gate into life leads, Rosenzweig tells us that in the very *first* words of the very same book: "From death"—or rather, as Rosenzweig himself immediately adds in correction, "from the *fear* of death" (1985, p. 3, emphasis added, translation modified to accord with German original). The "redemption" which is the topic of the third and final part of the book, the part that ends with the gate "into life," is no escape from death itself. It is, rather, the liberation from the *fear* of death—the fear of that final trauma that begins to traumatize us from the moment we are born, or at least born into the awareness that we are mortal, and to rob us of our own capacity fully to live life itself now, today.

By the account Rosenzweig gives in the rest of his introduction to the first part of *The Star*, what immediately arises "from death, from the fear of death" is nothing other than philosophy itself. At least that is so for all philosophy "under the figure of Socrates," as I have put it elsewhere (Seeburger, 2014). I will use that figure, the figure of Socrates, to explain what Rosenzweig is saying.

The Socrates at issue is the one Plato presents in his dialogues, above all in the *Phaedo*, which shows us Socrates on the day of his death. In his depiction Plato also shows Socrates off to us, as it were. He presents him, precisely, as the hero who will slay the monster of the fear of death that holds youth in its thrall, just as the Theseus of Greek myth once slew the Minotaur at the heart of the Labyrinth in Crete, to free Athens from the curse of recurrently having to sacrifice the best of its youth to that beast.

Millennia later, however, Rosenzweig will have none of that. Instead, as he presents it in *The Star*, philosophy under the figure of such a Socrates is nothing short of a form of suicide, that form namely in which one resigns and consigns oneself to living a mere shadow of genuine life, denying the terms of the problem death sets one by fleeing to the realm of the Ideas or Forms—that is, into just the sort of supposedly "true" world above and beyond this one that Nietzsche pilloried in his "History of an Error."

Then, too, there is Heidegger, born in 1889, 3 years after Rosenzweig, and whose own magnum opus *Being and Time* (1962) first appeared just 2 years prior to the latter's death in 1929 from Atromyotrophic Lateral Sclerosis (ALS). Heidegger reads the entire history of philosophy as the obscuration and forgetting of what he characterizes in *Being and Time* as "the question about the meaning [or sense: German *Sinn*] of Being" (the question of just what this says: "to be"), an obscuration and forgetting that can only be salvaged in a "repetition" (*Wiederholung*, the same word that Freud uses in speaking of the "repetition compulsion," *Wiederholungszwang*) of that whole history wherein that meaning or sense is at last retrieved. Seen within the context of Heidegger's whole opus, that retrieval, however, is no dragging forth of Being out of hiding, as it were, and demanding it tell us what sense it makes. Rather, it is a recalling of Being precisely as the unending interplay of revelation and withdrawal, sending and withholding, disclosure and hiding. Such a retrieval or repetition is an event-ful *letting Being be*, rather than attacking it with just the right "method" for establishing "control and dominion" over it, to borrow terms and ideas from Descartes' *Discourse on Method*. Thus, in Heidegger's thought, as in both Nietzsche's and Rosenzweig's, the story of philosophy is told as a story of the flight *from* trauma at last turning around into learning to live *with* it—and the lesson is delivered that living with it is really the only way to become fully alive in the first place.

Telling the history of philosophy as a tale of trauma, even if not called by that name, did not pass away with Nietzsche, Rosenzweig, and Heidegger—who did not die till 1976. That same story has continued to be told in various versions since then, by numerous later philosophers.

Heidegger's version of that tale had honored Nietzsche, but nevertheless placed the latter still within the ongoing obscuration and forgetting of Being, before the final "turn" into a retrieving recovery of the story as a whole. Emanuel Levinas, one of Heidegger's students, who was at least as heavily influenced by Rosenzweig's *Star* as he was by Heidegger, pulled the same thing on Heidegger that the latter had pulled on Nietzsche. In *Totality and Infinity* (1969) and other works, Levinas told the story of philosophy as a recurrent, persistent movement to incorporate the infinity of "the Other" into the totality of "the Same," and he ranked Heidegger among the totalizers.

Contemporary French philosopher Alain Badiou has more recently done the same (if not the Same) to Levinas as Levinas did to Heidegger, who did it to Nietzsche. Himself effecting what he perceives to be a retrieving repetition of Plato against the critique of him from Nietzsche on, Badiou sees Levinasian emphasis on "the Other" as the contemporary continuation of a flight from the disruptive eruption of truth itself, which he conceives no longer as "being" but as "event." For Badiou, the event of truth, that is, the event as which truth itself occurs or literally takes place, is no less a lightening-bolt of in-sight than it is in Heidegger. Heidegger's version of the traumatic tale of philosophy has truth striking humanity out of the mold of the "subject" and into that of what he calls "*Dasein*," the "there" (*da*) of "Being" (*Sein*), like a coin being struck from ore at a mint. In Badiou's (2001) version the "human animal" is struck out of itself and into the "subject of a truth," a subject whose whole and sole ethical responsibility is to be faithful to the truth that has so struck. By either version, however, being struck by lightening, most especially by the lightening of truth, remains traumatic. So, too, does the relation to the whole history of philosophy as the story of just such trauma.

I could easily go on. Go on, for one, to Giorgio Agamben (1998), the contemporary Italian philosopher who tells the traumatic tale of philosophy yet again differently, as one that culminates in the going-global of the Nazi death-camp system—which is surely trauma enough to jolt even the most jaded. Before Agamben, there was Jacques Derrida, in whom philosophy embodied itself as a patient Penelope at night, unweaving the tapestry she had woven during the preceding 2500-year-long day. There is also Jean-François Lyotard, whose own meta-narrative in *The Postmodern Condition* (1984) told the traumatic tale of the emergence of philosophical "postmodernity" from the death of all philosophical "meta-narratives," ending a long process from Plato to Wittgenstein—who is yet another traumatic figure from the first half of the twentieth century. In Wittgenstein's later works he broke the silence to which philosophy itself had led him, and itself, at the end of his *Tractatus Logico-Philosophicus*, published shortly after World War I. The later Wittgenstein treated philosophy itself, including his own earlier thought, as one long, uniquely peculiar misunderstanding, as it were, and said that what he ended up doing was just to try to show the philosophical fly the way out of the philosophical fly-bottle.

There are yet others to whom I could keep going on, but I have surely already gone on long enough to make credible my claim that one can discern a convergence worth noting between much of recent philosophy, on the one hand, and the even more recent study of trauma. It also suffices to allow me to draw my discussion to an end by suggesting that looking at philosophy itself through the lens of trauma can permit us to see that, as befits trauma as such, trauma has actually been there in philosophy itself all along. Guided by that vision, we can construct a plausible account—as, in fact, we can already find in such recent philosophers as Nietzsche, Rosenzweig, and Heidegger—in accordance with which philosophy itself is not only born in and from trauma, but then also follows a traumatic trajectory until, at last, philosophy today is challenged to assume responsibility for its own traumatic provenance and nature. By rising to that challenge philosophy would only be following the advice of one of its own: Nietzsche's advice to become who one is, and has indeed always been, but only as always still to be.

Thus does trauma come to be the trauma of—and for—philosophy.

11.8 Conclusion

In the opening paragraph of this chapter, I wrote that when I put philosophy in dialogue with trauma in my own thought, the term trauma eventually came to suggest itself to me as what I there called "a crucial trope for philosophy itself." In the just-completed sixth and final section of this chapter, I have, in effect, used that very figure or trope to retell the tale of philosophy as a number of important recent philosophers have themselves already told it. Telling the tale of philosophy—that is, recounting the history of philosophy itself—as such a tale of trauma can help philosophers in more than one way. At least that is true for me as a philosopher.

For one thing, telling philosophy's history as a tale of trauma allows the philosopher to hear an underlying accord sounding through what otherwise sounds like no more than discord between the major voices of recent and contemporary philosophy that I mention in the final section. As different as Nietzsche, Rosenzweig, Heidegger, Levinas, Badiou, Agamben, Derrida, Lyotard, and Wittgenstein may be—and have taken themselves to be, as they certainly have—they can all be brought under that same trope or sign of trauma. All tell a tale of the history of philosophy, and of their own place in it, that can be retold as a tale of trauma. Hearing the traumatic harmony, as it were, of such a rich diversity of voices does not in the least detract from hearing the individual voices themselves, any more than the harmony of instrumental voices in a well-wrought musical symphony does. To the contrary, the harmony lets the brilliance of the individual voices sound all the more clearly in their individuality. That is no small gain.

For another thing, telling the history of philosophy as a tale of trauma can also help to free philosophers from just compulsively repeating that history, and free them to find new, hitherto unheard of, ways of continuing tell the philosophical tale. Those new possibilities, whatever they might turn out to be, would have to emerge from philosophy heeding, in effect, Rosenzweig's admonition to stop being driven by the *fear* of death, that universal human trauma, and instead to turn and face it. That is, philosophy would need to stop running along the path of the *avoidance* of trauma, and it would instead need to turn and pass "through" the trauma—to find what has all along been waiting there, *in* that trauma as it were.

Such philosophy would no longer be under what I have called the figure of Socrates, which means, at least as Rosenzweig tells the story of philosophy, a figure of *suicide*. Instead, it would come under the figure of what might be called, following but adding to Rosenzweig, a figure of genuine *recovery*. Seen in such a literally transfigured way, the whole, long story of philosophy becomes a tale of how the compulsively repetitious avoidance of a defining trauma culminates finally by turning, after many centuries and altogether unexpectedly, into recovery in the face of it.

As such, the story of philosophy can offer itself, in turn, as a model for thinking about trauma as such. From the story of philosophy told as a tale of trauma, the traumatized and those who study and try to help them may then be able to draw important resources, as I indicated already in my fifth section on the "irremediability" of trauma above, for gaining greater clarity about just what would constitute true "recovery" from trauma, whatever that trauma may be.

By offering such a resource for recovery from trauma, philosophy for its own part can be seen as doing no more than repaying its debt to trauma, as it were, for the rich, enriching challenges that it puts to philosophy. In paying its debt to trauma by rising to those challenges, philosophy would just be continuing its own process of ongoing transfiguration. Thus, in paying its debt to trauma, and thereby enriching trauma studies and endeavors to assist trauma survivors, philosophy would not be losing any riches of its own. Rather, the more philosophy repaid, the more it would gain it all back again new, like Job at the end of his own story. It would thereby continue to receive, and give thanks for, the *gift* of trauma.

References

Agamben, G. (1993). *The coming community*. Minneapolis: University of Minnesota Press.

Agamben, G. (1998). *Homo sacer: Sovereign power and bare life*. Stanford: Stanford University Press.

Agamben, G. (1999). *Remnants of Auschwitz: The witness and the archive*. New York: Zone Books.

Alcoholics Anonymous. (2001). *Alcoholics anonymous* (4th ed.). New York: A.A. World Services.

Badiou, A. (2001). *Ethics: An essay on the understanding of evil*. London and New York: Verso.

Blanchot, M. (1986). *The writing of the disaster*. Lincoln: University of Nebraska Press.

Borradori, G. (2003). *Philosophy in a time of terror: Dialogues with Jürgen Habermas and Jacques Derrida*. Chicago: University of Chicago Press.

Brison, S. J. (2002). *Aftermath: Violence and the remaking of a self*. Princeton: Princeton University Press.

Butler, J. (2004). *Precarious life: The powers of mourning and violence*. London and New York: Verso.

Butler, J. (2009). *Frames of war: When is life grievable?* London and New York: Verso.

Camus, A. (1955). *The myth of Sisyphus and other essays*. New York: Alfred A. Knopf.

Caruth, C. (Ed.). (1995). *Trauma: Explorations in memory*. Baltimore: Johns Hopkins University Press.

Caruth, C. (Ed.). (1996). *Unclaimed experience: Trauma, narrative, and history*. Baltimore: Johns Hopkins University Press.

Chrétien, J. L. (2002). *The unforgettable and the unhoped for*. New York: Fordham University Press.

Derrida, J. (2005). *Rogues: Two essays on reason*. Stanford: Stanford University Press.

Fassin, D., & Rechtman, R. (2009). *The empire of trauma: An inquiry into the condition of victimhood*. Princeton: Princeton University Press.

Faulkner, W. (1950). *Requiem for a nun*. New York: Random House.

Felman, S., & Laub, D. (1992). *Testimony: Crisis of witnessing in literature, psycho-analysis, and history*. London and New York: Routledge.

Freud, S. (1950). *Beyond the pleasure principle (J. Strachey, Trans.)*. New York, NY: Liveright. Original work published 1920.

Glassner, M. I., & Krell, R. (Eds.). (2006). *And life is changed forever: Holocaust childhoods remembered*. Detroit: Wayne State University Press.

Heidegger, M. (1962). *Being and time*. New York: Harper.

Heidegger, M. (1968). *What is called thinking?* New York: Harper.

Heidegger, M. (1969). *Identity and difference*. New York: Harper.

Heidegger, M. (1971). *On the way to language*. New York: Harper.

Heidegger, M. (1998). Letter on humanism. In *Pathmarks*. Cambridge: Cambridge University Press.

Heraclitus (1964). In M. C. Nahm, (Ed.), *Selections from early Greek philosophy*. New York: Appleton-Century Crofts.

Herman, J. (1992). *Trauma and recovery: The aftermath of violence—from domestic abuse to political terror*. New York: Basic Books.

Laplanche, J., & Pontalis, J. P. (1973). *The language of psychoanalysis*. New York: W. W. Norton.

Laub, D., & Auerhahn, N. C. (1995). *Knowing and not knowing: Psychoanalytic inquiry, 5.1.*. London and New York: Routledge.

Levinas, E. (1969). *Totality and infinity: An essay on exteriority*. Pittsburgh: Duquesne University Press.

Lifton, R. J. (1979). *The broken connection: On death and the continuity of life*. New York: Simon and Schuster.

Lipman, M. (1984). The cultivating of reasoning through philosophy. *Educational Leadership, 42*(1), 51–56.

Lipman, M., Sharp, A. M., & Oscanyan, F. S. (1980). *Philosophy in the classroom*. Philadelphia: Temple University Press.

Lyotard, J. F. (1984). *The postmodern condition*. Minneapolis: University of Minnesota Press.

Nietzsche, F. (1954). *The portable Nietzsche*. New York: The Viking Press.

Ricoeur, P. (1992). *Oneself as another*. Chicago: University of Chicago Press.

Rosenzweig, F. (1985). *The star of redemption*. Notre Dame: University of Notre Dame Press.

Seeburger, F. (2013). *The open wound: Trauma, identity, and community*. Seattle: CreateSpace.

Seeburger, F. (2014). *God, prayer, suicide, and philosophy: Reflections on some of the issues of life*. Seattle: CreateSpace.

Žižek, S. (2002). *Welcome to the desert of the real: Five essays on September 11 and related dates*. London and New York: Verso.

Irresponsible Nonsense: An Epistemological and Ethical Critique of Postmodern Trauma Theory

12

Anne Rothe

12.1 Introduction

The trauma concept rose to discursive dominance in literary and cultural studies with Shoshana Felman and Dori Laub's *Testimonies: Crisis of Witnessing in Literature, Psychoanalysis, and History* (1992), which "headed the boom in the transformation of Yale Deconstruction into trauma theory" (Luckhurst, 2008, p. 8). The process was reinforced by Cathy Caruth's edited volume *Trauma: Explorations in Memory* (1995) and her monograph *Unclaimed Experience: Trauma, Narrative, and History* (1996). These three texts established the research paradigm for the new discipline of trauma studies that quickly penetrated the humanities and rose to the status of master narrative, not least because it both reflected and reinforced the trauma culture zeitgeist of the 1990s (Luckhurst, 2003; Rothe, 2011).

While trauma studies scholarship has moved above and beyond these foundational texts over the past two decades, my radical critique, which expands on the arguments of Ruth Leys (2000), Wulf Kansteiner (2004, 2008), and Harald Weilnböck (2008), challenges trauma theory as a research paradigm because it was built on such a deeply flawed foundation. The following argument is thus part of what I would characterize as an external critique of postmodern trauma theory generated by scholars who themselves do not partake in the discourse they analyze.[1] As such, it is a fundamental critique that essentially rejects trauma theory and does not seek to reform and advance any of the arguments made in the three inaugural texts cited above. Moreover, the discursive mode of this external critique could be described as polemical, which I take to reflect an emotional response to a discourse that is not only epistemologically untenable but also and especially ethically irresponsible.[2] It thus differs significantly from internal critiques of trauma theory offered by scholars like Karyn Ball, Stef Craps, Geoffrey Hartman, Dominick LaCapra, and

A. Rothe, Ph.D. (✉)
Department of Classical and Modern Languages, Literatures, and Cultures, Wayne State University, 487 Manoogian Hall, Detroit, MI 48202, USA
e-mail: au8313@wayne.edu

[1] Leys' socio-culturally contextualized intellectual history of the trauma concept does not employ any of the arguments made in the three inaugural texts of postmodern trauma theory. Moreover, the last two chapters in which she radically critiques both van der Kolk's arguments and their reception in trauma theory as well as Caruth's arguments differ significantly in their discursive mode of polemical argument from the predominantly descriptive and narrative mode employed in the previous chapters. Therefore, I consider her critique like Kansteiner's, Weilnböck's, and my own to reflect a discursive position that is external rather than internal to trauma theory.

[2] Kansteiner (2004) is a notable exception. However, in the essay he coauthored with Weilnböck, the authors do employ polemical discourse in order to radically critique the notion of trauma as conceptualized in postmodern theory.

Y. Ataria et al. (eds.), *Interdisciplinary Handbook of Trauma and Culture*,
DOI 10.1007/978-3-319-29404-9_12

Susannah Radstone who seek to revise and develop trauma theory despite their often substantial critique of the foundational texts and the diversity of their arguments.

A second scholarly tradition within which my argument is rooted is the radical critique of the misuse of scientific research in postmodern theory. In *Fashionable Nonsense: Postmodern Intellectuals' Abuse of Science*, physicists Alan Sokal and Jean Bricmont (1998) expanded the critique of postmodern appropriations of scientific concepts from Sokal's (1994) (in)famous *Social Text* essay while changing the discursive mode from simulation to empirical analysis. My essay title explicitly invokes their monograph because I will argue that a similarly nonsensical appropriation of scientific research was generated in postmodern trauma theory. Substituting the qualifying adjective indicates that the likewise fashionable transformation of the trauma concept from signifying the psychological aftereffects of extreme violence into a metaphor for a stipulated postmodern crisis of signification is not only epistemologically untenable but also ethically irresponsible.

12.2 Interdisciplinary Gestures

Rather than indicative of the extent to which Caruth's theory is flawed, Roger Luckhurst (2008, p. 13) argues that, paradoxically, "the length of Leys' critique acts as a strange sort of monument to its importance." In defense of Caruth and trauma theory at large, he invokes sociologist of science Bruno Latour's (1987, p. 201) notion that knowledge is structured in multidimensional networks and the significance and explanatory power ascribed to a concept are determined by its degree of associative power to bind heterogeneous ideas (Luckhurst, 2008, p. 14). While Latour developed his argument by analyzing the research generated via complex social interactions among teams of scientists and engineers, it may be applicable to the emergence and rise to discursive prominence of scholarly discourse at large, including the ascent of trauma studies. However, Latour remains neutral with regard to the validity of the scientific findings. Seeking to defend Caruthian trauma studies, Luckhurst appropriates Latour's *de*scription of how ideas emerge and become dominant in scientific discourse as a *pre*scription for evaluating their validity. Luckhurst's argument is thus structurally analogous to Caruth's own misleading interpretations of ideas from disciplines like psychoanalysis, deconstruction, trauma therapy, and the cognitive sciences used to authorize her claims.

Latour argued that, regardless of its empirical validity, the discursive success of a scientific hypothesis is determined by the number, length, and strength of associative links it generates between previously disparate ideas, both within its own and other disciplines. Hence, by invoking Latour to defend Caruth's theory, Luckhurst suggests that the links established between the postmodern trauma concept and its conceptualization in the disciplines she references are vast, strong, and deep. He thus inadvertently echoes and extends Leys' (2000) notion of close ties between Caruth's postmodern theory and the trauma concept generated by psychiatrist and neuroscientist Bessel van der Kolk. However, as Gary Weissman (2004, p. 236) argued, despite the fact that Caruth included van der Kolk's coauthored essay in *Trauma: Explorations in Memory* (van der Kolk & van der Hart 1995, pp. 158–182) and both scholars cite a couple of each other's publications, Leys overestimated the discursive depth and strength of the cross-references. Although Caruth seeks to relate her theory to the trauma concept developed in the cognitive sciences, her references are brief, sporadic, and superficial. Rather than engaging in a truly interdisciplinary endeavor, Caruth selectively references van der Kolk to authorize her own argument via the aura of hard science. While this reflects her positivist understanding of scientific research, mistaking his largely speculative ideas for established facts furthermore indicates her limited engagement with cognitive science scholarship. Caruth's interdisciplinary gestures could fulfill their authorizing function because van der Kolk's research lies outside humanities discourse—even the fact that much of it is speculative and contested among cognitive scientists is little known—and literary studies scholars could neither adequately evaluate its explanatory value nor realize that Caruth moreover employed it selectively, superficially, and figuratively. While van der Kolk seeks to minimize the scientific status of his core claims as unverified hypotheses, he carefully phrases his findings to allow this understanding while actively inviting the reading, paradigmatic for Caruth and trauma studies scholars generally, that they are based on verifiable empirical results (Leys, 2000, p. 239).[3]

In fact, Caruth's and van der Kolk's trauma concepts share only two causally related core axioms: Memories of traumatizing experiences are retained and recalled via categorically different cognitive processes than memories of ordinary events. The reason for categorically differentiating memories of traumatic and ordinary events is that when the former are encoded in the mind they supposedly bypass consciousness and therefore remain absolutely veridical since they are unencumbered by mimetic processes and dissociated from all other memories. However, the two scholars differ about the specifics. Van der Kolk does argue that traumatic events are cognitively processed via different mechanisms and remain accurate and unaffected by the processes of selection and interpretation that govern the perception of ordinary events as well as by the decay of memory traces. However, he also maintains that the memories only remain in their uninterpreted and dissociated state until they are recalled and represented for the first time and hence their supposed quasi-mystical absolute truth remains inherently inaccessible. Caruth (1996, p. 59) further expands this inherently unverifiable idea into the hyperbolic claim that because "the outside has gone inside without any mediation" not only the subjective experience of the traumatic event entered and is retained veridically in the mind but also—using her key word (which van der Kolk does not employ)—a *literal* copy of the event itself. Furthermore, unlike van der Kolk, Caruth splits traumatic memory into a dichotomy of trauma and memory as she defines trauma in opposition to memory as that which was not experienced and thus cannot be (consciously) remembered (Weissman, 2004, pp. 133–134).[4] Last but not least, unlike Caruth who argues that trauma cannot be remembered and thus not represented, as a psychiatrist, van der Kolk does consider the recall and representation of traumatic memories possible and necessary.

Caruth furthermore seeks to generate interdisciplinary links to psychotherapeutic trauma discourse in order to support her theory. In her interview with psychiatrist Robert Lifton, who treated Japanese survivors of the American atomic attacks and American Vietnam War veterans, she tries to elicit confirmation of her core thesis that trauma is inherently unknowable and unrepresentable from him three times (Caruth, 1995b, pp. 134, 135, 141). However, each time he only stresses the initial difficulty of recollection and representation because, after all, remembering and representing traumatizing experiences constitute the *raison d'être* of trauma therapy. Caruth's axiom that trauma cannot be known and her prohibition evocative of the second commandment that it must not be represented is thus inherently antithetical to therapeutic discourse. Hence, as Harald Weilnböck (2008,

[3]At least once, van der Kolk (1996, 297) does however admit, if only in a footnote, that after more than two decades of research and a plethora of publications, he had been unable to empirically verify his core hypotheses: "The question of whether the brain is able to 'take pictures,' and whether some smells, images, sounds, or physical sensations may be etched onto the mind and remain unaltered by subsequent experience and by the passage of time, still remains to be answered."

[4]According to Gary Weissman (2004, 236), "in the preface and two introductory essays she wrote for *Trauma: Explorations in Memory*, Caruth refers to traumatic experience, traumatic events, the traumatic reexperience of the event, traumatic symptoms, the traumatic occurrence, the traumatic nightmare, traumatic dreams and flashbacks, traumatic reenactment, traumatic recall, traumatic recollection, traumatic suffering, traumatic pasts, and traumatic history. Not once, however, does she refer to traumatic memory or traumatic memories." And although she employs both "trauma" and "memory" in the title of her edited volume and in two chapter titles of her monograph, "the word scarcely appears elsewhere in its pages. In fact, the book's index includes only two page reference for 'memory,' one of them in error."

para. 5) argued, clinical psychologists will not "be able to understand what most humanities scholars who speak about trauma really mean by that term" and that the closer they look at "what humanities scholars say about trauma, the stranger it will seem—to the point of being nonsensical."

Caruth moreover employs Freud's "brand" name to support her thesis of trauma's return in non-symbolic literality. Although she uses his term *Nachträglichkeit* (belatedness), she redefines the concept in an inherently un-Freudian manner. According to Freud, it signified the retroactive conferral of meaning on memories of early childhood sexual experiences, i.e., their delayed interpretation as traumatic (Leys, 2000, p. 270). As the understanding of all memories changes over time and is only accessible in inherently symbolic representations, for Freud, "there can be no unreworked return of the origin" (Kansteiner, 2004, p. 203). However, Caruth redefines *Nachträglichkeit* as indicating that because the trauma can be neither located in the time-space of the event nor in the belated realization of its traumatic nature, it returns in non-symbolic literal form. According to Wulf Kansteiner (2004, p. 203), "although Caruth goes to impressive lengths to find passages in Freud's large, complex and contradictory oeuvre which confirm her assumptions, the very notion that there is such a thing as a non-symbolic, non-reworked, literal memory of key emotional events in a person's life is a fundamentally un-Freudian idea."

In order to justify her claim that trauma can neither be located in past reality nor in its supposed belated, literal, and unmediated return in the present, Caruth argues that it was not consciously experienced. Since only Freud's train accident model can be appropriated to argue that the experience could not enter consciousness because train accidents happen unexpectedly and extremely fast, Caruth (1996, p. 6) casts this, rather than the Oedipal model, as the dominant trauma paradigm in both Freud's and her own theory (Leys, 2000, p. 278). However, it is the Oedipal model of repressed sexual childhood memories and their belated return as symbolic representations that constitutes Freud's core trauma paradigm. The train accident model is also least suited to understand experiences of extreme violence like torture, genocidal persecution, and physical and sexual violence, as they are not only intentionally and gratuitously inflicted but also often occur repeatedly and over long periods of time.

Caruth furthermore appropriates Freud to authorize her own argument in her discussion of his late essay *Moses and Monotheism*. Her interpretation focuses less on the speculative argument developed in the essay—that Moses was an Egyptian and murdered by the Israelites as an Other and that Jewish history was haunted by the return of this repressed murder—than on the temporal gap between its two prefaces. They are dated "before March 1938" and "June 1938." During this period, Freud fled from Nazi persecution in Austria to England. Caruth connects the two dates by generating a narrative in which they serve as the signposts that signify a temporal gap which she, furthermore, casts as a void and thus the site of the trauma of Freud's flight into exile, which is only present in its absence and in Freud's silence between the prefaces precisely because, according to Caruth (1996, p. 20), trauma cannot be grasped or represented (Leys, 2000, pp. 286–288). In other words, she uses Freud's authority to sanction her own theory by ascribing its performative enactment to him.

While Luckhurst (2008) stresses the associative power of Caruth's trauma concept to defend her theory and, indeed, she references several and rather diverse discourses, the interdisciplinary links she establishes are weak and shallow. After all, her foundational axioms are antithetical to the core ideas of the discourses she appropriates: In order to expand her claims from the level of individual cognition, Caruth invokes Jean-Francois Lyotard's postmodernism and Paul de Man's deconstruction and expands on Shoshana Felman's (1992) translation of the latter into a theory of trauma constructed around a crisis of witnessing. However, the idea that trauma marks a quasi-sacred origin for a stipulated crisis of signification is inherently antithetical to the venerable postmodern project precisely because the latter sought to deconstruct the notion of essences and origins. And while the rise of trauma theory to a disciplinary master discourse in the humanities reflects that, ironically, postmodernism became a master discourse itself, it contradicts the postmodern idea of deconstructing master discourses. Moreover, despite the fact that Caruth appropriated ideas from Freudian and, to a lesser extent, Lacanian psychoanalysis, trauma theory is not only inherently anti-analytical but also its Caruthian core axiom of trauma's non-symbolic literality is intrinsically anti-Freudian. Furthermore, in its insistence that trauma cannot and must not be remembered and represented because this will destroy its quasi-sacred literality, trauma theory contradicts the core therapeutic notion that traumatic memories must be integrated via narration to minimize psychological dysfunction. Last but not least, since Caruth casts trauma and memory as a dichotomy, trauma theory is intrinsically antithetical to empirical studies of traumatic memory in the cognitive sciences. Consequently, Caruthian trauma theory effaces the vast scholarship on traumatic memory from neurobiology to cognitive psychology, including most of van der Kolk's research.

It was the claim to have generated extensive and strong interdisciplinary links between the understanding of trauma in postmodern theory, the cognitive sciences, psychiatry, clinical psychology, trauma therapy, and psychoanalysis as well as the resulting appearance of its explanatory omnipotence that postmodern trauma studies rose to the level of a master discourse in the humanities. However, the links to the trauma concepts generated in these other disciplines are not only weak but also limited in number. For instance, of the vast research in the cognitive sciences, Caruth and trauma studies scholars generally—the articles in *Acts of Memory* (1999) edited by Mieke Bal, Jonathan Crewe, and Leo Spitzer are paradigmatic—not only limit their references largely to van der Kolk, but also of his many publications only cite the essay included in Caruth's (1995) edited volume to invoke the authority of hard science. In his defense of Caruth and trauma studies generally, Luckhurst (2008) thus significantly overestimates the number and strength of interdisciplinary links generated between the rather diverse notions of trauma in postmodern theory and other disciplines. As the core notions of trauma theory are antithetical to those in the referenced disciplines, it is inherently unable to participate in a truly interdisciplinary discourse on trauma. The superficial and selective interdisciplinary gestures of trauma studies scholarship instead appropriate ideas from other disciplines to authorize untenable claims via the aura of hard science and the simulation of interdisciplinarity. As such, trauma theory reflects a similar tendency in postmodern theory at large. As Sokal and Bricmont famously argued in *Fashionable Nonsense*, postmodernists like Lacan, Kristeva, Baudrillard, Deleuze, and Virillio extensively referenced scientific concepts in pseudo-interdisciplinary gestures to authorize their arguments but transformed them into metaphors that are nonsensical in the scientific discourse from which they were appropriated.

12.3 Sacred Truths

Although trauma theory engages in close discursive interaction with Holocaust studies, this does not constitute an interdisciplinary endeavor because the subjects are intertwined to the extent of constituting the same field of inquiry. Central to Holocaust studies is the notion, introduced by Elie Wiesel, that the genocide of European Jewry constitutes a historically unique and inherently incomprehensible event. According to its most prominent and influential American interpreter, as Novick (1999, p. 201) described Wiesel, the Holocaust "lies outside, if not beyond, history," "defies both knowledge and description," "negates all answers," "cannot be explained or visualized," and is "never to be comprehended or transmitted" (Wiesel cited in Finkelstein, 2000, p. 45). Wiesel furthermore cast the Holocaust as a sacred mystery and based his uniqueness claim on an analogy to Jewish religious chosenness rather than historical analysis (Fackenheim, Steiner, Popkin, & Wiesel, 1967, pp. 266–299; Chaumont, 2001, pp. 89–120). However, his axioms are untenable not least because asserting

Holocaust uniqueness based on Jewish chosenness creates a structural analogy between God and the Nazis. And despite Wiesel's repeated assertion to the contrary, it also constitutes a claim to "permanent possession of the gold medal in the Victimization Olympics," as Peter Novick (1999, p. 195) put it bluntly, because claiming uniqueness means that "your catastrophe, unlike ours, is ordinary; unlike ours is comprehensible; unlike ours is representable" (Novick, 1999, pp. 8–9). Although Wiesel cast the Holocaust as singular and unfathomable, paradoxically, the mystery must nevertheless be divined because it holds universally significant lessons. The privileged authority to do so is solely attributed to the survivor (Novick, 1999, p. 201) who thus functions as "both priest and prophet of this new religion" (Seidman, 1996, p. 2) and constitutes the "American Jewish equivalent of saints and relics" (Wieseltier cited in Novick, 1999, p. 201). Survivor testimony is ascribed the status of mystical revelations and thus cast as rationally impenetrable and therefore exempt from empirical verification and the rules of logic and causality.

Although it seems nonsensical for a scholarly discipline to define its object *a priori* as sacrosanct and unknowable, trauma studies echo the core notions of Holocaust sanctity and incomprehensibility and thus cast trauma not as an object of empirical analysis and theoretical reflection but rather as "a sacred item and object of quasi-religious veneration," as Harald Weilnböck (2008, para. 54) put it. According to Weilnböck (2008, para. 45), trauma studies discourse is moreover characterized by a "certain ontological and even clerical sound" which indicates that it "cannot be understood [...] but instead demands that its readers believe in it as one believes in a religion." As trauma theory ascribes its object of veneration the status of the sacred, trauma is also defined as the site of ontological truth. Likewise analogous to Wieselesque Holocaust mysticism, it is cast as inherently inaccessible, unknowable, and unrepresentable and hence all attempts at rational understanding and representation are considered blasphemous. Trauma theory displays a disdain for and an almost paranoid fear of all forms of representation, which it thus seeks to prohibit, analogous to the Second Commandment, because representation distorts and hence destroys trauma's supposed absolute but unknowable truth (Kansteiner & Weilnböck, 2008, p. 237).

Trauma theory's core axiom that its quasi-sacred object of adoration is inherently unknowable and unrepresentable also reflects Dori Laub's (1995, p. 65) claim that the Holocaust constitutes "an event without a witness." Neither survivor testimony nor "diaries kept by victims, photographs secretly taken by prisoners, and reports from messengers and those who escaped the camps" (Weissman, 2004, p. 236) constitute acts of witness because, as Laub (1995, p. 66) stipulates, the experience of genocidal persecution overwhelmed the victims' minds and they thus lack "an independent frame of reference through which the event could be observed." Consequently, "the historical imperative to bear witness could essentially not be met during the actual occurrence" and the Holocaust therefore cannot be known (Laub, 1995, p. 68).[5] However, empirical research in the cognitive sciences has demonstrated that the perception, encoding, storage, and retrieval of traumatic experiences only differ in degree and not in kind from the processes involved in the generation and recollection of other memories (McNally, 2003; Schacter, 1996). And therapists like Robert Lifton likewise noted only a relative difficulty and not an absolute inability among traumatized individuals to recall and narrate their experiences (Caruth 1995b). The vast number of Holocaust memoirs and video testimonies, in the gathering of some Laub was even actively involved, also indicate the invalidity of his axiom that the lived experience of Holocaust survivors could not be wit-

[5] While Laub shares the trauma theory axiom of the supposed impossibility of experiencing trauma at the time of occurrence, as a practicing psychoanalyst, he does believe that narration, and representation more generally, are possible and necessary in order to work through the traumatizing experience. For Laub, testimony thus has a therapeutic function. However, the fact that he does not share the axiom that trauma cannot and must not be represented central to Felman and Caruth is largely effaced both in his own essays and their references to them.

nessed and thus remains unknowable. Moreover, while the Holocaust obviously cannot be represented *in toto* either as lived experience or as historical event, this is not due to the extremity of the event but simply reflects the mimesis problem that representations are inherently partial as completeness would essentially require them to be the object or event. Contrary to Laub's claims, then, the fact that no one experienced the Holocaust *in toto* means neither that there were no witnesses who can testify to their personal experiences nor that the genocide is unrepresentable as a historical event (Weissman, 2004).

Laub and Wiesel differ with regard to whom they ascribe the ultimate authority to divine the supposed mystery of the Holocaust as each ascribes it to (someone like) himself, the therapist-interlocutor or the survivor, respectively. However, they share both the conflation of the genocide as historical event with its personal experience and the notion that this composite entity constitutes the core embodiment of the negative sublime whose ontological truth will and must remain inexplicable and unrepresentable despite, or paradoxically rather because, it must be invoked ubiquitously. Felman and Caruth merged Wiesel's Holocaust mysticism and Laub's notion that the genocide had no witnesses with Paul de Man's deconstructionism, particularly his obscure axiom that signs are only referential in crises of signification, to argue that not only past traumas but all history can solely be known via the failure of representation. As the past can never be known in its ontological totality, the argument goes, it cannot be known at all because not only trauma testimony but also all signification constitutes a misrepresentation and is thus inherently traumatic (Caruth, 1996, p. 90). However, as Wulf Kansteiner (2004, p. 205) aptly critiqued, "while it is appropriate to insist on a troubling element of undecidability in all processes of communication, it is neither necessary nor advisable to express this essential dilemma of representation through the metaphor of trauma. Just because trauma is inevitably a problem of representation in memory and communication does not imply the reverse, i.e., that problems of representation are always partaking in the traumatic."

The argument for trauma's supposed quasi-sacred ontological truth moreover slips and slides between the incongruous epistemologies of cognitive science and postmodern theory but cannot even be convincingly theorized, let alone empirically supported, in either. Trauma theory employs pseudo-scientific rhetoric to assert its core axioms—for instance, that "trauma stands outside representation" (Caruth, 1996, p. 17) and remains "absolutely true to the event" (Caruth, 1995, p. 5)—as scientifically valid by arguing that memory and trauma constitute a dichotomy and the mind retains traumatic experiences in literal but inaccessible totality. However, such arguments not only tautologically restate what should be explored theoretically and empirically but they are moreover contradicted by cognitive science research. Moreover, the quasi-religious notion of trauma's ontological truth, which is unencumbered by cognitive or mimetic processes, remains in literality, and is intrinsically inaccessible and incomprehensible, is not only antithetical to scientific discourse, and, given its anti-representational stance, to trauma therapy but, ironically, also to such core postmodern ideas as the existence of extra-representational essences.

12.4 Cloning Witnesses

The trauma concepts developed in disciplines ranging from neuroscience to cognitive psychology and clinical psychology, psychoanalysis and psychiatry are, then, antithetical to the dominant ideas in postmodern trauma theory, which nevertheless and despite its supposed interdisciplinarity upholds its axioms unencumbered by these discrepancies. Beyond the claim of its ontological truth, they include the stipulation that trauma is transmitted in its literality not through the interpretative practice of representation but via inadvertent processes metaphorically cast as contagion (Caruth, 1995, p. 10).

Echoing de Man's specious stipulation that only when language enacts a failure of representation is it referential, Caruth (1995, 1996) and Felman and Laub (1992) argue that trauma is unwittingly encoded in the aporias and absences not only of survivor testimony (co-)generated in face-to-face interviews and mediated accounts like diaries, memoirs, and video testimony, but also of canonical fiction, films, and even some of Freud's essays. The cultural artifacts are said to performatively re-present the trauma in its literality via their paradoxes and silences and inadvertently infect audiences with it, precisely through the representational failure of language. Caruth sought to demonstrate these ideas by recourse to canonical literature (Duras and Kleist), film (Resnais), and psychoanalysis (Freud and Lacan). Felman employed more complex interpretations of canonical literature (Camus' *The Fall*) and films (Lanzmann's *Shoah*) and argued that she had observed the contagion first-hand in her graduate course when her students were supposedly infected with the trauma unwittingly encoded in the texts and films assigned for the class.

Caruth and Felman thus conflate the reception experience of some highbrow texts and films and the actual experience of traumatizing events based on the empirically nonsensical claim that in both the immediate and the mediated experiences the trauma enters the mind in a manner that bypasses consciousness and circumvents mimesis. The cultural artifacts into which trauma was supposedly encoded unwittingly via paradoxes and silences are thus ascribed the capacity to duplicate or, to use an apt metaphor, clone trauma in literal totality because their reception is said to have the same effect on the audience as the traumatizing event had on the victim in immediate reality. Dominick LaCapra (2001, pp. 102–103) critiqued this notion, which also dominates Holocaust studies, arguing that the "major difference between the experience of camp inmates or Holocaust survivors and that of the viewer of testimony videos" is "blatantly obvious." Yet, he still maintained that because viewing Holocaust video testimony may cause some of the ever-increasing PTSD symptoms, such as recurring nightmares, "the possibility of secondary trauma cannot be discounted" (see also Weissman, 2004, p. 220). However, claims that media representations can traumatize audiences, whether by infecting them with trauma in its literal totality, as Caruth suggests, or in a muted version of secondary trauma, as LaCapra hypothesizes, are antithetical to empirical media studies research. Reception analyses of media violence by scholars like Goldstein (1998) and Bryant and Zillmann (1991) have demonstrated that media consumption does not traumatize the audience.[6]

Conflating the reception of mediated violence and its immediate experience relies not only on the axiom that witnessing trauma is inherently impossible but also requires the vast metaphorical extension of witnessing to encompass the face-to-face reception of testimony and even the media reception of canonical texts and films. Caruth and Felman merged their deconstructionist axiom that trauma signifies a failure of representation with Laub's obscure claim that Holocaust survivors can only become witnesses to their experience of genocidal persecution with the help of a therapist-interlocutor like himself because "the listener (or the interviewer) becomes the Holocaust witness before the [survivor-]narrator does" (1992, p. 85).[7] As Gary Weissman (2004, p. 137) critiqued, for Laub the interlocutor is thus "more essential to the process of bearing witness to the Holocaust than the survivor." However, according to Elie Wiesel's contrary notion, only survivors have experiential knowledge, are thus witnesses, and can testify to their personal experience of victimization as well as to the Holocaust as divine mystery. The survivors' signifying power moreover supersedes the professional expertise of their interlocutors, includ-

[6] Only previously traumatized individuals and very young children, who have not yet acquired the cognitive maturity to clearly distinguish between reality and representation, may be (re)traumatized by the consumption of media violence.

[7] The essay was reprinted as "Truth and Testimony: The Process and the Struggle" in Caruth (1995, pp. 61–75). Laub's notion of generating the witness in the discursive interaction between a therapist-interlocutor and a survivor implicitly excludes all non-surviving victims from witness status and their diaries and other documentation from constituting testimony. Despite the fact that the claim that traumatic events are categorically impossible to experience and that only in narrating them can survivors therefore become witnesses is untenable and unethical, it is central to trauma theory. It was taken up and expanded, for instance, by Kali Tal (1995) and Thomas Trezise (2013).

ing "the scholars and philosophers of every genre," since "Auschwitz, by definition, is beyond their vocabulary" (cited in Weissman, 2004, p. 48). While Wiesel thus restricts the moral capital of divining the Holocaust's sacred mystery to the new priesthood of survivors, he also argued that "whoever reads or listens to a witness becomes a witness" (cited in Minzesheimer, 2009, p. 1D), in other words, that witnesses can be duplicated or cloned. Wiesel, then, ascribes primary witness status to survivors whereas according to Laub's obscure anachronism, this subject position is rather occupied by the interlocutor. Moreover, Laub attributes (primary) witness status only to the survivor's immediate interlocutor while Wiesel includes audiences of video testimony and readers of memoirs in his notion of (secondary) witnesses. Despite their antithetical views with regard to who constitutes primary or secondary witnesses, both Laub and Wiesel expanded the notion of witnessing to the reception of testimony. And although the epistemology of this rhetorical maneuver is dubious, not least because it obscures the significant discrepancies between Laub's and Wiesel's respective understanding of witnessing, Caruth and Felman incorporated it into trauma theory.

The metaphorical notion of witnessing was further extended via the postmemory concept introduced by Marianne Hirsch (1997, 2008) and Andrea Liss (1998). For Hirsch, it signifies the simultaneity of intimate closeness and ultimate distance to the Holocaust memories of her parents. However, projecting her own intense interest in her parents' experience of genocidal persecution onto all children of survivors via the postmemory concept is untenable. According to clinical psychologist Aaron Hass (1996, p. 157), who is himself the son of Holocaust survivors, the current understanding of the so-called second generation is based on very limited empirical data that is moreover one-sided as it was largely derived from the cultural products generated by those children of survivors who are actively engaged in addressing their parents' past. Hass writes that most of the adult children of Holocaust survivors he encountered in his practice and research had little knowledge of the genocide and little interest in its commemoration. Moreover, Hirsch not only merges parental Holocaust memories and childhood memories of their stories but also implies a metaphorical extension of witness status to the second generation, both of which is empirically and ethically unsustainable. Nevertheless, she subsequently extended the postmemory concept and the witness position even further to anyone who has a close interest in personal experiences of the Holocaust in order to merge her own theory with Andrea Liss's. However, while "postmemory" may be a useful concept when restricted to express the personal connection some among the so-called second generation feel to their parents' past, any concept that is extended to be virtually all-inclusive loses its explanatory power. The creation of a plethora of related concepts—including "secondary memory," "prosthetic memory," "vicarious memory," "vicarious witness," "secondary witness," "retrospective witness," "witness's witness," "witness by adoption," and "witness through the imagination"—further reinforced the blurring between memories of lived experiences and familiarity with Holocaust narratives as well as the metaphorical extension of the witness position (Weissman, 2004, p. 92).

However, the most dubious expansion of the subject position of witness and the rhetorical act of testimony was generated by Michael Bernard-Donals (2001).[8] Taking recourse to trauma theory tropes from Felman and Caruth, Laub, and Hirsch, he argued in the eminent *PMLA*, that Holocaust survivors could not witness and thus cannot intentionally testify to but only inadvertently infect others with their trauma, which is contained in literal totality in "stutters, breaks and impossible juxtapositions of images" (p. 1308). Consequently, not the survivors but the audience, whom they inadvertently infected with their trauma, constitute Holocaust witnesses. Bernard-Donals nonsensically and unethically argues that a delusional impostor like Bruno Dössekker, who claimed to be a child survivor named Binjamin Wilkomirski, constitutes the preeminent Holocaust witness and his

[8] My critique is informed by Gross and Hoffman (2004).

horror kitsch fantasies are the ultimate Holocaust testimony. Dössekker had spent three decades consuming some 2000 books on the Holocaust and twice as many survivor testimonies as well as traveled to Holocaust sites in Poland and Latvia in search of an identity he could embrace before he wrote his false memoir *Bruchstücke: Aus einer Kindheit 1939–1948*, published in English as *Fragments: Memories of a Wartime Childhood* (Maechler, 2001, p. 67). According to Bernard-Donals, Dössekker is the preeminent witness and his fake memoir the ultimate Holocaust testimony precisely because he had not experienced the genocide but rather been infected with others' traumas encoded in the supposed silences and paradoxes of the thousands of testimonies and other Holocaust media products he consumed. Trauma theory thus enabled Dössekker's absurd recasting from the ultimate Holocaust spectator and delusional confabulator into the paramount witness and of his false memoir into the paradigmatic testimony.

While Bernard-Donals' claim that testimony communicates "what lies beyond what can be logically understood, beyond what makes sense" (p. 1305) does not contribute to an understanding of this mode of discourse, it aptly, if inadvertently, captures the epistemology not only of his own argument but also of trauma theory at large. And since its axioms and arguments lie beyond what makes sense and can be logically understood, they must be embraced analogous to religious beliefs, as Weilnböck (2008, para. 45) aptly noted, a rather dubious epistemology for a scholarly discipline.

12.5 Postmodern Ethics

Although postmodernism's rejection of master discourses and embrace of alterity reinforced the critique of oppression, persecution, and disenfranchisement, its emphasis on the constructedness of subjectivity and experience simultaneously threatened identity politics by collapsing its empirical foundations into a slippage of signifiers (Ball, 2000, pp. 6–7). The introduction of Holocaust aesthetics into postmodern theory and subsequent transformation of Yale deconstruction into trauma studies indicates that the notion that signification is arbitrary became increasingly unacceptable, especially after the posthumous revelation of de Man's latently pro-Nazi journalism. However, the result was not a critique of postmodernism's extreme relativism but the nonsensical and unethical transformation of the Holocaust into a rhetorical figure. Trauma theory thus reflects and reinforces the transformation of the genocide into metaphor and metonymy and its appropriation for epistemological purposes other than understanding the historical event itself by postmodernists like Jean-Francois Lyotard and Hayden White. While for White (1992, pp. 37–53) the Holocaust functioned as a kind of litmus test that led him to partly revise his claim that history is infinitely emplotable,[9] Lyotard likewise employed it figuratively to substantiate his radical critique of foundational, totalizing discourses (Kansteiner, 2004, pp. 199–202). Despite some venerable intentions,[10] postmodern theory thus transformed the genocide of European Jewry into a "free-floating metaphor of a severe, unrepresentable (and perhaps unverifiable) collective trauma, which is easily attached to all kinds of issues and agendas" (Kansteiner, 2004, p. 202).

Stripped of empirically specific victimization and suffering, the notion of trauma was radically redefined from signifying the destructive, potentially long-term aftereffects of extreme violence into a metaphor that served to theorize a supposed

[9] White still sought to safeguard his dubious notion that history is infinitely emplottable by ascribing special epistemological status to a small number of so-called limit events, of which the Holocaust constitutes the paradigmatic instance, and only conceded that such limit events are not infinitely emplottable because certain modes of emplotment, such as comedy or pastoral, would not constitute adequate emplotments. Contrary to White, I would argue that such modes of emplotting the Holocaust are currently ethically unacceptable but they are not inherently less veridical or historically reliable.

[10] Even as acerbic a critic as Harald Weilnböck acknowledged that trauma theory is "permeated by signs of the utmost respect and compassion for those who suffered (in the Holocaust and/or other atrocities), as well as indications of a vocation to help maintain the legacy of the victims" (2008, para. 87).

postmodern crisis of signification. With this drastic change in denotation, the negative connotations were likewise fundamentally altered. Though stipulated to be unknowable, trauma was increasingly idealized and celebrated in a rhetoric full of pathos and quasi-religious fervor "as providing unprecedented insight into the human condition" and "a welcome disruption of existing frameworks of social and institutional incorporation" (Kansteiner & Weilnböck, 2008, p. 234). Given its paradigmatic irreverence for logical and verifiable arguments and embrace of paradoxical speculations, trauma theory ascribes the utmost epistemological value to its object of veneration precisely because it cannot be known. The celebration of trauma as a quasi-sacred icon of ontological but inherently unknowable truth is not only nonsensical but also unethical as it effaces the very real past and present experiences of persecution, victimization, and violence.

Moreover, when trauma is defined as inherently unknowable, victims are cast as incapable of testifying and thus dispossessed of the socially significant subject position of witness. In trauma theory, only those who know how to listen for the silences and paradoxes not only in immediate survivor speech but also and especially in literary texts and films that supposedly constitute re-presentations of trauma in its literality, are ascribed witness status. In other words, victims and survivors are deprived of their witness position and their narratives of testimony status so that Holocaust and trauma studies scholars, whom Gary Weissman (2004, p. 20) emphatically dubbed nonwitnesses, can ascribe the former to themselves and the latter to their postmodern speculations. The core question is thus not only or even primarily "how knowledge of extreme experiences is possible" (Hartman, 1995, p. 544) but rather who is ascribed the discursive power to divine trauma's supposed ontological truth. While the attempt to reassert the discursive dominance of experts by usurping the witness position may be an inadvertent reaction to the transition of interpretive authority from the critical discourse of scholarship to the experiential knowledge of testimony in what Annette Wieviorka (2006) described as the era the witness, it is nevertheless unethical.

Beyond engaging in what Weissman (2004, pp. 26–27) characterized as self-aggrandizing fantasies of witnessing, trauma studies scholars moreover confuse and conflate the distinct subject positions of victim and perpetrator. The absurd axiom that victims can only inadvertently communicate their trauma by generating an exact duplicate in another's mind via a mystical process metaphorically described as infection means that they must traumatize their interlocutors and thus generate a structural analogy between victims and perpetrators. Caruth, moreover, ascribes not only the perpetrator position to victims but also victim characteristics to perpetrators, most importantly the status of traumatized individual. In her discussion of Freud's interpretation of Tasso's *Gerusalemme Liberata* in *Beyond the Pleasure Principle*, Caruth focuses on the scenes when Tancred kills Clorinda because he did not recognize the beloved in the armor of an enemy soldier and upon his realization flees into a magic forest where in despair he cuts a tree with his sword only to learn that he had killed Clorinda again when her blood and voice appear from the tree's wound. Although Caruth (1996, pp. 1–9) invokes *Beyond the Pleasure Principle* to authorize her own reading of Tasso, she interprets Tancred's second act of violence as a literal re-presentation of his unrecognized trauma and therefore antithetically to Freud's notion that it constitutes the symbolic return of the repressed enacted as repetition compulsion. Caruth likewise conflates the subject positions of victim and perpetrator by ascribing the status of traumatized party to the perpetrator in her reading of *Moses and Monotheism*. Freud had provocatively speculated that Moses was an Egyptian and killed by the ancient Israelites as an outsider, thus casting the latter as perpetrators of a crime that was repressed but would return throughout Jewish history and come to dominate it. Analogous to Tancred's killing of Clorinda, Caruth argues that the Israelites likewise did not experience their supposed perpetrator trauma of murdering Moses.

However, Caruth's interpretations of Freud's essays are not only tenuous but also ethically flawed. Stressing Tancred's supposed perpetrator trauma effaces Clorinda's victim trauma while claiming that Clorinda's voice testifies to his rather than her own experience redefines victim testimony as signifying the perpetrators' supposed trauma. As Caruth repeatedly refers to Tancred as a survivor, she even absurdly conflates the subject positions of survivor and perpetrator. And while her analogous casting of the ancient Israelites as traumatized is more in sync with the construction of secular Jewish identity around the untenable notion of vicarious Holocaust victimhood than with Freud's speculation that they are perpetrators of a suppressed murder, Caruth's interpretation of *Moses and Monotheism* is both nonsensical and unethical, not least because it has chilling implications. If the Israelites were not only traumatized but paradoxically committed murder without experiencing it, one could analogously argue that the Nazis were traumatized by their murder of European Jews which they likewise did not experience. Both Leys (2000, p. 297) and Kansteiner (2004, p. 205) have made a similar argument with regard to Caruth's ascription of trauma status to Tancred's killing of Clorinda and her voice as testifying to his perpetrator trauma rather than her own victim trauma. By analogy, the status of traumatized individual could be ascribed to the Nazis and the testimony of Holocaust victims and survivors could be understood as relating not to their own traumatic experiences but the supposed perpetrator trauma of their murderers. While the analogy is only a partial one since Tancred's killing of Clorinda was unintentional and Caruth's interpretation of Freud's hypostatized murder of Moses by the Israelites thus constitutes a closer analogy, both of her readings are unethical as they ascribe the status of traumatized party to perpetrators and thus merge their position with that of their victims.

Caruth's dubious interpretations of Freud's essays rely on the axiom that trauma cannot be witnessed and re-presented. However, this does not constitute an ontological impossibility but rather an ethical and aesthetic question of what is deemed appropriate public discourse in a particular culture. As Gary Weissman (2004, p. 167) put it with regard to *Schindler's List*, Spielberg depicted "enough horror to avoid revising or distorting history, but not so much as to alienate or repel viewers." According to Geoffrey Hartman (1997, p. 63), it is thus "a question of should not rather than cannot" and the ethical decision of what should be represented "does not have to be aggravated by a quasi-theological dogma with the force of the Second Commandment." Postmodern trauma theory's decidedly anti-representational stance of defining its object of veneration as unknowable and even prohibiting representation as essentially sacrilegious thus constitutes an absurd premise for a scholarly discipline and is moreover deeply unethical. It deprives victims and survivors of the witness position only to ascribe it to trauma studies scholars. It effaces the categorical distinction between perpetrator and victim by ascribing trauma status to the perpetrator's experience and casting victims in the perpetrator position because they can supposedly only convey their own trauma by traumatizing others. Moreover, the idea that what Michael Roth dubbed "narrative lust" (cited in Weilnböck, 2008, para. 48) must be resisted because representation transforms the quasi-mystical entity and thus constitutes what Caruth terms "a sacrilege to the trauma" (cited in Weilnböck, 2008, para. 52) is antithetical to the therapeutic imperative that representation is necessary, possible, and beneficial.

12.6 Conclusion

Trauma theory transforms empirical instances of persecution, disenfranchisement, and subjugation, for which the Holocaust has become paradigmatic, into a rhetorical figure to theorize a supposed postmodern crisis of signification. In order to do so, the empirically unsustainable arguments are authorized by simulating interdisciplinarity, defining the object of study as one of veneration rather than critical analysis, and prohibiting its representation as sacrilegious. Moreover, trauma theorists dispossess victims and survivors of the subject position of witness in order to ascribe it to themselves and the status of testimony to their self-aggrandizing speculations. In order to further empower the latter, they seek to prevent critique by simulating sacred discourse that cannot be critically analyzed based on rational arguments and empirical evidence but must simply be believed. The representational authority of survivors is further lessened by unethically confusing and conflating their subject position with that of the perpetrator because trauma can supposedly only be communicated via infection and thus by traumatizing others, both immediate interlocutors and media audiences alike. Postmodern trauma theory thus systematically minimizes the authority of those who experienced extreme violence, persecution, and oppression and recasts the notion of trauma from signifying its psychological effects into a floating signifier of the postmodern condition. Given the extensive and deeply rooted epistemological and ethical flaws intrinsic to the three inaugural publications of postmodern trauma theory and the fact that its core axioms could, moreover, be employed to argue that the horror kitsch phantasies of Holocaust survival in Wilkomirski's fake memoir constitute the ultimate Holocaust testimony and the delusional author its preeminent witness, I consider this discourse to be both nonsensical and irresponsible.

References

Bal, M., Crewe, J., & Spitzer, L. (1999). *Acts of memory: Cultural recall in the present*. Hanover: University Press of New England.

Ball, K. (2000). Introduction: Trauma and its institutional destinies. *Cultural Critique, 46*, 124–152.

Bernard-Donals, M. (2001). Beyond the question of authenticity: Witness and testimony in the *Fragments* controversy. *PMLA, 116*(5), 1302–1315.

Bryant, J., & Zillmann, D. (Eds.). (1991). *Responding to the screen: Reception and reaction processes*. Hillsdale, NJ: Lawrence Erlbaum Publishers.

Caruth, C. (Ed.). (1995a). *Trauma. Explorations in memory*. Baltimore: Johns Hopkins University Press.

Caruth, C. (1995b). An Interview with Robert Jay Lifton. In Caruth, C. (Ed.). (1995). *Trauma. Explorations in memory* (pp. 128–149). Baltimore: Johns Hopkins University Press.

Caruth, C. (1996). *Unclaimed experience. Trauma, narrative, and history*. Baltimore: Johns Hopkins University Press.

Chaumont, J.-M. (2001). *Die Konkurrenz der Opfer: Genozid, Identität und Anerkennung*. Lüneburg: Zu Klampen.

Fackenheim, E., Steiner, G., Popkin, R., & Wiesel, E. (1967). Jewish values in the post-holocaust future: A symposium. *Judaism, 3*, 266–299.

Felman, S., & Laub, D. (1992). *Testimony. Crises of witnessing in literature, psychoanalysis and history*. New York: Routledge.

Finkelstein, N. (2000). *The holocaust industry: Reflections of the exploitation of Jewish suffering*. London: Verso.

Goldstein, J. (Ed.). (1998). *Why we watch. The attractions of violent entertainment*. Oxford: Oxford University Press.

Gross, A., & Hoffman, M. (2004). Memory, authority, and identity: Holocaust studies in light of the Wilkomirski debate. Biography *17*(1), 25–47.

Hartman, G. (1995). On traumatic knowledge and literary studies. *New Literary History, 26*(3), 537–563.

Hartman, G. (1997). The cinema animal. In Y. Loshitzky (Ed.), *Spielberg's Holocaust: Critical perspectives on Schindler's list* (pp. 77–103). Bloomington: Indiana University Press.

Hass, A. (1996). *In the shadow of the Holocaust*. Cambridge: Cambridge University Press.

Hirsch, M. (1997). *Family frames: Photography, narrative, and postmemory*. Cambridge: Harvard University Press.

Hirsch, M. (2008). The generation of postmemory. *Poetics Today, 29*(1), 103–128.

Kansteiner, W. (2004). Genealogy of a category mistake. A critical intellectual history of the cultural trauma metaphor. *Rethinking History, 8*(2), 193–221.

Kansteiner, W., & Weilnböck, H. (2008). Against the concept of cultural trauma. In A. Erll & A. Nünning (Eds.), *Cultural memory studies. An international and interdisciplinary handbook* (pp. 229–240). Berlin: de Gruyter.

LaCapra, D. (2001). *Writing history, writing trauma*. Baltimore: Johns Hopkins University Press.

Latour, B. (1987). *Science in action. How to follow scientists and engineers through society*. Cambridge: Harvard University Press.

Laub, D. (1992a). Bearing witness or the vicissitudes of listening. In S. Felman & D. Laub (Eds.), *Testimony. Crises of witnessing in literature, psychoanalysis, and history* (pp. 57–74). New York: Routledge.

Laub, D. (1992b). An event without a witness: Truth, testimony, and survival. In S. Felman & D. Laub (Eds.), *Testimony. Crises of witnessing in literature, psychoanalysis, and history* (pp. 74–82). New York: Routledge.

Laub, D. (1995). Truth and testimony: The process and the struggle. In C. Caruth (Ed.), *Trauma: Explorations in memory* (pp. 61–75). Baltimore: Johns Hopkins University Press.

Leys, R. (2000). *Trauma. A genealogy*. Chicago: University of Chicago Press.

Liss, A. (1998). *Trespassing through shadows: Memory, photography, and the holocaust*. Minneapolis: University of Minnesota Press.

Luckhurst, R. (2003). Traumaculture. *New Formations, 50*, 28–47.

Luckhurst, R. (2008). *The trauma question*. New York: Routledge.

Maechler, S. (2001). *The Wilkomirski affair: A study in biographical truth*. New York: Schocken.

McNally, R. (2003). *Remembering trauma*. Cambridge: The Belknap Press.

Minzesheimer, B. (2009). Wiesel again rebuilds on ruins. *USA Today*, 1D.

Novick, P. (1999). *The holocaust in American life*. Boston: Houghton Mifflin.

Rothe, A. (2011). *Popular trauma culture: Selling the pain of others in the mass media*. New Brunswick: Rutgers University Press.

Schacter, D. (1996). *Searching for memory. The brain, the mind, and the past*. New York: Basic Books.

Seidman, N. (1996). Elie Wiesel and the scandal of Jewish rage. *Jewish Social Studies, 3*(1), 1–19.

Sokal, Alan (1994). Transgressing the Boundaries: Towards a Transformative Hermeneutics of Quantum Gravity. *Social Text* 46/47 (spring/summer 1996), pp. 217–252.

Sokal, A., & Bricmont, J. (1998). *Fashionable nonsense: Postmodern intellectuals' abuse of science*. New York: Picador.

Tal, K. (1995). *Worlds of hurt: Reading literatures of trauma*. Cambridge: Cambridge University Press.

Trezise, T. (2013). *Witnessing witnessing: On the reception of Holocaust survivor testimony*. New York: Fordham University Press.

van der Kolk, B. (1996). Trauma and memory. In B. van der Kolk, A. McFarlane, & L. Weisath (Eds.), *Traumatic stress: The effects of overwhelming experiences on mind, body, and society* (pp. 279–302). New York: Guilford Press.

van der Kolk, B., & van der Hart, O. (1995). The intrusive past: The flexibility of memory and the engraving of trauma. In C. Caruth (Ed.), *Trauma. Explorations in memory* (pp. 158–182). Baltimore: Johns Hopkins University Press.

Weilnböck, H. (2008). The trauma must remain inaccessible to memory: Trauma melancholia and other (ab-) uses of trauma concepts in literary theory. Retrieved August 1, 2009 from http://www.eurozine.com/articles/2008-03-19-weilnbock-en.html.

Weissman, G. (2004). *Fantasies of witnessing. Postwar efforts to experience the holocaust*. Ithaca: Cornell University Press.

White, H. (1992). Historical emplotment and the problem of truth. In S. Friedlander (Ed.), *Probing the limits of representation* (pp. 37–53). Cambridge: Harvard University Press.

Wieviorka, A. (2006). *The era of the witness*. Ithaca: Cornell University Press.

13 The Death of the Witness in the Era of Testimony: Primo Levi and Georges Perec

Yochai Ataria

13.1 Introduction

13.1.1 The Holocaust and the Question of Bearing Witness

Dori Laub (Felman & Laub, 1992) describes an encounter between historians and the testimony of a female holocaust survivor who told about four chimneys that went up in smoke during the revolt at Auschwitz in October 1944. From a purely factual perspective this event did not occur. In addition, the same survivor did not remember having been in the Canadian section of the camp where the murdered prisoners' belongings were sorted and stored. This was enough for the historians to reject her entire testimony—because a testimony that is not accurate cannot be relied upon as historical documentation. Yet Dori Laub is not concerned by this. From his perspective what is important is the act of giving the testimony. Telling the story enables the witness to break free of an awful silence (Laub, 1995).

The issue of bearing witness is known to be problematic (Loftus, 2003; 1993). And it becomes especially difficult when discussed in the context of trauma (Brewin, 2007; Caruth, 1995; Douglass & Vogler, 2003). Indeed this issue goes back the the birth of of psychoanalysis. This is even more so in the case of the testimony of Holocaust victims (Douglass & Vogler, 2003; Langer, 1991; Laub, 1995). By its very nature the Holocaust is an event that negates the notion of bearing witness to the point that from a purely historical perspective we can, therefore, say there were no witnesses to the Holocaust: neither from within all that transpired nor from testimony coming from outside of what happened (Felman & Laub, 1992)

On the one hand, a story that is told over and over becomes automatic and in many senses loses its authenticity, ceases to be tied to the event itself, and turns into a recitation of sorts (Ataria, 2014a). Yet on the other hand, an authentic story, as Dori Laub (1995) asserts, is not necessarily tied to the facts. Thus, at the extremum, that is, at the extreme point at which, in the context of the Holocaust there can be no point more distant from the norm, the expected, the understood, is that it is impossible to differentiate between authentic memory on the one hand and dreams or mere fantasy on the other. At such a point it is impossible to distinguish between a witness *who*

This chapter was written following a conversation with Yuval Neria and several friends during the Shivah mourning period for his father. The chapter is dedicated to those who know something but out of love and compassion choose not to tell about it, even at a great personal price.

Y. Ataria (✉)
Department of Neurobiology, Weizmann Institute of Science, Rechovot, Israel
e-mail: yochai.ataria@gmail.com

Y. Ataria et al. (eds.), *Interdisciplinary Handbook of Trauma and Culture*,
DOI 10.1007/978-3-319-29404-9_13

was there, like Primo Levi, and an imposter like Binjamin Wilkomirski whose book *Fragments: Memories of a Wartime Childhood 1939–1948* (Wilkomirski, (1996) was ultimately revealed as a fabrication divorced from historical reality. It goes without saying that in the final analysis such a case deals a mortal blow to the institution of bearing witness.

13.1.2 The Witness as His Own Historian

In a brilliant and landmark article, historian Pierre Nora (1989), a representative of the Nouvelle Histoire school, describes a situation in which memory and history become two separate and totally contradictory entities. Nora (1989) further argues that in practice memory no longer exists, for we are living in an era in which memory has been converted into memorial sites, archives, museums and the like. We have relinquished the memory that is tied to life itself and to the subjective experience in favor of history that is an intellectual act. Historical criticism of memory is indeed radical. As such, not only is memory always suspect from the historical perspective, so that in certain respects the role of the historian is to distance and repress memory, but in many ways history actually seeks to annul the institution of memory as something that brings the "contaminating" subjective experience to the historical discourse. In its tendency to cancel the very notion of memory, history replaces it with documents and certificates accumulating in infinite numbers of archives, often with no filtering, without distinguishing between what is important and what is not. Nora (1989) is of the opinion that the process of annulling memory has succeeded, so that paradoxically what remains today is history that is nothing more than a collection of stories or a central narrative surrounded by stories that corroborate it—a closed circle. Yet this is not the primary and authentic story of the traumatic experience. That is, stories of this kind cannot be treated as authentic memories. As opposed to spontaneous memory, historical memory is in essence serious, controlled and conscious, and it is thus cut off from the subject telling about it. Because historians are firmly grounded in the various archives (the regions of memory), in effect they too become regions of memory. Thus, the witness as historian also turns into a region of memory.

In the current era in which survivors feel an obligation to document their stories, the documentation of memory becomes everything except the spontaneous story tied to the primal experience. The testimony is always part of a larger conservation project for the next generation to KNOW. As a result, the roots of the testimony regarding the traumatic event are not always connected to the survivor's individual experience. Survivor witnesses become their own historians. Under such circumstances the memory becomes a well-defined testimony and in return the testimony turns into a disk in a huge bank of data. At the extremum, individuals relinquish their authentic memories in exchange for a historical description of their lives. Survivors appropriate a history for themselves and all that remains of the authentic memory are fragments that the history did not manage to vanquish and dismiss (Nora, 1989).

Yet, as Stone emphasizes (1979), in the process of annulling memory, we have not been given a true and objective history. Of course there is also no accepted and agreed upon history. At the extreme is the radical constructivism approach, according to which historical description by historians tells us only about the distorted image of the historians themselves (LaCapra, 2001). With this in mind it is important to stress that in the current era all intellectuals with a sense of historical consciousness are not only historians of sorts, but also subjects conscious of the fact that they are the subject of history and create history in the way they tell it (Huizinga, 1959).

Thus, within the framework of Nouvelle Histoire, which is primarily narrative, it is not possible to disregard the problems inherent in every story. This is especially true for the story of the posttraumatic survivor. Nouvelle Histoire, in the best case, is a collection of complementary and competing narratives, and it adds a layer to the attempt to describe history more objectively—scientific-concrete history. In the worst case this is a school that does not teach us anything about what was in the past. Rather, it informs us only about the way in which we always analyze the past relative to the political present in which we live, that is, always within the context of interests that are sometimes openly revealed and expressed and sometimes hidden and repressed.

Clearly, history, as a scientific discipline is in a state of crisis, especially when it comes to trauma (Caruth, 1996). With this in mind, the question of the survivor who becomes a witness as an historical source is fundamental.

13.1.3 Aims and Goals

It is incumbent upon us to examine the role of the witness. How does bearing witness affect the way history is shaped? Can testimony be relied upon in the writing of history? These are the questions that this chapter examines.

In the next section I consider the witness Primo Levi, who examines these questions in his book *The Drowned and the Saved (I sommersi e i salvati) (1993)* and in a series of interviews collected by Belpoliti in a book titled *The Voice of Memory: Interviews 1961–1987* (2001). After that I discuss Georges Perec in the context of his book *W, or the Memory of Childhood* (2003), in which, in addition to telling the story of the island of W, Perec casts doubt on one's ability to reliably bear witness based on memories of the past. In considering these works I compare Levi and Perec in order to examine this complex issue in depth with respect to the witness as narrator, the witness as storyteller and the witness as historian. After that I also discuss the writing process itself, as well as the motivation behind this process from the perspective of Levi and Perec. I conclude with two different and authentic models for bearing witness that Levi and Perec propose, each in his own way.

13.2 Primo Levi and the Question of Witnessing

13.2.1 The Identity of the Witness

In his book *The Drowned and the Saved* (1993) Primo Levi focuses on, among other issues, the problematics of memory. When it comes to the Holocaust, this appears to be a particularly complex issue. The Nazis destroyed the evidence not merely to eliminate the actual proof of what they had done but also as part of larger plan to silence the annihilation and maybe even more importantly to obliterate the methods they used. Many Jews, on the other hand, in many cases were almost obsessively engaged in historical documentation, as is clear, for example, from the diaries of the Sonderkommando, which describe the process of destruction in the greatest of detail. It is essential to understand that the Nazis' approach was quite radical. They believed that destroying the material evidence would be sufficient for no one would believe what happened. And indeed the survivors of the camps had a hard time convincing the outside world that people had been gassed and burned on such a large scale (Friedländer, 2007).

Levi's perspective (1993), according to which the most solid material for reconstructing the truth about the camps is based on the memories of the survivors, should be treated with this in mind. Namely, Levi's approach that the survivors' stories are true and reliable in its very essence opposes the Nazis' notion. Interestingly, however, at the same time in various interviews, Levi stresses that his stories are not historical stories or a substitute for historical stories (Belpoliti, 2001).

Clearly, the notion that the most solid material for reconstructing the truth about the camps is based on the memories of the survivors raises a fundamental problem with respect to bearing witness. The victims themselves, those who were burned or drowned or destroyed, are no longer among the living and are therefore not able to tell what happened. Only the ones who remained alive are left, in descending order of the importance of their testimony: (a) the hangmen, (b) the prisoners who were part of the mechanism of destruction and thus situated in a gray zone, and (c) "ordinary" prisoners (without extra privileges) who constituted the majority of those in the concentration and death camps, only a few of whom survived. This however raises an inherent problem: The closer the perspective of the witnesses is to that of the hangman (without passing judgement on how prisoners attempted to survive), the greater the possibility these witnesses can testify regarding what happened with respect to the amount of information, the perspective and the mental ability (due to the preferential physical conditions) and to make distinctions regarding what went on at the concentration camps. Yet at the same time and correspondingly, it is clear that their reliability as witnesses decreases for they are clearly motivated to conceal substantial parts of the story. Indeed, because they are repulsed by their own actions these people prefer to distance themselves from their original memories and to create a more comfortable reality (Levi, 1993). Thus, it is not surprising that those with clear privileges, that is, those who acquired privileges by enslaving themselves to the camp authorities, did not testify at all, for obvious reasons. Alternatively, their testimonies were deficient, distorted or totally fabricated (Levi, 1993). The prisoners who had no extra privileges were in a situation in which it was often difficult for them to testify regarding broader processes beyond their individual experience, which occurred under extreme circumstances. Due to the nature of the experience, some of the prisoners became unable to make distinctions and their ability to bear witness was damaged for good. This may explain why Levi over and again repeats that he is testifying only to what he himself experienced.

13.2.2 The Leakage of Memory

Another problem is that as the years go by and the victims get older, their memory is liable to be impaired (Nadel & Jacobs, 1998; Peace et al., 2008; Porter & Birt, 2001; Shobe & Kihlstrom, 1997). Often the victims are influenced by information they learned in retrospect from reading or from the stories of other victims (Levi, 1993). It is clear to Levi that even though memory has many virtues, in many cases it eventually becomes deceptive. Memories are not fixed. They tend to be erased and to change over time, and often foreign elements are added to them (Levi, 1993). As I have noted elsewhere (Ataria, 2014a), a major problem in the testimony of trauma victims is that the reliable story is in effect an automatic story, a cooked-up, made-to-order story, at the expense of the authentic memory. Such circumstances are marked by a gradual leakage of memories and their replacement by a fabricated and semi-automatic description. Indeed, according to Levi (1993) the story is nothing more than a formulated and ornamented form brought to completion which focuses on the role of crude memory and grows at its expense. Ultimately, Levi is concerned about the preference for the convenient truth over the authentic memory. In another paper Ataria (Ataria, 2014a, 2014b), Traumatic memories as black holes: A qualitative-phenomenological approach explained that individuals must be capable of living with their past. The purpose of the story is not to describe "what really was" but rather to enable victims to live their lives in peace. Indeed trauma victims who remember well often yearn for lack of memory they want to be able to forget (Semprún, 1998). Thus, if the victimizer wants to deny what he did (or what he knows was done), the victim wants to avoid and forget the particularly difficult and painful experiences. As a consequence, these events remain clouded in fog for years (Laub, 1995). Despite these reservations Levi believes that, at least for himself, even if some of his memories have somewhat faded with time, they are in a deeper and more essential sense appropriate to the background and are neither grating nor have they been more than just slightly damaged (Levi, 1993).

13.2.3 The Desire to Become the Ultimate Witness

In an interview with Rosellina Balbi in 1982, as in many other interviews, Levi describes his strong desire to tell:

> The need to tell our story was so strong in us that I began to write the book right there, in that German laboratory, frozen, heavy with war and with spying

> eyes. I knew that I had no way of preserving those scribbled notes because, if they had found them on me, they would have cost me my life. But I wrote the book as soon as I returned, in a few short months, the memory burning within me (Belpoliti, 2001, p. 103).[1]

Thus, Levi's most famous work, *If This Is a Man* (United States title: *Survival in Auschwitz*) is directly connected to his memories. For example, Levi describes how he wrote the chapter titled "The Canto of Ulysses" in half an hour in an ongoing trance state (Belpoliti, 2001). It was important to Levi that his book *If This Is a Man* (1959) serves as a reliable and extremely accurate testimony. In effect, Levi saw the book as a legal act and himself as a witness. This testimony brings a fundamental insight to Levi's writings: Levi's manifest purpose is to be the ultimate witness. In his books about the time he spent in the camps, Levi is not a writer and does not want to be a writer. On the contrary, Levi the witness takes over the role of narrator, with the role of Levi the writer consciously rejected. As emerges in the interview with Giuseppe Grassano (1979), Levi believes this ability to testify precisely to what happened there is what made his books so valuable: "Galileo was a very great writer precisely because he was not a writer at all. He simply wanted to expound what he had seen" (Belpoliti, 2001, p. 126). Hence it is important to Levi to stress the fact that he does not consider his book *If This is a Man* to be a literary work but rather a form of testimony, similar to the way in which Galileo provides testimony about his observations during his experiments.

The comparison to Galileo is perhaps the most critical in all of Levi's writings. A scientist should report on observations and Galileo, as one of the most important scientists, adheres to observations and objectively describes the results of his experiments and observations. Levi is convinced that he too acts, or at least strives to act, in a similar manner. Possibly this is how we can understand his statement that when he was a prisoner in the camp he was already preparing himself to be a witness', as he stated in his interview with Marco Vigevani in 1984: "For some reason that I cannot fathom, something anomalous happened to me, almost an unconscious preparation for the task of bearing witness" (Belpoliti, 2001, p. 255). Levi felt capable of describing reality objectively, as if he were a tape recorder: "Even today, after so many years, I have preserved a visual and acoustic memory of my experiences there that I cannot explain," and he goes on to say: "Not only that: I also still remember, as if recorded on to tape, phrases in languages I do not know, Polish or Hungarian ..." (Belpoliti, 2001, p. 255). For this reason Levi believes that he can "tell the story of what I saw truthfully, with accuracy" (Belpoliti, 2001, p. 255).

Levi is, then, a witness who tells his story, as he explains in an interview with Giuseppe Grassano: "I came back from the camp with a narrative impulse that was pathological" (Belpoliti, 2001, p. 129). Yet due to this fact, the process in which he told his stories over and over before writing them down caused them to be constructed in a certain way and changed them from a raw recording to a particular narrative. To put this another way, the raw material was sent to the editing room and turned into a story, as Levi himself explains in the same interview: "on the train [editing room] I remember telling my stories to whoever I found myself with" (Belpoliti, 2001, p. 170).

As with Galileo and his objective reporting of his observations, in every scientific work a distinction must be made between the results section that is intended as an objective report on the findings and the discussion section that is open to interpretation and speculation. Accordingly, a distinction must be made between the initial testimony that the victim "vomits" out practically without any control (the results) and the organized and structured narrative (the discussion). A good scientist will always clearly and distinctly separate between the results and the discussion. Introducing elements into the results that are compatible with the initial hypothesis could be construed as fabrication. Levi's attempt to explain confuses these sections. Paradoxically, however, it is Levi's attempt to be the Galileo of the *lager* (Auschwitz concentration camp) that probably made him such a great writer.

[1] Belpoliti edited the collection of interviews and conversations with Primo Levi. Before each quotation or set of related quotations I note the name of the interviewer and the date of the interview (or its publication date).

13.2.4 Witness–Storyteller–Writer–Historian

Levi is well aware of the issue of the reliability and authenticity of testimony and he discusses this openly in a conversation with Giuseppe Grassano in 1979:

> This problem of being a counterfeiter, of feeling false, worries me. Often I ask myself questions. For example, this subject that I want to deal with, revisiting the *Lager*, I would have to talk about events seen 35 years ago. But am I sure they all happened and am I obliged to tell them exactly as they were? Couldn't I, for example, change them a little to serve my purpose, or even invent them from scratch? (Belpoliti, 2001, p. 133).

Levi well understands the difficulties of a writer who is also a witness, of a witness who is a writer, of a writer who is a historian, of a historian who is a writer, and finally of a witness who is a storyteller who is a writer who is a historian. Hence it seems that ultimately, despite the attempt to disrupt this formula, every witness who relinquishes silence is also a storyteller, a writer and a historian.

Levi attempts to deconstruct this equation, and in the same interview with Grassano he asks whether "there's a clear difference between telling stories you claim are true, demanding to be believed to the letter, and telling stories like Boccaccio, for another purpose, not to record facts" (Belpoliti, 2001, p. 175). Levi would have liked to be able to answer *yes* to this rhetorical question, but it seems to be not so simple an assignment. In the case of Levi's books the question is even more difficult, for Levi, as he describes in an interview with Federico De Melis in 1983, seeks explanations: "I have always taken a different route in my books. I began writing about the camps and I carried on writing about things that happened to me, but always trying to explain, to resolve problems. I have been reproached for this tendency towards the didactic" (Belpoliti, 2001, p. 157).

Thus, Levi also adds philosopher to the witness–storyteller–writer–historian equation. As can be understood from the title of his book *If This Is a Man*, at the extremum Levi attempts to understand the nature of humankind—nothing less. Here we must return to the issue that disturbs Levi himself: Does testimony seek to explain, or should it describe events with an accuracy that is as close to reality as possible? What would we expect of Galileo? Was it the description of the findings only that turned Galileo into a myth, or was it the story (the theory and the interpretation) surrounding these findings that turned him into a myth? Levi, it seems, mixes the discussion section with the results section. It is unclear to what extent Galileo would have agreed to such a step. Yet it is very hard to find a scientist who does not fall into this trap. Still, one should remember that evidence without a theory to arrange it is meaningless (Popper, 1959).

A historian seeking the objective truth would likely prefer testimony that does not attempt to interpret but rather describes without bias. In a 1987 interview with Roberto di Caro, Levi states that his declared purpose, in his book *The Drowned and the Saved* (1993) is: "an immense need to put things in order, to put order back into a world of chaos, to explain to myself and to others." He goes on by saying: "Writing is a way of creating order. It's the best way I know, even if I don't know many" (Belpoliti, 2001, p. 174). Perhaps this is what Levi meant by stating that the only way to be saved is to tell. Not only does the story release the victim from the sense of unease, it puts him into deeper contact with the other. It also enables the victim to create order and maybe even make the situation seem reasonable.

It is interesting to see that on the one hand Levi speaks of the need for order, while on the other hand he speaks of bearing witness in terms of chaos, as vomit. He states that he wrote from instinct and that he felt a need to get things out, like someone who has vomited undigested food (Belpoliti, 2001). Yet the purpose of bearing witness is not to explain but rather to describe. The book *If This Is a Man* should be considered as testimony and not literature. In an interview with Marco Vigevani in 1984, Levi stated: "when I wrote the book, almost 40 years ago now, I had one precise idea in mind, and *it was certainly not to write a work of literature. It was rather to bear witness* … I wanted to recount what I had seen" (Belpoliti, 2001, p. 250, my emphasis). Yet Levi's attempt to understand and explain can harm his testimony if he is incapable of absolutely distinguishing between the results (the testimony) and the discussion (attempt to explain and understand).

13.2.5 Political Historian as Storyteller Witness

Years after his liberation, Levi describes the difficulty in reconstructing his primal experience as a prisoner. In an interview with Marco Vigevani (1984), Levi states: "Now, after so many years, it is hard even for me to return to the state of mind of the prisoner of that time, of myself back then" (Belpoliti, 2001, p. 251). Thus, it appears that from Levi's perspective the book *If This Is a Man,* completed in December 1946 and first published in 1947 in Italian, has itself turned into an artificial memory. "In particular, writing the book has worked for me as a sort of 'prosthesis', an external memory set up like a barrier between my life today and my life then" (Belpoliti, 2001, p. 251). In order to return to the experience of the prisoner at Auschwitz, Levi returns to his book as the source of the experience itself: "Today I relive those events through what I have written" (Belpoliti, 2001, p. 251). Similarly in an interview with Milara Spadi in September 1986 for a West German radio station, Levi stressed that his story is absolutely anomalous because he is separated from his experiences by books that serve as artificial memory, substitute memory. He stated that had he not written *If This Is a Man* he would certainly have forgotten many things. He noted that he gave many interviews, and that in them he distinguishes between the actual experience and today. Levi is also aware of the fact that his story has taken control over him, in a way has imprisoned him and detached him from the primal experience.

If we consider Levi's statement to Risa Sodi in a 1987 interview that bearing witness is an extremely political act, the focus on this problem becomes much sharper. How is it possible to bridge the gap between Levi as an automatic, inhuman tape recorder and Levi who is aware that his testimony is a political act? In other words, how is it possible to bridge the gap between Levi as the ultimate witness and Levi as a witness with clear political interests? In my view, there is only one possible solution. Levi, perhaps like other witnesses, turned himself into a documenting historian during the time he was a prisoner. This is a political act. In order to become a tape recorder, while he was a prisoner Levi abandoned the human perspective. In other words, Levi contends that in order to be a reliable witness, the victim must renounce the human perspective (Ataria, 2014c). This unconscious preparation to become a witness is a process of relinquishing one's humanity, at least during the period of imprisonment, in order to be capable of documenting, as a historian that is present at a turning point in history. In this sense, Levi, like other witnesses, is first and foremost a historian and only after that a witness who tells a story while attempting not to be a writer.

Yet as part of the role of historian and part of the political game, the witness must at least externally remain a storytelling witness. Thus, Levi, as someone who was there, admits to the intensity of his testimony. In a 1995 interview with Milara Spadi he states that hearing about these things from a third party, a stranger who did not experience them, is not like hearing them from someone like him, who has a number tattooed on his arm. This leads us to suggest that Levi is a political historian who is consciously aware of his role as witness–storyteller. He states that he became a professional survivor, almost a mercenary.

13.2.6 Interim Summary: Primo Levi

Even though Levi is aware of the problems, he feels his testimony is reliable and authentic. The purpose of this chapter is not to undermine or disagree with this, but rather to present the problems Levi raises that are relevant to any witness whoever he or she may be.

1. There is a discrepancy between a story that is vomited out, the initial and authentic story that is connected by an umbilical cord to the primal memory of the traumatic experience, and the constructed story that is told over and over again until it becomes automatic.
2. It is difficult to see how a witness who is aware of themselves cannot be their own historian, writer and storyteller.
3. Memories fade with time and often the story itself becomes the source of the memory and replaces the experience.

These problems are relevant to any testimony. For Levi additional problems arise:

1. His attempt to explain and understand harms the authentic story and confuses the results section with the discussion session.
2. Before Levi wrote *If This Is a Man* he told his story to anyone who wanted to hear it. In so doing, he appears to have consolidated the story and subjected it to some form of editing.
3. As Levi admits, *If This Is a Man* turned into an artificial memory and he experiences his days in captivity through this book. The fact that Levi became a "professional witness" apparently exacerbated this problem.

Against this background I now move on to *W, or the Memory of Childhood* by Georges Perec.

13.3 Georges Perec: W, or the Memory of Childhood

13.3.1 Two Series in One Collection: Technical Introduction

Before beginning my analysis of the book *W, or the Memory of Childhood* by Georges Perec (2003) it is important to note that this book incorporates two parallel "stories." The first story, hereafter referred to as the *First Series*, describes Gaspard Winckler's decision to look for a child whose identity he assumes after he deserts the army. This story appears in the odd numbered chapters (1–11) in the first part of the book and in the even numbered chapters (12–36) in the second part of the book, which describe life on the Island of W. The second story, hereinafter referred to as the *Second Series*, is Perec's own story. The even numbered chapters in the first part (2–10) tell the story of his childhood and his family from the perspective of the adult Perec. In the odd numbered chapters in the second part (13–37), Perec the boy writes about his life at various boarding houses after his mother was sent to Auschwitz in 1943.

13.3.2 Up to His Mother's Death

The *First Series* tells the story of Gaspard Winckler: a soldier, deserter, writer, witness; a counterfeiter; an imaginary character on the therapist's couch. Perhaps this is nothing more than the story of Perec himself, with all these characters incorporated within him. Perhaps not. In any case, everything is ambiguous. The *First Series* is written by Gaspard Winckler in the first person: "Today, impelled by a commanding necessity and convinced that the events to *which I was witness* must be revealed and brought to light, I resolve to defer it no longer" (Perec, 2003, p. 9, First Series—my emphasis). Like many other survivors, Gaspard Winckler (though at this point we do not yet know this is Gaspard Winckler), the main character in the *First Series*, remained silent for an extended period of time: "For years I wished to keep the secret of what I had seen" (ibid, p. 9, First Series), but eventually he gave in and told his story. The fact that Gaspard Winckler, the witness, is the last person on earth who can *tell what happened there* is the motivation: "Whatever may happen now, whatever I may now do, I was the sole depository, *the only living memory*, the only vestige of that world. That, more than any other consideration, was what made me decide to write" (ibid, p. 10, First Series—my emphasis).

Even though the opening appears to be testimony of the "ordinary type" in which the witness, for example Primo Levi or Elie Wiesel, feels compelled to be an emissary and to bear witness to what happened "there," Perec does not intend to allow us to become submerged in a naïve and noncritical reading of his testimony: "For years I sought out traces of my history, looking up maps and directories and piles of archives. I found nothing, and it sometimes seemed as though I had dreamt, that there had been only an unforgettable nightmare" (ibid, p. 9, First Series). This statement on Perec's part leaves us facing a difficult problem that is often posed by major researchers in the era of bearing witness: the problem of the inner world of the witness who gives testimony and at the same time admits to knowing nothing, admits to being a counterfeiter, to telling *an imaginary story that is real* or to *bearing witness to what cannot be said or told,* therefore remaining, within the very definition itself, blocked and closed off. In this sense, indeed somewhat paradoxically, the witness must impersonate somebody else in order to tell what *really* happened. It is interesting that this impersonation is what enables Perec to expose a truth that is greater than any testimony anchored in fact.

Gaspard Winckler testifies that he cannot say whether what he saw was a dream or whether those things really did take place. Later it becomes clear to us that W is a story Perec himself wrote when he was only 13 years old, yet here is what Gaspard Winckler says: "I wish to adopt the cold, impassive tone of the ethnologist: I visited this sunken world and this is what I saw there" (ibid, p. 10, First Series). If we read Gaspard Winckler's story without any empathy and compassion, as historians force us to, we must reject Gaspard Winckler's testimony for we know (or at the very least suspect) that this testimony is in fact based not on his own memories of the events but rather on a story written by a 13-year-old. Hence even if the 13-year-old child's story is based upon real experience (later on we see this is not the case), Gaspard Winckler's story cannot be trusted for it is rooted not in his memories but rather in an external device—the book he (or maybe someone else) wrote when he was 13 years old. Nevertheless this is not the case, for it is indeed almost impossible for us as readers to reject testimony that should be rejected. At this point we are exposed as wanting to believe despite being told explicitly that we are being lied to. We yearn to identify and we cannot reject the "testimony."

Alongside Gaspard Winckler's story, we are also exposed to the story of Perec's own life. In this case the cold truth, and it is indeed frozen and cruel, is presented immediately at the beginning of the chapter in the first part that opens the *Second Series*: "I have no childhood memories. Up to my 12th year or thereabouts, my story comes to barely a couple of lines." He continues: "I lost my father at four, my mother at six; I spent the war in various boarding houses at Villard-de-Lans. In 1945, my father's sister and her husband adopted me (ibid, p. 13, Second Series). This is the real story of Georges Perec, a Jewish boy whose parents came from Poland.

In addition, Perec's life story is told in detail in Chaps. 6 and 8 of the first part (both chapters are part of the *Second Series*). Yet when we delve more deeply, it is impossible to disregard the unique writing method on these pages. The chapters are full of marginal notations, almost ad nauseam. Beyond providing an intentionally exhausting reading experience, the role of the marginal notations is to fundamentally undermine the ostensible historical reliability of the "autobiography." In a deeper sense, there appears to be disparagement of the notion that it is possible to base autobiography on facts. In this section Perec dryly describes his history and the history of his family. LaCapra (2001) notes that, ideally, in academic research writing each sentence should be supported by a reference that points to the source and whether the source is original (testimony, documents and the like) or another type of source. Perec's purpose is to make fun of this method, and LaCapra is indeed well aware of this possibility.

At the end of the first part of the book we are confronted with two types of testimony that by their very nature invalidate each other. The story of W is fabricated and forgotten:

> When I was 13 I made up a story which I told and drew in pictures. Later I forgot it. Seven years ago, one evening, in Venice, I suddenly remembered that this story was called W and that it was, in a way, if not the story of my childhood, then at least a story of my childhood (Perec, 2003, p. 13, Second Series).

In referring to the sentence *Later I forgot it,* those among us who are romantics and perhaps those who are psychoanalysts would say that this is the truth, that Perec represses what happened to him and that W describes Perec's traumatic and impossible experiences between 1939 and 1945. Yet this is a naïve view, for later in the *First Series*, in Chap. 3 (the second testimony), it becomes clear that the man who sets out on the journey and whose identity we do not yet know is a soldier who has deserted. If so, he is not the only survivor. He is the last witness, though this too, it seems, is not really true for later we learn that someone else survived, someone who Gaspard Winckler meets by chance. Whether Gaspard Winckler is his real name or a made-up, invented name, he was, even if against his will, part of the machinery of death. He was not a victim in the basic sense of the word.

In the following discussion, I refer to the adult character as Gaspard and to the child as Winckler. Gaspard was sent in search of an 8-year-old boy who was thought to be dead, and after deserting Gaspard adopted the boy's identity. We can assume that Gaspard and the boy are actually one and the same character and that the doctor who asks Gaspard to search for the boy is a therapist of sorts. In effect the soldier (Gaspard) and the boy (Winckler) are the same character. The *First Series* describes Gaspard's attempt to preserve his childhood memories, if not his childhood itself, when he sets out to save Winckler who has been stranded in the middle of the ocean—at least metaphorically. At this point it is clear that the two series carry out a dialogue between one another. In the first part of the book he writes: "My childhood belongs to those things which *I know I don't know* much about. It is behind me; yet it is the ground on which I grew, and it once belonged to me, however obstinately I assert that it no longer does" (ibid p. 19, *Second Series*—my emphasis).

Perec describes a man who is fleeing his childhood and who, at the same time, is being pursued by absent memories. In this sense, at least, this represents adoption of the Freudian model of forgotten trauma (which might by illusionary) pursuing the victim (Freud, 1939). This then is the relationship between Gaspard and Winckler, and the feeling becomes intensified considering that the child Winckler is deaf and dumb. Trauma has often been known to cause deafness and dumbness (Myers, 1940). The trauma here can be attributed to the death of his mother in 1943 when Perec was 6 years old. Perec is well aware of the psychoanalytic discourse, surrounding this issue and was even in analysis for 5 years at the time he wrote this book (Bellos, 1993). He notes the following with respect to deafness and dumbness:

> ... since all the doctors they had consulted were quite clear on this point: there was no internal injury, no inherited disorder, no anatomical or physiological deformity to account for the boy being deaf and dumb; this could only be ascribed to some infantile trauma whose precise configuration unfortunately remained obscure despite examinations by numerous psychiatrists (Perec, 2003, p. 33, First Series).

The miracle is in the cessation of the dumbness of Winckler the boy, or the discovery of the memory that served as an anchor for Perec himself. That is, the *First Series* represents the voyage in which the adult Perec attempts in the *Second Series* to rescue his childhood, or at least some of his childhood memories. But this is not possible. It is only a misconception fostered by the psychological discourse as part of the therapeutic industry we live with today: "each of them clings to this illusion, until one day, off Tierra del Fuego, they are hit by one of those sudden cyclones[2] which are everyday occurrences in those parts, and the boat sinks" (ibid p. 33, First Series). In any case if we return to the deafness and dumbness of the child Winckler, we can claim that this is also a metaphor for the link between the adult Gaspard and his childhood, a child who hears nothing and says nothing. He is cut off, separated, and it is impossible to make contact with him. Even though Perec finds a way to describe his childhood, he incarcerates the description in deafness and dumbness. In the second section, the description of Perec's childhood is based on "yellowing snapshots, a handful of

[2] On the other hand, this cyclone can be interpreted as an outburst of traumatic memory. Indeed, with Perec anything is possible.

eyewitness accounts and a few paltry documents to prop up my implausible memories" (ibid p. 19, Second Series).

Thus, the Island of W, which is based on the fabricated story of a 13-year-old boy, is meant to tell us something *real* about Perec's childhood, while the other story, which is based on historical documents, is an extremely fragile story. It seems that Perec himself summarizes this paradox perfectly by reflecting on the nature of the entire "book" and perhaps on the possibility of writing anything at all about trauma:

> I do not know whether I have anything to say, I know that I am saying nothing; I do not know if what I might have to say is unsaid because it is unsayable (the unsayable is not buried inside writing, it is what prompted it in the first place); I know that what I say is blank, is neutral, is a sign, once and for all, of a once-and-for-all annihilation (ibid p. 47, Second Series).

Nonetheless, indeed quite surprisingly, the chapter ends on an optimistic note:

> I am not writing in order to say that I shall say nothing, I am not writing to say that I have nothing to say. I write: I write because we lived together, because I was one amongst them, a shadow amongst their shadows, a body close to their bodies. I write because they left in me their indelible mark, whose trace is writing. Their memory is dead in writing; writing is the memory of their death and the assertion of my life (ibid pp. 47–48, Second Series).

13.3.3 After His Mother's Death

While the first part of the book describes Perec's life until he was separated from his mother in 1943, when she was sent to Auschwitz. The second part describes Perec's life in various institutions (written in the first person) and continues the *First Series* about life on the island of W (written in an informative style). Both parts look back at the past albeit in different ways.

Perec again writes about the difficulty of anchoring his thoughts: "What marks this period especially is the absence of landmarks; these memories are scraps of life snatched from the void. No mooring. Nothing to anchor them or hold them down. Almost no way of ratifying them. No sequence in time, except as I have reconstructed it arbitrarily over the years" (ibid p. 73, Second Series). Indeed the memories appear to be the opposite of what really happened. In the first part of the book Perec's memory from the boarding house of a little girl who was locked up and was hurt because a medal was torn off her actually conceals a contrary memory: not of a medal that was torn off but of a yellow Magen David patch affixed by a pin. Yet it is essential to note that Perec never wore a yellow patch. In the second part of the book memories describe events that did not happen to him but that he was *witness* to. In this sense adopting someone else's story shows the reader, the listener who adopts Perec's story of the witness, the extent to which such an act can be problematic.

An example of a story that Perec adopts is about his sledding accident and breaking his shoulder. Even though no one remembers this accident, the accident did take place. But it was not Perec who was injured. Instead, this happened to another boy named Philippe. "The thing happened, a little later or a little earlier, and I was not its heroic victim but *just a witness*" (ibid p. 83, Second Series, my emphasis).

Perec also describes other events in this way and casts doubt upon them. It seems that even returning later to the scene of events does not arouse any memory whatsoever:

> The children's home we moved into was much smaller than Collège Turenne. I cannot remember its name or what it looked like and when I returned to Lans I tried but failed to identify it, as either I lacked any sense of familiarity anywhere or, on the other hand, I would decide that any old chalet was it and strain to winkle out of some architectural detail, out of the presence of a slide or an eave or a gate, the material of a memory (ibid p. 129, Second Series).

Interestingly, Perec's first novel, which was originally titled *Gaspard Is Not Dead,* and after that *Le Condottière,* begins with the description of another incident, an injury that caused a scar on his upper lip that became the mark by which he identified himself. The hero of the book *(Le Condottière)* is Gaspard Winckler, the same Gaspard who sets out to search for the boy from the *First Series* in the first section of "the book." This would not be so upsetting if Gaspard from *Le Condottière* were not such a brilliant counterfeiter. This upsetting fact compels us to read the entire book, or at least the half representing the *First Series*, which is printed in italic font and describes the life of Gaspard Winckler from the perspective that Winckler is a swindler, a liar and a counterfeiter. Nothing less. For this reason we must at the very least wonder whether Winckler is a deserting soldier and whether he is as naïve as he describes himself. Or perhaps, as emerges in the autobiographical description in this book when the boy protests his innocence in various cases, he indeed did what was claimed. For example, Perec states that one day a girl was found confined in a locked broom closet. Everyone blamed the boy and demanded that he admit to having locked her up, even if unintentionally. All the *evidence* indicates that "I was the only person who could have locked up the little girl. But I knew perfectly well that I hadn't done it, on purpose or not" (ibid p. 130, Second Series). Yet a bee sting turns things upside down: "For all my classmates, and *especially for me,* this sting was *proof* that I had locked up the little girl: the Good Lord had punished me" (ibid p. 130, Second Series, my emphasis). The bee sting resembles his scar from another story:

> One day one of my skis slipped from my hand and accidentally grazed the face of the boy putting his skis away next to me and he, in a mad fury, picked up one of his ski-sticks and hit me with it on the face, with the spike end, cutting open my upper lip (ibid p. 109, First Series).

To Perec this scar is of prime importance as a "distinguishing mark" and it is "so as not to hide it that I do not wear a moustache" (ibid p. 109, First Series). This mark, if I correctly interpret what I have difficulty defining as a "book" (and therefore put in quotation marks), is meant to represent the bogus innocence of Perec, the boy who constantly protests his innocence. The fact that Gaspard Winckler in Perec's first book *(Le Condottière)* has a similar scar and murders a man out of his personal failure to forge a painting that was commissioned from him testifies to the lie behind Gaspard's ostensible "innocence."

A shocking picture emerges from the description of Perec's childhood after the loss of his mother. He renounced his memories and replaced them with books:

> a hundred other episodes, whole chunks of story or mere turns of phrase which feel not only as if I had always known them but, much more, as if they were, to my mind, *virtually part of history*; an inexhaustible fount of memory, of material for rumination and of a kind of certainty (ibid p. 144, Second Series—my emphasis).

Perec rereads books, or parts of books, again and again and this rereading creates within him "an enjoyment of complicity, of collusion, or more especially, and in addition, of having in the end found kin again" (ibid p. 144, Second Series), just as looking at old family pictures brings up childhood memories.

Like Perec, we also tend to adopt history that is not ours. This, perhaps, is the source of collective history and maybe even of collective trauma. Perec reveals this practice in a ridiculous light: he adopts cheap fiction. While on the other hand, we do this by relying upon dependable historical sources, yet I would likd to suggest that both of these processes are identical. Essentially, as Schacter (2001) argues, one of the strongest difficulties of human memory is to remember the source of memory. The story of W must be approached from the perspective of this insight. Perec mentions the book *Michael, the Circus Dog* and notes that

> at least one of whose episodes *imprinted itself in my memory*: an *athlete* is about to be drawn asunder by four horses, but in actual fact the horses are pulling not on the athlete's limbs but on four steel cables crossed over in an *X and camouflaged by the athlete's costume*; *he smiles under this fake torture*, but the circus director demands that he make a show of the most excruciating pain (Perec, 2003, p. 143, Second Series, my emphasis).

We must take this description into account, particularly in view of the fact that (ibid p. 77 in the Second Series) we understand that X and W are identical signs. That is, the entire description of what happens on the island of W is imaginary, the result of forgery, of cheap fiction, of show, while at the same time it is a frighteningly accurate description of a concentration camp—for the sign X is also identical to the Nazi symbol, the swastika—卐. Essentially, each of these signs is meaningful and hollow in the same time.

Indeed it is shocking that not only does a book stand at the core of the story of W, but once again a story that based on a fraud, for the athlete smiles under this *fake torture* in a way Perec presents here a new alternative to read Kafka's story "In the penal colony".[3] Yet it is even more shocking that even this piece of information does not lead us to reject the whole story as nothing more than a fraud.

13.4 Levi, Perec and the Question of Bearing Witness

13.4.1 Introduction

According to Felman, the age in which we live can be defined as the age of testimony, and testimony by definition is derived from human memory. We saw in the introduction that one of the main questions in contemporary historical discourse is how to treat the testimony and memory of the individual when it comes to understanding and writing about events. This issue becomes much more difficult when memory refers to a traumatic event.

In the second part of this chapter I describe and examine the testimony of Primo Levi. Clearly, Primo Levi is one of the central witnesses of our time. Not only has reshaped discourse regarding life in the concentration camps, he has also influenced our attitude of the very concept of testimony. In the third part of this chapter I discuss a different kind of testimony, that of Georges Perec. Undoubtedly, and we must keep this in mind, the experiences of Levi and of Perec are not identical. Levi was born in 1919 and was sent to Auschwitz in February 1944 together with another 650 Italian Jews. After 11 months the camp was liberated by the Red Army, and only 20 survivors were left from Levi's transport. Perec, in contrast, a French Jew born in 1936, had an entirely different experience. His father was drafted into the French army and was killed in 1940, and his mother was murdered in Auschwitz in 1943.

Though Levi and Perec differ in many ways, on a deeper level they conduct a linked discourse regarding the role of the witness as storyteller, writer and historian, both on the individual level and also with respect to the association between memory and history. In this section I seek to show that ultimately Levi and Perec write in order to respectively differentiate themselves from the living (Levi) and the dead (Perec). I believe that the points of congruence between these two should be examined against the backdrop of the clear disparity between them.

13.4.2 The Witness's Fear of Being a Counterfeiter

As indicated in the third part of this chapter, Perec feels like a counterfeiter, which manifests in several ways. First, Gaspard Winckler, the deserter soldier who becomes a witness in the book *W, or the Memory of Childhood*, is not exactly an innocent witness. At the very least this is a man who was deep in the gray zone and perhaps even among the victimizers (murderers). Second, Gaspard Winckler is the hero of Perec's first book, in which he is engaged in forging paintings. This fact should cast doubts upon his testimony, but quite surprisingly this does not seems to happen. Indeed we are exposed to a subject who wants to be believed at any price (on this issue see: Žižek, 2003).

It appears impossible to really distinguish between Gaspard Winckler and Perec himself. Perec sees himself as a counterfeiter, and the imaginary yet precise description of the Island of W, which symbolizes concentration camps (or forced labor camps), in essence originates in the book that Perec wrote when he was only 13 years old—*When I was 13 I made up a story which I told and drew in pictures.*[4] Yet Perec admits

[3] Kafka, F. (2011). In the penal colony. Penguin UK.

[4] In the following sections, quotations that were previously given are presented in italics without indicating the page number.

remembering practically nothing from that period of his life. In this sense, for Perec, the book has turned into an artificial memory. Perec's memories are nothing more than the story of events from the period of his childhood that happened to other people and that he has adopted as his own story. Not only are Perec's "memories" borrowed, but the entire story of the Island of W, in fact, is the result of novels Perec read in his childhood and whose plots became substitutes for his own childhood memories.

Perec is also a counterfeiter on a much deeper level, for he has absolutely betrayed the unwritten contract between the witness/storyteller and the listener/reader. So, similar to real testimony, Perec's is convincing to the point that the reader believes the story despite knowing that it is false and nothing more than the fruit of the teller's imagination. It should be considered, however, that in cases of severe traumatic experiences there is no other way to tell the untellable rather than by adopting different kinds of techniques that allow the victim telling what really has happened by inventing imaginary story in kind. Indeed Semprun (1998) discus this possibility in his book Literature or life. Essentially, the problem in this case is how to avoid kitsch (Friedlander, 1984).

This is not the case with Primo Levi. For him, the character of the counterfeiter cannot exist. Nevertheless, the question arises as to why, in his first book, *The Wrench,*[5] which he does not write as a witness, he refers to himself in terms of a counterfeiter. Is it because in truth he cannot take upon himself the role of writer? As he claims in an interview with Pier Maria Paoletti in 1963: "But I realized I was a foreign body" (Belpoliti, 2001, p. 80). Or perhaps he was concerned or even terrified that he had turned bearing witness into a profession and therefore his testimony was nothing more than an automatic story, that he had experienced the period of the camps by means of books and was cut off at least to some extent from the events themselves. In this sense, in the following quotation from an interview with Luca Lamberti in 1971 if we convert the word "create" to the phrase "bear witness" we can see that Levi was in fact terrified that he was nothing more than a counterfeiter: "All we can ask of those who create [bear witness] is that they should be neither servile nor false" (Belpoliti, 2001, p. 80).

Perec is linked to the deepest anxieties of survivors who become witnesses. And yes, I intentionally use the word "become" because there is a shift here from survivor to witness (Laub, 1995). Levi describes the fear of many concentration camp prisoners that *even if we tell what happened no one will believe us* (Belpoliti, 2001; Levi, 1993; 1959). In order to deal with this fear Levi, like many other prisoners, had already turned himself into a historian while he was imprisoned, in order to become a historical documentation machine in real time. In the age of testimony after the Second World War, the survivor is terrified of inaccuracies. To be more precise, the witness who acts as historian does so out of a desire (whether conscious or unconscious) to corroborate his testimony through solid historical facts. The witness feels threatened by history and hence often adopts his story to the historical story.

Thus, when the witness takes on the role of writer he fears becoming a counterfeiter. Additionally, the witness feels like a counterfeiter when he adapts his testimony to the historical knowledge he acquired after the traumatic event so that his testimony will not contradict the "historical truth." In the age of testimony there can no longer be an innocent witness.

13.4.3 The Death of the Innocent Witness

Levi stresses the discrepancy between the testimony of survivors who had no privileges, those who survived due to special privileges (the gray zone) and the victimizers themselves. Note that—survivors who had privileges are not the same as those who were themselves victimizers and oppressors. Nor must we fail to differentiate between the survivors who had privileges and those who did not. Perec shockingly demonstrates how easy it is for us to see the oppressor, Gaspard Winckler, as a victim.

[5]First published as La Chiave a Stella by Einaudi in 1978, the book was written after Levi had retired from SIVA. Published in English in 1987.

In the posttrauma era we recognize that everyone has been traumatized, including the victimizers/oppressors, and we are willing to forgive and forget. Everyone has undergone trauma, perhaps even as part of the modern condition (Luckhurst, 2008; Seltzer, 1997), everyone carries a trauma: we must listen to everyone, have mercy and forgive. Clearly such a process ultimately harms the victims of actual trauma. If in the past the trauma of the victims was not recognized, today we no longer recognize the unique nature of their trauma because "everyone has been traumatized." Hence we prefer to see Gaspard Winckler as a victim and not as part of the industry of murder.

And we must ask whether it is still possible to talk about an *innocent witness*. Certainly not all the survivors had privileges and not all of them were part of that gray zone. Yet in the Kafkaesque era saturated with feelings of guilt, is it possible to talk in terms of an *innocent witness*? That is, even if we assume that at the time of the event itself the witness was innocent, does the witness in the attempt to forget, in order to recover, still remain innocent today? Has bearing witness become a political act or even an act of rebellion? Can we still treat testimony as something innocent and impartial?

There is another problem here as well. Terr (1984) describes a situation in which, due to the need to feel in control rather than totally helpless at the time of the trauma, the victims of trauma assume responsibility regarding things that were out of their control. In this sense it seems that as part of the coping process the victims assume an active role, and in many cases this is a negative role with respect to the traumatic event. This is a kind of defense mechanism. Survivors have ceased to be *innocent witnesses,* among other things because they prefer to be a partner to the act rather than to admit to themselves that they live in a world of absolute chaos.

While Primo Levi seeks to discriminate unequivocally between the types of testimony, Perec demonstrates for us how difficult it is in practice for us not to identify with the witness even if we know that he had special privileges or even was part of the group of oppressors. Through the case of the little girl who was locked up, Perec even demonstrates for us how in certain cases the witness describes himself as an *innocent witness* while in fact he was an active participant in the crime. On this point Levi and Perec appear to agree. Witnesses with privileges and those who were oppressors (again without confusing these two groups) prefer to conceal their active role in the crime and as a result are perceived as victims in their testimony. Moreover, Levi's and Perec's reflections on the very process of bearing witness prevent us from speaking in terms of an *innocent witness.* In this sense we may be in the era of testimony, but this is an era devoid of witnesses.

13.4.4 Testimony as Scientific Work

As Gaspard Winckler notes in the "book" his purpose is to tell about what he saw with "the cold, impassive tone of the ethnologist: I visited this sunken world and this is what I saw there" (Perec, 2003, p. 10, First Series). In many ways this is also Levi's purpose. Thus, sometimes Levi's descriptions come out of his mouth as if he has surrendered his humanity so that he can record what he has seen. The model of Galileo as the objective reporter of his observations is the desired model for the witness from the historical-factual perspective. In turn, Levi describes an unconscious process of already preparing to bear witness during his time in the concentration camp and of his attempts to renounce the human perspective and to become a historian in real time. Perec pokes fun at this option. According to him, because of the loss of the human perspective in this process we can adopt the experience of someone else and at the extremum abandon our personal memories in favor of stories originating in books. Perec does not propose a new option, though he takes this to the extreme by giving up his lost memories in favor of adopting "memories" from the books he has read. Clearly, Levi is fully aware of this possibility. In the answer to a question posed by Aurelio Andreoli in a 1981 interview, he states that he originally wanted to give his book *La ricerca delle radici (The Search for Roots)* the title *Another Way of Saying I.* In this book Levi examines what influenced him from the literary perspective and wonders: "How much of what we write comes from what we read?" (Belpoliti, 2001, p. 99). It is fascinating that Levi defines this book as a personal anthology and even as "a form of autobiography" (Belpoliti, 2001, p. 98). That is, he is aware of the possibility that, at least to some extent, we adopt content from the world of literature.

Despite the attempt to show that testimony is scientific work that requires preparation during the time of the trauma itself, when witnesses stop being human and turn themselves into scientific tape recorders, this type of work in effect is impossible and indeed may have radical implications in the opposite direction. Not only is it impossible for witnesses to scientifically bear witness to what was. What in fact happens is that they adopt an entirely different story.

In the introduction I state that we are in an era in which human beings are their own historians and history defers to memory. Here we see the extreme implications of this process. The elements comprising the autobiographical story of each individual may originate in the memories, testimonies and even novels of others; Perec describes his own autobiographical history as a "hundred other episodes, whole chunks of story or mere turns of phrase which feel not only as if I had always known them but, much more, as if they were, to my mind, virtually part of history; an inexhaustible fount of memory, of material for rumination and of a kind of certainty" (Perec, 2003 p. 144, Second Series).

If we accept this possibility, we can argue that we can embrace memories that are not our own and, in turn, even live someone else's life. One justification is that the facts do not correspond to the memories or to what individuals think they know about their lives. Indeed, when Perec attempts to describe his past in a factual and dry manner he makes use of marginal notes over and over again that negate or at the very least cast doubt upon what was stated in the original text. Perec demonstrates for us that it is impossible to create an accurate and proven autobiographical history. The other side of this idea is that it is indeed possible to embrace someone else's memory.

13.4.5 A Built-In Trap

Many people who have experienced ongoing traumas suffer from dissociation, structural memory problems, and cognitive problems among other issues. In some cases the victims of such traumas, especially those that occurred during childhood (van der Kolk et al., 1991) suffer from split and fragmented personalities and structural dissociation (Nijenhuis et al., 2010; van der Hart et al., 2004). The result of severe and ongoing trauma may be the generation of two personalities that attempt to destroy one another. Perec describes this condition precisely—a situation in which an individual flees the memories of his childhood while at the same time pursues them; an individual who attempts to deny his past while at the same time his past pursues him; an individual who attempts to exchange his childhood memories for literature. The result is that on the Island of W. Perec portrays the witness as he truly is—a posttraumatic storyteller, a broken individual in dispute with himself, filled with paradoxes that cannot be bridged.

Referring to the witness who has become his own historian as a posttraumatic figure leads us to rethink not only the institution of bearing witness, but also historical discourse itself. In extreme cases of complex and intransigent trauma (Herman, 1992) the posttraumatic individual has difficulty separating the present from the past (LaCapra, 2001). Without this ability, a situation is created in which the witness is unable to testify and experiences the trauma in the present. This is a Catch-22, since such a witness, who is confused, perplexed and divided within himself, is the one who can describe the primal experience of the moment of trauma (Ataria, 2014b). Yet it is precisely this possibility that prevents such individuals from being witnesses, for to become a witness they must observe the event from a distance and be a historian. Perec reveals the ultimate witness to us. Yet, paradoxically, it is impossible to believe such witnesses, even if they are absolutely innocent. What makes this case a Catch-22 is that this is the witness we deeply want to believe.

Perec admits that, if the truth be told, his testimony bears witness only to one thing—the total emptiness of the posttraumatic figure: *I know that what I say is blank, is neutral, is a sign, once and for all, of a once-and-for-all annihilation*. Perec is Gaspard Winckler and at the same time is the child himself. It is impossible to separate these characters even though they deny any acquaintance. This reality also is not far from that of Levi's. In an interview with Edoardo Fadini in 1966 he states: "I am split in two… they are two halves of my brain… they are two parts of me that exist so distinctly that I cannot bring the second" (Belpoliti, 2001, p. 85). Every witness, it appears, is caught in a built-in trap, an inherent contradiction. As soon as such witnesses are capable of telling about the trauma, the story becomes disconnected from the experience itself, for the traumatic experience is found on many levels that are beyond words, beyond language.

13.4.6 To Write in Order to Live

The ultimate question is this: Why should the witness tell his story or write at all? Like many other witnesses, Levi comments on the uncontrollable and pathological need to tell. In a 1987 interview with Roberto Di Caro, Levi states: "Recounting them [recounting those experiences] was a need, you would need strength not to write or to talk about them" (Belpoliti, 2001, p. 174). Levi, like many others, also describes writing as a process of recovery, telling Silvia Giacomini in a 1979 interview that he stopped acting like a survivor when he began writing. In a 1970 interview with Giuseppe Grassano, Levi describes the liberating joy that fills him when he tells a story. Essentially it is because Levi feels that if he did not write he would feel cursed. Thus, Levi's writing is ultimately intended for someone else, as he states in an interview with Roberto Di Caro in 1987: "My books have been written for an audience" (Belpoliti, 2001, p. 169). It is true that Levi is writing for the Italian reader. But even more than that he is writing for the German reader (Levi, 1993, Chaper 8). For Levi, bearing witness is a political act. He also seeks to contest the accusations that the Jews were helpless, passive and went like sheep to the slaughter. On this point it seems that Levi has accepted the notion that a story has healing powers.

Yet Levi admits that the need to bear witness is not the most important reason for writing. It appears there is a more important and deeper reason. As Levi states in an interview in 1980 with Ernesto Olivero (Belpoliti, 2001), it is more important for him to prove, to confirm and to clarify that he is *different from the other*; that he has experienced something the other did not experience and therefore that he is *on a higher plane than the other*, that is, on a higher level from those who had not been in the concentration camps.

On this point, it seems, Levi and Perec are in agreement. Despite the major differences between them, they both write in order to individualize themselves. But while Levi does this in order to differentiate himself from the other people around him, and perhaps especially from those who had special privileges and survived, Perec does this in order to differentiate himself from those who died—"writing is the memory of their death and the assertion of my life" (Perec, 2003, p. 48, Second Series).

In sum, Levi and Perec both write in order to live. Levi writes about the living, while Perec writes about the dead. To put it another way, while Levi writes about *what is*, Perec writes about what is *absent*.

13.5 Primo Levi and Georges Perec: Two Authentic (and Contradictory) Models of the Witness

13.5.1 Levi's Approach: Insisting on Mini-narrative While Acknowledging its Limitations

As we see in the second part of this chapter, in his book *The Drowned and the Saved* (1993) and in various interviews (Belpoliti, 2001) Levi openly and soberly discusses the problems of bearing witness. He describes general and specific problems he had to cope with, reveals his interests and his background, and explains how he consciously transformed himself into a transparent witness.

In addition, Levi adopts the approach of the historian who knows that it is impossible to create a meta-narrative without the transgression of some inaccuracy and that it is impossible to turn history into pure scientific research. He shapes his testimony according to this principle while acknowledging its limitations.

Among other things Levi fully understands that eventually even the historian cannot avoid telling a story (Stone, 1979). Indeed, in his book *If This Is a Man* (1959) Levi wishes to testify, yet he understands that his final product is in fact a story—that it is not a testimony in the classic sense. Obviously Levi is not merely a witness telling what happened; he is also a *writer.* Levi understands that this step is unavoidable—he cannot avoid being both a witness and a writer. For this reason Levi chooses to focus on the mini-narrative without pretensions of providing a historical description and without attempting to produce a meta-narrative.

By focusing on the mini-narrative on the one hand and acknowledging its unavoidable limitations on the other hand, Levi becomes the "ultimate witness," the Galileo of his era, expressing how lost faith in the subjective experience is something that can be measured. His role is to tell what happened, as best he can, while being true to what he really saw, and what he experienced.

13.5.2 Perec's Approach: Exposing the Inability to Testify

Perec takes the exposure of limitations to the extreme. As we see in the third part of this chapter, even though we cannot rely upon Perec's story, as readers we cannot help but identify with him, even if we are unable even to determine with whom he identifies in the book. Perec's testimony creates the paradox of the liar—a liar who openly states he is lying. At this point, when there is not the shadow of a doubt that we must be skeptical, Perec describes the Island of W, which he compares to the death camps (manipulating the letter W turns it into a swastika—see page 77). This description, as we will see, is extremely accurate, without containing even one fact that can tie the Island of W to the death camps.

What, then, is the Island of W? A place without any geographic point of reference that does not appear on any map. White men from Western countries founded it, though "it doesn't make much difference whether W was founded by outlaws or sportsmen" (Perec, 2003, p. 67, First Series). In any case "W, today, is a land where Sport is king, a nation of athletes where Sport and life unite in a single magnificent effort" (ibid, p. 67, First Series). Any violation of the rules, "intentional or unwitting—a meaningless distinction on W—leads to automatic disqualification" (ibid p. 71, First Series). "The rules of Sport are harsh and life on W makes them harsher still" (ibid p. 110, First Series). Most of the laws of W are "normally so laconic, and whose very silence is a mortal threat to the Athletes under its yoke" (ibid, p. 152, First Series). "But we know the world of W well enough to grasp that its most lenient Laws are but the expression of a greater and more savage irony" (ibid, p. 154, First Series).

Yet despite all this, obedience to the rules does not help the athletes, for the reality on W is a reality governed "by arbitrary decisions, by aberrant umpiring, by abuses of power, by the liberties taken and the almost outrageous partiality constantly displayed by the Judges" (ibid, p. 112, First Series). Thus, the "Athlete must know that nothing is certain … Decisions concerning him, whether they be trivial or vital, are taken without reference to him" (ibid, p. 117, First Series). For example, "he may well believe that his task, as a sportsman, is to win … but he may come last, and still be declared the Winner: someone, somewhere, decided that that race, on that day, would be run that way" (ibid, p. 117, First Series). Thus, in effect "it is more important to be lucky than to be deserving" (ibid, p. 118, First Series). This arbitrariness is part of the desire "to give everyone a chance" (ibid, p. 118, First Series).

On the Island of W four villages compete against each other. It soon becomes clear that these competitions are in facts "selections" (ibid, p. 73, First Series) that apparently take place each and every day, just like in the concentration camps. The precise and accurate screening of the athletes "reduces checking procedures to a minimum" (ibid, p. 83, First Series). The selection does the work for the authorities. In order to understand the nature of these competitions on W it is enough to describe the Atlantiads competitions (one of the competitions on the island) "that are placed under the sign of total liberty" (ibid, p. 130, First Series). The purpose of these competitions is to reach women who, for this event, have been removed from the closed areas where they live and afterwards must run for their lives because "as a rule it is right in front of the podium, either on the cinder track or on the grass, that they get raped" (ibid, p. 125, First Series). In this competition the competitors, "like the women they pursue, should be entirely naked" (ibid p. 127, First Series). Due to the nature of the competition it seems that at least one-third of the competitors were "knocked out and are lying unconscious on the ground" (ibid, p. 130, First Series) either while in the battle arena or before: "Pitched battles break out at night in the dormitories. Athletes are drowned in sinks and lavatory pans" (ibid, p. 133, First Series).

The further we read in the *First Series* in the second part, the clearer it becomes that W is not an island where people are engaged in sport but rather a death camp where "the survival of the fittest is the law of this land" (ibid, p. 89, First Series). As expected, the results are poor, the contests are bogus and "the pentathlon and decathlon contestants enter the stadium dressed as clowns, wearing outrageous make-up, and each event is used as a pretext for mockery" (ibid, p. 85, First Series). The losers are unlikely to remain alive, for the result is "the death of the man who came last" (ibid, p. 110, First Series). If the contest does not end in death, the loser must pay the usual price: "he will probably save his skin and undergo only the same punishment as the other losers," namely, "like them, he will have to strip naked and run the gauntlet of Judges armed with sticks and crops; like them, he will be put in the stocks, then paraded around the villages with a heavy, nail-studded, wooden yoke on his neck" (ibid, p. 111, First Series).

The "winners" are of course rewarded with an additional meal. This is part of the "dietary system of W" (ibid, p. 91, First Series) that results in "the vast majority of Athletes … therefore be[ing] chronically undernourished" (ibid, p. 91, First Series). In turn, when the losers return, "exhausted, ashen-faced Athletes tottering under the weight of oaken yokes" (ibid, p. 139, First Series), they begin "tearing each other to pieces for a scrap of salami, a drop of water, a puff at a cigarette" (ibid, p. 139, First Series).

Until the age of 14 children are kept in separate areas, and then they are brought to one of the four villages and referred to as novices. "Novices have no names" (ibid, p. 99, First Series), just as "practicing Athletes have no names" (ibid, p. 99, First Series). During the first few months the novices are held in detention. Their hands and feet are tied, their mouths muzzled, and at night they are chained to their beds. Indeed, life on the Island of W is terrifying. The most important thing for novices to learn in order to survive, however, is that "the Law is implacable, but the Law is unpredictable. The law must be known by all, but the Law cannot be known" (ibid, p. 117, First Series). Thus, in practice, in order to survive, the novice must understand that "what he is seeing is not anything horrific, not a nightmare, not something he will suddenly wake from, something he can rid his mind of." Yet "[h]ow can you explain that this is life, real life, this is what there'll be every day, this is what there is, and nothing else." Indeed on W "you have to fight to live. There is no alternative… it is not possible to say no. There's no recourse, no mercy, no salvation to be had from anyone. There's not even any hope that time will sort things out" thus essentially "that is the only thing that will turn out to be true" (ibid, pp. 139-140, First Series). Not surprisingly then, after six months, when the novices are freed from their chains, there is only one way for them to survive and that is to become the servant of one of the champions and to provide him with commercial and sexual services. This is the abridged format of the social structure on the Island of W—the relationship of the dominator to the dominated in which there is no access to the masters while the slaves tear each other apart. In sum, life on W is as follows:

> Submerged in a world unchecked, with no knowledge of the Laws that crush him, a torturer or a victim of his co-villagers, under the scornful and sarcastic eyes of the Judges, the W Athlete does not know where his real enemies are, does not know that he could beat them or that such a win would be the only true Victory he could score, the

> only one which would liberate him. But his own life and death seem to him ineluctable, inscribed once and for all in an unspeakable fate (ibid, pp. 159-160, First Series).

Clearly in his description of the Island of W Perec succeeds in capturing the essence of the concentration and death camps. Perec appears to present a different model of the witness—the witness who does not remember. Perhaps he really did forget, perhaps he repressed his memories or perhaps he does not want to remember. More than anything else, Perec is the witness who describes the forgetting, the annihilation, the severance from childhood memories and from traumatic memories. Perec is the opposite side of the witness who has turned himself into a historian (Levi). Perec represents the broken, defeated witness who is perhaps guilty and perhaps not. He does not want to remember but he does not manage to forget. He tries to remember but is trapped in his loss of memory. Perec is the most reliable witness, the one trapped in the paradox of the liar who traps us with him in a paradox, in a state of limbo. Perec is the witness who testifies to the disintegration of memory and through this disintegration he captures the very essence of the concentration camp. This is an authentic model for bearing witness: the witness who does not attempt to describe what he saw from a historical perspective, the witness who adopts the experiences of other people and openly admits this. Perec is the model of the dismantled witness, the post-traumatic witness who is embroiled in a dispute with himself, who without hiding anything exposes his authentic inability to testify.

In sum, Perec is the witness who is totally aware of the paradox of the liar and his testimony stems from this paradox. Thus, paradoxically, this actually reveals him as an authentic witness who, in a certain, sense salvages the human experience.

13.5.3 Witnesses' Obligation to be True to Themselves

Can the most reliable witness (e.g., the one whose testimony corresponds exactly to the historical facts) cause advocates of the revisionist movement who openly claim that the Nazi death camps were a fraud to withdraw their claim? This is, indeed, a fundamental question, but the answer is a resounding no!

Having said this, a critical point remains. We must understand that witnesses do not have to cope with Holocaust deniers. That is simply not their role. The evidence is strong and objective and the findings cannot be denied. In a certain sense Holocaust deniers are denying reality itself, denying not only the past but also the very notion of any factual information. This is an almost metaphysical denial that abolishes the gap between reality and imagination. Thus, it is important to understand that ultimately all the testimonies about a particular event, as Tolstoy suggests, do not enable us to know everything about the event. Furthermore, collecting evidence such as documents and photographs and cross-referencing these with living witnesses will not be sufficient for those who deny reality itself. Essentially, the lone witness cannot face up to those who choose to deny. This is true in every field. Nothing can convince a total skeptic. The fear of absolute skepticism and radical relativism seems to have led certain historians to quantify history and turn it into an exact science. Yet as Lawrence Stone (1979) puts it, the quantitative method ultimately proved to be hollow and useless.

Witnesses can never replace the historian. That is not their job, nor is it their job to cope with those who deny reality. A witness describes another layer of what was, not at the expense of anything else. It is indeed true that in a reality where historians find themselves in a profound crisis and engaged in meta-scientific discussions regarding the nature of their work, witnesses are pushed to the side and therefore attempt to turn their personal story into a historical story. Under such circumstances the unique nature of the witness is lost. Yet witnesses should not be part of this game, and the crisis of history should not bother witnesses. Accordingly, it is not the witnesses' job to handle these issues. Instead, a witness needs to obey different kinds of rules and to find a way to be authentic, nothing more and nothing less. Levi and Perec are doing just this, each in his own way.

Levi and Perec represent two contradictory models of the witness. They are situated at the two ends of the spectrum. Levi already took on the role of the historian while he was in the camps and turned into an obsessive documenter in an attempt to be the Galileo of the concentration camps. Time has proven that he succeeded at this. Perec, on the other hand, represents the authentic witness who gave up on and renounced the historical perspective. The book *W, or the Memory of Childhood* is not an actual story. Hence, based on this book it is not clear who Perec really is—a writer or a storyteller. Ultimately he is a witness who is an anti-storyteller, anti-writer, anti-historian. He is what he is: a posttraumatic witness, self-embroiled, disintegrated, broken. He is a witness who wants to forget but cannot, who wants to remember but has lost contact with the childhood memories that are paradoxically chasing him in their absence.

13.6 Concluding Remarks

In order to preserve the institution of testimony witnesses must be allowed to be what in fact they are—no more and no less: people who were there and who saw the atrocities and who are now describing what they saw and what they heard and what they felt. They describe their subjective experience in a way that is not dependent upon any outside factor, without taking the historian or historical facts into consideration. In their own unique ways both Levi and Perec offer authentic models of bearing witness.

References

Ataria, Y. (2013). Traumatic silence [Hebrew]. *History & Theory: The Protocols, 29*, http://bezalel.secured.co.il/8/ataria29.htm.

Ataria, Y. (2014a). Acute Peritraumatic Dissociation: In Favor of a Phenomenological Inquiry. *Journal of Trauma & Dissociation, 15*(3), 332–347. doi:10.1080/15299732.2013.853722.

Ataria, Y. (2014b). Traumatic memories as black holes: A qualitative-phenomenological approach. *Qualitative Psychology, 1*(2), 123–140. doi:10.1037/qup0000009.

Ataria, Y. (2014c). Trauma as a Black Hole in the Heart of Culture [Hebrew]. *Ma'arag, 5*, 239–270.

Bellos, D. (1993). *Georges Perec: A life in words*. Boston: David R. Godine.

Belpoliti, M. (Ed.). (2001). *The voice of memory: interviews 1961–1987*. (R. Gordon, Trans.) New York: New Press.

Brewin, C. R. (2007). Autobiographical memory for trauma: Update on four controversies. *Memory, 15*(3), 227–48. doi:10.1080/09658210701256423.

Caruth, C. (Ed.). (1995). *Trauma: Explorations in memory*. Baltimore, MD: Johns Hopkins University Press.

Caruth, C. (1996). *Unclaimed experience: Trauma, narrative, and history*. Baltimore, MD: Johns Hopkins University Press.

Douglass, A., & Vogler, T. A. (2003). Introduction. In A. Douglass & T. A. Vogler (Eds.), *Witness and memory: the discourse of trauma* (pp. 1–53). New York: Routledge.

Felman, S., & Laub, D. (1992). *Testimony: Crises of witnessing in literature, psychoanalysis, and history*. Florence, KY: Taylor & Frances/Routledge.

Freud, S. (1939). *Moses and monotheism*. (K. Jones, Trans.) New York: Vintage Books.

Friedländer, S. (2007). *The years of extermination: Nazi Germany and the Jews, 1939–1945*. New York, NY: Harper Collins.

Reflections of Nazism: an essay on Kitsch and death /Saul Friedlander; translated from the French by Thomas Weyr. New York: Harper and Row, 1984.

Herman, J. L. (1992). Complex PTSD: A syndrome in survivors of prolonged and repeated trauma. *Journal of Traumatic Stress, 5*(3), 377–391. doi:10.1002/jts.2490050305.

Huizinga, J. (1959). The Task of Cultural History. In J. S. Holmes, & H. van Marle (Eds.), *Men and Ideas* (pp. 17-76). New York.

LaCapra, D. (2001). *Writing history, writing trauma*. Baltimore, MD: Johns Hopkins University Press.

Langer, L. (1991). *Holocaust testimonies: The ruins of memory*. New Haven: Yale University Press.

Laub, D. (1995). Truth and Testimony: The Process and the Struggle. In C. Caruth (Ed.), *Trauma: Explorations in memory* (pp. 61–45). Baltimore, MD: The Johns Hopkins University Press.

Levi, P. (1959). *If this is a man*. (S. Woolf, Trans.) New York: The Orion Press.

Levi, P. (1993). *The drowned and the saved*. (R. Rosenthal, Trans.) London: Abacus.

Loftus, E. (1993). The reality of repressed memories. *American Psychologist, 48*, 560–572.

Loftus, E. (2003). Our changeable memories: legal and practical implications. *Nature Reviews Neuroscience, 4*, 231–4.

Luckhurst, R. (2008). *The trauma question*. London: Routledge.

Myers, C. (1940). *Shell shock in France 1914-18*. Cambridge: Cambridge University Press.

Nadel, L., & Jacobs, W. J. (1998). Traumatic memory is special. *Current Directions in Psychological Science, 7*, 154–7.

Nijenhuis, E., van der Hart, O., & Steele, K. (2010). Trauma-related Structural Dissociation of the Personality. *Activitas Nervosa Superior, 52*(1), 1–23.

Nora, P. (1989). Between Memory and History. *Representations, 26*, 7–24. http://www.timeandspace.lviv.ua/files/session/Nora_105.pdf.

Peace, K. A., Porter, S., & ten Brinke, L. (2008). Are memories for sexually traumatic events "special"? A within-subjects investigation of trauma and memory in a clinical sample. *Memory, 16*(1), 10–21. doi:10.1080/09658210701363583.

Perec, G. (2003). *W, or, the memory of childhood.* (D. Bellos, Trans.) Boston: David R. Godine.

Popper, K. (1959). *The Logic of Scientific Discovery*. London: Hutchinson.

Porter, S., & Birt, A. R. (2001). Is traumatic memory special? A comparison of traumatic memory characteristics with memory for other emotional life experiences. *Applied Cognitive Psychology, 15*(7), 101–117. doi:10.1002/acp.766.

Schacter, D. (2001). *The seven sins of memory*. Boston: Houghton Mifflin.

Seltzer, M. (1997). Wound culture: Trauma in the pathological public sphere. *October, 80*, 3–26.

Semprun, J. (1998). Literature or life. New York: Penguin Books. Trans. Linda Coverdale.

Shobe, K. K., & Kihlstrom, J. F. (1997). Is traumatic memory special? *Current Directions in Psychological Science, 6*, 70–74.

Stone, L. (1979). The Revival of Narrative: Reflections on a New Old History. *Past & Present, 85*, 3–24.

Terr, L. (1984). Time and Trauma. *Psychoanalytic Study of the Child, 39*, 633–665.

van der Hart, O., Nijenhuis, E., Steele, K., & Brown, D. (2004). Trauma-related dissociation: conceptual clarity lost and found. *Australian and New Zealand Journal of Psychiatry, 38*, 906–914. doi:10.1111/j.1440-1614.2004.01480.x.

van der Kolk, B. A., Perry, C., & Herman, J. L. (1991). Childhood origins of self-destructive behavior. *American Journal of Psychiatry, 148*(12), 1665–1671. doi:10.1176/ajp.148.12.1665.

Wilkomirski, B. (1996). *Fragments: Memories of a wartime childhood.* (C. B. Janeway, Trans.) New York: Schocken Books.

Žižek, S. (2003). The puppet and the dwarf: The perverse core of Christianity. Cambridge, Mass. MIT Press.

14 Walking, Walking Out, and Walking Through: Transitional Space and Traumatic Time

Haviva Pedaya

14.1 Introduction

In the following pages I will try to propose a multidisciplinary way of looking at walking and trauma, combining several points of view: anthropological, religious, historical, and phenomenological. Walking in itself has been and still is the subject of well-known literary and philosophical discussions, most notably in Walter Benjamin's essay, "The Return of the Flâneur,"[1] as well as important scholarly works such as the essays of De Certeau[2] and others; in the framework of his discussion of the practice of everyday life De Certeau discusses walking in words inspired by and echoing Benjamin. Walking has also inspired important works of art, such as the sound-art projects of Janet Cardiff.[3] The survey of walking tropes here is part of a larger research project, elaborated in my book "Walking Through Trauma" (Pedaya, 2011). It involves different eras as well as transitions through space: the twelfth century and the early Renaissance; sixteenth century—the expanding world-picture; and twentieth century—Modernism.

In this study I present and discuss walking within the boundaries of Jewish mysticism as a practice of exile.[4] Walking as ritual is a case of a-nomistic practice, that is, practice and ritual that are not included in the ritual and legal corpus of Judaism (*halakha*). I follow stages of processing trauma and as they correlate phenomenologically with walking and the categories of the discussion of trauma.

I will portray walking as capable of being a symptom of each of the components of a traumatic state as a whole: (a) the presence of the memory of the trauma itself, the memory of the expulsion; (b) the presence of Acting-out; (c) the presence of Working-through; (d) the additional possibility—and this will be one of the foci that I will propose here—that walking builds a transitional space[5] in which the a-nomistic ritual constitutes a framework that gradually makes

[1] A portrayal of the wandering boulevardier (flâneur) as the face of modernity is offered in Walter Benjamin's "The Return of the Flâneur" (1999, pp. 416–455).

[2] Michel De Certeau (2011) offers a description of the impact of ambulating.

[3] See Christov-Bakargiev (2003), pp. 14–15.

[4] Walking is discussed in Eliot Wolfson's study of walking as a redemptive act, concentrating on late Kabbalistic sources and Hassidism. See Wolfson's (1997) discussion of walking as a redemptive act in Jewish modern sources.

[5] The concept of transitional space is related to the transitional object of Winnicott, *Playing and Reality* (1971). For the application and development in poetic contexts of Winnicott's theory of space as a transitional object see Mishori (2005).

H. Pedaya (✉)
Ben-Gurion University of the Negev, Jewish History Department, Elyachar Center for Sephardi Heritage, Ben-Gurion University, Beer-Sheva, Israel
e-mail: haviva.pedaya@gmail.com

Y. Ataria et al. (eds.), *Interdisciplinary Handbook of Trauma and Culture*,
DOI 10.1007/978-3-319-29404-9_14

possible the transitional space in which Acting-out transmutes into Working-through; (e) the additional stage is a stage of working-through; and (f) projection of the trauma onto the symbolic level, a stage that is bound up with the construction of space and with the attribution of symbolic meaning to the act of walking. This last aspect is exemplified in the generation following the expulsion from Spain with the philosophers and mystics of sixteenth-century Jewry.

At this stage there are a number of additional aspects, including what I will call the spatialization of time, where concepts of walking and space are projected onto the larger historical time and processes within divinity and its symbolic structure; the walking in the concrete world is understood as activating, changing, representing, and catalyzing process in the invisible symbolic structure of the wandering/walking Jew.[6] Another important facet of the view offered here is that of cross-generational transmission of trauma, where the different generations make sense of displacement, detached existence, and otherness in developing ways and modes of life.

14.2 The Context of Jewish Culture

In a situation of acute exile, that is—where a person is driven out of his place—he often breaks immediately, running or walking, into the journey of a captive or a refugee, or into a journey of flight from invaders, murderers, soldiers, and fighters. Walking is part of the representation of the trauma itself; thus the memory of the trauma is etched on the person who experiences it. This is the starting-point of our investigation.[7]

Walking is carried out immediately and it is itself part of the traumatic expulsion which has just occurred. Sometimes walking develops as a form of reaction to trauma; this is likely to happen whether the person is expelled or not. This walking reflects Acting-out and is largely the result of a split in the structure of the dynamics of the personality, which appears first of all as a break in the continuity of time which is expressed on the axis of place. There are cases in which the main part of the trauma is in the realm of the psychological-familial territory—a person's first abstract unit of place—i.e., situations of betrayal, desire, widowhood, and orphanhood. There are situations in which the main part of the trauma developed in the relation to one's first physical territory, the body, and afterward the house. These traumatic situations cause the person to abandon ***the place that was*** and to go to ***emptiness***, to the ***no-place***, to ***the place that will not be***. The consciousness of destruction compounds the loss of what was together with the loss of what could be hoped for. Sometimes there is no pain from the destruction of what was to be. The future has been blocked off. The person is flooded by a sense of hopelessness. In the most extreme form of traumatic walking, the walking of acting-out, it is often accompanied by muteness. This walking is directed toward emptiness, toward the lack of place, toward the place that ***will not be***. A modern model of this walking is incorporated in the opening scene of the film *Paris, Texas* by Wim Wenders[8] where the obsessive walking is meaningless to the viewer. Present-day and recent films are also flooded with traumatic walk-

[6]The relation between the human realm (specifically the Jewish historical reality) and the mystical dimension received explicit expression in the work of Gershom Sholem. See Gershom Scholem (1975, 1975a). Scholem, with influences of the Hegelian-Marxist tradition, saw an inverse relationship between the degree of possession of a piece of reality and the shrinking or growth of the symbolic level. Although this cannot be regarded as an exclusive model, it is doubtless one of the central models in the history of Judaism. See also Pedaya (1991).

[7]See Kanafani (2001).

[8]See Wenders (1984). This is a portrayal of the different wanderings of the father and the son as an odyssey between Europe and the USA. Much has been written about this film. I will mention especially the in-depth study of Avner Faingulernt (2009), pp. 120–149. In his dissertation he discusses the structures of nomadic and father-son relationships in American cinema while distinguishing between the types of odysseys they produce.

ing, like the Polish film *Ida*,[9] which depicts the traumatic breakout into walking at the end of the film. The third type of walking is walking as a prolonged process of Working through the trauma, in the framework of religion and the experience of exile as an established experience in Jewish religion, which occurs through ritual development of walking in which ritual walking heals and compensates for traumatic walking. We shall find such rituals for the most part in the generation of the expulsion from Spain and its descendants.

Previous scholarship dealing with the link between the expulsion from Spain and the responses to it in the Kabbalah, as developed by Gershom Scholem, focused on the question of the theoretical and mythic-speculative processing of the event and the idea of exile. On many occasions, Moshe Idel polemicized with Scholem's view of *tzimtzum* (contraction) as an expression of God's exile within Himself.[10] Here I suggest a new, as-yet un-researched response to exile—that practices of walking and expulsion[11] are a reflection of the climate of expulsion and are intensified by the expulsion. I suggest that these rituals be examined at the moment they come into being and be seen as a process which seeks to relive the traumatic event, but in a structured and controlled way. Moreover, the ritual is a process of Acting-out which seeks to liberate the trauma from the terrestrial-social context (the horizontal, social axis) and place it on the transcendental, vertical axis of man-God relationships.

The reading I will propose below is that of the expulsion from Spain as a trauma and of the descendants of the expulsion as a prominent test case of the transfer of trauma—and of its working-through—to the intergenerational axis. That is to say, we shall examine the descendants of the generation of the Spanish expulsion over the continuity and crossing of two axes: the axis of the trauma and the intergenerational axis. The a-nomistic ritual of walking which developed intensively in the generation of the expulsion makes it possible to paint a broad picture—from *acting-out*, the walking of the expulsion (a traumatic walking), building up to the processing which creates a space beyond the present and a space of *working-through* of the trauma. The *Acting-out* is transformed into *Working-through* and into a feeling of fortification and healing.

Walking as an activity that converses with society is a going-outward—out from the dwelling-places, from cities, houses, villages, or countries. Walking can be a symptom of society's punitive act—exile or expulsion—or an act of self-punishment in which self-exile develops from the wish to atone, to repair or perhaps even redeem.

The shift in the act of walking—from a practice that represents exile to that of redemption—occurs chiefly around the eighteenth century and is connected with the characteristics of the late modernism of the eighteenth century, while early modernism, which for the Jews included the trauma of the expulsion, opened with an acute structuring of walking as a practice designating exile together with the eruption of Messianic apocalyptic hopes.[12]

14.3 Hands and Feet: Walking and Writing

Part of the ritual practices of walking consciously mirror a reflective relation to the match between walking and writing.[13] It seems that all the basic

[9]Pawlikowski (2014).

[10]For M. Idel's approach, who disagrees with Scholem on various bases and frameworks, see Idel (1992). Also see Idel, 1998a, Idel, 1998b, Idel, 2000. Regarding Gershom Scholem on Kabbalistic structures, Messianic moments, and the connection with historical dynamics, see Scholem (1975, 1975a).

[11]My colleague, Jackie Feldman, in response to my work, suggests calling this phenomenon a "theodicy of practice."

[12]Walking as both a manifestation of diasporic uprootedness (Galut) and the process of returned and rejuvenated existence (*Ge'ula*). Eliot Wolfson (1997) traces the outlines of the model of walking as redemption in Hasidism and other mystical traditions in Judaism. See Pedaya (2011a, 2011b) "Walking through Trauma", pp. 158–159.

[13]Henry Thoreau expressed this impression in his journals: "Methinks that the moment my legs begin to move, my thoughts begin to flow." Thomas De Quincy surmised that Wordsworth walked more than 180,000 miles, miles that are woven into his work (Solnit, 2001). On the link between walking and writing in the context of the modern city, see for example Orna Coussin's blog "To write by the water? And more on Shaun Levin's writing maps,"

parallels between man and beast and, as it were, all the muffled memory of the parallelism between hands and feet are expressed by some writers in a connection of the experience of walking with the feet with the experience of writing with the hands.

Walking is one of the more important characteristics that define and unite a culture and its characteristics—of wealth or poverty, rural or urban, antiquity or modernity, detachment or representation, practice, and art.[14] Walking in space, when it is correlative to "walking" in consciousness, becomes a field of concentration or scattering of thoughts, an activity in which the emphasis is on association or dissociation.

Two practices meet at this junction, however dissimilar they appear: writing and walking. In the field of Jewish mysticism, mystics appear not only as walkers, but as expressing the walking of a further agency—transcendental or Messianic—which they make present as part of what is to come;[15] it is here that the symbolic and the temporal spaces meet.

October 25, 2012 (Hebrew). Coussin explains that Levin's ideas "rely on the principle that writing at its best is connected with walking, that is, that writing is something like swallowing the distance on foot." In a similar vein, the poet Amir Gilboa wanted to walk from Russia to Israel.

[14]Modern masterpieces depicting this connection include Italo Calvino's *Invisible Cities* (1978, p. 13): "You walk for days among trees and among stones. Rarely does the eye light on a thing, and then only when it has recognized that thing as the sign of another thing: a print· in the sand indicates the tiger's passage; a marsh announces a vein of water; the hibiscus flower, the end of winter. All the rest is silent and interchangeable; trees and stones are only what they are"; De Certeau (2011, p. 117): "thus the street geometrically defined by urban planning is transformed into a space by walkers. In the same way, an act of reading is the space produced by the practice of a particular place: a written text, i.e., a place constituted by a system of signs." Also see Benjamin (1999). Also see Solnit (2001) and Derrida (1972, 1977) who connects walking and writing in their transgressional aspects.

[15]See the Ba'al HaTurim's Pentateuch commentary, Exodus 2: "And a man went ... That is, and a man went from the house of Levi. And elsewhere and a man went from Beit Lechem in Judah" (Ruth 1:11). To say by means of this walking came the first redeemer and by means of the same walking will come the last redeemer who is the Messiah son of David, may he come speedily in our day.

14.4 Initial Definitions: Space, Time, History, Nation/People, Messianism

Beginning with a certain timing about which it is possible to argue—whether we start before the exile of the First Temple or after it—the Jewish historic experience turns into an experience and consciousness of exile. To put it crudely and briefly, Exile (*Galut*) *means grasping yourself as exterior to your home, a dislocation from the place where you belong—physically and spiritually*. True, exile as a collective experience of the consciousness of a people, in which generation after generation experiences itself as a native to and at home in the place where one was born, is more complicated.

To be outside place—and in the encounter of place with the concept of transferring desire from the temporal to the spatial—indicates messianism. With the beginning of the trauma and exile the Jewish consciousness of several mystic seers and interpreters formed the image and likeness of a subject which expresses the entirety of history for the collective it represents. The Messiah, at least in apocalyptic consciousness, was grasped as a walker. There were exegetic-homiletic stories and parables (midrashim) of the sages which described the Shekhinah (the divine presence, with a feminine aspect) as a source of holiness that wanders with the dislocated people, wherever they go.[16] Though they were not the center of the historical depiction, in the enormous transition that was carried out between the apocalyptic literature and the literature of the Kabbalah one significant displacement occurred: the Shekhinah took over the central place of the Messiah as the representation of Jewish history.[17]

This dramatic *Galut* is also a displacement of gender, from a masculine to a feminine subject. Spiritually it is a shift from a human to a divine entity. Thus the representative subject of Jewish history, which in ancient Judaism was the Messiah, has become—with the ascendancy of the Kabbala—the *Shekhinah*.

[16]Talmud Bavli Trachtate Megilla 29a. See Pedaya (2013a), and Hasan-Rokem (1986, 2008, 2009).

[17]See Pedaya (2012, 2013, 2015a, 2015b).

This shift in the gender of the divine presence (who is now also the carrier of Jewish destiny) has consequences from the viewpoint of the historic body and with regard to the definition of *walking as a practice*: whether and how the walkers relate to the body that walks history. The trace of the walking can be a foot, a shoe, a crutch, a bird, a tracker of footsteps, and forgotten garments. On the larger scope explored by the great thinkers and mystics having adopted the feminine and temporal modes—the trace is of the mother's presence or the tracks of what is not yet inscribed.[18]

This distinction is important, for trauma in the symbolic collective memory is not only inscribed in details but also represented in an overarching metaphor which expresses the essence of the trauma. This overarching metaphor is for the most part a picture of the humiliation of the Divine female, her fall or breaking, as we shall see below in the work of Rabbi Yitzchak Luria (henceforth—"Luria")[19] and Rabbi Moses Cordovero (henceforth "Cordovero")[20] regarding the Shekhinah. We shall discuss different depictions of the Shekhinah as representing a different of Walking-working-out trauma.

14.5 Walking and Consciousness

The phenomenon of ambulation and thought is well known as far back as the Greek academy—peripatetic philosophers walk and teach and converse, the work is created while walking; there are strong affinities also to the Oral Torah.[21] The legs do the walking, the hands do the writing, and gradually there arises in force the typical model of ambulations in the Zohar, similar to the pastoral ambulations in nature, in which there are conversations that are written down after the fact and document revelations, whether these are the fruit of actual ambulations or not. Later comes the ambulatory model of *Tikkunei haZohar* in which the mystics walk in the footsteps of the exiled Shekhinah and have no nest, no resting ground except in the book which they themselves are composing.[22]

In early modern times one of the descendants of the generation of the expulsion, Cordovero describes walking which expels itself outside the city as a practice of scattering the feet (springing from an identification with the Shekhinah, which is the scattered holiness of God[23]) which causes a flow of sporadic innovations to the consciousness, resulting indeed in brief sayings. In late modernism the Grand Rabbi of Piaseczno,[24] who was sitting in the Warsaw ghetto, the heart of traumatic events, caught at the burning point, describes consciousness as a field on which fall good thoughts, of which precisely the associative

[18]See Roi (2011), Pedaya (2014a).

[19]Rabbi Yitzchak Luria Ashkenazi (Hebrew acronym: Ha'ARI Hakadosh, Jerusalem 1534-Safed 1572), one of the greatest Kabbalists in the history of Jewish mysticism. He was raised and educated in Jerusalem and in Egypt. In Safed he became known as the focus of Kabbalistic study. His doctrine of the "tsimsum (contraction)" and the detailed system of the hidden and revealed worlds deeply influenced Judaism when it entered the modern world.

[20]Rabbi Moses Cordovero (1533–1570): a Safed kabbalist (the name testifies to his Spanish origins). Until the arrival of Rabbi Yitzhak Luria in Safed, Rabbi Moses Cordovero was considered the greatest Kabbalist. He devoted much effort to the interpretation of the Zohar. Many of the distinctions in the body of this essay have to do with the typological characterizations of Rabbi Cordovero as opposed to Rabbi Luria.

[21]The word Halacha is often interpreted as related to "walking in the footsteps of the Lord" (as in Duet. 28, 6) or as a metonym for "walking all the way to the end" (Nathan ben Jehiel of Rome in his Aruch Hashalem).

[22]In the atmosphere of *Tikkunei HaZohar* and *Ra'aya Mehemna,* when a situation of walking is described, the atmosphere is dark and the extraterritorial consciousness is an inseparable part of it. The exile of the Shekhinah is a kind of super-narrative with which the ceremonies of exile are connected in one way or another, though this is not expressed in the same way by every thinker or mystic. This narrative is sometimes activated from an assimilation to or identification with the Shekhinah on the part of the mystic, as in the *Zohar* and the *Tikkunei haZohar.*

[23]This motion of the Shekhina mirrors that of the People of Israel, as in the famous saying of the Talmud (tractate Megillah 29a): "Wheresoever they were exiled, the Shekinah went with them."

[24]Rabbi Kalonymus Kalman Shapira (1889–1943), a Hasidic Grand Rabbi who made significant innovations in the field of Hasidism and education (for instance *The Students' Responsibility)* with a pronounced existentialist slant. Under the German conquest in World War II he continued to be active in the Warsaw ghetto.

aspect which breaks up the continuity of ordinary consciousness contains in itself a message more significant than routine consciousness. In the Piaseczno Rebbe's world, it is the evil that is the backdrop, the standard, and the given. Flashes of inspiration, from the beyond, are the good. That is a distinct and deep difference in world-picture from earlier Hasidic thought.

The closer we get to modernism, the more we find a striking parallelism between what formulates itself within the boundaries of mystical creativity and what formulates itself in the *stream of consciousness* in the level of the ars-poetical concept. Such a parallelism reveals itself to a quick glance on other levels.[25] But in this framework we shall concern ourselves with modernism at its height.

Concentration or scattering as a cognitive and physical practice can create either congruence or asymmetry in the consciousness of the individual. Similarly, sometimes they embody the individual's finding pleasure amid the existential pain of his collective punishment, whether through the oppression of exile (scattering) or through the punishments of sequestering (concentration) in a place with no possible mobility.

14.6 The Context of Jewish Culture

Earlier stages of the nomadic and ambulatory consciousness such as Cain and the Levites are explored in my work "Walking through Trauma" and only briefly mentioned here.[26] The Promised Land is inseparable from the promise of exile, of displacement.[27] There is a homicidal element at the interstice between the stages of nomadic life, agriculture, and urbanism. Wandering and walking as a form of punishment appear in the biblical myth (we will not discuss the more ancient nomadic foundations of the near-east[28]) chiefly in connection with Cain, the first murderer and the builder of the first city. The city is, as it were, both the punishment and its circumvention, for the city is detached from natural as well as agricultural land. The city is essentially a kind of wandering, paradoxically bringing together society as the heritage of he who is forever not a part of the natural nor the human realm. It is a manifestation of the myth that culture begins with trauma; murder is at the root of civilization and the changes in the conception of the city. Christian theology of the Church Fathers gave great weight to the tie woven by Biblical myth between Cain as punished with exile and Cain as the founder of the first city. Augustine laid the theological foundation for the development of two cities, which becomes two parallel lines: the historical city and the city of God. We might say that Cain's city is identified with the course of human history. Augustine makes this conceptual move along with the detachment from apocalyptic thinking. Henceforth, the spatial dual city is translated to the temporal: two kinds of time and a depiction of life as a kind of voyage toward the City of God; history, on the other hand, the earthly city, is the stage of Cain's wandering.

The city is a particular and formative focus of civilization. Walking as a practice anchored in concrete situations of exile nevertheless can rebuild symbolic reality. This process is already described by the prophet Ezekiel (Yehezkel), who as prophet and priest embodied the collective Jewish situation—through rituals and performances of exile—to his small audience in Babylon.[29]

[25] Mark (2015), Chapter Three—The Stream of Mystical Consciousness: The Character of Mystical Experience and the Way that it is Shaped as Literature in "The Guest Who Came In" pp. 90–137.

[26] See Knohl, 2008, regarding the nomadic origin and nature of the Levites. Also see Gruenvald, 2003, pp. 88–93, who characterizes the Cain story as it unfolds into the Hebrew ethos, and eventually also into the forced ethnic nomadism (p. 87).

[27] For more on exile and place, see Gurevitch and Aran, 1994; Gurevitch, 2007; Hirschfeld, 2000; Eisen, 1986; Pedaya, 2011a; Sagi, 2015.

[28] See Hooke, 1958, pp. 64, 98, 108–110.

[29] Yehezkel in fact organizes a "public event" which strives to reach a specific goal in the world and a change in reality. See Don Handelman (1990). Handelman deals with the anthropology of public events and proposes a paradigm of play and ritual. He distinguishes between exemplary ritual (model), reflective ritual, and representative ritual, and locates them in the framework of the system of the "lived-in-world." The paradigm which he proposes regarding an event of the type of the model fits the exemplary ceremony that I am talking about.

Following this short introduction to the city, and with a sharp transition the High Middle ages and with the focus on the city as an area of refuge, especially among the Jews of Germany, practices of walking were means of exile outside the cities, of social punishment and personal penance. The function of punishment is to stimulate the going-out into a liminal process. Exile as a practice of walking is a ceremony whose character is that of a pilgrimage to nowhere,[30] or basically to a reconstruction of the I-Self relations, whereby wandering and detachment stimulate the disintegration of the ego (or "the I"—associated with the territorial), unraveling it and through the extraterritorial connecting it, or in this case reconnecting it, to the (social) self.

In contrast, beginning with the thirteenth century we hear that among mystics among the Jews of Spain (and apparently not without connection to the Christian mystical orders) practices of walking were instituted that expressed detachment from this world and connection to a heavenly spiritual territory whose real land is the book. In these cases the I-Self axis is unraveled and rebuilt in a liminal transitional space; it has to do not with social punishment, but with the longing for ecstasy and revelation, or at most with self-"punishment."

Two prevailing dimensions—the real and the symbolic—map out the mystical contemplation of the world. These are also seen in Jewish mysticism as two realms: the real and the spiritual. They have undergone constant fluctuation from the standpoint of power relations among them. The subject of being tossed about between levels of real and symbolic time and place is a key subject when it comes to understanding turning points in collective Jewish history; in the life of the exiled community it is a principal problem of the relations between the concrete layer of reality and the symbolic layer in the life of the exiled community. These layers—as long as we are talking about walking as a means of movement in space—are represented both on the horizontal axis and the vertical axis; from the standpoint of the exiled subject, departure from the actual city is a movement in the space of concrete reality which strengthens the connection to the spiritual place on the transcendental axis.

These patterns have continued to serve in the modern period, but from the early modern period on we notice a fundamental change of all the systems to new forms and molds. From now on, departure and isolation can exist in the center of the city, rather than outside it; and this correlates with many important changes that occurred in European culture and in its political reality, and with many developments that occurred in the definition of the center, outside and anti-center (with the ascendancy of the concept of the state as opposed to the previous dominance of the city). I will survey the turn that occurred from within the Jewish perspective. The abandonment of place in favor of wandering is always accompanied by a feeling of connection to one axis: either to a symbolic place or to the true or lost "self."

The modern detachment from the medieval city as a temple of culture and religion is a severance from all that constitutes classic life forms. Today departure from the city in the merely territorial sense is not yet a departure from culture—the practice of urban ambulation is carried on online. The socioeconomic factor is significant: The poorer the person is, the larger the role of the center-periphery side of theirs. The contemporary version of this self-exile is found in the economic and political refugees from Africa and the Middle East toward Europe, rushing the West as a besieged city.

The spontaneous practice of walking outside cities expresses detachment from the medieval city as a form of self-punishment on the axis of atonement (primarily in Germany and the North of France), and as a mode of expression of an aspiration toward revelation on the axis of ecstasy (primarily in Spain).

[30]The phenomenon of non-arrival at a real physical place is connected to a strong feeling of a metaphysical center which is itself in motion. Even in the framework of pilgrimage there are examples in which the feeling of pilgrimage is attained without reaching any specific place but through movement itself. See C. Bawa Yamba (1995, pp. 6- 12).

In my book *Walking Through Trauma*[31] I show that the movement of departure is in dialogue with movement of other connection and is thus similar to ceremonies of transition and to the liminal process as described in three stages—departure, intermediate area, and connection. However, this space is a space of new movement and restructuring of identity. Thus the territorial and the extraterritorial may represent the tension between ego and my self.[32]

The expulsion from Spain crossed with the phenomenon of the strengthening of spiritual and symbolic space. This space was at the peak of its process of expansion since the inheritance of the *Zohar* and the *Tikkunei HaZohar* and served in many senses as a counter-territory (in accordance with the ancient dynamic of the earthly and heavenly Jerusalem). The mystic wanderings and ambulations were grasped as a way of connecting with that invisible spiritual territory, and served the Jew's feeling that he was extraterritorial to the culture in which he had felt at home in the recent past. At the same time, this tension is also represented on the vertical and horizontal axes. The extraterritorial or vertical is the self, while the territorial and the horizontal are the ego, which is sometimes under pressure of social punishment and sometimes under pressure of mystical practices toward for a new birth from within the "self."

14.7 The Sixteenth Century: Reorganization of Reality After the Expulsion from Spain: Rabbi Isaac Luria and Rabbi Moses Cordovero

Luria, the Kabbalist from Egypt who went to Safed and taught there for 2 years, offered to the Jewish world, after a great crisis and on the cusp of a new era gaining recognition in Christendom, a complete theological system that could only be understood as destined to reorganize reality, the picture of the Divine, and material universe together, in the face of the great trauma of the expulsion from Spain and the remapping of the world as a result of the discovery of previously unknown territories (America). While the discovery of the New World proposed a remapping to the Christian world, Luria occupied himself with remapping the Jewish world, the picture of the spiritual world, or, to put it another way, a new symbolic order which from now on sheds a different light on the order of the concrete world. He in fact proposed a radically new form of organization of Jewish identity in a shifting context.[33]

[31] Pedaya (2009, pp. 30–32).

[32] For the tension between "I" and "myself" as concept and as experience there are many expressions in philosophy and scholarship. For a description that is not beholden to a specific scholarly position see the remarks of Gideon Efrat (2000, pp. 49–55): "The ego and the self are two poles of the soul. The ego would like to live in the house of the self, to be with itself. The self is like a 'native land,' thus a fixed place, roots, harmony, a place in which components of the self-acquire meaning for the ego and at the same time put themselves together in a unity of meaning and feeling: the unity of one who 'feels at home.' The I, as one who lives in the native country of the self or is expelled from it, is, in the light of what has been said, an image of consciousness (an image of the self), that is flimsy, vague, deficient, lacking in unity and meaning, as long as it is not fed and nursed by the covenant with the self. The self is the solid 'bedrock' of the I, the house. From the standpoint of psychology, the self is the space of the various subconscious data that build personality on various levels of consciousness, while the ego is the conscious reflection on this space and the behavioral obedience to it (obedience to the self-image), reflection of relationship or distance, of unity (domesticity) or dichotomy (exile). The ego in exile clings to this alien self (evidently, the ego has no choice but to cling to some self), with which it cannot form a unity. The redemption of the ego is its return from its exile. Its return home: the exchange of an alienated, dismantled and rickety self-image for an 'authentic' personality and, accordingly, connection to a new I that is unified, solid and meaningful."

[33] In my book *Walking Through Trauma* (Pedaya 2011a, 2011b) I displace the focus of the discussion from the dispute about whether there is a connection between Luria's idea of the tsimtsum (which Gershom Scholem presents as the idea of the exile of God within himself (Moshe Idel disputes this)) and the expulsion from Spain, to a discussion of a new sort, a discussion of the question of the connection between exile as a practice and the expulsion from Spain. The shifting of the center of gravity to practice makes it possible not only to propose an examination in a new light of the plethora of walking ceremonies in the sixteenth century, but also to begin for the first time, by means of the category of ritual, the significant discussion of the expulsion from Spain as a trauma whose traces are recognized in Jewish mystical literature. I also shift the center of gravity from the question of *tsimtsum* to the question of the breaking *(Shevirah)*, since the breaking is likely to be among other things a reflection of the scattering of the Jews in the world after the expulsion. See Scholem (1975, 1975a) and in contrast see the approach of Idel (1998, 1998a, 1998b, 2000).

The emphasis in the new world view proposed by Luria is not an interpretation and sorting of the streams of knowledge that were before him in the style typical of Cordovero, who in his panoramic writings proposed a systematization of a kind with dictionaries and encyclopedias (which are also a kind of scattering). The aim of Luria was the creative systematization of a certain body of knowledge which relied on a few principal exemplary works and a limited corpus, such as the *Zohar*, the teachings of Nachmanides,[34] and the writings of Yosef ben Shalom Ashkenazi,[35] the interpreter of the Sefer Yetsirah. Luria's work aimed at instituting a complete system of divinity and reality as a whole, a system that creates and activates myths and founding metaphors. When Luria institutes this encompassing system and sets it up as an organization of a world view, he expresses a fundamental transformation in the Kabbalistic and interpretive materials. Such thinkers as Luria, who particularly experience breakdown or displacement, create a writing that contains not only a past, but a future. Luria—whether or not this was his intention—established a new conceptual spiritual and metaphysical index that impacted all of modern Judaism, often more than some people were willing to admit. In the perspective of distance from the subject of the expulsion and the trauma, which nevertheless is still there in the background, this index was inseparable from a metaphorics of space and movement. When we study the history of ideas it is not only a question of finding the source or component of one idea or another, but the question is always about the structural causes and the problems that drive a given (cultural, religious, social) institution.

The relation between walking and writing, related to here in a narrower sense, can be illuminated in a broader context as well; Cordovero, on the apparently literary level, occupied himself with collecting, and thus created anthologies that contained and encompassed everything. In fact the conscious principle that Cordovero employed—from his ecstatic work in the *Book of Banishments* (*Sefer Gerushin*)[36] to the conscious interpretive character of the rest of his work—is to make the scattering, the spreading-out of all that is latent in the works of Kabbalistic Judaism, possible. This is in accordance with his central principle of the scattering of consciousness; that is, he grants legitimacy to products of the creative spirit of the mystical collective, and similarly to fruits of the spirit of the mystical individual, even to scattered associations.

Luria occupied himself on the literary level with the isolation and rejection of many sources. This apparently stands in opposition to the idea of *gathering*[37]—but if we keep in mind that his *gathering* is directed to a single goal and particular signification, we can understand that the project of *unification* and *contraction* is reflected in his hermeneutic conception. It expresses itself in his canonical project, which does away with a considerable portion of the mystical literature. This also occurs in his *piyyutim* (liturgical poems) work, which focuses on a few key *piyyutim* and rejects many others.

[34]Rabbi Moshe ben Nachman (Gerona 1194-Israel 1270), also known as Nachmanides. One of the greatest rabbis of Israel in medieval times, in both the esoteric and the exoteric fields, an interpreter of Scripture, a Talmud sage, a philosopher, and Kabbalist.

[35]Rabbi Yosef ben Shalom Ashkenazi ("the Tall"), author of a commentary on the *Sefer Yetsirah* (attributed by the printers to the Raava"d—Rabbi Avraham ben David of Posquières).

[36]This book contains Kabbalistic commentaries and insights related to 99 biblical passages. These are the result of his self-banishment (as a practice shared with others) outside his Safed home, to the fields. This exile, banishment, was perceived both as a personal practice and as a communion with a displaced reality, a fundamental rift existing between the masculine and feminine in the divine realm.

[37]The *gathering the sparks* means—given variations in the particular interpretive mode—a process of redeeming the divine light as it is spread, scattered in a reality in the state of Galut. The pure divinity has contracted to allow the existence of the world, and in that world in its current form (with a complex genealogy and process leading up to this point) there are remnants of this original purity that are imbedded deep in the non-divine and await collection and reabsorption.

Both Luria and Cordovero can be assessed from the angle of canonization. Canonization is essentially bound up with actions of concentration—gathering, and these occurred contemporaneously with processes that took place in *halakha*.[38]

Rabbi Yehudah Loew of Prague,[39]with his distance from the experience of actual breakdown, created a polished focusing of consciousness, which organized and defined the separateness of the Jewish people.[40] In contrast, Luria created one key principle, whose force was like a sharp needle that pierced every idea, every traditional picture, and reshaped them in relation to the new reality.

14.8 Perspectives of the Traumatic Rift: Close and Distant, Earthly and Divine

History's judgment is that Cordovero, who occupied himself more with the formulation of a systematic organization of all the Kabbalistic literature and the formation of the trauma on the immediate level by means of ceremonies of expulsion as we have interpreted them, was absorbed to a lesser extent as a systematic organizer in the literature of the generations that came after him. Cordovero proposed a hidden apocalyptic answer, but it tended toward regression. It expected a continuation of the catastrophe, and—put in other terminology—it was entirely directed toward the second catastrophe. However Luria, whose teaching as it written down by his students is much harder to read and to comprehend than the writings of Cordovero, was absorbed into the consciousness of following generations as an organizing factor even though most of his writings were too difficult to read. The reason for this is that Luria supplied an answer for an entire generation, an organizing system which was gradually included and absorbed into the systematic thinking of subsequent generations. This system crystallized the schema of crisis and repair, whether or not that purpose was formulated explicitly or even consciously. Another reason for this is that the gargantuan spiritual enterprise provided a clear and distinct ritual expression, making them organic for the Jewish form of life, more readily absorbable by the general Jewish public than arcane teachings on their own.

This influence of Luria is noticeable afterward also in Sabbatianism and in Hasidism, with the modern psychophysical split. It operates at the first seam-line of developing a discipline of the self, introducing a new version of theory and practice.[41] From the point of view of older theological structures—specifically those coming out of the school of Nachmanides—God could be construed as indifferent to history and catastrophe. The Lurianic crisis reinvolves the divine into reality, if only by its own crisis, splintering and dispersion in the world. In any case, I would argue, different forms of combination and synthesis, not only of hermeneutic structures but also of structures in the mystical experience, are of the essence of modernism from its early beginnings, and in increasing measure from the eighteenth century on. Therefore it is no longer possible to argue for the exclusivity of one line—whereas it was easy in medieval times to sketch the relation of ideational and mystical structures to schools and individuals in a distinct typological manner. And so it is necessary to define in each time anew the nature of the combination under discussion, together with a well-defined terminology. That which served as a repository for a given mystical model in medieval times no longer constitutes an adequate and exclusive instrument.

Although the method of Luria is complicated and almost hermetically closed to many, at the same time it is very accessible and communicative from the standpoint of the deep metaphoric codes which organize it and from the standpoint

[38]Elon (1973) part III, the chapter on Rabbi Yosef Karo (pp. 1089–1092).

[39]Rabbi Judah Loew ben Bezalel, seventeenth century, Poznań-Prague, rabbi and author, philosopher, and commentator who forms a bridge between the Jewish world and Renaissance thought. The most important Ashkenazic thinker of the early modern period, and one of the most important figures in Jewish theology as a whole.

[40]See the development of the concept of the transcendent, Sorotskin (2006).

[41]See Pedaya, 2005; Pedaya 2015a, 2015b, 2015c, 2015d, 2015e.

of the answers that it gives to a suffering and wounded generation. The key attribute of this reality that has priority over all others is the structural-existential-ontological fracture. With the close connection between practice and theory, Luria proposed answers and methods that had no spiritual substitutes, a crisis-theology for a generation undergoing a crisis.

14.9 In-Between Worlds: Crisis Theologies and Modernity

In Christian culture, positions that could be defined as crisis theology were formulated by Pascal and received new life in the nineteenth century by Kirkegaard (with an emphasis on action) and in the twentieth century after the two World Wars,[42] and are sometimes mentioned as relevant in postmodernism.[43] The communicative value of these metaphors was enormous. Its very identification is decisive for an understanding of the influence of Luria on the Kabbalah of the seventeenth century, on Rabbi Israel Sarug[44] and through Sarug on Europe as a whole, and on the Hasidism of Poland on the one hand and on philosophies like that of Franz Rosenzweig on the other.[45] The dialectic structure suggested by Gershom Scholem for the fluctuations of Jewish mysticism between the concrete and the spiritual is of indispensable importance even when one is aware of its parallelism to the historical authority of the workshop of Hegel-Marx; but it is necessary to restrict this depiction and to define exactly the domain of its validity.[46] In fact this is a sketch on the diachronic axis which seeks to reflect one type of problematic—Messianism; in order to get a full picture and a better understanding of Jewish history one must fence it off, and also deepen the discussion of it by setting up a more complex synchronous system opposite and beside it, for dissection with additional axes.[47]

14.10 The Extraterritorial: Standing Outside Time—Walking to the Promised Land

With the expulsion, and since we are speaking of a collective that was not only pushed out to a domain extraterritorial to Spain, but also as it were to a domain outside history, the displacements of identity move between counter-formation, absolute exodus to the "outside," and identity formation as an attempt at ingress; this dialectic structure is critical.

In the seventeenth century, alongside the development and deepening of Lurianic Kabbalah by the students of Rabbi Israel Sarug, the ascendancy of Sabbatianism is not only a way of turning to the dimensions of actual reality in comparison to the previous concentration on symbolic dimensions,[48] but also (from within the prism which I proposed above) a turning of the energies of walking toward the land of Israel, toward a specific place as a destination. Conversely, Yaakov Frank's fixation on Poland precedes the Hassidic abandonment of the territorial.[49] As a direct continuation of the direction

[42]On crisis theology, see the spate of books on the subject in the atmosphere between the two World Wars and after World War II. However the term here is not limited to that of Karl Barth's "theology of Krisis" where the antinomy is between the limited reality and the ultimate divine, the crisis of a person's shortcomings in the face of pure aspirations. Crisis here denotes a larger scale of discontinuity, break, and fracture that engulfs entire civilizations.

[43]Tomlin (1997).

[44]Rabbi Israel Sarug (sixteenth to seventeenth centuries) was a Kabbalist and a spreader of the Kabbalah of Luria in Italia, whence it was diffused to Europe.

[45]On the influence of Lurianic Kabbalah on Rosenzweig see Idel (1988), Horwitz (2007) (her essay surveys the spectrum of personages and books by means of which Rosenzweig could have been exposed to Kabbalah); see in addition her discussions in her collection of essays (Horwitz, 2010). See also Wolfson Horwitz (2010) and Pedaya, "Fathers and Sons: The Mirror Community and the Image Community," in Pedaya (2011a, Part 3, 232–242).

[46]Note the concept of Messianism according to Scholem (1975a), and Idel's (1998a) criticism thereof.

[47]See Pedaya (2011a).

[48]See Scholem (1975a).

[49]Jacob Frank (Poland, 1726–1790) was a false messiah in Poland of the eighteenth century, styled as a continuer of Sabbati Zevi, and his sect of believers were called the "Frankists." In the autumn of 1759 he converted to Christianity with a group of his disciples.

of Jews to a *no-place*—to the sea, to the extraterritorial—the Jews seek to arrive at *the* place, the absolute place. This feature of messianism and locality will follow the wandering Jewish people through their various circumstances.

Charged messianism, when it radicalizes by its very nature, makes it necessary to skip over time, and its meaning is the immediate liquidation of history and focusing on a specific destination. Modernism brought with it from its beginning models that appear in combination and fall apart one beside the other. This is also the case in mysticism and in the conception of history and locality.

Rabbi Moshe Haim Luzzato (henceforth—Luzzato),[50] for example, expresses the mixture of these domains, since it is possible to characterize him on the one hand as a "pilgrim" to the land of Israel and on the other hand as someone who flees to the land of Israel as a place of refuge. The dynamics of excommunication from which he suffers become more and more acute, but he still naïvely thinks or hopes that by being within the boundaries of the city of Padua he will not be subject to the rabbinic court of Venice, that is, he still is thinking in terms of cities, while his persecutor, Rabbi Moshe Hagiz,[51] formulates the rule that "all the Jews are one city," a rule that is still in dialogue with the medieval tradition in the face of Christianity. In the end Luzzato withdraws into himself as the smallest unit of the city, seeing himself as a fortified town, and arrives in the land of Israel.

[50]Moshe Haim Luzzato, also known by the acronym Ramchal (1707–1746), eighteenth-century rabbi, Kabbalist, writer, rhetorician, and poet. In his lifetime his teachings and Kabbalistic doctrines were controversial because of the many revelations he received and his messianic and historiosophic conceptions; he was suspected of Sabbatianism, but after his death he became a revered figure to most currents of Judaism. Regarding his role in Jewish and general Modernism, see Garb (2014).

[51]Rabbi Moshe Hagiz, one of the sages of Jerusalem in the eighteenth century, was one of the chief fighters against Sabbatianism. As part of his struggle against Sabbatianism he sought to forbid the study of the Kabbala. See Carlebach (1990), Pedaya (2011a, p. 201).

14.11 The Times In Between: History and Place in Transition

Fernand Braudel proposes (Braudel, 2005)—in the domain of general history and from the economic viewpoint—to characterize European history centennially, and argues that the beginning of the development of the West is in the course of those 400 years from the fifteenth century (especially the second half) until the eighteenth century, in which the economic and commercial center shifted from fairs and markets to stores and the stock market and there were fierce struggles among commercial cities.[52] Foucault defined the seventeenth century as the century which constructed the institutional penal systems, with large prisons, and changed the patterns of punishment through concentration in the cities. The renovated organization of the city also determined who could be punished within and who, by means of rejection to the outside. The renewed organization of the ghettoes is clearly also connected with this moment.[53]

If we apply to Judaism the thinking in terms of the characteristics of centuries, we shall say that if the sixteenth century represents scattering and is the great century of walking to the *unknown* or to *nowhere*, to assimilation, Sabbatianism, and self-loss and absorption into different communities and cities, the seventeenth century will be remembered as the one that fanned the fiery impulse to *walk to one place—the land of Israel*, while the eighteenth century will be depicted as the one that picks up the pieces of the messianic walk to the land of Israel, the place defined as the one destination. The actualization of the urge to walk to a specific, defined place will be characterized as a walking defined by the impetus toward redemption (in Sabbatianism, and later in some of the currents of Hasidism). In contrast, walking in a place defined by its liminality is a walking of exile (practiced in the beginning of Hasidism, surfacing again in different ways throughout the history of Hasidism).

[52]Braudel, Capitalism (1985/2005).

[53]On the rise of the structure of the ghetto see David Sorotskin (2004, 2006, 2007 chapters 1–2, 2011). Also Weinstein (1999).

As stated above, already in the sixteenth century Luria connected the two meanings by portraying the whole world as the liminal place of exile, with all of history as a liminal event. The walks that take place in exile, even if aimless and scattered, are part of the project of *gathering*, and thus in a *final analysis* they are steps which build up the process of the redemptive walking. This completes the chronological projection of the spatial trauma. Time, again spatialized as traumatic, becomes the subject of Jewish modernism in its various forms, with shades of modern Jewish nationalism included in this dynamic.

There are thinkers whose centrality can be characterized as illumining anew and in detail all the thinking of the period that may be placed vis-à-vis them; the teaching of Luria was of this kind. In relation to him one can place any thinker who can be defined as someone who formulated a voice of the period and distinguish between them, and from these comparisons and distinctions one can deepen the discussion of the entire period. For instance, we can compare Luria with Rabbi David HaReuveni.[54] HaReuveni is himself a conceptual keystone for the age: the great expulsion of the Jews from Spain and Portugal, on the one hand, and the attempt at a great voluntary importation of Jews to Spain and Portugal on the other hand, occur in mutual relation and open the early modern period with the attempt to combine the opening of the horizons of the New World with the apocalyptic message that still fluctuates between the impetus of the past and a renewed directedness toward the future. The activity of HaReuveni can be seen as an impetus to replenish the traumatic loss, to restore the object that was ejected out to its ancient state, and this attempted on the physically and historically concrete level.[55]

14.12 Utopian Stumblings on the Way to the Promised Land

Just as in the wake of the expulsion it is possible to find the sharpest formulations for the relocation of the Jews outside time (outside history), so there are also very sharp formulations of the Jewish location outside space. The tension between the "no-place" as the representation of the extraterritorial in the trauma of the expulsion and the "no-place" as the (quite literal) representation the ultimate good place is that of the dual meaning of the very term *Utopia* itself. The tension is enormous; yet the two appear together in the Judaism of the generation of the expulsion.

In contrast, this must be compared to basic phenomena in general culture in which the impetus awakens to search for and locate the ideal unknown—paralleled to revelation and the exposure, as it were, of the territorial unknown. That is, one must read Thomas More's *Utopia*[56] as a textual event corresponding to Columbus's discovery of the real American continent—thus, the geographical (at least potential) liquidation of the unknown radiates to the general liquidation of mystery. Thomas More's Utopia is a place without hiding places, without mystery. The lack of theological mystery tends toward the removal of social or political mystery. [57]

These phenomena, of the real discovery of a "new place" which until lately had been a "no-place" (not part of human consciousness), are expressed in a variety of compositions that have a visionary aspect, as though the discovery of "the place that was not" changes the order of things, producing an acceleration of the drive to create an additional symbolic place that will dominate the existing order or even expose or nullify it. Thus we must locate all the new compositions on the subject of Utopia. On the one hand they express the hope and the desire for the unknown factor, the "no-place," and on the other hand they

[54] David HaReuveni (end of the fifteenth century–beginning of the sixteenth century) was a Jewish traveler who initiated contacts with the Christian elite in the era of the expulsion from Spain and Portugal for the advancement of his military plans for the redemption of Israel and the establishment of a state for the Jews in the land of Israel. The different layers of his plans (which brought forth a redemption movement that caused bloodshed amid the Jewish and Marrano populations), his origins, and his colorful and mysterious personality have not been deciphered to this day. He probably came from the Arabian peninsula or from Yemen.

[55] On the Reuveni himself and the Ten Tribes see Ben-Dor (2009).

[56] See Chen-Morris's in-depth preface to Ayelet Even-Ezra's Hebrew translation of More's Utopia (More, 2002; Chen-Morris, 2008).

[57] See More's *Utopia* (2002). Also it is necessary to read HaReuveni opposite the loss of Spain in the reality of its Jews.

represent certainty about the existence of a new order and a new place whose imaginary founding or discovery represents what will change the social and symbolic order of the place and will reconstruct on the symbolic level the shock of the general world at the discovery of America.

Along with the new processes of centralization, those of European consciousness in the wake of the discovery, and the change of relations between the mystery and location in the real and the symbolic, Judaism also underwent a renewed centralization; the expulsion of the Jews, from the Jewish point of view, also opened an era of a new order, though from the standpoint of the Jew and Judaism the establishment of the order of the new world is founded on crisis and exile. Simultaneously with the discovery of the New World, the Jewish resident of Spain loses his foothold in the Old World and turns into an ex-territorial. The early modern age has its foundation in trauma. Judaism extracts from the trauma—as part of the battle of these forces and as a priming of even more far-reaching processes—conceptual and experiential structures capable of expressing and containing these spatial shocks.

14.13 Poles of Reality and Symbol: David HaReuveni and Luria

As we have started to describe above, Luria, the great designer of the new symbolic order in the early modern period as expressed in Judaism, did this by drawing the Godhead in the first stages of its revelation in spatial concepts, instead of its older traditional design, the fruit of the Neoplatonic heritage as developed in the Kabbalah, in concepts of time. In this system, the entire system of commandments rests on the principle of healing the rupture of cosmic exile, collecting the fractured shards of divine light spread in the world.[58] In contrast, Rabbi David HaReuveni is the principal and most significant representative of the attempt to institute a new symbolic order whose expression would be in concrete reality; precisely at the time of the scattering and distancing of the Jews there arises in HaReuveni the will to *represent, find, and discover the remnants*, the ancient survivors of the Jewish people in a procedure that promises to re-enlarge the volume of the Jewish people.

14.14 Messianism and Crisis Theology

Besides defining the procedure of Luria as opposed to the composition of Utopias in the general culture—these require a paradigmatic place in concrete reality, whereas he shapes from the foundation the metaphysical place and renews it—we must also point to the oppositional parallelism to the organizing concept. If we posit for instance as point of relation Hobbes' *Leviathan*,[59] then I propose a comparison, in the context of a Christian Europe undergoing processes of secularization and struggling with the significance of the modern state, between what happens on the level of metaphoric "organization" on the level of the state and what occurs on the level of symbolic organization on the plane of the Godhead.[60]

The link between the idea of the Leviathan and the wanderer expelled outside it is suggested by Galit Hasan Rokem by reading together the idea of the Leviathan as a state and the idea of the Wandering Jew, the wanderer without political representation, while relating to an additional, later textual focus, namely the famous work by Carl Schmitt.[61]

Some of these statements will acquire great significance after the concept of the community arises in the Hasidism of the eighteenth century.

[58] I dilate on this in my forthcoming book, *Judaism and the Picture of the World* (2016).

[59] Thomas Hobbes, 1990 *Leviathan*.

[60] On the two distinct conceptions of the relation between the myth of Leviathan and history, as identified with the historic cycle within the Godhead or as acting with relation to external history (in both conceptions Leviathan represents chaos, but the concept of chaos is different) see Pedaya (2003); for the sake of the discussion focused on the Leviathan and on the snake in relation to millenarism and the state see Pedaya (2012, 2013a).

[61] See Hasan-Rokem (2008, 2009); Pedaya (2015b). I propose the link between the accelerated formation of the Leviathan on the Divine symbolic level of the Jew and the Leviathan on the political level of the Christian, in my essay "The Sixth Millennium"—Pedaya (2012).

Luria established the critical concepts, which are all key concepts in the theory of consciousness and the modern Jewish soul; they are all deep, symbolic, and anchored in ancient, even Gnostic myths.[62] However this does not negate another description of them, namely that at the same time all of them contain, despite their abstractionism, a deep echo of the crisis, and therefore it is impossible to refrain from reading Luria's schema as a schema of crisis, trauma, and overcoming on all levels, and from finding in it a reflection, historical even though the general tendency of the pattern he suggests is not toward history but beyond it.

If Hobbes claims explicitly—in the framework of philosophical writing—that only the community has freedom, Luria, who writes in a mystical framework, formulates a reworking of the reasons for the commandments in Jewish law (*mitzvot*): the gathering of the sparks, the unification of divine masculine and feminine aspects, as well as the community of Israel with the *Torah*—totality of the *mitzvot*. Luria in fact expresses, though indirectly, the conception that a common project of redemption is likely to become reality only by means of a community. The community, like a single individual, has a single mission, which in future will free it, and freedom is redemption.

I do not find trauma reflected in one concept—the *tsimtsum*[63]—rather I think that we are dealing with at least four concepts: *tsimtsim, shevirah* (breaking), *tikkun* (repair), and *reshimu* (impression)[64] which build together a theology of crisis. They need to be examined together, since as a comprehensive structure they contain the concepts of diminution, contraction *(tsimtsum),* walking, scattering *(shevirah),* the remnants *(reshimu)*, and the gathering and (re)assembling *(tikkun).*

Above all these things there still stands one concept that is apparently not mentioned but it is also a principle of the process of new symbolic order in the sixteenth to seventeenth centuries, the concept of *space*.[65] The divine is described in a spatial symbolic framework, and not in a system of immanence like time, which is the classic Neoplatonic model (which also existed in the Far East) with which the structures of early Kabbalah are stamped. The transition from the thinking of "time" to the thinking of "place" is congruent at the same time with the central event of the period, whose echoes are relevant to the new mythic process, and with the spirit of early modernism in general.

With such a view, I contend that Luria created a framework, a language, and a method with which the dynamics of the entire Godhead is a dynamics of crisis and trauma. He attains the "lacuna" that was left behind by the receding divine, and gradually turns it into an object of striving toward the transition. That is to say, this is also a way of coping with the empty space; the essence of the *tsimtsum,* the contraction or withdrawal, is the establishment of *absence* and the *empty point*; it too is apt at times to be grasped as a lacuna, and is yet to function also as an object of

[62] Also see my recent book on Kabbalah and Psychoanalysis (Pedaya, 2015d).

[63] The process of Tzimtzum was a point of contention between Idel and Scholem. See Scholem in his "Toward an understanding of the Messianic idea in Israel " (Scholem, 1975) and Idel's consequent publications, especially in his "Concerning the Concept of Tsimtsum in Kabbalah and in Scholarship" (Idel, 1992). The argument surrounding the primacy of Lurianic Tzimtzum or older concepts of this sort is not central to my approach, since it is not necessary for Luria to be the originator of the concept in order to organize a system around it. Also, I place a stronger emphasis on *shvira* as scattering.

[64] The tsimtsum (contraction or constriction) is the act of the primal distinction, the separation of the infinite Creator in a way that creates space and makes possible an existence separate from him, a duality built into the experience of reality; the laying-bare of what is found in the empty space to the Divine abundance cannot after all go easily, and there occurs a breaking of the vessels—the mechanisms which were supposed to sustain the contact with the Infinite. This is an event which is both cosmogonic and historical (through the sins of man and the people throughout the generations); the tikkun is a process of picking up the pieces left from the breakage and bringing them together to a state of completeness; the reshimu (i.e., the impression of the pattern of light even after its withdrawal) leaves even in space after the tsimtsum the border of the infinite, the potential and reality of the Divine presence—if only through its absence. See Baskin (2011).

[65] The sixteenth and seventeenth centuries are marked with this centrality of Galilean-Cartesian and Newtonian treatments of space.

desire to return to what is impenetrable, void, and inaccessible. Together with this, Luria abandoned the concepts of emanation as a process that occurs and embodies itself in time in favor of emanation as a process that occurs and embodies itself in space. In this I see the center of gravity of the change in the general picture of the world of the period as it irradiates his mysticism.[66]

14.15 The Sixteenth Century: Destruction and Historiography

In the sixteenth century there occurs a sketching of all the theological models and possibilities that became operative at the central intersections of Jewish existence in modernity: secularization, Haskalah, Hasidism, early Zionism, and the reformulation of theological and concrete stances in post-Shoah Judaism; modes of writing, hermeneutics, and canonization; in fact this is the broadest "historic moment," a moment of vibration of the open string, from the standpoint of representation of the range of different and varied historiographical modes.[67] In the context of this short essay I can relate only to Luria and to Cordovero; both of them reflect, in approximately the same short time span, in which their paths crossed in Safed, a gigantic literary and hermeneutic enterprise which gathers to it the creation of the *Zohar,* and together with this a completely different relation both to reality and to the literary canon. In this historic timing they mark two different possibilities of existence. True, in order to explain the choices of Cordovero and Luria we need to place them in a more inclusive and encompassing historical context.

The following significant elements of action and choice are here proposed as the dynamic At crucially challenging junctures of Jewish history of addressing the pressures of destruction and devastation (of temple or community), trauma, and loss (such as persecutions): The struggle of the Leadership (with the question of the new object of the communities' resources), Creation, Ingathering, and Canonization.[68]

14.16 The Work of the Present and The Images That Govern It

And from here we shift to the two significant choices and the representation of the two different directions at the crossroads of the sixteenth century. Luria, perhaps from a perspective of distance as opposed to the perspective connected with acute trauma which characterizes Cordovero, suggested a structural conceptualization of the trauma and in so doing opened the work of the present to the future, and transferred the frustrated desire onto a new focus, an idea of repair and building. All this he did by means of reorganization, both of method and world view and of the ritual system. In contrast, Cordovero, who was a direct descendant of a family that had been expelled, continued to give expression to the apocalyptic experience, the experience of the "end" to which the generation of the expulsion had been pushed, and gave strong expression in conceptualization and in image to the concept of history as decline in accordance with the feeling of destruction and the traumatic present that was still full of destructions. Accordingly, the practices that Cordovero suggests fluctuate between Acting-out and Working-through; the ceremonies of expulsion, especially, express the existence of anxiety. At the same time, these ceremonies aspire to find in the liminal space a potential for a transformational process, of assimilation transformation and development that makes it possi-

[66] Also elaborated on in Pedaya (2015a).

[67] A full-scale historiographical survey and catalog project was suggested by Ben-Zion Dinor but was never created (See Pedaya, 2011a, pp. 211, 287 ref. 479).

[68] To put it very briefly: what happens in the Second Temple period with the destruction and loss of the object of the Temple—two options are opened for the formulation of the destruction as a loss or as an absence, and the metamorphosis into loss is helped by the direction of the wandering energies to the literary canon. This takes place in the sixteenth century with the loss of space where the two options are formulated in mystical space, the space of emanation and time, while the canon is reorganized.

ble to transition from *acting-out* to *working-through*. It is interesting to look at the mythic pictures of time which govern the work of the present. In his commentary on the Zohar, *Ohr Yakar* (Precious Light), Cordovero wrote[69]:

> … And so the world was thus built and ruined over and over until the Temple was constructed; and in that hour the world attained its finest standing—not as in its origin but the highest level of perfection. It was from that point that the world began its stages of descent until the destruction of the temple, and in the construction of the second temple the building was not complete; indeed in the second temple's destruction a darkness overtook the entire world and since then it was that the world descended and with it the Shchina down through the Klipot and they rule, with every day more cursed than the last … And this is the Fallen Succah of David that is always *falling and descending*, with the end and *redemption hinging on its descent—once it is completed it [the Shchina] will rise all at once*. It is thus that the secret of redemption is *in the depths of the abyss and the corrupt halls*; he who is familiar with these depths and sees the fallen Shchina and how many more stages are left.

In a concept that is essentially apocalyptic there is a double concept of time; there is a revealed story and a hidden story of history. Thus the story of the descent of the Shekhinah is the hidden story and the true determinant of the "duration." And thus the hidden story—or the proper "conception of history that is in keeping with this insight"[70]—is the fall of the *Shekhina*, the feminine image, to the bottom of a pit, and only when she is on the lowest rung is the chapter of the fall completed and she ascends all at once, and thus history comes to an end. This is the absolute reverse of the way Luria conceives of revealed and hidden history as conducted both on the same principle. Here is not merely a tension between "progress" and "regression" in the world-picture of Luria—in the sense that is accepted in the discussion of progress in the framework of European history. Rather the coordination in the movement of the revealed and hidden story tends much more in the direction of progress, while the gap between the stories, the tension, and contradiction between them is the life breath of apocalypticism, as is the expectation of traumatic future, internalized as second nature from the lessons of the past.[71]

Well-known lines of thought in Lurianic Kabbalah can be described as a mode of regression; however, it seems that the emphasis is on the cosmic *scattering of the lights* at the beginning of being, that is, in the primordial past; and then the process of *gathering*, which is in fact a form of ascent, is the actual hidden story which explains the historical development.[72] In other words: There is indeed an expectation of a redeemed, healed future. The tension between the devastation of the past and the future (boding either solace or suffering is mediated through *ritual*); it is the bridge between the wounded past and the as-of-yet opaque future. For example, the walking rituals of Cordovero serve to "inoculate" the Self—fortifying and revitalizing it, functioning on the representational-identification level. In the system of Luria, walking the earth is the process of gathering the shards of divine light, acting on a cosmic scale.

If we compare the versions of the story of the hidden course of history, whose subject is the *Shekhinah* according to Luria and Cordovero, and by means of this they present the overarching metaphor of the collective trauma, then it seems that according to Cordovero the story of decline is the story of the time of "duration," while according to Luria the story of decline or crisis occurs immediately at the start of time, while the time of the "duration" is a time of building and ascent.

These two relationships to time are of course also two modes of experiencing time from the post-traumatic standpoint.

[69]*Ohr Yakar*, vol. 16, p. 84 [Translation: Israel Belfer].

[70]Benjamin (2011) p.257.

[71]From this standpoint it is interesting that some of the interpretations in this spirit are indeed connected to some extent with messianic apocalyptic midrashim as absorbed in the Zohar. I discuss the basic characteristics of this connection in my essay "The Sixth Millennium" (Pedaya, 2012); see also chapter 7, "*MiNeged Va'Avarim*" in Pedaya (2002a, 2002b). See also Zak (1992); Liebes (1982, p. 206 n. 406). For example, the apocalyptic atmosphere drives a regression to nihilistic action, such as the treatment of actual women by Frank.

[72]Compare the essays of Gershom Scholem, "The Messianic Idea in Israel", "The Idea of Redemption in Kabbalah" (1975, 1975a).

There is a difference between the depiction of the Shekhinah as a single, personified figure, for whom the course of existence is the complete descent, dramatically rising at the end, and the description of that figure of light as one that explodes at the cosmogonic moment, the course of existence being the duration of her regathering into a complete figure.[73]

It is probable that in this simile of exile, which governs the consciousness of Cordovero, there also lies an explanation for the preference of scattering (human, cosmological) as a "condition of redemption": if the *overarching image of time* is experienced as a fall into a kind of pit or narrow cage, then walking and scattering of consciousness are an action opposed to the state of being enclosed in a pit, a kind of ***iron cage*** of the Jew, the cage of the duration of falling.[74]

On the other hand, the governing image in the consciousness of Luria explains walking as *gathering*; in relation to the image of scattering and explosion, *tikkun* is the gathering and focusing of the scattered. There is also a coordination between the unification of the subject and the unification of the collective, and the placing of the present in a future continuity, for the trauma is primary and structural and is represented within the present only as a future-moving myth.

Within this image, Cordovero gave expression to the community of trauma; he was a living channel for the tradition of memory of the expelled, in which many elements of the trauma were living and present, as were, I would assume, elements of the Spanish interpretive tradition of the *Zohar* in an immediate way. Many elements of Cordovero's teaching were absorbed into the Kabbalah or subsequent generations, but it was Luria whose general organizing framework was of a deep significance, for already in its primal and extremely communicative foundations it contained future, it contained an image of repair.

For the community of his close associates and students, Cordovero was the one for whom the trauma was still present and echoing in his world. Thus in the sixteenth century Cordovero and Luria stood at the same crossroads at which the circle of the Zohar had stood in the thirteenth century, when the millennial aspirations collapsed. Rabbi Shimon bar Yochai (the Rashbi,[75] the literary protagonist of the *Zohar*, proposed an opening of the future as a new object of relation and as a step that would enable a community of memory that would move forward from the trauma, similar to the step taken by Rabbi Yochanan ben Zakkai[76] after the destruction of the second temple, for the rabbinic collective, as opposed to the apocalyptic stance adopted by others.

14.17 Community, Destruction and Identity, Time and Place

The sixteenth century is also characterized as a time that sketched all the models and theological possibilities of the combinations that can exist between structures of time and place, between structures of community, trauma, and identity, as also in the definition of the subject of the messianic process. They are again activated at every central juncture of Jewish existence in modern times: Secularization, Enlightenment and Hasidism, the beginnings of Zionism, and afterwards new theologies and reorganizations of theological and concrete positions after the Holocaust.

[73]For additional discussion of the cosmic process as a process of redemption see Liebes (1992), p. 165. For a basic comparison between Cordovero and Luria on the subject of sanctification of the name and the ten martyrs, including a discussion of messianism, the diminution of the moon, and prostration see Zak (1992).

[74]For a treatment of time as a pit, see (2011a, 2015c) where I elaborate on this trope in the context of Edgar Alan Poe's "The Pit and the Pendulum" (Poe, 1842), and Saul Bellow's "The Bellarosa Connection" (Bellow, 1989).

[75]One of the Tannaim in the second century C.E. In popular and rabbinic tradition the composition of the Zohar, in which he functions as a central figure, is attributed to him.

[76]One of the leaders of Pharisaic Judaism in the first century C.E.; in the years of the destruction of the Temple he led the process of preservation of Judaism through the move to Yavneh and the preservation of the oral Torah and the rabbinic tradition.

The theological system built by Luria opened two basic possibilities: one is the conceptualization of psychology and the other is the transfer of the messianic project to the process of the collective which is carried out in an active manner. In the system of Cordovero the subject of the messianic process is the Shekhinah and her continued falling, which is the hidden clock of messianic time—a process that is "tolerable" from his standpoint, that is, from the standpoint of the apocalyptic point of view, because of the feeling of the proximate location of the end of time, and thus of the chance of redemption. It seems that according to various calculations Cordovero located his generation as one generation before the revealed end, and according to him the chain of the signs (again similar to the apocalyptic approach) will lead to the end. For instance, he predicted that the resurrection of the dead would take place in the year 5408 (1648 in the Gregorian calendar).[77]

The system that Luria builds in relation to the crisis of the collective, to the expulsion in the framework of the sixteenth century, is a complex structure. On the one hand he builds an exact psychology and thus reflects the ascendancy of the subject in Judaism; in a whole system of practices this too undergoes conceptualization and crystallization into this process of structuring of the self. On the other hand he builds a teaching that crystallizes the whole Jewish collective as the subject of the messianic process and gives to the new subjective order the explanation that **there is a purpose in the walking**. In the dispersion to the four corners of the earth the Jews are the hidden logic of the cities; the cities are not what is obscured, but rather the secret of their existence is the exile that occurs among them. The movement of the expelled, their wanderings, their alien-ness, their dispersion, is the hidden reason for the external building of kingdoms and peoples. Mapping modern Jewish history is thus not concerned primarily with territory but with the motion of wandering.

[77]The *Zohar* with the interpretation of "Ohr Yakar", vol. 6, p. 53 (Shemot), and see in the *Sefer HaZohar,* part 2, p. 10a; also see Zak (1995), p. 274; Pedaya (2012).

14.18 Community, Destruction and Identity, Time and Place: Sabbatianism

This system that Luria constructed serves, in the hands of Nathan of Gaza,[78] as a central tool in the psychological interpretation of the Messiah. The Messiah is the ultimate subject who anticipates the appearance of the modern subject in Jewish mysticism. Luria formed the foundations of psychology, but he fixed it in a static form as a reflection of the Divine system; and significant for this structuring, besides the processes rooted in his soul and his mythic consciousness and its sources, is perhaps the fact that Luria's immediate biographic background—that which is connected to the course of his personal life—is not rooted in Christian Europe. In his structuring of the self and practice of the self Luria marks the opening of early modern times when he suggests an organized psychology and along with it a system of practices, all of them connected with the systematic aspect of the discipline of the self. [79] In contrast, in the medieval structures the discipline of the self was based in a deeper and broader way on the question of the coordination or lack of coordination with a relatively stable social order within its defined microcosm, so that castigation or expulsion was enough to awaken the impulse of return to order.[80]

When Nathan of Gaza and the Sabbatian system as a whole became active, we see how the European Jewish modus of walking outside the place changes to a tremendous impetus of walking to a place, a desire that was announced in the visions that came to the Marranos in Portugal in waves of prophecy among women under pressure from the Inquisition.[81] In this period of the seventeenth century the Messiah is the subject,

[78]Avraham Natan ben Elisha Haim HaLevi Ashkenazi (Jerusalem 1643-Skopje 1680).

[79]See Pedaya (2015a).

[80]The decline of ostracization as punishment (from Spinoza and Luzzato to Frank and Hassidism) is an essential part of the establishment of the modern Self in Judaism.

[81]See my essay "Land: time and place – apocalypses of the end and apocalypses of the beginning" (Pedaya, 2002a), in which I also mention the studies of Beinart concerning the Marranos.

he dwells above the established order, and in and through him the desire of the collective for a new order is expressed. The failure of the transformation between modes became a widespread process of voluntary assimilation of part of the Jewish collective into Islam or Christianity, as in the case of Jacob Fran: externally—the deliberate move to Poland, and internally—the transition into Christianity or Islam. In the wake of the constructions that Nathan of Gaza opened (or blazed) on the authority of Lurianic Kabbalah, walking into the identity of the other becomes the walking that ends the exilic situation.

14.19 Charisma and Messianism Reabsorbed: Hasidism

Against this backdrop the instigator of the modern Hasidic movement—Rabbi Israel ben Eliezer, the Baal Shem Tov ("the Besht"[82])—appears as the classic charismatic figure heralding a multifaceted (social, theological, psychological) turning, containing the old forms together with new structures, teaching and expressing the turn from the Hasid of the old type to the Hasid of the new type. Generally, Hasidism in its beginnings contained the whole spectrum of old and new practices, both in the narrow sense of the word and in the broad sense of the matter.

In the narrow sense of the word, the wandering Jews in Eastern Europe justify their walking as a practice both by means of an overarching structure of exile and by means of an overarching structure of redemption. More generally, the different possibilities that were disseminated in the sixteenth century continued to echo over the course of succeeding centuries and were disseminated strongly in the eighteenth century. Thus, for instance, messianism transitioned from an attempt to capture a turn to the ultimate holy place from a millennial point of view or a beginning of time and was transferred to man as the smallest unit of place, encouraging internal redemption. Another modus is the justification of the practice of exile through internalization of an inner story of atonement of the body (that is, no longer the body of society but the body of the person). Yet another modus is the justification of ambulation as identification with the *Shekhinah* in exile. The picture of walking the breadth of Europe contracts to be mainly a picture of preachers wandering throughout Eastern Europe, creating on the move. Urbanization and the process of capitalism were taking place more slowly there than in Western Europe. [83]This corresponds to the character of Eastern Europe, where, in comparison to the West, the old and the new are present together, with both at full strength. In Eastern Europe of the eighteenth century there is a certain similarity to the ferment of thirteenth-century Spain.

Historically, we are again witness to the strong tension that is latent among those men who lack a position in the communal structure, who have no fixed salary and no steady work, whose wanderings are necessitated by their occupation—they are the ones who mediate between the dimensions of the earthly and the concrete. Some of the transformations that affect Hasidism occur within the field of constructions and conduct that belong to the "old world," and this is incorporated in the personality of the Besht, for whom being a magician was a springboard connecting the old and the new world.

The Besht in the eighteenth century leads directly (and not entirely in line with his own character) to the decline of asceticism and visceral atonement connected with the image of the "scattering," and to the ascendancy of the concept of purification and the ecstasy of inclusion, and thus brings out the fact that within the steps of walking much fuel of redemption as a form of gathering remained latent; again the rationale of wandering as a rationale of gathering arises and crystallizes.[84]

[82]Rabbi Israel ben Eliezer, known as the Baal Shem Tov (eighteenth century, Galicia, and Poland), father of the Hasidic movement.

[83]See Braudel (1985/2005).

[84]On walking as redemptive practice see Wolfson, "Walking as a Sacred Duty."

14.20 Gaining a Foothold on the Imagination: On the Way to Eratz Israel

Thus to the practices of walking that grew in accelerated form in the traumatic generation of the expulsion from Spain. A different rationale was given in myths and rituals, but they often grew from the same basic experience of concrete traumatic wounding. They combined in different ways and they subverted and unraveled social and religious structures. To these structures of walking, whose mythic beginning is anchored in the Biblical myth of Cain, a myth of crime and punishment, they joined prophetic practices that modeled the punishment of exile to the community. These structures were absorbed into the Christian-Jewish dialogue because of the Christian blame for the Jewish murder of the Messiah. In the course of the Middle Ages it had sometimes happened that practices of walking picked up speed from the energy of messianic structures, not only in the character of the anti-Messiah of Christianity but also from the inner logic of Jewish thinking. Messianism expresses the place where exile and redemption are like the positive and negative in the process of development of the same picture.

These structures, in which walking is a practice connected with a rationale of punishment, exclusion or exile from a position outside a given system, received in the course of European Jewish history an additional impetus from expulsions, from judicial formulations on the status of the Jews, and also from the formation of the mythic place of the Jew vis-à-vis Christianity as eternal witness. The distance between the eternal witness and the eternal Jew is not great, and therefore while the central mythical occupation of the witness is walking, the social order of Christian Europe reflected this mythic-symbolic concept and preserved in different versions the concept of the Jew as alien to place. The expulsion from Spain as a crisis of the collective brought to the surface many practices and rituals of exile, whether focused on walking itself as a framework for *Acting-out* and *Working-through* or whether within a more general framework of the need to mourn. The conception of the land of Israel as a haven of destination grows gradually, from the visions of Marranos under stress to the visions of David HaReuveni and Shlomo Molcho. The visions of those who came out of the generation of expulsion, such as Alkabetz and Karo, also direct the descendents of the generation of the expelled to Israel as a territorial place identified with the Shekhinah, and after that Sabbatai Zevi[85] in his messianic vision under the direction of Nathan of Gaza—a figure who is counted among the mystics of the land of Israel. Luria reestablishes the mythic order and reconceptualizes the scattering of the Jews in a mythical logic that answers the situation of European Jewry like a heavenly voice.[86]

14.21 State of Emergency and Political Establishment

In modern times, the philosophical and theological discussion of the state of emergency reverts constantly to the theological-political document composed by Carl Schmitt and its famous assertion that Sovereign is he who decides on the state of emergency.[87] This very formulation was of course made possible by a thinking in which judicial hegemony is deeply reflexive, that is, formulated by one of the most important constitutional jurists in the Weimar republic, deliberating with and relying on the literature of jurists who preceded him and occupied themselves with defining sovereignty. When he states that the significance

[85] Sabbatai Zevi (1626–1676) was the one of the most famous false Messiahs of Jewish history. Founder of the Sabbatean movement.

[86] In the formulation of Bernard de Clairvaux, Catholic martyr, Letter to Eastern France and Bavaria Promoting the Second Crusade, 1146: "The Jews are for us the living words of scripture, for they remind us always of what our Lord Suffered. They are dispersed all over the world so that by expiating their crime they may be everywhere the living witnesses of our redemption. Hence the same Psalm (59) adds 'only let thy power disperse them'… If the Jews are utterly wiped out, what will become of our hope for the promised salvation, their eventual conversion?" (Carrol, 2002, p. 271).

[87] Carl Schmitt (2010), pp. 5–12.

of a state of emergency in jurisprudence is analogous to the significance of a miracle in theology, he creates a conceptual focal point—serving as a basic distinction for many kinds of discussion that will come after him and inspires systems of analogies to other theological systems that preceded him.[88]

From the different standpoints that I have expounded here I will add that we must speak of two aspects of relation to the state of emergency: *Sovereign* is he who can decide on the state of emergency of the state and he who has it in his power to merge and identify the normative law with the emergency statutes as much as he wishes. *Oppressed* is he who acts from the constant state of emergency of being the individual, the minority, limited in power and resources, and (inevitably) against the law of the sovereign that is directed against him.

Sovereign is he who can act constantly from a position of boundary-setting and the identification of law with power. Persecuted is he who seeks the ways of unraveling the symmetry between power and law, which creates the constant state of emergency for him as the oppressed. The Sovereign creates the state of emergency and unifies it with the extensions of his power and his constitution. The Persecuted finds himself in the Sovereign's (ruler-imposed) state of emergency and dreams of the true (reality-imposed) state of emergency; this, in other words, is the definition of the apocalyptic state of mind.

14.22 The Ultimate "Other Place": Present and Past Through the Holocaust

The difficulty of distinguishing and separating between theoretical tendencies, ideologies, messianism, and nationalism, and impulses of the collective moved by the force of post-traumatic existential experience, is in itself a distinguishing mark of a collective memory saturated with the trauma of the Holocaust. The concentration camp constituted the peak of processes of exile through concentration within a place and became a laboratory for collective annihilation, utterly nullifying the symbolic place that the Jewish People held in Europe. The ashes and smoke became the symbol of the liquidation in the most extreme place on earth. The dwelling place in heaven became the distinguishing mark of the poetry of Paul Celan, Dan Pagis, and Uri Zvi Greenberg who sought a more supernal or infernal place than the earth itself. It is not possible to separate the impetus of expansion according to place in the space of the land of Israel from the trauma of the annihilation of the absolute place, of the body of the people. It is likewise impossible to separate the trauma of the crematoria, whose symbolic representation is the exile to heaven, from the reliance—more pronounced than ever—on the symbolic space of messianic Judaism in the land of Israel, especially in the era of secularization in Israeli society.[89]

In this respect, the discussion of Zionism solely by the standards of post-colonialism is inadequate. It misses the essential perspective of European exile, expulsion, and annihilation on the history of the Jewish people, while the land of Israel constitutes the symbolic space which accompanies that movement. In this light the Holocaust and in its wake the establishment of the state of Israel are tightly coupled parts of this long history. In order to make sense of the immediate past and present, this larger scale must be appreciated.

Throughout this essay we have seen that practices of exile can sometimes be *Acting-out* or *Working-through* of the traumas of expulsion, and therefore a widening of the gaze to certain practices in the Israeli space (taking possession, claiming our heritage, settling) can illumine that these are not only practices of redemption, but are at the same time practices nourished by the symbolic space established by exile, expulsion,

[88] See the discussion proposed by David Sorotskin, "The Theology of the Transcendent" (2006), and for an expansion of the discussion on Carl Schmitt see Sorotskin (2011).

[89] On this whole topic of projection of time on the earth as a historical action that establishes Zionism see my book *Space and Place* (2011a, parts 1 and 4).

and concentrated extermination. Life outside the place in the European context acquired more significance because of the feeling of life outside *the* lost place, the land of Israel.

A complete description of the phenomenon of return to the place must include the fatality of impulses of activity—the force of inertia resisting a change of place, and the power of fear of lack of place. These impulses to action are likely to reappear unconsciously in the assemblage of the meanings of actions—which will be perceived in the framework of their conception as legitimate activities of a sovereign state fighting for its life—such as diminution of the place of the other, because of the weight of collective memory, the long memory, sealed by the experience of expulsion and by a *displaced* life. This is not a politically oriented stance, rather a widening of the view to elucidate the Israeli political paradigm of placing and subsisting in a territory as redemptive sitting (literally, from the root y.s.v—*yishuv, hit'yashvut*) vs. diasporic walking.

14.23 The Context of General Culture

Here I would like to add the dimension which is required by additional widespread processes that occur in modern European culture. Identity itself, as something stable and fixed, undergoes two decisive stages: in the modern stage a movement occurs in the direction of a universal existential identity, whose characteristics are the exile of the individual from the world as a whole; in the postmodern stage, when it is made clearer still that identity is momentary, sporadic, and changing, and the text is the world, exile no longer carries any negative charge of pain or suffering, but is itself the definition of the ideal of being unconnected, untethered.

Walking as a practice is also elevated to an ideal, with the great and essential difference that it is carried out within the city. Whereas the walkers from the High Middle Ages to early modern times—and in Judaism even in the eighteenth and nineteenth centuries—walked *outside* the cities (and, by means of the experience of the area that was extra-territorial to the city, experienced exile, actualized it, and made it present), from the eighteenth century on the modern walkers walk within and in the center of the city to make their curse (which is essentially also their blessing) present. In the modern and postmodern world, the detachment from the territorial boundaries of the city is not necessarily an abandonment of culture—the practice of urban ambulation can be replaced by surfing on the Internet. Thus, the movement of *detachment* is always a dialogue with other movements of *attachment*; these days, exile (in its wider sense of *Galut* as described out above) to the poor, those who aren't free to change their living situation and location, is limited in space. The opposite person, equipped with passport and credit card, can go to the airport. Even the backpackers who walk in the Far East, though they certainly do attempt to go out to the liminal domain,[90] like pilgrims walking to a holy place (in the center or in the margins) in order to reestablish an inner center within themselves, can return to their homes at any time they wish, and thus they are not caught in a state of exile.

14.24 The Transformation of Urban Space

We cannot separate the processes and evolution of the city, its growth, and the changes that have taken place in it from the revolution in the concept of the city. The Christian theology of the Church fathers attached great importance to the connection that the Biblical myth weaves between Cain punished by exile and Cain as the founder of the first city,[91] its establishment by the hand of a murderer. Augustine laid the theological groundwork for the foundation of two cities that are like two parallel lines that do not meet: the historical city and the city of God. One may

[90] A study on this has been written by Yehudah Herman under my direction.

[91] Regarding Cain and the founding of the city—in tradition, myth, and ritual—see Gruenwald (2003), 65.

say that the city of Cain is identified with the course of human history. Augustine carries out this course side by side with the detachment from an apocalyptic frame of mind, and translates the duality of the city to the temporal plane—two kinds of time. Augustine places the emphasis on life, as a kind of journey to the city of God, while history—the earthly city—is the stage for the wanderings of Cain.[92]

From the ninth to tenth centuries exile was punishment for murder and sexual transgressions in Christian society, in regions of Germany, France, and England. In Christianity, which is not a religion of praxis, like Judaism, there occurs a process (also on other levels) whereby myths become the basis for norms and laws. A myth that has an essentially normative tendency—the myth of Cain—indeed becomes the basis for the formation of practices of punishment. In the High Middle Ages and with the ascendancy of the city, the murderer is sent to wander outside the city. In a manner that is rather dialectic, religious Jewish society in Christian Europe, especially in the regions of France and Germany, is influenced by these practices of punishment and likewise internalizes them.[93]

Various scholars have tried to explain the historic dominance of punishment through exile; the explanation that I propose is that in Christian society it is directly connected with the ascendancy of the city and with the drawing of its distinct borders and cohesive territory, as a unit of place and culture, which made it possible to define the extraterritorial, the no-place, in relation to it. That is to say: in a rather paradoxical way, the murderer is cast out of the city because in the Middle Ages the city becomes a center of identity and a center of society. In relation to what is happening in Christian society in the urban system, a similar process occurs in the community system in urban European Jewish society (from here on my comparisons between Judaism and Christianity are essentially between city and community; the community is paralleled to the urban unit, as a sort of "city within the city"). In contrast, in the seventeenth century we witness practices of punishment as exile and exclusion *within* the city, which no longer serves as a distinct area of protection, distinguished physically from the outside.

The systems which we discussed flowed into modernism and were secularized from the beginning, principally through art, painting, and poetry. Foucault opens his discussion of discipline and punishment with the public ceremony of execution, which is pregnant with the components of punishment which we have discussed.[94] I add that from the viewpoint of exile and ceremonies of exile there is an additional revolution here: not only the transition from what is exposed to the eye to what is imprisoned in inner rooms, but also a transition from punishment as a scattering in a vast space to punishment as a contraction into a tiny cell. Clearly there is a strong connection between urban history and the change in the concept of the theater of exile. In the small, fortified medieval cities which were intimate cities of refuge and places of shelter, exile was outside the city; in a world that has undergone processes of industrialization and mechanization and has become distant from the rural (and wild) land, and with the accelerated growth of the city, the theater of the experience of alienation and the actualization of walking as a practice of exile has moved, paradoxically, to the center of the city. While those who grasp themselves as exiles walking the center of the city, others—the punished ones who were once perhaps condemned to walking outside the city—are shut up in closed rooms. Imprisonment is not only a substitute for the public spectacle of execution, but also an expression of immobility as replacing the punishment of constant walking. From there the historical road leads to the concentration camp as an extreme confluence of the model of forced spatial restriction and burning at the stake.

[92] St. Augustine (1984) book XV, ch. 1, 597, 600–601.

[93] Regarding banishment as punishment, see Kaplan (2000), pp. 61, 67, 175.

[94] Foucault (1995), pp. 32–33 (on banishment in the eighteenth century), p. 115 (transition to incarceration).

14.25 The Streets: Walking the City and Writing

In modernity there is walking for the sake of walking and the journey without destination takes place in the heart of the city and among the crowd (as one can see clearly in Baudelaire and Walter Benjamin, for example), but the basic myths and narratives continue to play their game. The three models reappear as three secularized models: the model of the wandering murderer Cain becomes the model of the "accursed poets" (Verlaine, Rimbaud, Baudelaire); the exemplar of the wandering prophet becomes the model of the artist and the writer (from stream of consciousness to Walter Benjamin, De Certeau, Jabès, and Derrida)[95]; and the apocalyptic model turns into the model of messianic poetry (Uri Zvi Greenberg) or writing that moves between image and flesh (Benjamin).

These models arose with the rise of the modern city and reappeared in the postmodern and post-urban age, with globalization. But in the Israeli sphere there is still the religious echo of the Promised Land. This country has raised children who have experienced a dual state of affairs, who have shared colonialism with the conqueror and with the conquered.

Colonialism, wherever it was, reactivated the systems of the ancient world: the enforcement of emigration and the enforcement of exile within one's own country: practices that were prevalent in the medieval city for the purpose of punishing murderers were activated in the colonial age for the sake of pushing those with built-in identity off to the side. The political exile who has been spat out of the state is the modern brother of the murderer who was removed from the city that was the vision of everything. Structures of exile within one's homeland have reactivated the model of two cities, and have again sharpened the will to internal emigration.

If we consider Baudelaire, who identifies himself and his friends with the "accursed," the seed of Cain, and who is also the author of the poetic manifesto of modernism, who sketches a new language and establishes walking in the city as a modern form of worship, we must relate this to the annulment of the ritual of ambulation outside the city as a religious practice of atonement and as the architectural construction of a space of non-identity and the formation of the liminal, and over against this, ambulation within the bounds of the city as a counter-practice, in which the "marked" create the sign that marks them with their own hands by establishing a new narrative of counter-aesthetics and counter-worship. While in the original religious practices exile, as the actualization of a liminal state in which the unraveling of identity or non-identity is conceptualized, served as a stage on the way to the reformation of identity—in the modern secularized situation, as Baudelaire already sketched (although he deliberately played with the concept of marking), the situation of non-identity is the desired situation, and is itself considered as self-fulfillment.

14.26 Images Governing Walking: Rabbi Yitzchak Luria, Rabbi Moses Cordovero, and Walter Benjamin

Our discussion of Cordovero and Luria brought out that beyond this or the other practice that they crystallized and proposed, and beyond these or the other myths that they adopted from the mystical and mythical tradition that preceded them, each of them proposes an enormous picture that governs their cosmogony, and the historical trajectory of the world. In various senses and in other contexts it is possible to sharply define the

[95] The writer Edmond Jabès, born in Cairo in 1912, fled to France in 1957, in his work (much influenced by mysticism) *The Book of Questions* discusses his way in walking as a principal practice that builds a world. The motif of walking also leads to the very act of posing the questions. In the opening of his book there are echoes of the Messiah who is delayed, of the wandering Jew, of those who walk in the footsteps of the Shekhinah who live in the book. See Jabès (1991).

function of this world picture within the mystical system, borrowing from Walter Benjamin's concept of history.[96]

This vast image that governs the system of messianic concepts and the practice connected with them also illuminates the difference between Luria and Cordovero—the former depicts the Shekhinah, which is in fact the image of light, as one whose absolute downfall occurred at the beginning of existence, leaving all later generations the task of gathering; the latter depicts the Shekhinah as continually falling, suffocating in the continuous fall until reaching the very bottom, thence she will turn around and rise up all at once; the former depicts progress and the latter regression. Luria gives reason and direction to the cyclical character of everyday and active practice, while Cordovero depicts boundedness to the cyclical character of gigantic time and a ritual practice with more passive characteristics.

It is probably also possible to examine Cordovero in the light of introverted mysticism and the manner in which it is likely at times to be bound up with characteristics of mourning and trauma.

14.27 Walter Benjamin: Regressive History as a Panoramic Journey: Flashes of Progress

Several thinkers who have proposed fascinating discussions of Benjamin have expressed opinions on the recurrence of voices, tendencies, and structures in his early and late works.[97] His work is characterized by increasing repetition of images and metaphors that are progressively deepened, annex new meanings, and become anchors that sketch the matrix of thinking as a whole. This phenomenon, which is basic to the character of his thinking and its contents, can also be illumined in light of his conscious attraction to the theme of the eternal return.[98] This axis of this thinking can be elucidated by means of relation to one of the cultural phenomena and games that he describes in the notes on his childhood, the imperial panorama:

> One of the great attractions of the travel scenes found in the Imperial Panorama was that it did not matter where you began the cycle. Because the viewing screen, with places to sit before it, was circular, each picture would pass through all the stations; from these you looked, each time, through a double window into the faintly tinted depths of the image. There was always a seat available. And especially toward the end of my childhood, when fashion was already turning its back on the Imperial Panorama, one got used to taking the tour in a half-empty room [...] Distant worlds were not always strange to these arts. And it so happened that the longing such worlds aroused spoke more to the home than to anything unknown.[99]

This axis of traveling while sitting still and of the cyclical return of images accompanied by a soft shade of nostalgia and melancholy crosses with another axis: the pedestrian's journey in the city. Through these two axes together the longitude and latitude of the existential journey are sketched in concepts of intellectual biography, even his concept of history which is a mirror image of this journey, as a journey composed on the one hand of flashes, fragments, and bursts and on the other hand of basic images that keep coming back; but in every turn of the circle the old images return with an accumulation of additional meanings and connections and are invaded by additional pieces of thought—sometimes the previous meanings are deepened and sometimes they are rejected and reorganized.

From the viewpoint of the history of walking, and the concept of history—as a walking—from the vantage point of the wanderer, I will try to illuminate the affinity between these two axes as

[96] Walter Benjamin, "Theses on the Concept of History" in Benjamin (2001), pp. 253–264. Also see Pedaya (2002a, 2003, ch. 1, pp. 63–65).

[97] As an example, see Azulay (2006), 11 (Hebrew); she notes that in the early text "The Metaphysics of Youth" there is an early echo of the later text, "Theses on the Concept of History" (ibid); also see Moses (2003), 106–107, on the image of the stars which precedes the halo and cuts under the surface through the whole of his work; Nieraad (1992).

[98] For a comparative discussion between Benjamin and Nietzsche on these themes see "Benjamin, Nietsche, and the idea of the eternal return," in Moses (2003, pp. 91–112).

[99] Benjamin (2006a, 2006b), pp. 42–44.

establishing some of the depth of constellations of Benjamin's thought.

The components of this affinity are walking, writing, flash, image, return, trauma, and destruction. These in turn can be organized into two basic constellations, two series that have between them a connection that is similar to the connection that stretches between the image of the journey while sitting down in front of the imperial panorama and the journey of walking in the street.

These constellations reveal the energy of movement and the strong static energy of Benjamin's thinking and together constitute a contrapuntal being.[100] The struggle that goes on within that being sometimes overpowers it. I want to emphasize that the earliest representation of these depth structures is rooted in childhood experiences that are connected with two different sorts of pleasure, with two different practices of journeying: the journey taken while sitting and looking at pictures that return, whereby the pleasure is from the known, with the interlocking of the past and the future in the impetus of return, in a cyclical fashion that produces an atmosphere of sentimental nostalgia, and on the other hand, a journey by walking that at any moment can open to the sudden attack of a sight, a situation, a thing, or an encounter with all the magic of foreignness, surprise, sometimes even temptation, and the Eros therein. The first is the basis for the latest structure of destructive images of a future that is being swept to its utter annihilation, and the second is the basis for the messianic concept of an open and seething present. In both cases the thinking is figurative. In the static eternal return, the destructiveness of regression is necessarily latent, and in the basis of aimless forward movement progress is rooted, not like that which moves forward in unitary fashion, but as a myriad of circumstances and gates that open in the present both to the past and to the future.

On these basic structures, which appear as early experiences of practices of life beginning with childhood, loops of thought and reflection and additional structures are fastened, and they reveal themselves both as tools that Benjamin activates when he discusses literature, urbanism, or history, and as forces that cast reflected light upon himself, on his psychological and intellectual structure. But throughout the length of Benjamin's psychological and intellectual biography a process occurs between them: if they can be set up as two forces or parallel lines that stabilize the system and interlock at its points of tension, then gradually, especially in the last decade of his life, these parallel lines encroach on each other, and get closer together until the inevitable point of collision—the situation of the duel, if one may seize on a further metaphor of his, in the framework of his discussion of Baudelaire.

Sometimes these two forces are historicism and historical materialism. [101]In the literary context this will be the tension between epic and quotation, between symbol and allegory, between the momentary and the total, between the abstract general and the manifestation of the concept into an image, the hieroglyph as opposed to writing. In the urban context this will be the tension between the frozen crowd, the automatons, the fictional characters, the passive spectator looking on from a window, and the active walker in the city; in the artistic context of photography: the tension between the flash and the radiance; in the historic context: the tension between time that is homogeneous and empty, and time that is full or the shock of the messianic arrest. In the context of secularization: the tension between theology and history.

Stephane Moses set up an opposition between Walter Benjamin and Gershom Scholem's concepts of exile.[102] I suggest that, in keeping with our discussion here, it is possible to parallel Benjamin's position on history and writing with that of Cordovero, and Scholem's position with that of Luria. The comparison will not be comprehensive and detailed, since Benjamin supplies a wider net of interlocking structures than does Scholem, and as they are different types—Benjamin was a creative thinker, and Scholem a

[100]A fundamental characteristic of exile as Edward Said formulated it in his description of the consciousness of exile. See Said (1984).

[101]Benjamin (2001), p. 262, "Historicism gives the 'eternal' image of the past; historical materialism supplies a unique experience with the past."

[102]Stephane Moses, "Between Paris and Jerusalem: the exile experience of Walter Benjamin and Gershom Scholem," in Moses (2003, pp. 113–123).

scholar whose research is open to philosophy, not himself a philosopher.

These structures do not necessarily appear in Benjamin as paired opposites of binary thought, but as two trunks that sometimes complement each other, and sometimes oppose each other, and are sometimes indistinguishably entwined. In their emotional dimensions they contain the hope of joy or happiness together with feelings of sadness and trauma. These fluctuations are without doubt bound up with the zeitgeist.[103]

There is a strong basis for parallelism between Benjamin and Cordovero. In Cordovero, too, there is a primal impetus bound up with the memory of a previous trauma, walking as a practice leading to brief and focused illuminations, flashes, the boiling-down of history to an overarching image, and an encompassing regressive feeling within which there are isolated instances of progress.

Both in Benjamin and in Cordovero there is a relation to trauma: With Benjamin it is a theoretic and conscious adoption, for his discussion of Baudelaire, of—relatively new—theories about trauma (Freud and Reik) that were published in his time. Benjamin's discussion of Baudelaire reveals his relation to the subject of trauma. Benjamin walks in the footsteps of distinctions made by Reik about the defense against trauma, setting a distinct point of time for the event.[104] With Cordovero it is an unconscious activity in which there is a muffled memory of a traumatic situation which undergoes formulation and sublimation by Cordovero. In both cases there is full coordination between walking, scattering of mind, and flash-like (poetic or ecstatic-revelatory) breakthroughs.

The structure in Benjamin, from the position of writing and walking, can be summarized thus: in three central stages of his thought Benjamin copies and duplicates the basic construction of his thought, which is continually deepened. The construction of scattering, cutting-off and the grasping of the particular, and the particular is what makes generalization possible. The stage of his literary discussion of allegory and German baroque drama, his discussion focusing on Paris, which is in fact a discussion of urbanism, his discussion of art through the discussion of photography, his discussion of history in the "Theses on History": On all these levels, amid significant developmental processes, the abandonment of surrealism and the movement toward the Marxist-societal approach, and in more or less calm states and in states of anxiety, emigration, and increasing stress, up to the taking of steps that cannot be separated from the experience of being a refugee, the construction of *fracture* develops and deepens until the actual breakage and the symbolic rupture meet in reality. From its beginnings the approach of scattering and the focus on the particular as point of departure toward the whole was inextricably bound up with his preference for the literary-social and at last with the preference which fixes both artistic form and the content of the messianic act in such a way that they are inseparable.

Benjamin portrayed the experience of modernism as that which allegory expresses better than the classic symbol.[105] While the latter is focused on nature, which it represents as redemption, modernism is closer to Baroque allegory as Benjamin understood and portrayed it: every particular case can bear an infinite number of meanings. Allegory

[103] See Pedaya 2002a.

[104] Benjamin, Baudelaire (2006), p. 161. "On some motifs in Baudelaire"; Theodor Reik (1999, ch. 20, especially pp. 168–170); Freud, (1948). For a discussion of Benjamin from the standpoint of consciousness and awakening of consciousness see Marder (2006); in this collection (Hanssen, 2006, 289), there are references to many of the important books on Benjamin that have been published recently in English. Marder's discussion, like many other studies of Benjamin, maintains a relationship of inspiration, as she herself testifies, to the work of Caruth (1996); see also Caruth (1995), 153; also see Andrew E. Benjamin (2005, pp. 77–79). Andrew Benjamin focuses on the fact that Freud's theory of trauma grew in the climate of World War I, and distinguishes between Benjamin's discussion of Baudelaire, which in his opinion is more influenced by Simmel on urbanism, and Benjamin's discussion of the work of art, which stands in a more prominent relation to Freud. See also Cadava (1997), which is organized according to concepts and offers on pp. 102–106 a discussion of the term "shock" in Benjamin.

[105] Benjamin, 1998, p. 176: "In the field of allegorical intuition the image is a fragment, a rune. Its beauty as a symbol evaporates when the light of divine learning falls upon it."

is a form open to different relationships between the sign and significance, and thus, in later stages of his thinking, time is represented as full and open. At the same time, in both cases there is an overarching narrative that is regressive.

Despite the flashes of redemption, the general organization of history is regressive, for a picture of retreat governs it (the angel in "Theses on History"),[106] and accordingly, from the beginning of his thought Benjamin claims that the writers of German tragedy saw nature as expressing an allegory of decline and death.

If in his writing at the beginning of the 1920s we see Benjamin applying these mental constructions to literature, while in the background is the understanding of the concept of history that is reflected in German tragedy, in his work on the Arcades Project—the thought of which originated on his visit to Paris in 1927 while the writing took place a decade later—and after the absorption of Marxism in his thought, Benjamin activates the principle of scattering, the focus on particulars, and seeks the unique brief minute that fuses the crystal of the inclusive event in the urban situation. The urban situation is the registration of countless images which have left traces. The city is built even as it is being destroyed, whether this is an emergency regime or whether these are the monuments of the bourgeoisie seen as "ruins even before they have crumbled."[107] From here he proceeds to the concept of photography as a moment of capturing the fragment that is inseparably bound up with shock, or to the concept of the emergency situation as formulating anew the intentional activation of shock.

For Benjamin, then, destruction, withering, and retreat are the initial position of the sudden flowerings of the artistic, the literary, the urban, and the historic, but even these flowerings in their full beauty are surrounded by the aura of their return to the point of departure, that is, to destruction.

[106]Benjamin, 2011, pp. 257–258.

[107]Benjamin, 1999, p. 11.

14.28 Summary

I do not think that Benjamin ever heard of Cordovero or the fundamental structures that characterize him. The parallelism is principally phenomenological, and I have hinted at it in the past when I compared Benjamin's concept of time with classic apocalypticism.[108] At the same time, he undoubtedly had heard of Luria from his friend Gershom Scholem, as it seems from the simile of the fragments and shards of messianic time that appears in his thinking in the framework of several comparisons between Benjamin and Luria.[109]

In light of the discussion I have developed here—and this became clear precisely through the effort to compare and to clarify the stance of Benjamin in relation to Cordovero or Luria—it appears that there could be room for further thought about the relation between the fragments in Luria and the illuminations of the gifts in Cordovero—and the fragmentariness of Benjamin.

For Luria, walking in the domain of reality as a whole, like all action, can sort out the fragments of Divine light (the exile of the Shekhinah) which are scattered everywhere—this is the Kabbalistic *gathering* as well as a progressive mode of action. For Cordovero the walking in the liminal domain (usually outside the city) which also represents the exile of the Shekhinah can lead to flashes of illumination and revelation that descend on consciousness like a gift from the Shekhinah in exile to those who imitate her.

Both in Benjamin and in Cordovero fragmentariness is linked to illumination; it is a brief verbal illumination of a statement that is fragmentary in character.

[108]Pedaya, (2002a, pp. 608–623).

[109]Andrew E. Benjamin and Charles Rice (2009); Handelman (1991). Recently Idel proposed an additional discussion on the subject of exile in Scholem in comparison with Heschel and Benjamin. He suggests that the concept of Luria is pessimistic and that Scholem and also Luria, although they were in the land of Israel, expounded a pessimistic, exilic view. Idel (2010), 216 ff. Idel's discussion is connected with the discussion offered by Maor (2010) and with his perception of the dispute in the Prague circle between positive and negative mysticism, correlated with the attitudes toward the land of Israel.

On this point the mysticism of Cordovero[110] corresponds to the structure of mourning, ecstasy, and passivity, introversion—receiving from the Shekhinah, while the mysticism of Luria corresponds to an active structure—gathering, giving, and acting in relation to the Shekhinah. Cordovero is close to Benjamin, since the domain of application is language and literary creation itself. He is close to him also because the constructions and creations occur in the domain of the overarching picture whose basic image is destruction; with Luria, on the other hand, the overarching picture is building, construction of the body of the Shekhinah.

The additional point that needs to be examined is the relation between walking's area and the act of walking, if we compare it to the tension that exists in Freud's description of consciousness (in the period of his topographic model). Consciousness defends itself from impressions and protects itself from stimuli that could be considered traumatic. The external energies threaten it with shock and devastation. Traumatic shock is the breach of the defense against stimuli, which Benjamin maintains as a correlation with the status of the particular moment and the separate impression in the creation, something that obliges the creator into presence: perhaps it is possible to see, in the end, that the unique function of defense against shock is to give the event—at the expense of the completeness of its content—an exact place in the temporality of consciousness.[111]

Parallel to the question of the emergency situation, which will come later, in his discussion on history,[112] Benjamin asks about the state of traumatic shock in relation to literature, "His poetry is founded in a sphere of *experience in* which the *shock experience has become a norm.*"[113]

This discussion makes still clearer the comparison with Cordovero: Instead of a traumatic breakthrough of the exile of the Shekhinah, he walks in her stead and waits for a breakthrough in the other direction, a creative shock, an experience that repairs and *works through*.

Cordovero acts and creates from a consciousness of trauma, but he is acting in the wake of a trauma that has already occurred. Benjamin exalts shock as a priming of creation, a primordial creative tension, but the conditions of his life and their reality bring him closer and closer to the state of actual trauma: exile in Paris, emigration, and finally suicide on Spanish soil. The two central pillars of his work, his thought and his life, increasingly bend toward each other till their capitals touch; the static and the returning meet with the messianic at every moment. The terror of the trauma ***that was*** becomes the terror of the trauma ***that will be***. From a psychoanalytic standpoint one can say in comparison to Winnicott's discussion of breakdown anxiety[114] and in connection with our discussion here of trauma that the conceptualization or portrayal of the overarching metaphor of the trauma (or the matching image) in Jewish history and by the Jewish subject who carries within him the neurosis of the generation moves in the tension between the breakdown ***that was*** (Luria) and/or the one ***that will be*** (Cordovero) and is sometimes crushed between the two at the moment of the disaster of the present, as happened to Walter Benjamin.

Being caught up in the pit, the vice of crushing past and future and losing the present is a figurative definition of trauma. Its understanding can be the key for healing but it can also be the driving force for apocalyptic outbursts that are taking place these days.

[110]This is not a generalization about the teaching of Cordovero or Luria, but an analysis of these teachings by means of the subject of walking.

[111]Benjamin, Baudelaire (2006), p. 168.

[112]His essays on walking in the city are early essays, while his historical theses are from the 1940s. The first essays on lyricism and literature have for the most part not been studied in Israel in connection with trauma. This is connected with the Hebrew translation for "shock." But Benjamin talks about trauma from the beginning, not like a wounded man; later his reporting is from the region of emergency.

[113]Benjamin, 2003, p. 318.

[114]Winnicott (1989)—written in 1963 and first published posthumously in 1974 (see Abram, 2007, pp. 174-177). One of his brilliant insights is that when a person suffers from anxiety about a future breakdown that threatens him, the source of the anxiety is a breakdown that has already occurred. The fear of the future is a reflection of the fear of the G past.

References

[Hebrew Translation: Braudel, F. (2005) *The dynamics of capitalism,* tr. Amots Giladi. Tel Aviv: Resling (Hebrew).]

Abram, J. (2007). *The language of Winnicott: a dictionary of Winnicott's use of words*. London: Karnac.

Azulay, A. (2006). *Once upon a time there was: photography after Walter Benjamin*. Ramat Gan: Bar Ilan University Press (Hebrew).

Baskin, J. (2011). Lurianic Kabbala. In J. Baskin (Ed.), *The Cambridge dictionary of Judaism and Jewish culture* (pp. 353–355). Cambridge: Cambridge University Press.

Bellow, S. (1989). *The bellarosa connection*. New York, NY: Penguin.

Ben-Dor, Z. (2009). *The ten lost tribes: a world history*. Oxford: Oxford University Press.

Benjamin, W. (1998). *The origin of German tragic drama*. London: Verso.

Benjamin, W. (1999). *The arcades project*. Cambridge, MA: Harvard University Press.

Benjamin, W. (2003). *Walter Benjamin: Selected writings, Vol. 4, 1938–1940*. Cambridge, MA: Belknap Press.

Benjamin, A. E. (2005). *Walter Benjamin and art*. London: Continuum.

Benjamin, W. (2006a). *The writer of modern life: Essays on Charles Baudelaire* (Nth ed.). Cambridge, MA: Belknap Press.

Benjamin, W. (2006b). *Imperial Panorama. Benjamin, Walter. Berlin Childhood around 1900* (pp. 42–44). Cambridge, MA: Belknap.

Benjamin, W. (2011). *Theses on the concept of history, Illuminations* (pp. 253–264). New York, NY: Random House.

Benjamin, A. E., & Rice, C. (Eds.). (2009). *Walter Benjamin and the architecture of modernity*. Melbourne: Re.press.

Braudel, F. (2005). *La dynamique du capitalisme*. Paris: Flammarion

Cadava, E. (1997). *Words of light: Theses on the photography of history*. Princeton, NJ: Princeton University Press.

Calvino, I. (1978). *Invisible cities*. New York, NY: Harcourt Brace Jovanovich.

Carlebach, E. (1990). *Pursuit of heresy: Rabbi Moses Hagiz and the Sabbatian controversies*. New York, NY: Columbia University Press.

Carroll, J. (2002). *Constantine's sword: The church and the Jews—a history*. New York, NY: Mariner Books.

Caruth, C. (1995). *Trauma: Explorations in memory*. Baltimore, MD: Johns Hopkins University Press.

Caruth, C. (1996). Traumatic Awakenings (Freud, Lacan, and the Ethics of Memory). In C. Caruth (Ed.), *Unclaimed experience: Trauma, narrative, and history* (pp. 91–112). Baltimore, MD: Johns Hopkins University Press.

Chen-Morris, R. (2008). The Invisible Island, or Remembering No-Place. More, T. *Utopia,* Tel Aviv: Resling pp. 7–32 (Hebrew).

Christov-Bakargiev, C. (2003). *Janet Cardiff: A survey of works including collaborations with George Bures miller*. New York, NY: P.S. 1 Contemporary Art Center.

De Certeau, M. (2011). *The practice of everyday life*. Berkeley, CA: University of California Press.

Derrida, J. (1977). *Of grammatology*. Baltimore, MD: The Johns Hopkins University Press.

Derrida, J., & Mehlman, J. (1972). Freud and the scene of writing. *Yale French Studies, 1972*, 74–117.

Efrat, G. (2000). *Shiv'hei Galut (In Praise of Exile)*. Jerusalem: Karta. (Hebrew).

Eisen, A. (1986). *Galut: Modern Jewish reflection on homelessness and homecoming*. Bloomington, IN: Indiana University Press.

Elon, M. (1973). *Jewish law*. Jerusalem: Magnes Press (Hebrew).

Faingulernt, A. (2009). *The fathers return in the Modern European Cinematic Odysseys*. PhD. Thesis. London: University of East London.

Foucault, M. (1995). *Discipline and punish: The birth of the prison*. New York, NY: Vintage Books.

Freud, S. (1948). *Beyond the pleasure principle*. London: Hogarth Press.

Garb, J. (2014). *Kabbalist in the heart of the storm: R. Moshe Hayyim Luzzatto*. Tel Aviv: Tel Aviv University Press. (Hebrew).

Gruenwald, I. (2003). *Rituals and ritual theory in ancient Israel*. Leiden & Boston, MA: Brill.

Gurevitch, Z. (2007). *Al Hamakom (On place/God)*. Am Oved (Hebrew): Tel Aviv.

Gurevitch, Z., & Aran, G. (1994). The Land of Israel: Myth and Phenomenon. In J. Frankel (Ed.), *Reshaping the Past: Jewish History and the Historians, Studies in Contemporary Jewry* (pp. 195–210). Oxford: Oxford University Press.

Handelman, D. (1990). *Models and mirrors: Towards an anthropology of public events*. Cambridge, MA: Cambridge University Press.

Handelman, S. A. (1991). *Fragments of redemption: Jewish thought and literary theory in Benjamin, Scholem, and Levinas*. Bloomington, IN: Indiana University Press.

Hanssen, B. (Ed.). (2006). *Walter Benjamin and the arcades project*. London: Continuum.

Hasan-Rokem, G. (2008). Carl Schmitt and Ahasver: The idea of the state and the wandering Jew. *Behemoth, A Journal on Civilization, 2*, 4–25.

Hasan-Rokem, G. (2009). Jews as postcards, or postcards as Jews: Mobility in a modern genre. *Jewish Quarterly Review, 99*, 505–546.

Hasan-Rokem, G., & Dundes, A. (1986). *The wandering Jew*. Bloomington, IN: Indiana University Press.

Hirschfeld, A. (2000). *Reshimot Al Ha'Makom*. Tel Aviv: Am Oved Publishers. (Hebrew).

Hobbes, T. (1900). *Leviathan*. London: Routledge.

Hooke, S. (1958). *Myth and ritual in the ancient near east*. London: Thames and Hudson.

Horwitz, R. (2007). From Hegelianism to a revolutionary understanding of Judaism: Franz Rosenzweig's attitude toward Kabbalah and myth. *Modern Judaism, 26*, 31–54.

Horwitz, R. (2010). *Franz Rosenzweig—the star and the man*. In A. Cohen (Ed.), Beer Sheva: Ben Gurion University.

Idel, M. (1988). Franz Rosenzweig and the Kabbalah. In P. Mendes-Flohr (Ed.), *The philosophy of Franz Rosenzweig* (pp. 162–171). Hanover, NH: University Press of New England for Brandeis University Press.

Idel, M. (1992). Concerning the concept of Tsimtsum in Kabbalah and in scholarship. *Mehqarei Yerushalayim, 10*, 59–112. Hebrew.

Idel, M. (1998a). *Messianic mystics*. New Haven: Yale University Press.

Idel, M. (1998b). The place of the symbol in the philosophy of Gershom Scholem. *Mada'ei Hayahadut, 38*, 43–78 (Hebrew).

Idel, M. (1998c). Subversive stimulants: Gnosticism and Messianism in Scholem's view of Jewish mysticism. *Zmanim, 61*, 64–76 (Hebrew).

Idel, M. (2010). *Old worlds, New mirrors: On Jewish mysticism and twentieth-century thought*. Philadelphia, PA: University of Pennsylvania Press.

Jabès, E. (1991). *The book of questions: Volume I*. (Rosmarie Waldrop. Rev. ed. Trans. from the French edition, Trans.). Hanover, NH: Wesleyan.

Kanafani, G. (2001). The return to Haifa. In A. Elad-Bouskila (Ed.), *The other rooms—three Palestinian novellas*. Or Yehudah: Maariv-Hed Artsi. (Hebrew).

Kaplan, Y. (2000). *An alternative path to modernity: The Sephardi diaspora in Western Europe*. Leiden: Brill.

Knohl, I. (2008). *Where are We from?: The genetic code of the bible*. Tel Aviv: Dvir Press. (Hebrew).

Libes, Y. (1982). The Messiah of the *Zohar*: on R. Simeon bar Yohai as a Messianic Figure. In *The Messianic Idea in Jewish Thought: A Study Conference in Honour of the Eightieth Birthday of Gershom Scholem*, pp. 87–236. Jerusalem. (Hebrew). (English version in *Studies in the Zohar*, pp. 1–84. Albany 1993)

Libes, Y., & Elior, R. (1992). *Terin Orzilin de-Aylata*' ('Two Young Roses of a Doe'): The Secret Sermon of Isaac Luria before his Death. In Y. Liebes (Ed.), *Lurianic Kabbalah—Jerusalem Studies in Jewish Thought* (Vol. 10, pp. 113–170). Jerusalem: Hebrew University, Mandel.

Maor, Z. (2010). *A New mystic teaching: spirituality, creativity and nationalism in the "Prague circle"*. Jerusalem: Zalman Shazar Publishers. (Hebrew).

Marder, E. (2006). *Walter Benjamin's Dream of 'Happiness.'* In Walter Benjamin and the Arcades Project, ed. Beatrice Hanssen. London: Continuum, 184–200.

Mark, Zvi. (2015). *The revealed and hidden writings of Rabbi Nachman of Bratslav: His worlds of revelation and rectification*. Transl. by Yaacov David Shulman. - Berlin; Boston, Mass. : De Gruyter Oldenbourg; Jerusalem: Magnes, 2015.

Mishori, E. (2005). *Tel Aviv—reality or Invention? The Representation of place in poetry as an expression of object-relation: Tel Aviv as Avot Yeshurun's Transitional Object.* Ph.D. dissertation: Tel Aviv University. (Hebrew).

More, T. (2002). *More: Utopia*. Cambridge, MA: Cambridge University Press.

Moses, S. (2003). *Walter Benjamin and the spirit of modernity*. Resling (Hebrew): Tel Aviv.

Nieraad, J. (1992). Afterword. In Benjamin, W. *Selected writings 1: The Walker*. Nieraad, J., & Kalderon, N., & Klinov, R. (Eds.). Tel Aviv: HaKibbutz Hameuchad. (Hebrew).

Peday, H. (2014). Shoe and body: Fertility and deification, life and death, victimization ad messianism. In G. Ventury, O. Bartal, & E. Lider (Eds.), *Put off thy shoes from off thy feet* (pp. 46–81). Jerusalem: Bezalel Academy. Resling. (Hebrew).

Pedaya, H. (1991). Land of spirit and land of reality: R. Ezra, R. Azriel and Nahmanides. In M. Halamish & A. Ravitzky (Eds.), *The land of Israel in medieval Jewish thought* (pp. 233–289). Jerusalem: Yad Ben Zvi. (Hebrew).

Pedaya, H. (2002a). *Vision and speech—the nature of the experience of revelation in Jewish mysticism*. Los Angeles: Kruv. (Hebrew).

Pedaya, H. (2003). *Hitallut, Zeman Mahazori Ve-teqst Qadosh [Nahmanides: Spiritual Elevation, Cyclical Time, and Holy Text]*. Tel Aviv: Am Oved. (Hebrew).

Pedaya, H. (2005). The mystical experience and the religious world in Hasidism, two types of ecstatic experience in Hasidism. *Daat, 55*, 73–108 (Hebrew).

Pedaya, H. (2011a). *Walking through trauma*. Tel Aviv: Resling. (Hebrew).

Pedaya, H. (2011b). *Space and Place: essay on the theological-political unconscious*. Tel Aviv: Hakibbutz Hameuchad. (Hebrew).

Pedaya, H. (2012). The Sixth Millennium—Millenarism and Messianism in the Zohar. *Daat, 72*, 51–98 (Hebrew).

Pedaya, H. (2013). 'And now we have no mother,' lines for the genealogy of the Shekhinah and the Mother, Appendix: The scholars of Babylon and the land of Israel. In B. Cohen (Ed.), *As a Perennial Spring: a Festschrift Honoring Rabbi Dr. Norman Lamm*. New York, 87–151.

Pedaya, H. (2013b). 'The wandering messiah and the wandering Jew: Judaism and Christianity as a two-headed structure and the myth of his feet and shoes. In G. Palmer & T. Brose (Eds.), *Religion und Politik; das Messianische in Theologien, Religionswissenschaften und Philosophien des zwanzigsten Jahrhunderts* (pp. 73–103). Tübingen: Mohr Siebeck.

Pedaya, H. (2014). Weeping history: the discipline of the self and the construction of Jewish historiography. In A. Ktzia (Ed.), *The East writes itself* (pp. 2–111). Tel Aviv: Gama.

Pedaya, H. (2015a). The crying history: Discipline of the self and constructing Jewish historiography. In K. Alon (Ed.), *The Est writes itself* (pp. 25–126). Tel-Aviv: Gamma. (Hebrew).

Pedaya, H. (2015a). The Messiah and the Wandering Jew. In *Festschrift for Moshe Halamish*, Ramat Gan: Bar Ilan University, forthcoming 2015 (Hebrew).

Pedaya, H. (2015b). *Kabbalah and psychoanalysis*. Tel Aviv: Yediot (Hebrew).

Pedaya, H. (2015c). In the midst of the Zoharic Secret [Bema'abe HaSod Shel HaZohar: Na'al, Ne'ila VeNe'elam—Sipuro Shel Hevel]. In: Elquayam, A. & Moalem, S. (eds.): *Shoshanat HaAyin*, Jerusalem: Magnes Press. (Hebrew).

Pedaya, H. (2016). *Judaism and the World-Picture*, forthcoming 2015 (Hebrew).

Poe, E. A. (1842). *The Pit and the Pendulum, in: The Gift, 1842*. Philadelphia: Carey & Hart.

Reik, T. (1999). *Surprise and the psycho-analyst: On the conjecture and comprehension of unconscious processes*. London: Routledge.

Roi, B. (2011). 'The Feet of the Shekhinah'—as an ethos-constructing ethos. *Kabbalah [Vol I], 22*, 181–218.

Sagi, A. (2015). Foreignness. Exile and sovereignty—investigations following the biblical tradition. *Democratic Culture, 16*, 219–275.

Said, E. (1984). The mind of winter: Reflection on life in exile. Harper's Magazine September pp. 49–55.

Schmitt, C. (2010). *Political theology: Four chapters on the concept of sovereignty*. Chicago, IL: University of Chicago Press.

Scholem, G. (1975). Toward an understanding of the Messianic idea in Israel. *Devarim BeGo, Tel Aviv: Am Oved, 5735*, 155–190 (Hebrew).

Scholem, Gershom. 5735 (1975a). The idea of redemption in the Kabbalah. In *Devarim BeGo*, pp. 191–216. Tel Aviv: Am Oved. (Hebrew).

Solnit, R. (2001). The legs of William Wordsworth. In *Wanderlust: A history of walking* (pp. 84–90). New York, NY: Penguin.

Sorotskin, D. (2004). Building the earthly destroying the heavenly. In A, Ravitzky (Ed.), *The land of Israel in the 20th century Jewish thought*. Jerusalem, pp. 133–167. Yad Yitzhak Ben-Zvi. (Hebrew)

Sorotskin, D. (2006). The theology of the transcendent: the Maharal of Prague and the growth of early Orthodox modernism in Jewish philosophy. *Kabbalah, 14*, 263–328 (Hebrew).

Sorotskin, D. (2007). The Timeless Community in an age of Change: The emergence of Conceptions of Time and the Collective as the Basis for the development of Jewish orthodoxy in early Modern and late Modern Europe, Ph.d. dissertation: Hebrew University. (Hebrew).

Sorotskin, D. (2011). *Orthodoxy and Modern Disciplination: The Production of the Jewish Tradition in Europe in Modern Times*. Tel Aviv: Ha-Kibutz Ha-Meuchad Press.

Sorotzkin, D. (2007). *Natural Law* and *Deviance*: The Problem of *Nature* and the Shaping of the Image of Judaism in Ideological Patterns in Early Modern Europe. In E. Meir & H. Pedaya (Eds.), *Judaism, Topics, Fragments, Faces, Identities: Jubilee Volume in Honor of Rivka Shats* (pp. 149–193). Beer Sheva: Bem Gurion Univesity. (Hebrew).

St. Augustine. (1984). *Concerning the City of God against the Pagans* (H. Bettenson, Trans.). London: Penguin.

Pedaya, H. (2002b). Land: time and place—apocalypses of the end and apocalypses of the beginning. In A. Ravitski (Ed.), *The land of Israel in the Philosophy of the Twentieth Century* (pp. 560–623). Jerusalem: Yad Ben Zvi. (Hebrew).

Tomlin, G. (1997). The theology of the cross: Subversive theology for a postmodern world? *Themelios, 23*, 59–73.

Weinstein, R. (1999). The Jewish ghetto and the urban quarter in the Italian cities at the beginning of the modern period: Between distance and nearness. *Zmanim, 67*, 12–21 (Hebrew).

Winnicott, D. W. (1971). *Playing and reality*. London: Tavistock Publications.

Winnicott, D. W. (1989). Fear of breakdown. *Psychoanalytic Explorations, 93*, 87–95.

Wolfson, E. R. (1997). Walking as a sacred duty: Theological transformation of social reality in early Hasidism. In A. Rapoport-Albert (Ed.), *Hasidism reappraised* (pp. 180–207). London: Littman Library of Jewish Civilization.

Wolfson, E. R. (2010). Light does not talk but shines: Apophasis and vision in Rosenzweig's theopoetic temporality. In A. W. Hughes & E. R. Wolfson (Eds.), *New directions in Jewish philosophy* (pp. 87–148). Bloomington, IN: Indiana University Press.

Yamba, C. B. (1995). *Permanent pilgrims: The role of pilgrimage in the lives of West African Muslims in Sudan*. Edinburgh: Edinburgh University Press.

Zak, B. (1992). Cordovero and Luria. In R. Elior & Y. Libes (Eds.), *The International Conference on Jewish Mysticism, 4: Lurianic Kabbalah* (pp. 316–319). Jerusalem: Hebrew University. Hebrew.

Zak, B. (1995). *At the gates of the Kabbalah of Rabbi Moshe Cordovero*. Beer Sheva (Hebrew): Ben Gurion University.

Primary Judaic Sources

Ba'al HaTurim (1639). *Pentateuch Commentary*, Hannover.

Cordovero, M. (1962). *Ohr Yakar [Precious Light]* (Vol. 16). Jerusalem: Achuzat Yisrael.

Sefer HaZohar [*Book of Splendor*], Korets 5538 (1778).

Online Sources

Coussin, O. (2012). *To write by the water? And more on Shaun Levin's writing maps*. Blog for October 25, 2012 http://ornacoussin.co.il/2012/10/25/ Retrieved August 31, 2015 (Hebrew).

Levin, S. (2015). Writing Maps. http://writearoundtown.com. Retrieved August 31, 2015.

Film

Pawlikowski, P. (2014). *Ida*. Poland, Denmark, France, UK.

Wenders, W. (1984). *Paris, Texas*. West Germany, France, UK. USA.

15 Trauma and Monotheism: Sigmund Freud's *Moses and Monotheism* and the Possibility of Writing a Traumatic History of Religion

Koji Yamashiro

15.1 Sigmund Freud's *Moses and Monotheism*

Until today various approaches have been used to read Sigmund Freud's *Moses and Monotheism* (Freud, 1939). While most, if not all, of the arguments Freud offered were blankly rejected both by biblical scholarship and anthropology of religion as lacking a foundation, this book was justifiably regarded as a psychological document of Freud's inner life (Yerushalmi, 1991, p. 2). It is not my purpose in the present chapter to review scholarly literature on Freud and his psychoanalysis in general or *Moses and Monotheism* in particular.

Rather, I would like to use Freud's book in order to sharpen our problematic: to rewrite the birth, development and death of the monotheistic religions as a traumatic history.[1] So far as I know, such an attempt seems to have never been seriously made. And indeed, some of the subsidiary observations given by Freud seem to be more meaningful than his main thesis just because of the problems they open up on the relation between trauma and monotheism.

It might be preferable to briefly summarize, first of all, the contents of *Moses and Monotheism*. A historical premise for the psychoanalytic inquiry can be virtually reduced to two main hypotheses (cf. Freud, 1939, p. 58):

1. In contradiction with the biblical accounts Moses was an Egyptian.
2. Moses was killed by his own people, who had rejected his monotheistic doctrine and fell into idolatry (this is in essence the adoption of Ernst Sellin's conjecture upon the end of Moses; cf Yerushalmi, 1991, pp. 25–27).

[1] I use the term Monotheism in its "standard" meaning, i.e., a religious model which is based on the belief in the single god and all of whose different forms can be considered to be derived, in the final analysis, from ancient Judaism. Some examples of the monotheistic reinterpretation of polytheistic religions, among others in Egypt and Iran, are outside the scope of the present chapter, though they are of some interest from the phenomenological point of view. Guy Stroumsa (2011) proposes the use of the alternative term Abrahamic religions, emphasizing the genetic relationship between Judaism, Christianity, and Islam and their branches, for which the idea of monotheism is not always central.

K. Yamashiro, Ph.D. (✉)
Faculty of Humanities, Hebrew University of Jerusalem, The Reznik Dorms Building 13 Room 153 Mount Scopus, Jeruslaem 97665, Israel
e-mail: koji.yamashiro@gmail.com

Y. Ataria et al. (eds.), *Interdisciplinary Handbook of Trauma and Culture*,
DOI 10.1007/978-3-319-29404-9_15

Both of the hypotheses are supported by a number of speculations and minor hypotheses, the examination of which will not specifically interest us here. In any case, Freud, with the help of these hypotheses, constructs the following narrative: Moses was an fervent adherent of the monotheism of Aten initiated by the Egyptian Pharaoh Ikhnaton; upon the latter's death and the subsequent oppression of the new cult, he chose the Israelites for the preservation of the true religion (the exodus), which, however, ends with a tragic result; thereafter the original teaching which Moses gave them merged into the worship of Yahweh, while the memory of the murder of Moses was repressed; however, over a period of centuries the forgotten faith gained more and more power until Yahweh was finally transformed into the God of Moses (Freud, 1939, pp. 7–53, 59–66, 105–111).

At this point, Freud observes that "religious phenomena are only to be understood on the pattern of the individual neurotic symptoms familiar to us—as the return of long since forgotten, important events in the primaeval history of the human family—and that they have to thank precisely this origin for their compulsive character and that, accordingly, they are effective on human beings by force of the historical truth of their content" (Freud, 1939, p. 58). Therefore, Freud's method is in essence applied psychoanalysis, or an "analogous" interpretation of religion (Ricoeur, 1970, pp. 159–254).

The pattern of the development of an individual neurosis is as follows. The experiences or impressions[2] early suffered and later forgotten, which have the decisive role in the etiology of the neuroses, are called traumas.[3] The effects of traumas are classified into two types: positive and negative, i.e., compulsions to repeat and defensive reactions, both of which can be regarded as fixations to the trauma. It should be noted that the phenomenon of a latency between the first reactions to the trauma and the later outbreak of the illness is typical. Thus the whole process is completed by the return of the repressed, though partial and distorted (Freud, 1939, pp. 72–80, 124–127).

Now, according to Freud, it is possible to uncover, on the basis of his own theory in *Totem and Taboo* (Freud, 1913), the forgotten traumas in a prehistory of the human race, "which after a long latency came into effect and created phenomena similar to symptoms in their structure and purpose" (Freud, 1939, p. 80). This primal scene can be reconstructed as composed of three phases: (1) the violent rule of the strong male, lord and father of the entire horde, who monopolized all the females (2) the patricide by the expelled sons, who devoured the father raw (3) the period of the struggles between the brothers and the subsequent social contract (the taboo on incest and the injunction to exogamy). The ambivalent relation to the totem (the totem worship/the totem feast) reflects the deferred obedience to the father on the one hand and the disguised triumph over the father on the other (Freud, 1939, pp. 80–84, 130–133; cf. Ricoeur, 1970, pp. 201–211, 237–244).

Then how could this forgotten trauma be transmitted in the course of thousands of years? Freud's ingenious answer is that an impression of the past is retained in unconscious memory-traces according to the phylogenetic model[4] (Freud, 1939, pp. 93–102, 129). As he puts it, "men have always known (in this special way) that they once possessed a primal father and killed him" (Freud, 1939, p. 101). The forgotten memory-trace can be decisively awoken by "a recent real repetition of the event." Therefore, the murder of Moses by his Jewish people is "an important link between the forgotten event of primeval times and its later emergence in the form of the monotheist religions" (Freud, 1939, p. 89). In other words, the advance from totemism to monotheism, which could be called the advance in intellectuality,[5] is the gradual return of the repressed (cf. Ricoeur, 1970, pp. 244–254).

[2] Freud does not distinguish between these two terms.

[3] For the analysis of the conception of trauma in Freud's psychoanalysis in general and in *Moses and Monotheism* in particular, see Caruth (1996, pp. 1–9, 10–24, 57–72), Ginsburg (2006).

[4] On Freud's Lamarckism, see Yerushalmi, 1991, pp. 29–33, 86–90, 123, n. 44; cf. Derrida, 1996, pp. 34–36.

[5] On this concept see the recent discussions of Assmann (2006), Schäfer (2006).

It should be added that Freud quite briefly discusses the possibility of applying his thesis to the monotheistic religions other than ancient Judaism: Except for his famous formulation of Christianity as "a son-religion" (Freud, 1939, pp. 85–90, 135–136), Freud makes only two passing remarks on Islam (Freud, 1939, pp. 92–93) and Rabbinic Judaism (Freud, 1939, p. 115). In other words, as Freud himself admits (Freud, 1939, p. 92), the validity of his theory is examined merely in one particular case of the Mosaic religion, while he seems to believe that all religious phenomena can be explained as the repetition of the primal patricide.[6]

15.2 Truth

The dazzling construction of countless hypotheses and speculations in *Moses and Monotheism* might seem to compel us to put into doubt our naïve conception of truth. In fact, the conception of truth can be regarded as a hidden motif of his enigmatic book. The expression "historical truth" already appears in the first essay "Moses an Egyptian" (Freud, 1939, p. 16), which had been published separately in 1937, and recurs time and again all through the book down to the last few pages. In the following passage, Freud explains in some detail this conception (Freud, 1939, p. 85):

> It is worth specially stressing the fact that each portion which returns from oblivion asserts itself with peculiar force, exercises an incomparably powerful influence on people in the mass, and raises an irresistible claim to truth against which logical objections remain powerless: a kind of "*credo quia absurdum*." This remarkable feature can only be understood on the pattern of the delusions of psychotics. We have long understood that a portion of forgotten truth lies hidden in delusional ideas, that when this returns it has to put up with distortions and misunderstandings, and that the compulsive conviction which attaches to the delusion arises from this core of truth and spreads out on to the errors that wrap it round. We must grant an ingredient such as this of what may be called historical truth to the dogmas of religion as well, which, it is true, bear the character of psychotic symptoms but which, as group phenomena, escape the curse of isolation.

In other words, the aim of *Moses and Monotheism* is to reveal in the pattern of the individual neurotic symptoms this "historical truth" in the particular case of Judaism, i.e., the return of forgotten events in the primeval history of the human family.

Freud's *écriture* is much more complex than this general statement suggests, however. In spite of his conviction in the correctness of the final conclusion (Freud, 1939, pp. 58, 101), he is aware of the uncertainty of a long series of logically invalid propositions which he likens to "a bronze statue with feet of clay" (Freud, 1939, p. 17) or "a dancer balancing on the tip of one toe" (Freud, 1939, p. 58). Indeed, as often pointed out, most of his hypotheses and speculations can hardly stand up to scrutiny. Thus, quite strangely, distortions and misunderstandings which, according to Freud, forgotten truth has to put up with when it returns, as it were, characterize his own psychoanalysis of the Mosaic religion: Paradoxically enough, the complete unreliability of Freud's discourse most convincingly proves the intensity of forgotten truth which he, at least in his opinion, found.

Certainly Freud himself will not readily admit our observation. However, the idea of the "historical truth" wrapped up in religious distortions and misunderstandings and uncovered by untenable psychoanalytical conjectures seems to imply, rather, the fatal flaw of Freud's own approach to the problem of the relation between trauma and monotheism. Whether his strange conviction of the "historical truth" is derived from psychoanalytical dogmatism[7] or from a peculiar kind of "deferred obedience" to Judaism[8] does not concern us here. Of crucial importance is the fact that the structure of *Moses and Monotheism* exactly repeats that of the religions

[6] In this brief summary I omitted several important topics which are not directly relevant to the present purpose, including Freud's interpretation of anti-Semitism. Meanwhile, some subsidiary points will be deal with later for the sake of convenience.

[7] As Derrida (1996, p. 95) says, "in life as in his works, in his theoretical theses as in the compulsion of his institutionalizing strategy, Freud repeated the patriarchal logic."

[8] See the discussion of Yerushalmi (1991, pp. 57–79).

which it analyses, i.e., the truth wrapped by distortions and misunderstandings.

Distortions and misunderstandings revealed in the dogmas of religion seem to be nothing other than the mirror image of the psychoanalysis of religion, while the primal scene of the patricide is repeatedly performed each time Freud "uncovers" the "historical truth" under the veil of monotheism. This certainly indicates that Freud's psychoanalysis of religion itself is nothing but a myth. In other words, the archaeological desire for establishing the traumatic *archē* of religion determines the mythical structure of Freud's theory.[9] In this connection, it is intriguing to note that in one place Freud, rather unexpectedly, expresses his thesis as "a fact which we have derived from the history of the Jewish religion or, if you like, have introduced into it" (p. 124). Thus *Moses and Monotheism* unintentionally hints at the unusual nature of writing the history of the monotheistic religions as a traumatic history.

The necessary process of mythologization is essential here. This might be called the trauma-salvation dialectic: It posits a decisive traumatic experience at the origin, which determines the course of salvation history (*Heilsgeschichte*), while this primeval trauma can be interpreted only by the promise of salvation. Although Freud's intuition, in my opinion correctly, discerned that dogmas of religion necessarily hide traumatic experiences under the code of myth, his psychoanalytic interpretation of religion itself turned out to be an "atheistic" variation of the "return of the repressed" because of its own inherent salvation narrative, i.e., the implicit teleology of Freudian psychoanalysis.[10]

The crucial question, then, is: How can we write down a traumatic history against a temptation to mythologize? Dominick LaCapra (2001, p. 42) depicts the possibility of writing a historiography of trauma as a "middle voice" between the documentary research model and radical constructivism in the following way:

> Such a coming-to-terms (i.e. with the wounds and scars of the past) would seek knowledge whose truth claims are not one-dimensionally objectifying or narrowly cognitive but involve affect and may empathetically expose the self to an unsettlement, if not a secondary trauma, which should not be glorified or fixated upon but addressed in a manner that strives to be cognitively and ethically responsible as well as open to the challenge of utopian aspiration.

However, in his penetrating treatment of this subject, Ataria (2014b) points out that LaCapra's approach overlooks the essential nature of trauma: It is a limit experience which is beyond the possibility of conceptualization, symbolization, and representation; every attempt of working through (narrative) is forced to erase its uniqueness; therefore, silence remains as a single impossibility after a traumatic experience, where the impossibility of writing could become "fragments of silence and representations of silence."

Therefore, the historiography of trauma seems to be possible only in an interminable iconoclasm of illusions, i.e., the uncompromising demolition of discourses which hide the traumatic experiences. Thus we are not allowed to simply treat of the monotheistic *Heilsgeschichte* (salvation history) as direct testimonies on traumas, even in case that it records its own historical tragedies in detail. Rather we must, without expecting any salvation, gaze on the moment when injures and wounds are encoded under the veil of the dogmas of religion and therewith expose innumerable traumas, though unfathomable in themselves, in the history of the monotheistic religions. Only then, can the birth, development and death of the

[9] Freud himself compares his method to archaeology (1896, p. 192): "He may have brought picks, shovels and shades with him, and he may set the inhabitants to work with these implements. Together with them he may start upon the ruins, clear away the rubbish, and beginning from the visible remains, uncover what is buried. If his work is crowned with success, the discoveries are self-explanatory … *Saxa loquuntur*!" Cf. Derrida (1996, p. 92): "Freud was incessantly tempted to redirect the original interest he had for the psychic archive toward archaeology." For the analysis of the archaeology of Freudian psychoanalysis in general, see Ricoeur (1970), pp. 419–458.

[10] On the teleology of Freudian psychoanalysis in general, see Ricoeur (1970), pp. 459–551. Cf. Yerushalmi (1991, pp. 96–100) on "a godless Judaism" of Freud.

monotheistic religions be described as the history of the encoding of injuries and wounds, which might be always structuralized anew according to each and every traumatic experience.

15.3 The Execution Machine

In his *In the Penal Colony* Franz Kafka (1971, pp. 140–167) depicts a strange execution machine. This machine is composed of three main parts: the Bed, the Harrow, and the Designer. The condemned man is laid naked on the Bed. The shape of the Harrow corresponds to the human form. As the Harrow quivers, the points of the needles pierce the skin of the body. Thus it keeps on writing deeper and deeper for 12 h. The Designer controls the movements of the Harrow with the help of the cogwheels according to the inscription demanded by the sentence. The condemned man does not know his sentence; he does not even know that he has been sentenced. In the first 6 h he suffers only pain. Then he loses all desire to eat and he no longer has the strength to scream. And little by little the sufferer begins to understand the inscription; he deciphers it with his wounds for the remaining 6 h. Thus redemption is promised for the man, on whose face a look of transfiguration will appear at his death.

The script which is impressed on the skin is unreadable, something like "a labyrinth of lines crossing and recrossing each other, which covered the paper so thickly that it was difficult to discern the blank spaces between them" (Kafka, 1971, p.148). Exactly in the same way traumas are engraved into the body; they are nonverbal wounds.[11] Moreover, the sufferer's inability to eat or to scream after 6 h of tortures definitely reminds us of that of the *Muselmann* ("muslim"), an argot used for denoting a captive of the Nazi concentration camps who showed a complete apathy to his own life as a result of extreme starvation and exhaustion[12]; and if the analysis that Ataria and Gallagher (2015) present is correct, a *Muselmann*, in the situation of extreme trauma, must have developed total disownership towards the body. Therefore, what we read in Kafka's story can be interpreted as the scene of the engraving of traumas on the separated body.

At first the condemned man does not know his sentence, even that he has been sentenced. Only after having suffered pain, he begins to interpret the Law with his wounds. For the condemned man redemption can be achieved only by recognition of sin.

Thus any traumatic experience precedes the act of deciphering. This *Nachträglichkeit* (afterwardness) is not merely chronological; it indicates that traumatic events suddenly unveil the bare face of incomprehensible reality, fate or even death itself, in front of the victim and all injuries and wounds are only *retrospectively* understood by the encoding of these *signes*, a promise of salvation.

Then it is possible to say that the archive for the Law is the body, on which traumatic traces are left by death.[13] The situation is rather paradoxical: The body serves as a repository of the Law against the destruction of death just owing to injuries and wounds made by its violence. In other words, death, i.e., eternal oblivion, alone makes remembrance possible. This paradox seems to determine the essential nature of the

[11] For the extensive discussion on somatic memories of traumatic events see Rothschild (2000) and van der Kolk (1994). Cf. Caruth (1996, pp. 1–9) on a voice crying out through the wound.

[12] On this phenomenon see the penetrating analysis of Agamben (1998, pp. 166–188, 1999, pp. 41–86).

[13] Derrida's excellent book on *Archive fever* (1996) fails to duly note on this point. However, some of his remarks seem to resonate with the idea of the body as an archive. In a rather *dogmatic* way Derrida repeatedly emphasizes the hypomnesic (material) nature of the archive (cf. Derrida, 2006, pp. 246–291) and its inherent tendency to death (destruction). And he adds that "there is no archive without a place of consignation, without a technique of repetition, and without a certain exteriority. No archive without outside" (Derrida, 1996, p. 11).

Meanwhile, Derrida's formulation: "As soon as there is the One, there is murder, wounding, traumatism." (Derrida, 1996, p. 78) is rather trivial, if he intends that the archive as the principle of gathering into itself of the One necessarily accompanies violence to the Other. It is more important to ask how, first of all, the engraving of traumas constitutes the essence of the archive.

transmission of the Law: Remembrance of the Law is made possible only by a chain of the engravings of traumas, which always tacitly presupposes the presence of death. And death, as it were, seeks for a new place of dwelling for the eternal persistence of the Law while one's body perishes. Thus, the script on one's body is endlessly copied on that of another through the execution machine. In this meaning, it might be possible to say that each and every trauma on one's body integrates the *Urgeschichte* (prehistory) of injuries and wounds.

These observations will return us back to the confrontation with Freud. In fact, at the end of Part I of *Moses and Monotheism*, he raises two difficulties for his thesis, one of which is formulated as follows: "… in what form the operative tradition in the life of peoples is present—a question which does not occur with individuals, since there it is solved by the existence in the unconscious of memory-traces of the past" (Freud, 1939, p. 93). As we have seen above, Freud's answer is phylogenetic: An impression of the primal patricide is retained in unconscious memory-traces.

However, some of his own arguments relevant to this subject might point in a different direction. Freud observes that "when we study the reactions to early traumas,[14] we are quite often surprised to find that they are not strictly limited to what the subject himself has really experienced but diverge from it in a way which fits in much better with the model of a phylogenetic event and, in general, can be explained by such an influence" (Freud, 1939, p. 99). Yet we should rather think that this typical pattern of the cultural responses to traumas indicates the existence of the fixed encoding of injuries and wounds which is shared among a certain group, community or society.[15] Our insight could be corroborated by a passing remark on the universality of symbolism in language, which Freud (1939) makes immediately before the above quotation: "It might be said that we are dealing with thought-connections between ideas—connections which had been established during the historical development of speech and which have to be repeated now every time the development of speech has to be gone through in an individual" (p. 99). Even if Freud himself rejects this explanation as insufficient, doesn't it hint at the way in which traumatic experiences are always interpreted only by a given encoding?

As we have seen above, in *Totem and Taboo* Freud reconstructed as the result of the primal patricide the period of the struggles between the brothers and the subsequent social contract (the taboo on incest and the injunction to exogamy). Ricoeur (1970) clearly exposes the hidden structure of this discourse: "With this renunciation of violence, under the goad of discord, there is given the necessary condition for the birth of social organization: the true problem of law is not patricide but fratricide; in the symbol of the brothers' covenant Freud encountered the basic requisite of analytic explanation" (p. 211). In other words, the primal patricide by itself cannot explain the formation of society.[16] This insight seems to indicate that the violent rule of the father, who monopolized all the females, is nothing but a caricature of the Law which imposes on all the members of the society the taboo on incest and the injunction to exogamy, a fiction which was necessary for Freud

[14] In this context Freud seems to use the term reaction not in the sense of pathological symptom but in the sense of "cultural" behavior.

[15] Cf. the drastic criticism of Freud's familianism by Deleuze and Guattari (1977), for example the following remark: "It is in one and the same movement that the repressive social production is replaced by the repressing family, and that the latter offers a displaced image of desiring-production that represents the repressed as incestuous familial drives" (p. 119).

[16] Cf. Deleuze and Guattari (1977, p. 80): "It seems that Freud himself was acutely aware of Oedipus's inseparability from a double impasse into which he was precipitating the unconscious. … This becomes even clearer when Freud elaborated the entire historico-mythical series: at one end the Oedipal bond is established by the murderous identification, at the other end it is reinforced by the restoration and internalization of paternal authority ('revival of the old state of things at a new level'). Between the two there is latency—the celebrated latency—which is without doubt the greatest psychoanalytic mystification: this society of 'brothers' who forbid themselves the fruits of the crime, and spend all the time necessary for internalizing. But we are warned: the society of brothers is very dejected, unstable, and dangerous, it must prepare the way for the rediscovery of an equivalent to parental authority, it must cause us to pass over to the other pole."

to connect the Oedipus complex to the state of nature (the City *tanquam dissoluta*).[17] Therefore, Freud's reconstruction of the primal scene tacitly replaces the problem of the origin of the Law with the supposition of the violence of the strong male, lord and father of the entire horde towards his sons. In this sense, Freud's interpretation of the conclusion of the social contract between the brothers as the deferred obedience to the father could be understood as the mirror image of an endless chain of executions, symbolically expressed by that of the son by the father.[18]

The repetitive construction of Freud's historiography of religion, i.e., the endless return of the primal patricide should be reread as a cyclic process of the execution machine through which the script on one's body is copied on that of another. However, the continuous chain of executions itself, by definition, inherently poses the problem of the origin. In other words, the Law must by nature presuppose the primal scene of the execution, the originary engraving of traumas.

Therefore, as the first working hypothesis I would like to suggest that a mode of encoding of wounds and injuries as a system of coordinates includes the attempt to structuralize traumatic symptoms according to the variable of time (history); however, in this mode of encoding the moment of the originary engraving of traumas will be remembered in "a compulsive, repetitive, and nostalgic desire for the archive, an irrepressible desire to return to the origin, a homesickness, a nostalgia for the return to the most archaic place of absolute commencement" (Derrida, 1996, p. 91).

At the same time, we should note that the interminable cycle of the execution machine has another important aspect, i.e., the formation of the Corpus. Here the crucial question is how a community can be envisaged as something analogous to the body. As is well known, the Latin word *corpus* means (1) "body of a person" and (2) "collection of writings." However, as far as I know, no treatment of this subject has correctly grasped the following point, which is essential for the understanding of the semantic structure of the word: The engraving of trauma is made on the separated body, which in its turn serves as the archive for the Law. In other words, the disownership towards one's body during traumatic experiences constitutes the necessary condition for the notion of the externality, i.e., the collective body (Corpus) on which the mode of encoding of traumas is registered.

And this externality should be spatially located, as Derrida (1996, p. 2) succinctly puts it: "It is thus, in this domiciliation, in this house arrest, that archives take place," since the archive is "the principle according to the law, *there* where men and gods *command*, *there* where authority, social order are exercised, *in this place* from which *order* is given—nomological principle" (Derrida, 1996, p. 1). We should add, however, that this archive has a limit which distinguishes between inside and outside: The mode of encoding of traumas is valid only inside the Corpus, the exclusive place where a condemned member of the community is saved by execution of the Law as a system of truth.

Then, as the second working hypothesis I would like to suggest that a mode of encoding of wounds and injuries as a system of coordinates must necessarily include the attempt to structuralize traumatic symptoms according to the variable of place (map).[19]

[17] Curiously, to my best knowledge, there is no serious treatment of the significance of the state of nature in Freudian psychoanalysis.

[18] The persistence in the model of the primal patricide seems to have prevented Freud from analyzing religious phenomena by his conception of the death instinct (*thanatos*) constantly developed since the publication of *Beyond the Pleasure Principle* (1920). The fact that Freud could not easily connect the metapsychological theory to his interpretation of religion might be observed in his discussion on the renunciation of instinct in obedience to the superego in *Moses and Monotheism* (Freud, 1939, pp. 116–122), where he fails to mention the death instinct, which he had already integrated into this structural model of the psyche in *The Ego and the Id* (1923). However, the destructiveness of the superego is one of the main motifs of Freud's late writings on culture (cf. Ricoeur, 1970, pp. 281–338).

[19] Here might be the place to make a preliminary note on a methodological issue. Ataria (2014c), in my opinion correctly, proposes a phenomenological approach to trauma based on the dissociation model. Then, the important question is whether it is possible to bridge the gap between phenomenology and structuralism by way of trauma studies owing to an original perspective which they can give on voice and script. Cf. Ricoeur's comparison between Freudian psychoanalysis and phenomenology (1970,

Thus, the body as the archive for the Law (corpus) is epistemologically determined by time (history) and place (map). Then, the following question should be asked: What is this execution machine through which the script on one's body is copied on that of another? Now, developing Friedrich Nietzsche's insight into the origin of the institution of punishment, Deleuze and Guattari (1977, pp. 144–145) remark that:

> It is a matter of creating a memory for man; and man, who was constituted by means of an active faculty of forgetting (*oubli*), by means of a repression of biological memory, must create an*other* memory, one that is collective, a memory of words (*paroles*) and no longer a memory of things, a memory of signs and no longer of effects. This organization, which traces its signs directly on the body, constitutes a system of cruelty, a terrible alphabet.

In other words, the difference between man and animal is created by the execution machine, which represses biological memory and creates collective memory. However, we might suspect that this differentiation is at the same time the necessary condition for the initiation of the cycle of the execution machine.

It is Giorgio Agamben who uncovered in the most profound way the significance of the anthropogenesis (hominization), i.e., the becoming human of the living being, for the understanding of the problem of biopolitics, which he discerns from the very beginning of political life (Agamben, 1998, 2004).[20] According to his thesis, the ban (the state of exception) is the essential structure of sovereignty in which man is abandoned, "that is, exposed and threatened on the threshold in which life and law, outside and inside, become indistinguishable" (Agamben, 1998, p. 28). This is the production of bare life, life exposed to death, that of *homo sacer*, who may be killed and yet not sacrificed. Thus sacredness is nothing but the originary form of the inclusion of bare life into the juridical order (Agamben, 1998, pp. 71–86).

His insight should be elaborated on in a separate study. Here I would like to briefly discuss the following point alone: Although Agamben brilliantly elucidates the political structure of sacredness, it seems that he fails to explain why the inclusion of bare life into the juridical order makes it possible for man to discover the notion of sacredness. Perhaps, we can imagine that the secret of sacredness is hidden in the moment of anthropogenesis at which traumas in the biological life are given a completely new meaning. Now, in his *Duino Elegies* Rainer Maria Rilke writes as follows (Rilke, 1955, p. 714, in my translation):

> With all the eyes the creature beholds the Open. Only our eyes, as though reversed, encircle it absolutely, like pitfalls set round its exit to freedom. What is outside, we know from the brute's face alone; for a small child we turn round, by force, that *it* look backwards at Formation, not the Open so deep within the brute's face. Free from Death. We only see Death; the free brute has its downfall perpetually behind it and God in front, and when it moves, it moves into eternity, like running springs.

Recognition of death, therefore, separates man from absolute freedom[21] and exposes him to bare life, reality without face, the nothingness between life and death. Then, conformation must be the work of deciphering traumas in bare life. It seems that sacredness was discovered as something lost in the empty point, the place of abandonment, where nature becomes the outside. Meanwhile, the initiation of the cyclic process of the execution machine can be identified with the encoding of wounds and injuries in bare life,

pp. 375–418), which could be a good starting point for such an investigation.

[20] Although Agamben limits the scope of his investigation to the problem of Western politics, his conclusions need to be, *mutatis mutandis*, extended into the analysis of political thought in general. Incidentally, it might be noted that Agamben seems to introduce "the West" in a somewhat transcendental manner: For one thing, he never delves into the analysis of Indian and Iranian texts, whose genetic relation to the Western political thought is rather apparent; in a similar way, the lack of serious treatment of the Abrahamic religions makes Agamben's study insufficient. Needless to say, it is not my intention to blur the peculiarities of sovereign power which developed in European context, on whose metaphysical structure Agamben (1998, pp. 44–48) offers an excellent explanation.

[21] For the analysis of Martin Heidegger's reversal interpretation of the open in Rilke see Agamben (2004 pp. 49–77). Cf. Agamben (2004) for the image of the animality in the eschatological vision.

i.e., its inclusion in the Law, which determines this lack of sacredness as guilt and therewith implicitly shows the existence of the way to expiation. Therefore, in place of regarding *homo sacer* as the figure which "before and beyond the religious, constitutes the first paradigm of the political realm" (Agamben, 1998, p. 9), it would be better to think that the inclusion of bare life into the Law itself is essentially rooted in the discovery of sacredness following recognition of death. And in this meaning, *homo sacer*, a life which may be killed and yet not sacrificed, should be reinterpreted as the being between the sacred and the Law, which would be structuralized as grace and justice in the monotheistic religions, as we shall see presently.

15.4 A Traumatic History

Below a brief sketch will be attempted for the composition of a traumatic history of monotheism as the cycle of the execution machine. Needless to say, in the scope of the present chapter our discussions are forced to be quite limited; here I would like to concentrate on two most basic schemes of the monotheistic *Heilsgeschichte* (salvation history): (1) time-space (2) corpus.

15.4.1 Time-Space

Let us begin with Ataria's important observations on the time-space dimensions of traumatic symptoms in his "Trauma: The Passage from Individual to Society" (Ataria, 2014a). According to him, at the moment of trauma time freezes and the spiral-regressive timeline splits from the linear timeline. At the same time, he pays attention to the disintegration of space by traumatic experiences, which he calls "a map without its territory." Thus the trauma is able to take place in the here and now, at least from the victim's perspective, as an event which cannot be positioned or fixed.

Now, according to the hypotheses advanced in the preceding section, a mode of encoding of wounds and injuries as a system of coordinates must necessarily include the attempt to structuralize traumatic symptoms according to the variables of time (history) and place (map). In the monotheistic traditions, as we shall see presently, two options are possible to solve the problem of the spiral-regressive timeline: to identify the frozen moment of trauma with (1) the beginning of the sacred history (the covenant) (2) the end of times (apocalypse). In a similar manner, there are two possible solutions for the disintegration of space, i.e., the movement towards (1) the promised land (the exodus) (2) the Paradise (utopia).

The Hebrew Bible begins, at least, twice: The first eleven chapters of the book of Genesis deal with the creation of the world and the general history of man; the second beginning is God's choice of Abraham (the covenant). In Genesis 12:1 God orders Abraham to leave his country and go to the land which will be shown him as his inheritance: "Go from your country, your people and your father's household to the land I will show you." In other words, the origin of the people of Israel concurs with the movement towards the promised land. Genesis 17:7–14 can be read as the summary of this point:

> I will establish my covenant as an everlasting covenant between me and you and your descendants after you for the generations to come, to be your God and the God of your descendants after you. The whole land of Canaan, where you are now alien, I will give as an everlasting possession to you; and I will be their God. ... As for you, you must keep my covenant, you and your descendants after you for the generations to come. This is my covenant with you and your descendants after you, the covenant you are to keep: Every male among you shall be circumcised. You are to undergo circumcision, and it will be the sign of the covenant between me and you. ... My covenant in your flesh is to be an everlasting covenant. Any uncircumcised male, who has not been circumcised in the flesh, will be cut off his people; he has broken my covenant.

Circumcision, the operation of removing the foreskin, is the sign of the covenant.[22] And perhaps, no matter what is the historical origin of this custom, in ancient Judaism this scar symbolically points to the frozen time of trauma, which must have been reinterpreted as the establishment of the covenant, the limit between the beginning

[22] On circumcision in general see, for example, Snowman (1971).

of the sacred history and the end of the prehistory of the forefathers and their gods. The salvation narrative hereafter advances between God's justice and mercy, which is expressed in terms of the exile from and the return to the promised land.

A topological shift which is most important for the subsequent development of the monotheistic religions can be summarized in two words: apocalypse and utopia. Below I would like to limit my analysis to a few typical examples. For example, in 2 Enoch the whole history of the cosmos is summarized as follows[23]:

> Before everything was, before all creation came to pass, the Lord established the Aeon of Creation. Thereafter he created all his creation, the visible and the invisible. After all that He created man in His image and put into him eyes to see and ears to hear, a heart to think and a mind to counsel. Then for the sake of man the Lord caused the Aeon to come forth and divided it into times and hours, so that man should reflect upon the changes and the ends of the times, and upon the beginnings and changes of the months, days and hours, and that he should calculate his (own) life and death. … when all the creation that was created by the Lord will come to an end, and every man will go to the Great Judgment of the Lord, then the times will perish, there will not be any more years, or months or days, the hours will not be counted any more, but the Aeon will be one. And all the righteous that will escape the Great Judgment of the Lord will join the great Aeon, and at the same time the Aeon will join the righteous, and they will be eternal. And there will not be in them any more either labour or suffering, or sadness or the expectation of violence; neither (will there be) the toil of the night or of the night or of the darkness, but they will have for always a great light and an indestructible wall, and they will have a Great Paradise, the shelter of an eternal habitation. Happy are the righteous who will escape the Great Judgment. For the faces will shine like the Sun.

According to *2 Enoch*, then, God created the Aeon of Creation and divided it, for the sake of man, into times, years, months, days, and hours; at the end of the creation, all these divisions will perish; there will be no more years, or months, or days or hours; there is only one time, the Great Aeon; all the righteous will escape the Great Judgment and join the Great Aeon living in the Paradise.

The notion of the two Aeons is indeed inherent in apocalypse, since the end of times is the limit between this Aeon and the Aeon to come. Thus, in 4 Ezra it is written: "But the day of judgment will be the end of this age and the beginning of the immortal age to come, in which corruption has passed away, sinful indulgence has come to an end, unbelief has been cut off, and righteousness has increased and truth has appeared" (Charlesworth, 1983, p. 541). Meanwhile, utopia is the *topos* of realized redemption, which is separated from this world, i.e., Paradise. On the Day of Judgment the wicked will be condemned to eternal punishment, while the righteous living, according to the will of God, will be introduced into the kingdom of God in eternal blessing as a reward for their good works during their lives in this Aeon (Scholem, 1971, pp. 1–36).

A new encoding of the time-space dimensions of traumatic symptoms seem to have been necessary to understand God's silence, incomprehensible injures and wounds of the Jews in the Second Temple Period, which ancient Judaism could not already decipher, as the author of 2 Baruch says: "Blessed is he who was not born, or he who was born and died. But we, the living, woe to us, because we have seen those afflictions of Zion, and that which has befallen Jerusalem" (Charlesworth, 1983, p. 624). Thus the identification of the frozen moment of trauma with the end of the times (apocalypse) brought a structural shift to the *Heilsgeschichte* (salvation history), i.e., the distinction between this Aeon and the Aeon to come.[24] In a similar way, the *topos* of salvation was shifted from the promised land to the Paradise (utopia), an apocalyptic version of the exodus. Thus, the monotheistic *Heilsgeschichte* (salvation history) is now determined by two horizons: the covenant/the

[23] According to the translation of Pines (1970), pp. 77–78, which is based on Vaillant's edition (the short recension).

[24] Cf. Ataria (2014a, p. 243): "The victim's need to insert the trauma into the sphere of time on the one hand and the inability to integrate (or plant) the trauma into the timeline of the 'past' on the other result in a situation in which the victim attempts to integrate the trauma into the present or future timeline as an apocalyptic possibility that creates a new horizon."

exodus as the archaeological horizon and apocalypse/utopia as the eschatological horizon.

15.4.2 Corpus

Let us now take a brief glance at two types of understanding of the engraving of traumas on the body, which developed respectively in rabbinic Judaism and Pauline Christianity.

In the Jewish communities, which rapidly became text-centered after the destruction of the Second Temple (A.D. 70) and the failure of the Bar Kokhba revolt (A.D. 132–135), the central issue was related to tradition and the canon (Halbertal, 1997). The basic assumption of rabbinic Judaism is that all legal teachings go back to Moses, which are divided into the Written Torah and the Oral Torah. In the Babylonian Talmud (Makkot 23b) Rabbi Simlai states that in the Written Torah "613 commandments were revealed to Moses at Mount Sinai, 365 being prohibitions equal in number to the solar days, and 248 being mandates corresponding in number to the limbs of the human body." In other words, the Written Torah is the year and the body of every Jew (Shabbat and the circumcision). Meanwhile, the Oral Torah is a collection of the teachings explaining and elaborating on the Written Torah, which has been passed down from generation to generation since Moses. It is the correspondence between the Written Torah and the Oral Torah, script and voice, that always guarantees the study of the Torah as the way to justice. Thus, virtually all the efforts of rabbinic Judaism were dedicated to the everlasting deciphering of traumas engraved on the body with the help of tradition: commentaries, controversies and canons.[25]

A completely different approach towards the engraving of traumas on the body is found in the New Testament.[26] In Romans 8:1–4 Paul formulates the significance of Jesus Christ in the salvation history as follows:

> Therefore, there is no condemnation for those who are in Christ Jesus, because through Christ Jesus the law of the Spirit of life set me free from the law of the sin and death. For what the law was powerless to do in that it was weakened by the sinful nature, God did by sending his own Son in the likeliness of sinful man to be a sin offering. And so he condemned a sin in sinful man, in order that the righteous requirements of the law might be met in us, who do not live according to the sinful nature but according to the Spirit.

God sacrificed his own Son as a sin offering for the believers who had been condemned to death by the Torah; however, this was made possible only by Jesus himself having been condemned as a sinner in place of them. Therefore, the resurrection of Jesus is interpreted as freedom from the slavery of sin (Jeremias, 1965, pp. 31–70; Strecker, 2000, pp. 116–178). The crucifixion and the resurrection of Jesus can be regarded as a structural shift which dramatically changed the significance of the engraving of traumas on the body in Judaism, as Paul proclaims in Romans 5:20–21: "The law was added so that the trespass might increase. But where sin increased, grace increased all the more, so that just as sin reigned in death, so also grace might reign through righteousness to bring eternal life through Jesus our

[25] Cf. Lorberbaum (2004, in particular, pp. 436–468), who argues that the destruction of the Temple gave impetus to the development of the notion of the presence of God on the body fulfilling the commandments.

[26] Strictly speaking, Gnosticism cannot be classified under the category of monotheism; moreover, it is even problematic to talk about Gnosticism as a unified phenomenon which can be clearly defined (Williams, 1996). However, it would be worth mentioning some interesting points relevant to our investigation. According to the Gnostic doctrine, this world and the human body were created by the evil demiurge, the God of the Jews, while the soul of the Gnostic, a divine spark, is derived from the Pleroma of light which belongs to the Supreme God; in parallel to this view, part of the Godhead itself is regarded as separated from its source and necessary to be restored; Gnosis, the secret knowledge of God, is the means for the attainment of salvation, i.e., the reintegration of the Godhead (Jonas, 1963; Rudolph, 1983). In this connection, it should be noted that there is good reason to suppose that the earliest Gnostic sects originated in certain Jewish groups who identified themselves with the seed of Seth, where the passage from the Jewish God to the Gnostic demiurge seems to have happened (see, for example, Stroumsa, 1984). The radical structural shift might be explained as based on the model of dissociation, the very traumatic symptom, one of the typical manifestations of which is an out of body experience, which could be interpreted as indicating the evil origin of this world and the body.

Lord." Then the repeated Binding of Isaac is God's act of mercy. Man can be saved not by endlessly deciphering traumas but by participation in the death of God's Son, i.e., his profound trauma, since thereby sin itself is disintegrated: "If we have been united with him like this in his death, we will certainly also be united with him in his resurrection. For we know that our old self was crucified with him so that the body of sin might be done away with, that we should no longer be slaves to sin—because anyone who has died has been freed from sin" (Romans 6:5–7).[27]

15.5 The Messianic Machine

The officer, the protagonist of *In the Penal Colony*, still believes the efficacy of the execution machine invented by the former Commandant. The great portion of the story progresses around the preparation for the execution of a soldier condemned to death by the sentence "Honor thy superior." However, having recognized that the whole procedure is convincing to no body, the officer releases the soldier and decides to execute himself by the sentence "Be just." During the execution, the machine goes to pieces and now "the Harrow was not writing, it was only jabbing, and the Bed was not turning the body over but only bringing it up quivering against the needles" (Kafka, 1971, p. 165). In the end, on the face of the dead officer "no sign was visible of the promised redemption, what the others had found in the machine the officer had not found" (Kafka, 1971, p. 166).

Does the execution machine cease to engrave traumas which can be deciphered? The situation exactly corresponds to Gerschom Scholem's definition of the Law in Kafka's *Trial* as "the Nothing of Revelation," i.e., "a state in which revelation appears to be without meaning, in which it still asserts itself, in which it has *validity* but no *significance*" (Benjamin and Scholem 1989, p. 142, cf. Agamben, 1998, pp. 49–51).[28] Now the script on one's body which is copied onto that of another by the execution machine is no more than "a labyrinth of lines," injuries and wounds which can never be given any significance but only endlessly transmit suffering.[29] The inability to decipher traumas seems to reflect the idea that modern life has lost the way to the Law with the disappearance of the sacred; the Law condemns the sinner as separated from sacredness but its retribution never expiates his guilt. In other words, the traumatic history of monotheism had already entered into a decisively new phase.

Walter Benjamin, who tends to think that "without the key that belongs to it, the Scripture is not Scripture, but life. Life as it is lived in the village at the foot of the hill on which the castle is built" (cf. Agamben, 1998, pp. 51–55; Benjamin & Scholem, 1989, p. 135),[30] describes

[27] Here I would like to add some brief comments on the place of Islam in the traumatic history of monotheism. The distinct historian John Wansbrough (2006) rightly supposes that the emergence of Islam as a dominant confessional expression can be seen as the response to interconfessional polemic ("sectarian milieu"), in which an appropriate set of monotheist symbols, *topoi* and *theologoumena* was (rather arbitrarily) selected by the membership of the clerical elite as its essential components. Now, most probably, the proto-Muslim communities formed their identity in their earliest stages in the context of Jewish and Jewish Christian missionary activities. In this meaning, it seems that Islam, in principle, adopted the mode of encoding of wounds and injuries which developed in Judaism and Jewish Christianity only with comparatively minor changes. However, some traumatic experience might be detected at the historical level. The members of the proto-Muslim communities believed that they were sons of Ishmael, who had been in the state of *jāhiliyya* (ignorance), but entered into that of *'ilm* (gnosis), when they abstained from the pagan environment and accepted the monotheistic faith under the instruction of their Jewish and Jewish-Christian mentors; however, at a certain point, Islam began to define itself as an independent religion with its authentic prophet and revelation (cf. Crone & Cook, 1977; Pines, 1990). I believe that the double separation from the pagan past and the monotheistic left a hidden trauma on Islam, which can be exposed in the theologico-historical construction of the Quran and other early Muslim literature, an issue which must, for technical reasons, be omitted in the scope of the present study.

[28] Cf. Benjamin and Scholem (1989, p. 126): "Kafka's world is the world of revelation, but of revelation seen of course from that perspective in which it is returned to its own nothingness."

[29] This should be compared with Ataria's analysis of trauma as a black hole in his "Trauma—A Black Hole in the Heart of Culture: The Passage from Individual to Society."

[30] Cf. Ataria's analysis (2013) of the world devoid of any possibility in Kafka's *The Castle* as a post-traumatic existence.

in detail the shock experiences in modernity, among others, in his "On Some Motifs in Baudelaire" (Benjamin, 1985, pp. 155–200). This essay is essentially based on the contrast between remembrance/*mémoire involontaire*/*Erfahrung* and recollection/*mémoire volontaire*/*Erlebnis*. Benjamin accepts Freud's suggestion in *Beyond the Pleasure Principle* that the function of consciousness is not to receive memory traces but to protect against stimuli. In this sense, traumatic shocks can be understood as breaking through the protection consciousness provides against stimuli. Therefore, "the greater the share of the shock factor in particular impressions, the more constantly consciousness has to be alert as a screen against stimuli; the more efficiently it does so, the less do these impressions enter experience (*Erfahrung*), tending to remain in the sphere of a certain hour in one's life (*Erlebnis*). Perhaps the special achievement of shock defense may be seen in its function of assigning to an incident a precise point in time in consciousness at the cost of the integrity of its content" (Benjamin, 1985, p. 163). Thus the shock, which is successfully defended, is incorporated in the registry of recollection, while the component of remembrance is what has not been consciously experienced.

It is in this context that Benjamin pays attention to the shock experiences of the big city crowd, i.e., a series of shocks involved in the traffic of a big city and the life of the worker at his machine along with a number of technological innovations and the development of advertisement. His description is not quite systematical. Nevertheless, it might be possible to distinguish two major aspects here: (1) the disintegration of the aura as "the unique manifestation of a distance" in remembrance (2) the automatic reaction to shocks as the result of adaptation to machines. Below, I would like to mainly discuss the latter, the point which is usually overlooked in the discussions on Benjamin's analysis of shock experiences of the big city crowd.

Perhaps this automatization of the body is the extreme form of manifestation of the cycle of the execution machine. However, the decisive point is that the formation of automatic responses to traumatic shocks is possible only when the key to decipher the Law is lost, since all the process is then devoid of any significance. Thus what we see in modern life is not the Corpus but the amorphous crowd, not eternity but the clock.[31] It should be noted that the automatization of the body corresponds with Agamben's description of modern biopolitics: "Together with the process by which the exception everywhere becomes the rule, the realm of bare life—which is originally situated at the margin of the political order—gradually begins to coincide with the political realm, and exclusion and inclusion, outside and inside, *bios* and *zōē*, right and fact, enter into a zone of irreducible indistinction" (Agamben, 1998, p. 9; cf. pp. 117–188, though he prefers to use the term "camp" there).

In my opinion, it is necessary to read Benjamin's *Theses on the Philosophy of History* in this connection, an approach which, as far as I know, has never been taken. The first thesis reads as follows (Benjamin, 1985, p. 253):

> The story is told of an automaton constructed in such a way that it could play a winning game of chess, answering each move of an opponent with a countermove. A puppet in Turkish attire and with a hookah in its mouth sat before a chessboard placed on a large table. A system of mirrors created the illusion that this table was transparent from all sides. Actually, a little hunchback who was an expert chess player sat inside and guided the puppet's hand by means of strings. One can imagine a philosophical counterpart to this device. The puppet called "historical materialism" is to win all the time. It can easily be a match for anyone if it enlists the services of theology, which today, as we know, is wizened and has to keep out of sight.

Benjamin might have read about this automaton in Edgar Allan Poe's "Maelzel's Chess Player" (1836).[32] However, the hidden motivation for this choice of the image seems to be found elsewhere; the puppet in Turkish attire reminds of Sabbatai Zevi, the Messiah of the Sabbatean

[31] In the scope of the present study, I omit the discussion on Benjamin's ambivalent attitude towards Henri Bergson's time theory.

[32] And, most probably, the reminiscence of E. T. Hoffmann's *Klein Zaches* can be also discerned here. I hope to deal with this point in detail elsewhere.

movement who, before the sultan, cast off his Jewish garb and put a Turkish turban on his head, a symbolical act of conversion to Islam.[33] (Benjamin must have heard about this extraordinary personality from Scholem, while the latter's *Sabbatai Sevi: The Mystical Messiah* (1973) was, I believe, written in response to the former's *Theses.*) Let us call this automaton, which is composed of the puppet (historical materialism) and a little hunchback (theology), the Messianic machine. His enemy is the Antichrist, as the subduer of whom the Messiah comes (Benjamin, 1985, p. 255). How, then, can he answer each move of his opponent with a countermove?

If the automatization of the body as the extreme form of manifestation of the cycle of the execution machine is the result of the adaptation to traumatic shocks, and therefore, the clock characterizes modern life for the amorphous crowd,[34] which has lost the key to decipher the Law, then the countermove of the Messianic machine is nothing but the shock of the arrest of thought: "Where thinking suddenly stops in a configuration pregnant with tensions, it gives that configuration a shock, by which it crystallizes into a monad. A historical materialist approaches a historical subject only where he encounters it as a monad. In this structure he recognizes the sign of a Messianic cessation of happening, or, put differently, a revolutionary chance in the fight for the oppressed past" (Benjamin, 1985, pp. 262–263). Here the notion of "a present which is not a transition, but in which time stands still and has come to a stop" (Benjamin, 1985, p. 262) is in sharp conflict with that of the clock, i.e., homogenous, empty time. How, then, can we break into pieces the continuum of history? By seeing in place of historical progress "one single catastrophe which keeps piling wreckage upon wreckage" (Benjamin, 1985, p. 257).

This catastrophe must be the figure of trauma. Therefore, the function of the Messianic machine is, in my opinion, to reverse with a countermove just the engraving of traumas made by the execution machine. And this is why the Messianic machine is "to win all the time," i.e., in its capacity to crystallize wounds and injuries into a single shock, the "divine violence" as the deposition of law,[35] which could open a fissure on the surface of the Law, when the past flashes up in remembrance[36] at the eternal present. Perhaps, the possibility of composing the birth, development and death of the monotheistic religions as a traumatic history can be found here: To gaze at the ungraspable moment of traumas which immediately disappears into the structure of religious dogmas and therewith to open "the strait gate through which the Messiah might enter" (Benjamin, 1985, p. 264). And this strait gate seems to be hidden in each and every trauma in our own life as integrating all wreckages in history. As if it were possible, in our age, to decipher the "revelation without God" for a *Muselmann* alone, for whom it is eternally forbidden to die as a Jew.[37]

Therefore, the composition of a traumatic history of the monotheistic religions will be possible only at the limit between truth and falsehood, where myth dissolves into nothing, by one who, having lost salvation, was banished outside, to such an extent that a Jew is called a Muslim. In this sense Freud's Moses and Monotheism at the same time uncovers and conceals the wounds and injuries inherent in monotheism by creating its own salvation myth. I would like to suggest

[33] Quite interestingly, for Sabbatai Zevi, as it seems, Muhammad, the prophet of Islām, was a shell (qelippah) of his messianic soul, as Jesus of Nazareth was so before his conversion. With this we might be able to compare the bizarre expression "husk-men" used by Levi for the description of the *Muselmänner*.

[34] Cf. the deep analysis by Gelili (2013) of the clock in Kafka's *Die Verwandlung*.

[35] Here I adopt Benjamin's insight into the "divine violence" as the breaking of the cycle of the "mythic violence" in his *Critique of Violence* (Benjamin, 1999, pp. 236–252), although he does not explicitly connect his idea to the Messianic context.

[36] Cf. the first paragraph of Paul Celan's Bremen prize speech: "Thinking (Denken) and thanking (Danke) in our language are words from one and the same source. Whoever follows their meaning betakes himself to the semantic field of: 'recollect,' 'bear in mind,' 'reminiscence,' 'devotion.' Please permit me, from here, to thank you" (Celan, 1983, p. 185, in my translation).

[37] "This word 'Muselmann,' I do not know why, was used by the old ones of the camp to describe the weak, the inept, those doomed to selection" (Levi, 1996, p. 88).

that the inclusion of bare life into the Law itself is essentially rooted in the discovery of sacredness following recognition of death, which could be identified as the lost terminus a quo *of the endless cycle of the execution machine. In other words, the notion of* homo sacer *should be reinterpreted as the being between the sacred and the Law, which would be structuralized as grace and justice in the monotheistic religions. In the age of the "revelation without God" the counter move of the Messianic machine is to crystallize wounds and injuries into a single shock and thus to open a strait gate on the surface of the Law.*

References

Agamben, G. (1998). *Homo sacer: Sovereign power and bare life*, Trans. D. Heller-Roazen. Stanford, CA: Stanford University Press.

Agamben, G. (1999). Remnants of Auschwitz: The witness and the archive, Trans. D. Heller-Roazen. New York: Zone Books.

Agamben, G. (2004). *The open: Man and animal*, translated by K. Attell. Stanford, CA: Stanford University Press.

Ataria, Y. (2014c). Towards the phenomenology of trauma. *Jewish Psychology*. http://www.hebpsy.net/articles.asp?id=3139 (in Hebrew).

Assmann, J. (2006). The advance in intellectuality: Freud's construction of Judaism. In R. Ginsburg & I. Pardes (Eds.), *New perspectives on Freud's Moses and Monotheism* (pp. 7–18). Tübingen: Max Niemeyer Verlag.

Ataria, Y. (2013). Kafka: A post-traumatic experience. In Z. Shamir, Y. Ataria, & H. Nagid (Eds.), *Kafka: New perspectives: Research and analysis* (pp. 304–321). Tel Aviv: Safra (in Hebrew).

Ataria, Y. (2014a). Trauma: The passage from individual to society. *Ma'arag, 5*, 239–270 (in Hebrew).

Ataria, Y. (2014b). Loyalty to silence. *History and Theory: Bezalel II, 29*. http://bezalel.secured.co.il/zope/home/he/1376936935/1388333556 (in Hebrew).

Ataria, Y., & Gallagher, S. (2015). Somatic apathy: Body disownership in the context of torture. *Journal of Phenomenological Psychology, 46*(1), 105–122.

Benjamin, W. (1985). *Illuminations*, edited and with an introduction by H. Arendt, Trans. H. Zohn. New York: Schocken Books.

Benjamin, W. (1999). In M. Bullock & M. W. Jennings (Eds.), *Selected writings* (Vol. 2). Cambridge, MA: Belknap Press.

Benjamin, W., & Scholem, G. (1989). In G. Scholem (Ed.), *The correspondence of Walter Benjamin and Gershom Scholem, 1932-1940*, translated from by G. Smith and A. Lefevere, with an introduction by A. Rabinbach. New York: Schocken Books.

Caruth, C. (1996). *Unclaimed experience: Trauma, narrative and history*. Baltimore & London: Johns Hopkins University Press.

Celan, P. (1983). *Gesammelte Werke* (Vol. 3). Frankfurt am Main: Suhrkamp Verlag.

Charlesworth, J. (Ed.) (1983). *The old testament pseudepigrapha* (Vol. 1). New York: Doubleday.

Crone, P., & Cook, M. (1977). *Hagarism: The making of the Islamic world*. Cambridge: Cambridge University Press.

Deleuze, G., & Guattari, F. (1977). In R. Hurley, S. Mark, & H. R. Lane (Eds.), *Anti-Oedipus: Capitalism and schizophrenia*. New York: Viking.

Derrida, J. (1996). *Archive fever: A Freudian impression*, Trans. E. Prenowitz. Chicago, IL: University of Chicago Press.

Derrida, J. (2006). Writing and difference, Trans. A. Bass. London: Routledge.

Freud, S. (1896). The aetiology of hysteria. *SE, 3*, 187–221.

Freud, S. (1913). Totem and Taboo. *SE, 13*, 1–162.

Freud, S. (1920). Beyond the pleasure principle. *SE, 18*, 1–64.

Freud, S. (1923). The Ego and the Ido. *SE, 19*, 1–66.

Freud, S. (1939). Moses and monotheism: Three essays. *SE, 23*, 1–137.

Gelili, S. (2013). The clock of Gregor Samsa. In Z. Shamir, Y. Ataria, & H. Nagid (Eds.), *Kafka: New perspectives: Research and analysis* (pp. 288–303). Tel Aviv: Safra (in Hebrew).

Ginsburg, R. (2006). In: R. Ginsburg & I. Pardes (Eds.), *New perspectives on Freud's "Moses and Monotheism,"* (pp. 77–91). Tübingen: Max Niemeyer Verlag.

Halbertal, M. (1997). *People of the book: Canon, meaning, and authority*. Cambridge, MA: Harvard University Press.

Jeremias, J. (1965). *The central message of the new testament*. London: SCM Press.

Jonas, H. (1963). *The Gnostic religion: The message of the alien god and the beginnings of Christianity* (2nd ed.). Boston: Beacon.

Kafka, F. (1971). In N. N. Glatzer (Ed.), *The complete stories*. New York: Schoken Books.

LaCapra, D. (2001). *Writing history, writing trauma*. Baltimore: Johns Hopkins University Press.

Levi, P. (1996). *Survival in Auschwitz: the Nazi assault on humanity*, Trans. S. Woolf, including "a conversation with P. Levi by Ph. Roth." New York, NY: A Touchstone Book.

Lorberbaum, Y. (2004). *Imago Dei: Halakhah and Aggadah*. Tel Aviv: Schoken Publishing House. in Hebrew.

Pines, S. (1970). Eschatology and the concept of time in the Slavonic Book of Enoch. In R. J. Zwi Werblowsky & C. J. Bleeker (Eds.), *Types of redemption*. Leiden: E. J. Brill.

Pines, S. (1990). Jāhiliyya and 'Ilm. *Jerusalem Studies in Arabic and Islam, 13*, 175–194.

Ricoeur, P. (1970). Freud and philosophy: An essay on interpretation, Trans. D. Savage. New Haven: Yale University Press.

Rilke, R. M. (1955). *Sämtliche Werke* (Vol. 1). Frankfurt am Main: Insel Verlag.

Rothschild, B. (2000). *The body remembers: The psychophysiology of trauma and trauma treatment.* New York: Norton.

Rudolph, K. (1983). *Gnosis: The Nature and History of Gnosticism*, Trans. Ed. by R. Mc. Wilson (2nd rev. ed.). San Francisco: Harper.

Schäfer, P. (2006). The triumph of pure spirituality: Sigmund Freud's *Moses and Monotheism*. In R. Ginsburg & I. Pardes (Eds.), *New perspectives on Freud's "Moses and Monotheism"* (pp. 19–43). Tübingen: Max Niemeyer Verlag.

Scholem, G. (1971). *The messianic idea in Judaism: And other essays on Jewish spirituality*. New York: Schocken Books.

Scholem, G. (1973). *Sabbatai Sevi: The Mystical Messiah, 1626-1676*, translated by R. J. Zwi Werblowsky. Princeton, NJ: Princeton University Press.

Snowman, L. V. (1971). Circumcision. *Encyclopedia Judaica, 5*, 567–575. Jerusalem: Encyclopedia Judaica.

Strecker, G. (2000). *Theology of the new testament*. German edition edited and completed by F. W. Horn, Trans. M. E. Boring. New York: W. de Gruyter.

Stroumsa, G. (1984). *Another seed: Studies in Gnostic mythology*. Leiden: Brill.

Stroumsa, G. (2011). From Abraham's religion to the Abrahamic religions. *Historia Religiorum, 3*, 11–22.

Van der Kolk, B. A. (1994). The body keeps the score: Memory and the evolving psychobiology of posttraumatic stress. *Harvard Review of Psychiatry, 1*(5), 253–265.

Wansbrough, J. (2006). *The sectarian milieu: Content and composition of Islamic salvation history*. Amherst, NY: Prometheus Books.

Williams, M. A. (1996). *Rethinking "Gnosticism": An argument for dismantling a dubious category*. Princeton, NJ: Princeton University Press.

Yerushalmi, Y. H. (1991). *Freud's Moses: Judaism terminable and interminable*. New Haven: Yale University Press.

16 The Crisis of Manhood

Yochai Ataria

The enemy . . . is anybody who's going to get you killed, no matter which side he's on. . . And don't you forget that, because the longer you remember it, the longer you might live

(Heller, 1961, p. 124).

16.1 Introduction: Men in the World of Post-trauma

After the Vietnam War, the white[1] man in the United States was defeated and humiliated. He experienced a fundamental trauma: the loss of the father and the collapse of the patriarchic system of values that the father symbolized. When the soldier returns, defeated and lost, he finds that his comrades in arms are no longer there, a situation defined by Morag as the collapse of fraternity (Morag, 2009). The soldier is left alone with his pain and solitude, full of violence, without the ability to communicate with his family or with women. He discovers that he is in captivity at home. In some cases he chooses to go back to what has become his real home (as in the movies *Apocalypse Now* and *The Deer Hunter*). In other cases he goes crazy and becomes unable to think of himself as a human being. When the soldier chooses to remain in his former home (the United States), he becomes a "taxi driver"—that is, a violent man without a father, without friends, someone who cannot engage in intimate relations with anyone, and certainly not with women.

At the onset of the twenty-first century, the defeated white man has metamorphosed into a shadow of his former self. He has surrendered his body to the shopping and porno channels, as for example the main character does in the movie *Fight Club* (Linson, Chaffin, Bell, & Fincher, 1999). This disintegrated man gladly submits to the insanity of Tyler Durden (in *Fight Club*), who is merely another incarnation of Kurtz *(Heart of Darkness/Apocalypse Now)*, Meursault *(The Stranger)* and Travis *(Taxi Driver)*.

The protagonists of the films *Apocalypse Now* (Coppola & Conrad, 1979), *The Deer Hunter* (Schrader & Scorsese, 1976) and *Fight Club* symbolize complex relations at several levels of meaning: between the conscious and unconscious, the father and son, the hunter and hunted, the captor and captive, the masculine and feminine; between nature and the city, the self and the other, the brother and the stranger, the prevaricating face shown to the world and the mask—the "genuine" mask which conceals the true identity. The postmodern era is marked by impossible and unbridgeable dualities that characterize the posttraumatic hero, who is very different both from the romantic hero as well as from the classic modern hero. Indeed the posttraumatic figure is split: on the surface he may appear normal yet beneath the surface, on the unconscious level, he is completely broken, frozen in the moment of trauma.

It is not for naught that Travis in the movie *Taxi Driver* (Schrader & Scorsese, 1976), Captain Willard (*Apocalypse Now*) and Michael (*The Deer Hunter*), each in their own way, reconstruct

[1] Clearly not only white men fought in the Vietnam War. The focus of the current paper, however, is on the status of the white man in America.

Y. Ataria, Ph.D. (✉)
Department of Neurobiology, Weizmann Institute of Science, Rechovot, Israel
e-mail: yochai.ataria@gmail.com

Y. Ataria et al. (eds.), *Interdisciplinary Handbook of Trauma and Culture*,
DOI 10.1007/978-3-319-29404-9_16

"the game" over and over again obsessively. The game is an uncontrolled repetition of the trauma that occurs as an attempt to fix what needs repair. Processes of adaptation are simply impossible for the posttraumatic individual. The end of the game is death. Indeed, death is what the posttraumatic hero longs for. Death is the only path to the purification that will never actually come. The community "back home" does indeed embrace these crazy masochistic men as the new heroes, but it is clear to the viewers and to the posttraumatic heroes themselves that death only sustains and maintains what is perverse and distorted.

The model of the father as a functional father, that is, as a figure who represents the law in the broadest sense, has collapsed. The brother-in-arms who was everything during battle has died or has dissipated into the past and disappeared. Over and over again it becomes clear that women do not constitute a possible solution. There is no comfort to be had, no consolation. Thus, on his date, Travis *(Taxi Driver)* goes to a pornographic movie intensifying his inability to achieve intimacy and to conceal his impotence, which has been converted into total violence. So long as the same game continues, the same impossible chronicle, there is no possibility of salvation. "We did not fight the enemy, we fought ourselves, and the enemy was in us," Chris remarks at the end of the movie *Platoon* (Kopelson & Stone, 1986). Yet murdering the unconscious within us, so it seems, is not the solution. In the postmodern era, salvation is unthinkable.

Vietnam represents the context of what can be defined as the collective post-trauma in the United States, the entry into the collective unconscious. This is an historical and archeological journey into the structure of the knowledge and the perceptions of white America, beginning with the murder of the first Native American through the dropping of the atom bomb on Japan and through the war fought in the humid jungles of Vietnam.

Fundamentally, then, Vietnam is not a place alien to Americans. The jungles of Vietnam reflect the image of the American inner world. The Vietnam War represents the eruption of the inner American discourse. Vietnam is the genuine space in which events happen, against the backdrop of the attempt to build and reshape the American model of masculinity (Hellman, 1982). In effect, Vietnam represents the posttraumatic part of the American experience. Therefore, the trauma of Vietnam is the product of the American narrative formulated over the course of more than 200 years. It is impossible to separate Vietnam from America, just as it is impossible to separate trauma from the posttraumatic individual and it is impossible to separate Barnes from Elias in the film *Platoon*. Vietnam is, in fact, the traumatic black hole of the United States. It represents the collective and essential constitutive trauma. Indeed, the Vietnam War is a turning point in the discourse on trauma and post-trauma (Herman, 1992).

The experience of captivity in Vietnam is the result of the fraudulent, baseless attempt to distinguish between "good" and "evil." Post-trauma is the product of the total collapse of the narrative that states that "if I am not good, I must certainly be bad." We can no longer color the world in two colors. We can no longer preserve these opposites. We can no longer continue to rule. We can no longer continue to silence the inner world. What the United States experienced in Vietnam is a replication of the *Akeda* story in which Abraham bound his own son for sacrifice while being controlled by an automatic and murderous mechanism.

Through an examination of the white post-Vietnam male in movies such as *Taxi Driver*, *The Deer Hunter*, and *Apocalypse Now*, the first section of this article attempts to reveal the very nature of the posttraumatic western figure. The second section examines how Kurtz (*Apocalypse Now*) on the one hand and Tyler Durden (*Fight Club*) on the other, deal with the crisis of manhood in the wake of trauma: by killing the father, both concretely and symbolically, both the real father and the very notion of fatherhood. In so doing, both approaches seek to destroy the very nature of law that is identified with the function of the father figure. Furthermore, as discussed in the third section, both approaches have something else in common. Both are ultimately apocalyptic in nature, involving either self-annihilation or killing the Other. These are the only alternatives remaining for the posttraumatic figure.

Hence, the final section of the article contends that the destruction of the father suggested by Kurtz and Tyler Durden is too violent and cruel and that ultimately what is preferable is the familiar, automatic cruel father in a reality in which anarchy controls everything.

16.2 The Posttraumatic Figure: Travis, Michael and Captain Willard

16.2.1 Taxi Driver—Travis

Travis, the soldier who has returned home from the Vietnam War, who is clearly traumatized and apparently a former prisoner of war as well, is steeped in violence. Travis is a solitary individual without a father, without even a friend in the world, lacking all ability to maintain intimate relations. At least at the level of meaning that is revealed, Travis is the figure that the United States chooses to define as its new hero. Indeed, he becomes a hero after his insane/messianic journey of revenge. He is the one who will rid New York City of its filth. Yet in effect Travis, a typical product of American culture, is interested in just a bit of blood in order to feel at home once again. Travis is not interested in cleansing and purifying the city of its filth. Rather, he wants to maintain his own inner contamination and decay, to preserve his sense of alienation, voyeurism, disparateness, distorted sexuality, and violence (Morag, 2009).

Travis is an orphan without a father or a mother. He is a psychopathic killer. Travis does in fact attempt to resuscitate his body and to restore his sense of self-efficacy. He does not do this however in order to recover his sense of self, but rather as part of a chronicle of psychopathology, indeed as part of a process of fixating upon the pathology. Travis does everything he can to sanctify, to enhance, to externalize, and mainly to stabilize the unconscious layers: the violence, alienation, messianism, distorted sexuality, and self-abhorrence, all this characteristic of an era lacking a God and lacking a father. When Travis sets out on his crazed journey, he seemingly removes the masks and decks himself out like a Mohawk Indian in order to return to a more primeval character, one that is pre-reflective and pre-Western. Travis wants to be reborn, not for the sake of inner purification but rather to preserve the horror and the trauma he has known. Travis does not "choose" to set out on a journey of killing, just like Kafka does not choose to write. He has no choice but to act as he does:

"The tremendous world I have inside my head. But how free myself and free it without being torn to pieces. And a thousand times rather be torn to pieces than retain it in me or bury it. That, indeed, is why I am here, that is quite clear to me" (Kafka, 1949, p. 288).

16.2.2 The Deer Hunter—Michael

The dialogue between Travis *(Taxi Driver)* and Michael *(The Deer Hunter)* is so straightforward that it cannot be ignored, and not only because these two characters are played by the same actor (Robert De Niro). Travis wants to be a hunter. Michael is a hunter by his very nature. Sometimes it seems that Travis is Michael in another incarnation, or that he is a fantasy in Michael's mind. Yet the difference between these two characters (Travis and Michael) is fundamental. Michael understands that the model of the father has collapsed and attempts to save the model of the brother, though this does not succeed with Nick, his old friend from back home who has become his brother-in-arms as well. He cannot go on with the game, cannot return to relations with a woman, to Nick's girlfriend Linda. Nick himself is incapable of talking to Linda, for "the surest of stubborn silences is not to hold one's tongue but to talk" (Kierkegaard cited in Camus, 1975, p. 19). He phones her from Vietnam but is incapable of talking. He no longer wants to talk. He knows that he belongs in the insane asylum with Steve, the third friend who was taken captive by the Vietcong. Returning to reality is impossible. Therefore Nick prefers to maintain his silence. This silence is reflected in the life of Michael when he totally fails to have intimate relations with Linda. Indeed, Nick and Michael are actually the same person living in two parallel dimensions, a condition that is quite typical of the posttraumatic experience in which the frozen element of time typifies the posttraumatic condition (Terr, 1984). It is important to understand that from the perspective of the posttraumatic man, the woman is not attainable; she is situated beyond the trauma, beyond the frozen time dimension of the traumatic subject.

Michael (the deer hunter) decides to return to Vietnam in order to release himself from the dybbuk[2] to return to his genuine home, to flee the captivity of the counterfeit homeland, or, in the words of Captain Willard from *Apocalypse Now:* "When I was here I wanted to be there. When I was there, all I could think of was getting back into the jungle" (Coppola & Conrad, 1979). Michael travels to save Nick in an attempt to save himself. His journey is a voyage into his own inner world. He does not want to relinquish the world, to give up on the other. He knows that only by rescuing Nick will he manage to save his own life. Yet the events that ensue are predictable and on a deeper level he cannot save Nick. Indeed, he must destroy Nick. Nick represents Michael's trauma, his scar. Nick is in fact Michael's inner world. Michael knows that in order to survive he must murder the inner voice that is Nick. (And we should keep in mind that the dominant trait of Kurtz in *Apocalypse Now* is his voice.) This is in fact a zero-sum game. Thus, by definition the posttraumatic condition is the zero-sum game one plays with oneself—the mind and the body becomes enemies. In the posttraumatic condition the mind and the body cannot continue to coexist hence one of then must cease to exist.

That being the case, what begins as a game turns into horrifying reality. Michael understands this and therefore he cannot tolerate Stan (one of their buddies who did not go to Vietnam) in the game with the pistol. In one of the most important scenes in the movie, Stan threatens to shoot Axel. Michael grabs the gun, puts a bullet into the chamber and recreates the game of Russian roulette that he, Steve, and Nick played while they were in captivity, uttering one of the movie's most important lines: "This is this, this isn't something else" (Coppola & Conrad, 1979). Here it seems that replaying the game of Russian roulette has become an obsession for Michael. That is, compulsive repetition turns into dominant reality. In this situation Michael is close to choosing his inner world over the world outside, and if he were to do so, his fate would be identical to that of Nick. Michael also recreates the threat posed to him by Stan, making it clear to the viewers, and mainly to himself, how games can turn into an impossible reality. This is the moment at which Michael understands that the only way to save Nick is to play yet another round of Russian roulette. In order to recover, the posttraumatic individual must play the game out to the end, just like Abraham played out the game with God (Benyamini, 2011).

16.2.3 Apocalypse Now—Captain Willard

On one level, Captain Willard's voyage is a journey through the American society represented by Captain Willard's crew. On another level, it is a journey to the depths of the American ideal represented by Kurtz—the father who has gone insane, the man who "knows what is good and, despite himself, does evil" (Camus, 1962a, p. 249). Ultimately Captain Willard must murder the myth. Yet paradoxically he does not do this because he wants to—"Kurtz was turning from a target into a goal"—but rather because this is what Kurtz wants him to do—"Everyone wanted me to do it, him most of all." It is interesting to discover in the movie that Captain Willard understands the true nature of Marlow's task in the book *The Heart of Darkness* (Conrad, 1990), upon which the movie was based. Kurtz wants to be murdered. He does not want to recover. He is not interested in indisputable facts and he certainly does not want to return "home" as a saint (like Travis). He is a graduate of the infinite games played by Michael *(The Deer Hunter)* and

[2]According to Jewish tradition, a dybbuk is a malicious spirit believed to be the dislocated soul of a dead person who possesses a living person and causes him to act in a certain way.

he understands that leaving the jungle will bring him back, just like Captain Willard, to the jaws of the dybbuk, to the trauma, to the recurring, infinite, and uncontrollable game. Kurtz knows that there is no place to return to and no point in returning: "Droll thing life is—that mysterious arrangement of merciless logic for a futile purpose" (Conrad, 1990, p. 65).

By nature Kurtz is not a violent sadist, and his uncontrolled outburst of violence stems from his humanity that is too large, from his ability to see the other in all of existence. Hence he can say the following to Captain Willard:

"I've seen horrors, horrors that you've seen. But you have no right to call me a murderer. You have a right to kill me. You have a right to do that, but you have no right to judge me. It's impossible for words to describe what is necessary to those who do not know what horror means" (Coppola & Conrad, 1979).

In Captain Willard's eyes Kurtz is a saint, even a martyr, because Kurtz has not ceased to be an ideal. In choosing to die at the hands of a soldier in the special forces who is like a son and a brother to him (both having served in the Green Beret Special Forces) Kurtz symbolizes the new God; the genuine superman who is saturated in trauma and in violence stemming from the other, from a perfect vision of the other within the self. Kurtz deals with the *Akeda*. But no less than that he also deals with the story of Cain and Abel in that he attempts, in his own twisted way, to make amends while wondering "What cry would ever trouble them?" (Camus, 1962a, p. 243).

Alternatively, if we want to claim that Kurtz preserves the model of Cain and Abel, we must then say that Abel yearns for death. Kurtz looks at the other and discovers the new God of anarchy within himself. In his life and in his death, Kurtz is in control of his fate, of nature. He does not judge himself according to Western values. He does not accept his guilt like Meursault in *The Stranger* (Camus, 1962b), and in the layer of meaning that is revealed he is far from a Kafkaesque character. He does not sink into himself like Clamence in *The Fall* (Camus, 2000). He is not convinced that he has a home on the faraway white continent. He is submerged in this very moment, in the present. He returns to his deeper roots and discovers the true ideal that accompanies the American narrative: "The horror! The horror!"

16.3 The New God of Anarchy: Kurtz versus Tyler Durden

16.3.1 The Binding of Isaac

Sarah laughed, Abraham understood, God did not, and since then the relations have been clear: Out of total insanity the father binds his son, and the mother remains silent and thus cooperates with the father and his craziness in a way that is absolutely bizarre. Insanity totally dominates our lives. The son is an orphan even while his parents are still alive. And perhaps he himself merely longs for death and his father has done his bidding. This is the way it is from generation to generation. Relationships are forced upon us. You love someone simply in order to sacrifice him out of an internal struggle, a dybbuk. This disease that has been discussed so much, perhaps even too much, does not loosen its grip—it remains relevant. For some time now this is not merely a matter of guilt as posited by Jaspers (2001). It is not merely a Christian or Jewish question, and no clear, unambiguous beginning or end point can be designated. Each of us is Isaac and also Abraham, but each of us is also and always Sarah—the one who understood God as a psychotic figure better than anyone else. The inner struggle creates the purest form of insanity that leads to automatic outbursts that cannot be controlled, as in the case of Sodom.

Today we know that Kafka himself wrote "In the Penal Colony" (2007) and we are relieved to learn that "one of us" (someone of flesh and blood) so accurately described the reality in which we live. Yet this is not the case with respect to the story of the *Akeda*. One could surmise that in another incarnation Kafka wrote the *Akeda*. But Kafka undoubtedly would not have allowed Isaac to remain alive in this story. And precisely here it seems that we are the butt of the joke—that the great parody is always at our expense. Leaving Isaac alive is worse than K's death like a dog in *The Trial* (Kafka, 2006). The biblical author however is much crueler than Kafka. He lets Isaac live and hence a culture that is absolutely traumatic was unleashed on the world: on Abraham for his willingness to butcher his son in order to take his revenge on God, on Isaac as the one who is bound for sacrifice and on his mother who said nothing. (And we have not mentioned Hagar and her son, Ishmael, who was banished merely for chuckling.) Sarah, the mother, disappeared and has yet to return because we all know where inappropriate laughter can lead. And indeed, she could have stopped Abraham from binding Isaac. The fact that Isaac remained alive enabled, in fact forced—as if from a dybbuk—the generation of the fathers to bind the generation of the sons over and over again.

Kurtz and Tyler Durden both understand, each in his own way, that there is only one way to be released from the burden of this difficult reality: to kill the father and all that he symbolizes, and to use Freud's (1939) words: "A hero is a man who stands up manfully against his father and in the end victoriously overcomes him" (p. 18).

16.3.2 Apocalypse Now—Kurtz

Kurtz understands very well that the father binds his son without any real choice. It is the father's inner dybbuk that leads him to sacrifice his son. Correspondingly, Kurtz no longer recognizes the system of values created by the white/Western/Christian world. He is not willing to be judged. He has no problem dying so long as he is put to death by a man who understands that the ethical system according to which we live has no validity. Perhaps it would be more accurate to say that Kurtz yearns to die but he is not willing to die at the hands of hypocrites who in the morning lecture on justice and morality and at night rape and plunder, who speak in terms of justice and act by dropping napalm bombs (the smell of victory).

It is clear that Kurtz wants to be released from life by dying. For once he wants to choose. Kurtz understands that in the existing system "man's greatest achievements were based on murder" (Houellebecq, 2000, p. 208). And he is able to choose his own death, as part of an idolatrous rather than a monotheistic setting, a system in which guilt is separate from redemption. More profound observation reveals that not only does Kurtz release himself, he also releases Captain Willard. From Kurtz's point of view, there is only one way to achieve release, and that is by binding his father according to the Freudian model (e.g., A hero is a man who stands up manfully against his father and in the end victoriously overcomes him). Kurtz is responding to the way that the Vietnam War is being conducted. He does this when he enters into a head-to-head confrontation, like Abraham with God, with the country that sent him to battle for "just causes." The impossible paradox is that we always believe that just causes require sacrifices. This is precisely the model at the basis of the experience of disaster in which we live. Kurtz received an assignment and demonstrated to his metaphysical fathers the significance of sticking to these objectives. He managed to meet every objective placed before him. But he did this without a mask, which he stressed by painting his face as if to say that this is who I really am. I removed all the masks. You wanted this . . . you got it. Kurtz follows in Abraham's footsteps. He takes matters to their most extreme conclusion, just to prove to the other side, to God, that words said and decisions made in air conditioned rooms while drinking a glass of red wine have repercussions, like at the Wannsee Conference where the Nazis decided upon the Final Solution.

Kurtz is obligated to humanity, not to God, obligated forever, and thus he allows Captain Willard to murder him. It would be more accurate to state that because he is obligated to humanity, he demands that Captain Willard murder him in order to release Captain Willard as well. Yet because Kurtz is the "first man" and the "rebellious man" at the same time, he demands that Captain Willard do this only after Willard himself has undergone a process of sobering and release, that is, a process enabling him "to learn to live and to die, and, in order to be a man, to refuse to be a

God" (Camus, 1962a, p. 245). Release always comes from inner insanity. Kurtz knows he must die, for "Lucifer also has died with God" (Camus, 1962a, p. 264). Kurtz has internalized the idea that he himself, by his very nature, constitutes the lesson of Western monotheistic culture. He sacrifices himself out of deep metaphysical insight. He is totally rational. He knows that the system, by its nature and its methods, has gone insane. It is important to stress that Kurtz is not a product of the system in the way that Private Leonard Lawrence (nicknamed "Gomer Pyle") in the movie *Full Metal Jacket* (Kubrick & Harlan, 1987) is a product of the system. Kurtz understands the system very well, indeed better than it understands itself. He understands the system in the way that Abraham understands God, or to be more precise, as Sarah understands God, and for that reason he places himself in a position of changing the system from within in the most radical way possible. Kurtz understands that reports like those he himself had written in the past, mere words, will not help. Just like God, the system needs blood, lots of blood, in order to change.

"In ancient times the blood of murder at least produced a religious horror and in this way sanctified the value of life. The real condemnation of the period we live in is, on the contrary, that it leads us to think that it is not bloodthirsty enough. Blood is no longer visible; it does not bespatter the faces of our pharisees visibly enough" (Camus, 1962a, pp. 243–244).

This is exactly what Kurtz intends to supply us. Every man who reaches Kurtz on his journey will discover along the way the extent to which the system has become faulty, has gone crazy. For Kurtz represents the collapse of the system. This is his goal—to reveal the absurdity of the system.

Thus, only when the individual who has come to kill Kurtz comes from a place of total refusal to be part of that automatic-mechanical-destructive system will Kurtz be willing to die at the hand of said individual. This *Akeda,* this self-sacrifice carried out by your son who is at the same time your brother in arm and who also understands the collapse of the overall system, is the height of the rebellion, because as Kurtz sees it, this *Akeda* releases both the binder and the one who is bound, thus setting a new starting point for human history.

Kurtz's vision is accurate. The posttraumatic individual is a cultural product. Thus he has forgotten how to speak using words and can only conduct himself in the system by means of games of death and killing, a system that can only speak in terms of bloodletting and the dead. Kurtz chooses to kill in the way that he does so that there will be no doubt. He knows (following the mass suicide of the Sicarii rebels at the Masada fortress) that fresh blood is the best way to talk to, and to arouse, God. Thus he attempts to beget a superman. Hence, in Kurtz's view, Captain Willard has been released from the chains of the system because Willard kills Kurtz out of abhorrence for the system and out of an understanding of its implications. On his journey Willard comes to understand that the generation of the fathers has betrayed him, and upon arrival at his destination, he is charged with the task of killing Abraham himself. Captain Willard, who in essence is the incarnation of Isaac, kills Abraham at the behest of Abraham (Kurtz). Thus Kurtz attempts to save himself in his death as well as to atone for Abraham's deeds. Kurtz attempts to restart history all over again. He attempts to save one soul, the soul of his son who is also his brother: Captain Willard. In this, Kurtz attempts to unify (and integrate) the model of Cain and Abel with the model of the father who sacrifices his son, and then he tries to dismantle both these models.

16.3.3 Fight Club—Tyler Durden

The movie *Fight Club* is an attempt to show how it is that insanity has become the only way to cope with what Marcuse (1964) refers to as the "one-dimensional man." Insanity and the one-dimensional man are two sides of the same coin. While the one-dimensional man represents the set of values that collapsed with the defeat of the white male, insanity represents the new story that has emerged out of the void. The author of *Fight Club* chooses to show us the conflict by means of the dialogue between the unnamed protagonist of the film and Tyler Durden, his alter ego. Like a prisoner in a concentration camp, the protagonist remains unnamed, and the only clue to his name is in sentences like "I am Jack's cold sweat." Durden says:

"The things you own end up owning you… You're not your job. You're not how much money you have in the bank. You're not the car you drive. You're not the contents of your wallet. You're not your fucking khakis. You're the all-singing, all-dancing crap of the world… It's only after we've lost everything that we're free to do anything…" (Linson et al., 1999)

Kurtz likely could have said the same thing: "Have you ever considered any real freedoms? Freedoms from the opinion of others… even the opinions of yourself?" Tyler Durden makes us confront that fact that even if we have not "murdered God"

"Our fathers were our models for God. If our fathers bailed, what does that tell you about God?… You have to consider the possibility that God does not like you. He never wanted you. In all probability, he hates you. This is not the worst thing that can happen… We don't need him!… Fuck damnation, man! Fuck redemption! We're God's unwanted children" (Linson et al., 1999).

Tyler exposes for us our one-dimensional and one-use reality. As the hero of the film (Edward Norton) says: "Tyler, you are by far the most interesting single-serving friend I've ever met" (Linson et al., 1999).

As Foucault (1965) claims, insanity grows from within. It stems from an alienated and hollow existence. Indeed Foucault goes on to say that there is insanity in all of us. Similarly, the hero of *Fight Club* says: "It was on the tip of everyone's tongue. Tyler and I just gave it a name." And indeed, on the journey into the horror of Vietnam, insanity is found in each of us. This cannot be denied—it is a result of living in the gray area in which each one of us can become the prey or the predator—or both (Agamben, 1998; Levi, 1959). The insane person states the truth: God, even if He exists, hates us. The alternatives we have created, the pornography and the shopping channels, are nothing but a choice of emptiness. We have simply forgotten what Sarah has always known—life (in particular if ruled by a psychotic God) is a form of black humor. Life has been planned in order to wreak havoc on everything that is important and to leave nothing of us behind. Even before we die we have already been turned into dust and ashes.

This being the case, in the beginning, Tyler Durden constitutes the model of ultimate release. He responds to the cries of a woman attempting to commit suicide (Marla), and in responding to the distress of another he ostensibly solves the problem put forth by Camus in *The Fall.* Yet even awareness that the only way to save oneself is to save another, does not help Clamence break out of his anemic, passive, and selfish condition and truly help someone else. At the end of the book Clamence admits to himself that even if the girl was to jump off the bridge again he would not jump in to save her. But the problem is more serious. Tyler (Brad Pitt) is the other side of the hero of the movie, someone who is at least partially insane. And despite the sense that Tyler is a model for life and for salvation, he is not real and the one who responds to the woman's cries for help is not a man who is level-headed in his thinking, but rather insane.

Like Kurtz, Tyler Durden wants to grant the world new hope. The hero of the movie, the narrator, ultimately does not want to destroy the world if the price is taking human lives. When Tyler erases the names of the members of the cult (the hero of the movie has no name while the crazy one does), the nameless hero of the film shouts out the name "Bob" after Bob has been shot. The duplications are inspired by Kafka's story, "In the Penal Colony" (2007): the exchange of roles between victim and accuser, the self-flagellation of the hero of the movie, the perpetrator who now becomes the one to be later sentenced—he is the judge, the prosecutor, and the mourner. Ultimately insanity becomes automatic (that is, with its source in the divine) and thus gains control over our lives.

The hero of *Fight Club*, a member of a generation that grew up with posttraumatic fathers (his father abandoned him when he was six) and that served in the Vietnam War, tries to revive his brother-in-arms. In doing so he discovers that this brother-in-arms, captive and shell-shocked, does not want to return to the existing system (e.g., Nick). He wants to destroy it and to begin again. In a certain sense this is the only option for him and for the posttraumatic survivor. The posttraumatic man in the postmodern era understands that he must respond to the other, yet this response is not according to the model of Levinas (2006). To respond to the other, to the stranger within you, is to return to your body and to return the body of the other to him, to return to a prereflective condition. To go back to being an animal. This is the way to dismantle the murderous traumatic mechanism.

To be a "rebellious individual" is first and foremost to rebel against yourself. To help the other means to help him discover the animal within him, the murderer within himself, the insanity within him—to awaken him from the coma of consumerism. Tyler understands this and thus makes the following statement:

"All the ways you wish you could be, that's me. I look like you wanna look, I fuck like you wanna fuck, I am smart, capable, and most importantly, I am free in all the ways that you are not" (Linson et al., 1999).

Tyler represents a state of mind according to which "it's only after we've lost everything that we're free to do anything."

At the end of the movie we understand that Tyler is the observer and the new God of anarchy. The protagonist of the movie, an ostensibly sane character, is a Don Quixote battling today's windmills: the credit card companies, the undisputed masters who are stronger than God and reason—the ones who determine what the truth is. We should remember that Don Quixote dies when he sees and recognizes reality as it is, but Tyler Durden offers us an alternative—one that is violent and whose price is human life. In this sense the difference between Tyler Durden and Franz Fanon (1968) becomes blurred, and the question is whether we are really interested in yet another violent revolution, for ultimately Tyler Durden does not oppose murder. Rather the opposite is true—he encourages it.

On another level we learn from the story of Tyler Durden how big and beautiful ideas ultimately lead to uncontrollable and uncontrolled acts of murder, like God's outburst in the story of Sodom. In view of the dominant posttraumatic experience, the problem is that it is not certain whether there is another choice, a nonviolent path for the posttraumatic individual to follow.

There is a great deal of similarity between Meursault *(The Stranger)* and Tyler Durden *(Fight Club)*. They both experience Kafkaesque emptiness. They both conduct their lives on the margins of society. They both are fed up with one-dimensionality and with hypocrisy. They both are totally authentic. And ultimately they both attempt to remove the mask, a crime whose punishment is death. Hence they both must be killed. Society has no other way of containing them. Yet can the machine in "The Penal Colony" decide what word to carve on their bodies? "courage," "daring," "innocence," "authenticity," or perhaps "misery" or simply "Mom." What should be carved on Kurtz, when all he can say is "the horror, the horror?" The machine does not know what to carve. Anarchy controls everything.

16.4 Cursed Duality: Self-Annihilation as Dybbuk

In the movie *Fight Club* we encounter its nameless protagonist: a man who slowly stops knowing when he is asleep and when he is awake, when he is himself and when he is Tyler, when he beats up on himself and when he is being beaten up by others, when he is alive and when he is dead, or when he is the victim and when he is the victimizer. Exactly like an individual who has undergone a trauma. After experiencing trauma, an individual lives in two separate and distinct dimensions that clash with one another. One of the characters always moves along the path of murderer and the other along that of the victim, though it is never clear "which is which and who is who" (Pink Floyd, 1973). As I claimed, this is the case with Captain Willard and Kurtz in *Apocalypse Now,* who are actually the same character. This is also the case with Michael and Nick in *The Deer Hunter.* That same eternal sense of sin binds the monotheistic individual, the one who constantly battles the accounts book, who must always be his own judge and constantly examine himself. Thus we are always accompanied by the same judge, the same hangman, and the same observer (the mirror in the opening scene of *Taxi Driver*). This incongruity erupts during trauma. Indeed trauma is the result of overdeveloped consciousness. That is, trauma is the illness of consciousness. In the traumatic condition we constantly examine life from afar and therefore never live life to the fullest. Absolute trauma contains only observation, without any point of reference, without an observer (Ataria, 2014; 2015; in press; Ataria & Gallagher, 2015). There is no body to grab onto, and it is clear that the sense of self has collapsed.

The hero of *Fight Club* does not attack himself but rather the one observing him. He attempts to rid himself of that judgmental character. Kurtz, too, is not willing to die at the hands of the judge. He is only willing to die at the hands of Captain Willard and only at the last minute does he totally identify with him. The posttraumatic character cannot go on living with this duality, with this sense that more than one person inhabits the same body – structural dissociation (Nijenhuis, van der Hart, & Steele, 2010). The posttraumatic condition is one in which the split has become too manifest, indeed insufferable from the point of view of the individual experiencing it. The solution is always the death of one of the characters. Thus, in *The Deer Hunter* the director gives us the impression that it is Michael who shoots Nick rather than Nick who is shooting himself (Morag, 2009). Yet they are the same character. Whether Nick shoots himself or Michael shoots Nick does not much matter. This same duality also represents the condition of the posttraumatic individual who is always embroiled in some sort of impossible conflict. This conflict is between the different characters within, characters whose desires diverge more and more as the conflict deepens, the gap widens and the two characters distance themselves one from the other more and more.

This era is characterized by an impossible inner conflict that is worsening each and every moment of our lives. This paradox, when it erupts, always does so in the form of an apocalyptic dybbuk. In the case of Travis in *Taxi Driver,* this is a semi-messianic act. In the case of Gregor Samsa in Kafka's *Metamorphosis,* the dybbuk erupts when the character turns into a cockroach and only ends when he relinquishes his "human" existence and remains only with the core truth—he is a cockroach: "We are transformed into the phantoms glimpsed yesterday evening" (Levi, 1959, p. 21).

Only death speaks to the posttraumatic individual, the one who cannot but see, who always finds himself at noontide and who knows that the attempt to cope with the judgmental system always leads to dying like a dog. The posttraumatic individual can only speak the language of blood and death. Michael, the hunter, understands this. He understands that words in themselves represent the prevaricating systems in which we are located and therefore he can only attempt to save Nick by playing Russian roulette.

Words have no meaning. Therefore, Meursault *(The Stranger)* chooses to remain silent during his trial. The posttraumatic individual understands that there is only one way—to return to the old playing board and not just to change the moves played but first and foremost to change the rules of the game. Michael, the hunter, attempts to do this and fails. Tyler Durden from *Fight Club* is convinced that by means of the collapse of the economic system this is possible; perhaps. He also knows that the only way to succeed in this assignment is to adopt God's techniques. Therefore, when the sane side of Tyler Durden (the character played by Edward Norton) attempts to stop the process, he cannot. Tyler predicted that his humanity would suddenly appear and therefore gave a specific order: From the moment the operation begins, it must not be stopped, even if he himself gives an order to that effect. Tyler Durden thus adopts God's automatic course. He understands that this is the only way to take matters to the end—with the indifference of the Kafkaesque machine. Meeting goals requires acting in a cold and emotionless manner "mass produced by dozens of careless hands" (Solzhenitsyn, 1968). Only thus is it possible to lead us back toward the Big Bang, to return to the starting point, to begin again.

From the perspective of the posttraumatic individual life itself has no meaning and therefore death has no meaning as well. Death is preferable to life without a home, a life of total alienation. When Travis, the taxi driver, returns "home" he understands this, and he cannot tolerate the inner filth. The filth on the streets of New York symbolizes his inner world as well as the collapse of the world of values he had once believed in. Like Captain Willard and like Kurtz, Travis returns to a bestial state. All the heroes understand that the human condition does not allow one to be human. It is necessary to take a step back, to a prehuman bestial state. In such a state violence is not a matter of choice but rather an uncontrollable dybbuk. In that world, there is no longer room for humanity. Clamence *(The Fall)* is proof of this. Clamence tells the story of human beings in this era, of self-consciousness that leads nowhere apart from impotence, thus resulting in the need for a total revolution. Slap does not help, nor does crying out (as in the case of Clamence). Only a pistol pointed at the temple. Only an unending stream of dead can generate any change whatsoever.

16.5 Patricide

In a world after Sarah was struck dumb, the male is helpless. He thinks that patricide will solve the problem, but it is not certain that this is what will happen. The main idea in this context appears in Kafka's short story, "The Judgment" (1971). From this story we learn that *even a horrible father is preferable to a world without any anchor*. Living in the shadow of a supreme authority, even though it is nothing more than a form of "divine justice" that is mechanical, technical, childish, and violent, is preferable to a reality in which the figure of the father in the broadest sense of the term (set of values, unwritten laws, divinity/tyranny) collapses, as it does, for example, in "The Penal Colony."

In a situation in which the father is no longer in the picture, a world in which the son has justifiably killed his father and God, the son is left with irreconcilable guilt feelings and an impossible guilt complex. This leads to the need to create a guilt that can be comprehended. This is a major and important turning point—killing the father does not help because on the macro level this patricide leaves you on the same playing field but without an anchor, a situation in which anarchy controls everything.

References

Agamben, G. (1998). *Homo Sacer: Sovereign Power and Bare Life*. Stanford: Stanford University Press.

Ataria, Y. (in press). When the Body Becomes the Enemy: Disownership toward the Body. *Philosophy, Psychiatry & Psychology*.

Ataria, Y. (2014). Acute peritraumatic dissociation: In favor of a phenomenological inquiry. *Journal of Trauma & Dissociation, 15*(3), 332–347. doi:10.1080/15299732.2013.853722.

Ataria, Y. (2015). Sense of ownership and sense of agency during trauma. *Phenomenology and the Cognitive Sciences, 14*(1), 199–212. doi:10.1007/s11097-013-9334-y.

Ataria, Y., & Gallagher, S. (2015). Somatic apathy: Body disownership in the context of torture. *Journal of Phenomenological Psychology, 46*(1), 105–122.

Benyamini, I. (2011). *Abraham's laughter [Hebrew]*. Tel-Aviv: Resling.

Camus, A. (1962a). *The Rebel*. (A. Bower, Trans.). Harmondsworth: Penguin Books.

Camus, A. (1962b). *The Stranger*. (S. Gilbert, Trans.). New York: Vitage Books.

Camus, A. (1975). *The myth of Sisyphus*. (J. O'Brien, Trans.). London: Penguin.

Camus, A. (2000). *The Fall*. (J. O'Brien, Trans.). London: Penguin.

Cimino, M. (Director). (1978). *The deer hunter* [Motion Picture].

Conrad, J. (1990). *Heart of darkness*. New York: Dover Publications.

Coppola, F. F. (Producer), Conrad, J. (Writer), & Coppola, F. F. (Director). (1979). *Apocalypse Now* [Motion Picture].

Fanon, F. (1968). *The Wretched of the Earth*. (C. Farrington, Trans.). New York: Grove Press.

Pink Floyd. (1973). Us and them. *On the dark side of the moon*. P. Floyd.

Foucault, M. (1965). *Madness and civilization*. New York: Pantheon Books.

Freud, S. (1939). *Moses and monotheism*. (K. Jones, Trans.). New York: Vintage Books.

Heller, J. (1961). *Catch-22*. New York: Simon & Schuster.

Hellman, J. (1982). Vietnam and the hollywood genre film: Inversions of American mythology in the deer hunter and apocalypse now. *American Quarterly, 34*(4), 418–439.

Herman, J. L. (1992). *Trauma and recovery*. New York: Basic Books.

Houellebecq, M. (2000). *The elementary particles*. (F. Wynne, Trans.). New York: Knopf.

Jaspers, K. (2001). *The question of German guilt*. (E. B. Ashton, Trans.). New York: Fordham University Press.

Kafka, F. (1949). *The diaries of Franz Kafka* (Vol. 1). (M. Brod, Ed., & J. Kresh, Trans.). New York: Schocken Books.

Kafka, F. (1971). The Judgment. In *The Complete Stories by Franz Kafka* (W. Muir, & E. Muir, Trans., pp. 101–113). New York: Schocken Books.

Kafka, F. (2006). *The Trial*. (D. Wyllie, Trans.) .Teddington: Echo Library.

Kafka, F. (2007). In the Penal Colony. In *Kafka's Selected Stories, Norton Critical Edition* (S. Corngold, Trans., pp. 35–59). New York: Norton.

Levi, P. (1959). *If this is a man*. (S. Woolf, Trans.) New York: The Orion Press.

Levinas, E. (2006). *Humanism of the other*. (N. Poller, Trans.) Urbana; Chicago: University of Illinois Press.

Linson, A., Chaffin, C., Bell, R. G. (Producers), & Fincher, D. (Director). (1999). *Fight Club* [Motion Picture].

Marcuse, H. (1964). *One-dimensional man*. Boston, MA: Beacon.

Morag, R. (2009). *Defeated masculinity: Post-traumatic cinema in the aftermath of war*. New York: P.I.E. Peter Lang.

Nijenhuis, E., van der Hart, O., & Steele, K. (2010). Trauma-related structural dissociation of the personality. *Activitas Nervosa Superior, 52*(1), 1–23.

Schrader, P. (Writer), & Scorsese, M. (Director). (1976). *Taxi Driver* [Motion Picture].

Solzhenitsyn, A. (1968). *The first circle*. (T. P. Whitney, Trans.). New York: Harper & Row.

Kopelson, A. (Producer), Stone, O. (Writer), & Stone, O. (Director). (1986). *Platoon* [Motion Picture].

Terr, L. (1984). Time and trauma. *Psychoanalytic Study of the Child, 39*, 633–665.

17 Laius Complex and Shocks of Maternality: With Franz Kafka and Sylvia Plath

Bracha Lichtenberg Ettinger

17.1 A Death Gift: From Abraham to Kafka's Father-Figure—The Delirium of Laius

> God is the name of the possibility I have of keeping a secret that is visible from the interior but not from the exterior. Once such a structure of conscience exists, of being-with-oneself, of speaking, that is, of producing invisible sense, once I have within me, *thanks to the invisible word as such*, a witness that others cannot see, and who is therefore at the same time *other than me and more intimate with me than myself*, once I have a secret relationship with myself and not tell everything, once there is a secrecy and secret witness within me, then what I call God exists [...] I call myself God [...] God calls me, if it is on that condition that I can call myself or that I am called in secret. God is in me, he is the absolute "me" or "self," he is that structure of absolute interiority that is called, in Kirkegaard's sense, subjectivity. And he is made manifest, he manifests his non-manifestation when, in the structures of the living or the entity, there appears in the course of phylo- and ontogenetic history, the possibility of secrecy, however differentiated, complex, plural and overdetermined it be, that is, when there appears the desire and power to render absolutely invisible and to constitute within oneself, a witness of that invisibility. That is the history of God, and of the name of God as the history of secrecy, a history that is at the same time secret and without any secrets. Such history is also an economy. (Derrida, 1996, pp. 108–109)

Let's think on Abraham first.

Sacrifice without sacrifice, according to Derrida, is the *History of men* only. Male-fathers–male-sons. Each time a son is lost then saved by the father, intended for sacrifice then saved by the father, pushed to fall, but then caught by the father alone—is it not an Abrahamic route?

Men's endless debt toward *sacrifice without sacrifice* of the finally saved son.

Derrida emphasizes that *death giving* to the son is a *men's only* affair. But is it not *a perverse* men's only affair when pushed to an edge where the son is not at all saved? A kind of *père*-version (*father*-version), to use Lacan's favorite expression? In perversion the objectivity of the other is affirmed and its vulnerability is denied.

The Kafkaesque son is oppressed by the *pretense of innocence* of the destructive father. Franz Kafka's father saw in his infant a true monster and thus became his tyrant. Kafka writes to the father whose game he will always lose: "From your armchair you ruled the world. Your opinion was correct, every other was mad, wild, *meshugge*, not normal" (Kafka, 1966, p. 35).

According to Walter Benjamin "[F]athers in Kafka's strange families batten on their sons, lying on top of them like giant parasites. They not

B.L. Ettinger, Ph.D. (✉)
Philosophy, Art & Critical Thought, European Graduate School (EGS), Saas-Fee, Switzerland
e-mail: brachastudio@gmail.com

Y. Ataria et al. (eds.), *Interdisciplinary Handbook of Trauma and Culture*,
DOI 10.1007/978-3-319-29404-9_17

only prey upon their strength, but gnaw away at the sons' right to exist. The fathers punish, but they are at the same time the accusers. The sin of which they accuse their sons seems to be a kind of original sin." "[O]ne is sentenced not only in innocence but also in ignorance" (Benjamin, 2007, p. 114). "In Kafka the written law is contained in books, but these are secret; by basing itself on them the prehistoric world exerts its rule all the more ruthlessly" (Benjamin, 2007, p. 115).

The Kafkaesque *perfect crime*, according to Jean-Francois Lyotard "does not consist in killing the victim or the witnesses" but rather "in obtaining the silence of the witnesses, the deafness of the judges, and the craziness (insanity) of the testimony" (Lyotard, 1996, p. 8). Jean-François Lyotard speaks of *the wrong* as the damage that goes together with the loss of the means to prove the part of the other in one's damaging oppressing. One loses these means, "for example, if the author of the damages turns out directly or indirectly to be one's judge." (Lyotard, 1996, p. 8). Ordinary communication is not enough for such a situation: a *differend*. One needs to invent "idioms."

How can a subject resist injustice when the father not only rules the system of justice but also appropriates the right to disobey it, occupying both positions, that of a narcissistic child and that of the Father? The machine is bigger than what Oedipus can contain. Deleuze and Guattari identify in their *Kafka—Toward a Minor Literature* an *exaggerated Oedipus* in action (Deleuze & Guattari, 1986, p. 9). But, in my view, it is not even an exaggerated Oedipus. Rather, it is a Laius. Unconscious or simply hidden. The son can discover the secret of Oedipus. After all, it is the subject-as-son who invented Oedipus. What the son cannot discover is the secret of Abraham. And perhaps, up to a point only. What the son can never discover is the secret of Laius. Such is precisely the material kept out of the son's reach. Isaac doesn't guess the intentions of Abraham, and if he does, he assumes for him the innocence he claims. But the son of Laius is not meant to survive. If he survives, his witnessing will enter the idiom of the differend. It will not be heard. The witness will be silenced, his testimony considered insane.

Behind the Kafkaesque power mechanisms of the Law, understood by Deleuze and Guattari as magnification and exaggeration of Oedipus Complex, a more powerful secret mechanism functions in the psychic and social field, originating in my view from a position of paternality in a Laius Complex. Secret father–son links are established under this père-version. When to the paternal "perfect crime" the son-Kafka replied with a seemingly Oedipus masquerade, it is perhaps because a son caught in the Laius delirium of a father can't discover his secret and truly live.

Let's talk about Laius.

Laius abducted and raped Chrysippus, the son of a king who was his host. In trying to escape Laius, Chrysippus fell or jumped from the top of a hill and was killed. When Laius' own son Oedipus was born, Laius ordered him killed on Mount Cithaeron.

The impulse of Laius is double. The first is envious erotic-aggressive: to seduce his friend's son and then rape him, to own his youth's treasures, his beauty, perhaps his creativity. This he cannot help: if another father's son jumps to his death—the real father's pain Laius doesn't share. Then follows a second impulse—to kill his own son. The abducted host's son was killed, the natural son was saved by a shepherd. The shepherd is the one who, like the mother preceding our birth, carries. The carrier feel-knows in the Real some secret that mothers, birthing or not birthing, already know. A value that Laius stands for its destruction.

A Laius delirium might fatally hit a father–son relation. If Abraham's is a secret *sacrifice without sacrifice*—Abraham seduced his son to death then saved him before he fell—Laius' is a *secret sacrifice per se*: the perfect crime.

When to Derrida's Abrahamic *death-gift* and to Kierkegaard's sacrifice I add the Laius secret delirium, the different nuances concern the *perfect crime* of *betrayal* combined with the *paternal pretense of innocence*. Laius' act doesn't enter the economy of "sacrifice-without-sacrifice" but a projective paranoid-narcissistic commerce of the enactment of symbolic death-giving to a son-object by way of a *seduction into death*. To avoid being succeeded by a creative son and to live the fantasy of surviving the son, the father seduces him to self-destruction. The symbolization of a Laius projective-paranoid scene is disguised by one prevailing law or by another, by some kind of social framing. Betrayal not only in the name of a rule fixed by the paternal figure but moreover, betrayal under the wings of the relationships' confidentiality; a secret betrayal.

Such a paternal desire for death-gift, kept secret by the rules of the father alone, a desire which originates in the becoming-father subjectivity of the father-analyst (and not from the infantile father-symbol and father-image that the son-analysand holds) is structured in a *Laius Complex* hidden behind the Oedipus Complex, masked by it, but entirely different from it. It is dyadic. It doesn't enter triangulation. This unique son is dangerous to me, he must be sacrificed to calm down some not-yet yet as-if symbolic paternality in a dyad that no m/Other can guess. The betrayal strike is enacted under some Law fulfilling mask. Laius hides himself behind some symbolically sustained paternal masquerade offered to the community.

When a patient is receptor of the analyst-Laius' direct projection or transference (disguised as a countertransferential reaction to the patient's unconscious)—a catastrophe might be solicited. The patient's psyche is perhaps invaded by a countertransferential delirium. Under the shock of betrayal, and too late in the sense of the earlier trusting that sustained the link, seduction into death occurs precisely at the site where the archaic maternal seduction into life is located, at the location of maternal response-ability to the trusting vulnerable infant. This paternal dyad abuses the primary trust that was once invested in the maternal dyad from which the son is paradoxically supposed to split itself with the help of this same paternal figure who fills the function of a symbolic father.

Derrida marks the difference between unknown as mystery, a forever secret, and unknown as simply hidden. The Laius death-gift, is, in my view, a well-hidden, well-kept, and unacknowledged secret. The son (patient, analysand) enters the realm of the sacrificed through the symbolic father's (analyst's) promise to offer the son some future love, i.e., through the analyst's assumed occupation of the locus of a maternal seduction into life. First weaving himself in the originary matrixial web, then tearing it apart—the betrayal of the trust that emerged in this stratum is a catastrophe to the "son's" psyche.

Can the awareness to the matrixial-maternal sphere moderate a Laius Delirium? In a subject-space of ethical carriance the economy of "it's either you or me" will fail; this calls for the introduction of ethics at the heart of the transferential field. The matrixial symbolic calls upon the father–son dyad to mark a space that will fail its economy of "it's either me, your father, or you, my son." Not only the Laius non-maternal yet dy*adic* economy must be revealed. We can also offer to try to transform it. Its alternative yet twin *triadic* pact, edifice and economy, that of the secret paternal *sacrifice without sacrifice*, the Abrahamic secret, can be opened to more daylight as well. "It's *either my* God or you *my* son" can also be transformed. The symbolic of (and sublimation from) corpo-real carriance can moderate the sacrificial delirious dyad and the imaginary triad (there where no woman-mother is represented either) if the foreclosed archaic maternality enters the structure of the subject.

The son's attempt to escape a Laius is doomed since this father-figure wears a masquerade of innocence. However, the projection of his delusions is the source, *not the reaction*, to the son's trouble born *during* the analysis. When a father figure dwells inside the disavowal of his Laius delirium (and imagines his projection to be *counter*transferential), the son's creativity is pathologized. The vulnerable son-patient who looks for the analyst-father's love in trust is psychoticized (the daughter hystericized). The Laius delirium enacts, to use Kafka's idiom: a "perfect crime." The analyst seems to offer Oedipal countertransferential interpretations (you, son, want to kill me, father, etc.). A Kafka-son, as we know, will assume his father's innocence, and start to exaggerate the Oedipus machine, to use a Deleuze and Guattari expression.

However, and unlike the analyst-father, Kafka's father was not just his symbolic and imaginary one but also his real one. The analyst can inhabit a father's position in the Symbolic and the Imaginary, without paying the price the Real father has to pay when the son jumps off the hill. Another father, not the analyst, will carry the parental pain, the parental sorrow. The analyst can replace the real father and triumph over him in the Symbolic; the structure, the setting, the theory and the practice of expressing direct countertransferential association invites this move. In case of a fall, the analytical son—unlike the real one—is always replaceable for a Laius figure.

It is now classical to talk about "negative transference." What about negative countertransference? What if a negative countertransference is not the reaction but the direct projection from the analyst's mind? What if it is an expression of frustration? The "negative countertransference" usually first flows toward the patient's intimate others—the analysand's past and present significant non-I(s): mother, father, environment. Laius ignores the possibility of the analysand's compassion toward its others. Ignoring the matrixial space itself is a trauma to the transubjective field produced during the analytic process itself.

The Oedipus Complex is a child-version of what *does the father want*. In the Oedipus Complex the Father is viewed from the infant's eyes. Yet other paternal possibilities are born with the arrival of parentality. Laius is one of the figures that mark a father-version of what a father wants. Here, by pere-version, the vulnerable infant is reduced to an object, and the mother is denied.

17.2 Carriance Envoided

The matrixial-maternal alliance, different from the mother–infant symbiosis, offers symbolic means to interfere with a delirious dyad. A principle of maternal intervention in a dyad streams from a sphere not only foreclosed but rather e*nvoided* in psychoanalysis. The ethics of carriance-in-compassion and wit(h)nessing that it entails supplies a resistance to Laius.

If, following Derrida, every father–son's sacrificial route is a between-men-only affair, what is radically disavowed, neither simply repressed nor just foreclosed, is in fact "mother" as a symbolic principle for meaning. Think via Sara the Abraham–Isaac triangle with God, think via the sorrow of Mary, think via the naming of Eve. The maternal-feminine-matrixial symbolic serves not only to interfere with a father–son hallucinatory dyad but suggests to it an outlet. In the move from Derrida's Abrahamic *sacrifice without sacrifice* where *women play no role* to the Laius sacrifice where women play no role *even more extremely*, inspired by the feminine-maternal-matrixial, I suggest to rethink the structure of the subject. *Subject as carrier*. I carry *therefore* I am. Moses is *Father* precisely because he carries like the mother carries infants. It is from this position that Moses expresses his trauma:

> And Moses said unto the LORD: 'Wherefore hast Thou dealt ill with Thy servant? and wherefore have I not found favour in Thy sight, that Thou layest the burden of all this people upon me? Have I conceived all this people? have I brought them forth [*gave them birth*], that Thou shouldest say unto me: Carry them in thy bosom, as a nursing-father [*nursing-mother*] carrieth the sucking child (*in brackets: my translation from the Hebrew*. Nubmers ch. 11, 11–12)

It is also from a similar subject position that Isaiah expresses his traumatic moment

> Even to old age I am the same, and even to hoar hairs will I carry you; I have made, and I will bear; yea, I will carry, and will deliver. (Isaiah 46, 4)

The "remedy" to paternal sacrificial delirium in a psychoticized dyad will not come from irony and amusement, which turn the son's relation to life and death into a game in which a Laius-father will always win. Is not the idea of the son-subject as being-toward-death related to the secret of the father's being-and-viewpoint of *subject-for-giving-death?* Can the feminine-maternal-matrix subject-space disentangle this hidden contractus? In a matrixial coemergence the becoming-mother encounters and witnesses the vulnerability of a subject whose *being-toward-birth-with-in-another* is to be accounted for too whenever a subject is being here, once the subject has already been born, when the other is a subject for the I, a vulnerable other in primordial trust.

A-priori envoided, a-posteriory invalidated, reapostasied as mystical—how to render effective this surplus, this more-than-repression, this more-than foreclosure, this not-exactly disavowal of *this* maternal thing? "Foreclosure" refers to the

Name of the Father and predestines to psychosis. Longing to the father's benediction, in the vestibule we wait. Shocks of maternality endure traumatically in the vestibule, and under silencing they grow, again and again silenced under the Symbolic and the Imaginary that serves Abraham and Laius through the tropes of Sacrifice. The env*oidance* of the maternal-matrixial subject-space is different from foreclosure, as here a disavowal is denied, and its object apostasied.

When Jacob renames his son Ben-Oni as Benjamin, the maternal shock of Rachel is invalidated, the trace of her real experience with her intimate other is disavowed and the meaning of her web of *sub*real strings is negated. Devoid of the symbolic potential impact of her experience as she is birthing-dying, the potential im-pact of her archaic alliance is envoided (Ettinger, 2013).

In a moderate form, a Laius paternal figure will destroy the son's creativity by means of its systematic reframing as pathological. In a countertransferential *father–son contractus* ruled by a Laius delirium the maternal becomes subjectless entity, replaced by a slogan, a ready-made pretext or alibi disguised as meaningful, a deus-ex-machina "cause" and retroactive source of just any psychic trouble. The offer of the mother-slogan is repetitive, and the repetition of the offering of such a figure-as-cause testifies to the work of the death-drive in the analytical space. We can easily recognize the *ready-made mother-monster* slogan; it is expressed via frozen ideas organized around one of the three primal mother-phantasies. Abandonment, Devouring, and Not-enoughness (Ettinger, 2010). To let the feminine-maternal inform subject, culture and politics, we have to first to recognize and then respect the shocks that fragilize her.

Knowledge of carriance indicates a process of co/in-habit(u)ation (Ettinger, 2006a, pp. 157–161) and announces the function of the implicated witness. Here, a space-subject appears in a subject-space of a-symmetrical coemergence and cofading.

The Ethics implied by the crossing between maternal *carriance, desire to give life and seduction into life*, and the *infant's primal trust* can, I hope, interfere with the desire of Laius. It can moderate the human Abrahamic *desire to give death*, to use an expression of Derrida, and the seduction into death I find in the *Laius delirium* I will present. With each enactment of a Laius delirium, the mode of compassion with-in carriance is more than denied. It is *envoided*.

If Laius, contrary to Oedipus, is a means to address some features of symbolic paternality as belonging to an originary adult-subject position when already-always subject and ethics are to be considered together, one way to think of this position passes through the relations that come as a shock to the becoming-father too, the relation to the other at its most vulnerable stage and position. The proximity to a vulnerable other without a passage through the maternal-matrixial corporeal shock, can be addressed in Levinas' ethical terms, when he recognizes that precisely in such relations *the impulse to kill* arises. Therefore, I-father shall not sacrifice! As an Abraham, indeed, the impulse to kill tempts me from the inside. The voice of Abraham seduces me from the inside to seduce my son onto death. But the eye of Cain looks at me from the grave. The eye of Cain orders me to disobey my desire to kill the vulnerable other. I have realized my force—I am becoming too strong—my impulse directs me toward a Laius' jouissance—I will resist it. Facing the vulnerable other, I will now allow the matrixial compassion to inform my desire. I shall fragilize myself. And if I failed, I will recognize my failure: I have failed to carry you. I suggest that to reach an ethical position of paternality where to have more power will mean to have more responsibility, not tyranny, we have to reach the paternal position by through acknowledgment of the maternal-matrixial Symbolic.

Being-with-oneself-with-in and in-resonance-with another: (m)othering-in-carriance, en-trusting. Being-with-non-self, looking in remembrance and still and yet *unturning* into a pillar of salt. I have failed to carry you. Still. *I must carry you.*

17.3 Shocks of Maternality and Mother–Daughter Knots

Young mothers are fragilized by the force of a sudden unexpected love, by sudden and irremediable response-ability and responsibility, by the enormous trust directed toward them by the infant, by the shock, sorrow, and jouissance of their care-carry mode of com-passion. Vulnerable, they are facing a new reality, realizing their deep transconnectedness to the vulnerable other. The weight of this carriance-and-trust estranges them in a world lacking the language to account for it, where affects, different from anxiety yet with similar resonance, lack recognition or value; a world where trust already expects a betrayal. The recognition of the Symbolic matrix can intervene to stop the performance of a potential betraying agency, to awaken self-awareness to one's own such power. This self-awareness is ethical. You shall not sacrifice the other. You shall not betray the trusting, vulnerable other. You shall be aware of your possible desire to perform a *seduction into death* and use your awareness to stop it.

To preserve trust as a human capacity needed for a life, for both ethical life and aesthetic enjoyment, means to perceive the potential for sacrificing the other, this kind of *potential for betrayal* in the adult. Carriance is the resistance to Sacrifice. Sacrifice is based on a certain prototype of the paternal that appears as neutral yet is a modus of betrayal, a secret perversion.

You carry, you wit(h)ness, you will give witness. The matrixial-maternal analyst-witness doesn't, or doesn't only, contain the carried in empathy (disguised as compassion yet narcissistic and Oedipal.) The witness carries in compassion, or in *empathy-within-compassion*, where the archaic significant others of my other are embraced in the process too. The *Laius figure* stands for the envoidance of the meaning of carriance. The kernel of a Laius' infanticide impulses dwells in the rejection of the life cycle that between generations is the timeline of difference-in-continuity. This impulse equals the rejection of the subject's future's creativity to which matrixial transconnectedness does attests. Motherhood traumatizes the mother-figure. Love fragilizes her. Self-fragilization, postpartum depression, psychosis, hypersensitivity, vulnerability, love-anxiety, care-anxiety. The hyper-response-ability, the shock of responsibility. And even the shock of the continual wit(h)nessing to-with one's non-I(s) and the weight of witnessing to the vulnerable other. Wit(h)nessing transforms witnessing. In compassion I shall witness. I will carry you.

Carriance is a symbol for the sublimation from the Real of maternal carrying. The Real of being carried by a female-maternal body-psyche absorbs its effects. This Real includes elements and a web of strings between elements from the subreal level, psychic traces of the contact between carrying elements and elements carried as well as unconscious traces of the experience of the maternal figure as a subject, not object, of carriance, transconnected to the I. Psychic traces of the links and of the exchanges on that transubjective level are inscribed in the archaic atmosphere where trust of an extremely vulnerable subject-infant is invested in the extremely fragile subject-mother. Primary carriance and trust labor in the depth-work of borderlinking at the level of the Subreal, where through strings and threads and resonance, interior kernels, the interiority of the self and the interiority of the other, open distances in proximity and become sensitive to the proximity in a distance. Imprints of the maternal carriance inform me as subject. But the moment of actual corporeality of carriance comes to me as mother as a shock. Traumatized then, precisely then—new buds of subjectivity emerge in me.

With the recognition of trans(sub)jectivity, certain psychic configurations—that otherwise manifest themselves in autist-like refusal, rebellion, and "hysteria," which hint at the pain that results from their foreclosure and envoidance on the level of culture, which hint at the disrecognition within this culture of the figure of the real mother *as subject*—find some symbolic relief.

A radical dimension of subjectivity emerges with the arrival of real, imaginary, and symbolic parentality. A new stratum of subjectivity emerges, for which not the infantile one is to be accounted. In adulthood it germinates for the first time; in adulthood it calls for responsibility. The private Laius impulse testifies to the inability to have compassion for the vulnerable non-I. Responsibility is informed by symbolizing intimate shocks of maternality.

Sub-symbolic, subreal corpo-real borderlinks between subject-infant and (m)Other find meaning outside Oedipus, Anti-Oedipus, and Laius complexities. The matrixial relief offer paths for rethinking the woman-to-woman, mother–daughter, mother–son, and finally subject-to-subject transmission. I was first triggered by the figure of Laius to discuss the expanse of the psychic foreclosure of the mother–daughter linkage in terms of a Jocasta Complex. Subjectivization processes that foreclosed the mother-Jocasta triggered Thanatos to turn the self against the other-inside-the-self (Ettinger, 2006c, pp. 216–217). Laius signified seduction into death. With the figures of Lol (Ettinger, 2006b) and Diotima (Ettinger, 2007) I proposed the *seduction into life* by maternal-matrixial Eros of borderlinking (*bordureliance*). Transconnectedness between individual "internal" kernels (internal is not to be confused with the narcissistic core) is recognized while the uniqueness of each individual psyche, of each subject as such, is respected.

The infant approaches the mother with primal phantasies. The Devouring Mother, the Abandoning Mother and the phantasmatic Maternal Not-enoughness are necessary for the infant as *primal* for endless experimentation with existential lacks and partial losses. The mother approaches her infant as subject, affected in the different zones of her potential shock: (1) In the time-space of pre-maternity and pregnancy (miscarriages, abortions, processes of adoption, tensions concerning pre-parentality, infertility, fertility, pregnancy, birthing, loss and mourning, barrenness, childlessness.) (2) In the event of Birthing. (3) In the long time-space of motherhood that spreads between birthing (or the arrival of the infant) until old age, until death (separation, loss, mourning.) The mother's shocks, with their joy and their sorrow, their traces, phantasies, their corresponding anxieties, the arousals that inhabit them, are all part of the maternal corporeality and of her psyche. The zones and the processes involving them are structural, even if any actual shock is existential, contingent and singular. The production of the "ready-made mother-monster" as object—object-cause-of suffering, object-basket for disposal of psychic toxic matter during therapeutic processes—its artificial production during countertransferential "interpretations"—hurts the maternal subject in her shocks.

Compassion arousal in her, as primary as the anxiety affect, contributes to the mother's self-fragilization as she is continually borderspacing-borderlinking, unconsciously performing for her infant the non-sexual seduction-into-life. She cares-carries. The third zone of shocks (from birthing onwards) is vast; there, contrary to the earlier zones, "mother" is not necessarily a female figure, and can stand for several (few, limited plural) figures, the same or different from the figure of the earlier zones. Shocks of maternality arrive in adult life as primal. Motherhood surprises. The space of trust-wonder-care associated with the mother's shocks is precious to the psyche. Empathy (to the patient-son, patient-daughter)-within-compassion (to her (m)others as subjects that went through shocks of maternality) is caring for one's potential future-I(s). The future of the subject, not its past is at stake here.

Daughter, son and mother are all subjects touched by the enigma of the trans-generational transmission of traces of trauma, all working-through the difficulties of each singular differenciation-jointness alongside the *symbiosis-proximity-separateness* axis, and of each differentiation-in-jointness alongside the *sameness-identity-otherness* axis: differenc/tiation with-in/from an archaic female-m/Other to begin with and later on from the mother as well as from others as subjects and transjects. Matrixial trans(sub)jectivity with its vibrating strings that attune transjectivity (subject-object) and transubjectivity (subject-subject) in resonance, dissonance, and consonance, is respected when the subject in-formed by the maternal carriance evades foreclosure and resists envoidance. These psychic processes are not limited to the maternal nor to pre-natality and pregnancy. They occur at any moment, in any relationships, in men and in women, in-between, all throughout life. Carriance is in the now of the relationships.

The subject wanders in an unconscious matrixial time-space and works through its strings and its threads all throughout life. Matrixial Eros is a principle of love invested in the subreal transconnectedness between invisible kernels. When primary phantasies of rejection and destruction, accompanied by anxiety and anger, arise, metramorphic processes work to balance them. In Freud, the I is subjectivized via repetitions of the mother's rejection. In Winnicott, the I is subjectivized via repetitions of her destruction, to which she survives. When Mother is conceived as the immemorial cause and aim of destruction and the principle of love is considered as reactive, the daughter's potential for future shocks in her own maternality *grows*.

Demeter (mother) is inside and outside Persephone (daughter). A Demeter-Persephone Complex (Ettinger, 2014) designates for the daughter and the mother particular routes, positions and parameters for self-recognition. In it, the role of the mother as subject and as subjectivizing agency is emphasized. The longing and the intuition of Sylvia Plath (*Journal*), the longing and the research of Adrienne Rich (*Of Woman Born*) leads both of them to the field of this myth. Rich believed that a Complex needs to be formulated to engage mother–daughter relations, and emphasized the lost ancient ceremonies of Demeter and the Eleusinian Mysteries. In our psyche, Demeter (each mother) was a Persephone (a daughter) once. With the mother as subject different ways open for rethinking sexuality, adolescence, the becoming-woman-m/Other, bodily transformations, desire and desirability, passion and com-passion and the passage from youth to old age. My non-I is sensed not as object or second or third entity but as subject and partial-subject intra-entangled with-in me. For that reason too my non-I (mother-subject) aspires to the respect of *my* analyst (parental figure): recognizing self and other over time along a Daughter-Mother/Non-mother-Crone continuity is respecting the potential or virtual other with-in the self which with its past already belongs to its own future. Future-I(s) and archaic maternal figure(s) are interwoven in all future trajectories.

When the analyst-mother channels each narcissistic rage toward the real mother she in the now "replaces" her rather then symbolically stand *at her side*. Such a substitution hurts the patient-daughter in her transubjectivity. She thus enters a vortex of retraumatization that might reach the "basic fault" (Balint, 1954). Psychoticization or "hysteria" might follow there where in other circumstances—in the circumstances of empathy-within-compassion—rebellion, pain, resistance, sorrow and joy could lead to compassion-*and*-resistance-*and*-creativity. If love by compassion is primary, and love by gratitude or following forgiveness is secondary, fascinance and trust in which a subject finds value and beauty in the Other precede envy of the other and can continue beyond the *mirror stage* and outside its parameters (Ettinger, 2005). The face of the m/Other is not only a mirror. From the start her face supplies the emerging subject with glimpses of non-abject otherness; from the start her delight not only in the infant but also in the world is a source of wonder and joy; from the start her relation to the outside and to others is a source of trust in the outside and in others. Shame and guilt accompany sudden collapses of ideal maternal figuralities, both during analysis and in daily life. Shame is the result of a humiliating attack on one's self-object and on one's transject. Careful different/ciation not rejection of the intimate others is called for. Compassion fragilizes, it even traumatizes thought in a non-malignant way: it traumatizes like love does. Compassion is as archaic as anxiety. Love, primary compassion, and trust arise as early as, and in parallel to, "schizoid-paranoid" sensibilities and anxieties, and they balance these anxieties. Primary reverance or awe balance fear and leads to respect. Primary compassion balances shame, and it balances the tendency of "perversion" that leans on the conception of the other as just object. Recognizing the early kinds of Mother-phantasies as *primal phantasies* when they reappear in regression moderates narcissistic-aggressive entitlement and balances rage, shame and guilt. Primary compassion combined with fascinance and primary awe combined with reverence and trust are the early human aesthetic, proto-ethical affects, carriers of ethical potentiality.

In the Symbolic, there is a crucial difference between (a): desire for rebirth as a desire to create a new passage from non-life to life in/for oneself and in/for the other, sometimes hidden behind death and rebirth metaphors, and (b): a desire for death hidden behind death and rebirth metaphors. Psychic representations of death fears and death drive, accompanied by phantasies of resurrection, might hide a desire not for death but for the renewal of the passage from non-life to life as entirely distinct from it. It might also hide a denied longing for the archaic (m)Other as matrixial, not as symbiotic. A suicidal wish might encompass and hide phantasmatic rebirthing—on behalf of the (now) adult subject, whose consciousness of sexuality bars his road to archaic (m/)Othernality that awaits a matrixial symbolization yet does meet only with Oedipal formulations that might sometimes hide a non-symbolized and unrecognized Laius impulse.

The passages into life occurred in coemergence with a female-maternal body-psyche whose sexuality is hard to admit. The Persephone-Demeter complexity reveals self and others as corpo-realized subjects whose sexuality and difference are recognized as long as their shareable web is recognized too. Recognizing "my" virtual and im/possible future-I(s) in "my" archaic (maternal) non-I(s) helps to reduce the pains of outer- and inter-generational conflicts and gives tools to work-through the enigma of—and the fear of, and the desire for—initiation and transmission. To work through the in-between variations along proximity-distance overtones (beyond the clear-cut states where the other is considered united, separated or rejected) and along resemblance-difference overtones (beyond the clear-cut positions where the other is considered same, stranger, abjected)—this is a process. It takes time—the duration of encounter-eventing in a passage-space. The patient's differenc/tiation with/from its others is a challenge for the analyst when he works to resist his own desire to over-identify with the rage or the disgust that the patient-daughter/son expresses (as infant) toward her intimate others, guided by the awareness that these affects will turn against the self in a deferred time. The archaic (m) other was subject/object of wondering and languishing, trust and fascinance, a transformational transject whose aesthetic effects are long lasting. If the analyst over-identifies with the daughter's rage then, in spite of momentary relief, her shame (in the mother, that posits *mother as abject*), her blame (of the mother, that posits *mother as rejected*), and her eventual guilt will in the future turn against herself. Compassion to the mother-figures is not at the cost of empathy to the patient; quite the contrary!

Persephone-Demeter strings (real) and threads (imaginary and symbolic) are unique in each trans(sub)jectivity. When their specificities disappear by metaphors of self-identity and get erased by fixed identity (including gender identities), the desire for non-life-coming-into-life—reflected in, and re-lived through the pains of youth coming into sexual adulthood and by the anxiety, shame and guilt aroused in regression while you are by now an already sexually adult figure—can be easily mistaken for death-drive. The analyst can become aware that s/he is entering a Laius position or attacking a maternal zone of maternal shock when she is tempted to invent an "explanation" by way of empathy-without-compassion.

Persephone (Daughter, also son) feel-knows with-in Demeter (past, present, future, potential, and lost Mother). Demeter feels-knows with-in Persephone. The analyst's symbolic space of carriance is opened as a subjectivising space that allows for psychic growth only inasmuch as it is interwoven with the archaic space in which the subject had already been desired enough so as to be carried into life—a decision that must belong to the mother in reality (whose decisions concerning her body we must respect in all circumstances.) When a patient says: "I hate" she expresses transient feeling. When the analyst formulates and establishes its "cause," playfulness stops; the transformational object becomes dangerous—retroactively, in the Imaginary, and grains of trauma might set in the now of the transference, even if its manifestation is deferred. Herself feeling at times not less "crazy" than her own (m)other(s)—the patient "knows" that s/he too, potentially, can become such an "object." The retroactive "cause" for anger, produced by such a process is a time-bomb.

Recognizing the three mother-phantasies (the mother who will "swollow" me (devouring), the mother who didn't love me well enough (not-enoughness), the mother who orphaned me (abandonment)) as basic and primal is not in contradiction to the recognition of traces of real traumatic events. As phantasies they must appears, with and without a real trauma. Here, a Lacanian view, that emphasizes—with diagrammatical positions inside structures and with topographical knots—the difference between the Real, the Imaginary, and the Symbolic, together with an inspiration from a Freudian source to discover primary phantasies and articulate them with mythologies, helps to perceive the difference between a real traumatic past event and a phantasmic organization, and to accordingly seize each for its own merit. When a transject is rejected in the web, our psyche, no matter what, bleeds. Whether or not trauma had occurred in the past, there is a lack in the structure, and the phantasmatic relations to it (Lacan's *object a*) are in the analysis retrieved. In the case of real trauma, we have to account for both kinds of phantasies, those rooted in the trauma and those who are free-floating and has become attached to primordial reality.

The analyst who psychologically substitutes itself to the split-off "good mother" object when he mirrors emphatically-without-compassion a daughterly complaint unknowingly acts as a socializing agent. With each rejection-abjection his imaginary daughter (patient) finds less value in becoming a woman, mother or non-mother "medusa" and later on old female "crone." Rejecting her potential-selves now directed to the archaic trans(sub)ject fracture interferes with the transmission and continuity-in-transformation. Deprived of the support of being carried by her archaic-m/Other's love, a daughter's rebellion enters the zone of death wishes.

In considering Otto Rank's concept *birth-trauma* Freud signals that "there is much more continuity between intra-uterine life and earliest infancy than the impressive caesura of the act of birth would have us believe." Every consideration of the fetal life, however, "can be accounted for *simply enough biologically* [...] the child's biological situation as a foetus is *replaced* for it [after birth] by a psychical *object*-relations to its mother" (Freud, 1926, p. 138). When Winnicott (1949) speaks of birth-trauma and acknowledges prenatal phantasy, and when Bion (1977) speaks of the caesura, what is still left not sensed enough is the mother-as-*subject*. The ideas of transitional object and space, like those of the "third," contribute to what I have come to recognize as trans(sub)jectivity. Its symbolic understanding—in-betweenness that is not a third or transitional space and object and met*r*amorphosis—demands metaphoric approximations. Caring for the patient's trans(sub)jectivity means recognizing the difference between anxiety and compassion, awe and wondering, and attending to the primary love that quite easily turns into shame, guilt and disgust, to the primary awe that quite easily turns into fear and contempt. Free response-ability is borne with the recognition of transjective *intra-intra* (kernel-to-kernel) psychic entanglement. Subjects *different/ciating-in-co-emergence* recognize degrees of resemblance. Their *intrados*, inside curves-caves as kernels, re-superimposed by resonance, join in trans(sub)jectivity while each individual subject emerges too. With the capacity to seize-feel-recognize the other as a desiring-*subject* the potential for wondering-caring grows.

Post-partum psychosis needs a matrixial analysis in which the differences from the parental same-sex figure are symbolized and imagined without splits, where the analyst recognizes and resists its own power, built into the setting, to triumph over the parental failures and its own narcissistic impulse to seduce via splitting. Since any instance of "positive" transference *is* nourished by the *(m/)Othernal* earlier *seduction into life*, the analyst will realize that in joining an already existing web he resides in besidedness and side-by-sideness, *at the side* of the other significant figures, and the space of analysis is nourished by this web.

The structure of psychoanalysis had been based on the foreclosure of trans(sub)jectivity and of the archaic (m)Other, on the denial of the mother *as subject* and on her *objectification.* This contributed to the difficulty to account for transformations that lean on the very archaic potential for transmission. Transmission along mental strings, vibrations in different frequencies and resonance, trans-inscription of affective and mental waves of psychic kernels both separate and entangled, and cross-inscription of traces of what forms psychic movements of borderlinking and borderspacing: the subject during/over time is thus a *trans*jectile.

The intra-side of the mother Demeter—her joy, shock, phantasm and trauma, sexuality, fragility and force is echoed, not mirrored, in the subject Persephone while the daughter's trauma reverberates in the mother. The subject—as daughter/son-infant, then and as adult, potential (non-)parent now—will traverse shocks of maternality (possibility of herself, and also, in any case partially those of her mother) in multiple ways. Persephone is concerned by the enigma of the desiring Demeter: What is mother? What is maternal love? Can a mother love, can she not-love her daughter? Could my mother *not* have loved me? Is mother a sexual *subject*? Each reply intends also her virtual and potential self: Will I remain attractive when I become adult, if I become mother? Will I remain subject when I become a child's *object*? Whatever her gender identity might be—on the matrixial dimension no subject can be totally Other to its m/Other. Disgust toward her induces future self-disgust. Blame toward her induces guilt and future self-blaming, humiliating her induces shame in the subject's virtual/future/past/potential selves. Splits induce addictive fixation of rage in a daughter's pole.

Through the prism of the three primal mother phantasies I can now re-frame Winnicott's enigmatic phrase: "it is a joy to be hidden but disaster not to be found" (Winnicott, 1963, p. 191). With his pleading to not look behind it (behind it there is nothing) this formula is his unique compound of primal mother-phantasies: "starting from no fixed place I soon came [...] to taking a claim, to my surprise, to the right not to communicate [...] a protest to the core of me to [...] the fantasy of being found" (Winnicott, 1963, p. 185). The thread of the *phantasmatic* abandoning mother registers feelings of psychic pain from different sources *including* the maternal source and helps to digest and elaborate the pain and find ways to understand and overcome it. Pain is amplified both by real abandonment and by other difficulties in differen*t/c*iation, which arise from different sources, internal and external. The thread of the *phantasmatic* devouring mother registers feelings of anxiety arising from different sources including the maternal source and helps to digest and elaborate the pain and find ways to understand and overcome it. Pain is amplified by real over-domineering as well as by difficulties in different/ciation arising from different sources. This primal phantasm digests and elaborates anxieties of being invaded, dominated, and penetrated; it is amplified by real parental impingements and overdomination. The *Not-enough mother* phantasy arises as a reply to the enigma of the repeated loss of harmony between the subject and *its* subject(s), object(s) and environment, and from difficulties to open distance in oneness-closeness, difficulties to find sufficient proximity in a separateness affected by rejection and to seize sufficient difference in a same/total-other combination affected by abjection. Apart from occurrences of real traumatic maternal abandonment and real traumatic maternal over-domineering (sources in the real), and apart from traumatic and dramatic disturbances in subject/subject/environment capacity for reattunement, it is *the failure to recognize* these three unconscious threads *as primal phantasies* that actively accounts, in and out of analysis, for the endless search after non-existing "causes" for those feelings, resulting in "replies" that *weakens* the matrixial Eros, thus creating an addictive vicious circle that exhausts the subject. *Re*construction (by the analyst) of unremembered early painful and joyful materials (brought up by the patient) should avoid retroactive *construction* of the archaic figures as the *cause* of anxiety; the meeting with such object-cause, according to Lacan, is illusionary. The Lacanian project to traverse one's phantasies means to admit their significant effects *as phantasies* even where and when the Real is/was indeed traumatic. The one doesn't exclude the other.

The Law in a society ruled by transparent paranoia disguised as the general norm might at such a fragile moment come as a shock to the matrixial mother–infant encounter-eventing and to the emerging maternal subject, since it doesn't take into account an ethics that could have corresponded to this fragility, ethics that could have been developed from the sublimation of the matrixial-maternal carriance and space.

Creativity related to the meeting between corpo-Real space of care-carry-*carriance* and fascinance-trust is symbolically indebted to the feminine-maternal subject. Betrayal of such a trust's core, whenever it will arise in the future, will come to the infant-subject-analysand in us as a shock: the shock of betrayal. It will turn the creative trust-fascinance into mortal fascinum. This shock might occur when the re-arousal of such vulnerability, trust and self-fragility in adulthood in reality is invited, then betrayed. It can therefore arise in the psychoanalytical relations that involve regression. The analysand is called by the analyst and the analytical setting to a regression, to dependency and trust. Betrayal by way of secret sacrificial tendencies on behalf of an analyst through, for example, the projection of a "father"-analyst's delirious psychotic countertransference on the analysand-"son" is a nameless horror.

17.4 A Love Gift: Scar in the Sky—Sylvia Plath (I)

Through Sylvia Plath I will explore some relations between the scene of trauma and phantasmatic scenarios, and will refer to potential for retraumatization by interpretations that ignores the matrixial. A mother-poet suffocates in her maternal love and shocks. I will attend here to Plath's *Journals* where she exposes threads from her analytical therapy, to reflect a possible turning against the self through the mother's devaluation. I will pay attention to her oscillations between her longing for a non-life and her death-wishes.

The *Journals* in-between life and art—like her poetry, it reads us. The *Journals* is part of her artistic endeavor, yet it is a *life* Journal: it reflects her permanent striving for truth-telling of real, traumatic and phantasmatic experiences. The diary and the poems reflect life, personal and non-personal, and a life's poetic engagement of which phantasy and mythology are a part. Life as source of poetry is not reduced to poetry, poetry as source of life is not reduced to life. Let's look at SP's account of her analytical therapy as an *auto-case-history*. The *Journals* tells me that strings to her matrixial-maternal real mother had been systematically symbolically devaluated.

When on January 15, 1956 Sylvia Plath writes her longing to be pregnant, she goes on associating thus: "I long for mother [...] I want to permeate the matter of this world." At this stage she counts her mother alongside those younger women in whose company she feels she can be a "wholly woman" (Plath, 2000, pp. 200, 201). On March 6, 1956, she associates to the terrible pains of love: "it hurts, father, it hurts, oh father I have never known; a father, even, *they* took from me" (Plath, 2000, p. 223). As to her intending lover she writes: "I want somehow to live with him always [...] to bear children to him: such heavenly pride to carry his child. My god [...] Oh someone, I run through names, thinking someone hear me, take me to your heart, be warm and let me cry and cry and cry. And help me be strong: oh Sue, Oh mr. Fisher, Oh Ruth Beuscher, oh mother." (Plath, 2000, p. 224). In this matrixial web, her therapist RB and the real mother still dwell side by side, transposed in their soothing function; the mother didn't take the father away, and RB doesn't substitute mother, both women-mother-figures represent warmth and strength. On March 8, 1956: "I rail and rage against the taking of my father [...] I would have loved him" (Plath, 2000, p. 230). The rage is addressed to nobody in particular; it is addressed to life, God, reality; its cause is destiny. Later on during the analytical session this rage is channeled toward the real mother. On February 24, 1958, Plath comments on Ted Hugh's "April" and her own "November" poems: "spring and winter in the moors, birth & death, or, rather, *reversing the order, death & resurrection*," which I interpret as an unconscious struggle to articulate how from *non-life*, and not *only* from death, new life can follow. *Non-life*'s symbolization includes death though.

Togetherness with the mother is problematic, it involves the father's death. "Togetherness" imagined through a phallic perspective creates the equation womb = symbiosis = psychic-death and, in a circular way, must be repulsed on the grounds of this same symbolic equation. The father's death reinforces Oedipal and Electra interpretations. Soon the therapist RB will personify the "good" mother, while the "bad mother" split-off facet will be projected onto the real mother who becomes, with the therapist's encouragement ("sanction" in SP's words), *the killer of the father* and an authority on the maternal deserve-ability of hate. In the *Journals*, December 12, 1958 we find:

> 'I hate her doctor'—I feel so terrific. In a smarmy matriarchy of togetherness it is hard to get a sanction to hate one's mother, especially a sanction *one believes in*. I believe in RB's because she is a

clever woman who knows her business & I admire her [...] What do I do? I don't imagine time will make me love her [mother]. I can pity her; she had a lousy life; she doesn't know she's a walking vampire. (Plath, 2000, p. 429)

Pity the abjected devouring monster—while all wondering and admiration are transferred to the therapist? The ideality of the mother has shrunk; disappointment, shame, and despair appear where the ideal imaginary cloth is stripped, but notice this: the signifiers of ideality (admire) seems to directly move from the mother to RB. Shame and despair in the maternal site grow, the meaning of the original maternal love is now lost, the mother figure is being replaced. SP describes why she hates the vampire; the description of what she now loathes risks to fit what the future might have prepared for her in a similar position in a frightening possible future: "she gave herself to her children," she married a "brut," she is "bleeding," left with 2 children to raise, with no time or attention to herself (Plath, 2000, pp. 429–430). "She'd had a lousy world" (Plath, 2000, p. 430). Now the mother is blamed for the loss of the father (a fate that might resemble hers as mother to children that would be left with her): "My mother killed the only man who'd loved me steady through life: came in one morning with tears of nobility in her eyes and told me he was gone for good. I hate her for that" (Plath, 2000, p. 431). Shame appears where admiration and trust once were located, rage is directed at the person who once belonged in the company of ideal women and represented love. Her figure is now shrunk. SP unknowingly seems to come to loath features that SP might identify later on as her own in her destiny as a woman. The mother non-I who receives "hate" under her therapist's "sanction," to use her own words, will resemble, over the matrixial time loop, her own I; her non-I stands for her potential future-I. Following SP's reading of Freud (according to her account) SP says about her attempted suicide: "I'd kill *her*, so I killed myself" (Plath, 2000, p. 433). "What to do with your hate for your mother [...] where do you look for a mother-person [...] who can tell you [...] about *facts of life like babies* and how to produce them? The *only* person I know and trust for this is RB" (Plath, 2000, p. 435)—therapeutic maternal *substitution and imaginary-symbolic replacement* occurred where I believe that side-by-sideness in "severality" would offer some healing. Signs of rage were channeled toward the mother who thus was retroactively established *as* the cause of trouble in accordance with the following idea that is paradigmatic and need to be rethought: "RB SAYS [...] If you are angry at someone else, and repress it, you get depressed. Who am I angry at? [Sylvia Plath]: *Myself.* [RB:] *No, not yourself. Who is it*? [SP:] *It is my mother and all the mothers I have known* who have wanted me to be what I have not felt like really being from my heart and at the society [...]" (Plath, 2000, p. 437.) All those mother figuralities are abstract results of patriarchal Western organization yet there was a real mother here *too*. The imaginary and symbolic devaluation was directed to the real mother, of her childhood and of the present. To be angry at her—or be angry at myself—or be angry at her, again—this vicious circle is reproduced with such interventions (though the real mother was a continual source of good-enough support according to SP's *Letters Home*.) Plath does realize, however, that hate to mother is a new problem of her life *now*. She continues: "Main Questions: What to do with hate for mother." The analytic formula keeps condensing her mother as cause-source of anger and now also of fear; shame and guilt could be the result of a sudden shrinking of ideality. SP reports her feeling of immediate happiness and relief when she is sanctioned to hate her mother, but soon after she reports of more anxiety and more depression. The analytic conclusion is reported by SP in the following terms: her mother *never loved her*, her mother did everything for herself *only*. Gradually the matrixial web disintegrates: *Journals*, December 27, 1958: "Hate of mother, jealousy of brother" (the person she otherwise reported to have loved the most in her life). "Yesterday had a session with Beuscher quite long, and very deep [...] I am experiencing a grief reaction for something I have only recently begun to admit isn't there: *a mother's love* [...] nothing I do can change her way of being with me which I experience as a *total absence of love*"

(Plath, 2000, p. 446). *Total* absence? And what will happen if I will resemble her? Or languish for her? And, if there is no Mother's Love, what about myself as a future Mother? The matrixial web is bleeding now. Roles and positions are there to be exchanged. The horror of Womanhood and Motherhood now more then ever lurks from the inside. In *Journals*, January 3, 1959 SP asks: "What do I expect or want from mother?" A scenario emerges:

> A great, stark, bloody play acting itself over and over again behind the sunny facade of our daily rituals, birth, marriage, death, behind parents and schools and beds and tables of food: the dark, cruel, murderous shades, the demon-animals, the Hungers [...] ASK ABOUT MOTHER-LOVE [...] I would probably interpret pain as a judgment: *birth-pain*, even a *deformed child. Magical fear mother will become a child, my child: an old hag child.* (Plath, 2000, p. 456)

On June 6, 1959, in a dream: ""Beuscher congratulating me. Mother turning away [...]" which shows, I think, that RB has *become* my mother" (Plath, 2000, p. 492). The *objectalized* Mother bleeds outside or inside herself? It's a time-bomb, a boomerang: when in Plath's own life the drama, not the societal but the corpo-real drama, her own ardent desire to bear children, emerged, immediately followed by fear of non-fertilization, anxiety of barrenness, worries concerning fertility, anxiety of and from pregnancies, and then abortions and then child-birthing—these loci of No Love are now hers: pre-maternality, birth-giving, motherhood, the idea of growing older, the idea that mother (once her, now you) is emptied of goods. The poet who kept asking *for the knowledge of the wise women about womanhood and motherhood*—received, I believe, an over-empathy to the raging child-girl-daughter in her. The mother-woman figure remained-and-became *frozen barren moon* with *marble womb*, devouring *medusa*, humiliated, *shameful old queen-bee*, exiled from *the engine that killed her*; her own maternal and female body is a bleeding flower. (S)mothered Mother-smother. When she gets pregnant (or have difficulties to get pregnant), when she experiences her menstrual bleeding, when a period arrives late, when she goes through non-conception, then miscarriage, birth-giving and miscarriage again, and birth-giving again—her self as female-adult-woman-mother has fallen like ashen smother, "a dead-end," dead mother and dead infant conglomerate. In SP's account of her therapy I didn't find signs of attribution of value to what seems to me as the archaic (m)Other-Woman-mother enigma that SP had posited all along: What is Mother as sexual subject *and* maternal subject *and* a birthing woman's-body? SP desires children, she experiences difficulties, she goes through shocks of maternality of the first zone, then of the second, and then of the third. She is unprepared. She writes (on what I see as a shock of the first zone), June 20, 1959:

> Everything has gone barren. I am part of the world's *ash*, something from which *nothing can grow, nothing can flower* or come to fruit. In the lovely words of 20th century medicine, I can't ovulate. Or don't [...] I would bear children until my change of life [...] I want to be an Earth Mother in the deepest richest sense [...] And what do I meet in myself? *Ash. Ash and more ash* [...] Suddenly everything is ominous, ironic, deadly. If I could not have children [...] I would be dead. Dead to my woman's body [...] a dead-end. (Plath, 2000, p. 500)

September 25, 1959:

> I woke from a bad dream. O I'm full of them [...] I gave birth, with one large cramp [...] I asked at the counter if it was alright [...] and the nurse said: "Oh, it has *nest of uterus* in its nose, but nothing is wrong with the heart [...] How is that. Symbolic of *smother in the womb*? Image of mother dead with the Eye Bank having cut her eyes out. Not a dream [which would mean a fantasy] but a vision [which means, an ill omen for a real future]. (Plath, 2000, p. 506)

A shock of the second zone?

November 15, 1959: "I lay in a morbid twit till the hollow dark of the morning full of evil dreams of *dying in childbirth* in a strange hospital unable to see Ted, or having a blue baby, or a deformed baby, which they wouldn't let me see" (Plath, 2000, p. 530) She is pregnant now, Frida will be born on the 1 April 1960. Who then is (was, going to be) the smothered/smothering mother? Later, alone with her small kids in London, overwhelmed, desperate, she writes to her mother following her lessons from her own therapy and from *reading* Freud, as she reports, that *psychologically* it will be a *mistake* if she accepted her help or a visit from her, that from a *psychological point of view* it is better that she will not see her. A woman-to-woman possible solidarity and continuity between the generations, between adult mother-Mother and adult daughter-Mother had collapsed? Suddenly, shockingly, if my-mother is No Love (deflated from authority and admiration with the encouragement of my substitute-mother-analyst), when me-mother is No Love I can't address my a mother. If my-mother is maddening and traumatizing, mother-me is/will-be maddening too. How to sustain then my shock at motherhood? One day, a "my"-self dwells in my Mother (Father) position. Who am *she* then for a *me*? Where in the world is Mother?

In her road to maternality SP had to face shock after shock; now she hurts in her own matrixial space; the Mother-site out-inside herself is abjected. Who in herself will have compassion for her shocks as a mother? How will she sustain together a maternal-and-sexual position? And finally, will me-mother too be blamed if my children's father would leave or pass away? "My mother killed the only man who'd loved me steady through life: came in one morning with tears of nobility in her eyes and told me he was gone for good. I hate her for that" (Plath, 2000, p. 431)...

Traces of love are hidden in the unconscious. These traces are to be discovered no less than those of hate. The hate of maternal figure overshadowed a love. If love, pain, and anger at the loss of the father are translated into anger at the mother then the other way round is important too: behind anger there is pain and behind pain there is love.

The literary-poetic persona *and* the actual person, both the girl, the woman and the poet, desired and enacted death. We can therefore ask, what happens to the now-mother-hating (and thus) self-orphaned girl-daughter poetic persona, and to the poet, when she enters pregnancy and motherhood? Sylvia Plath described by herself in the first-body of language is the persona of the subject-patient of the *Journals*, and RB is the persona of the therapist. Does the therapist-persona, admired and loved, offers-opens for the daughter-girl-poet person/persona a space for adulthood in potential motherhood? Would it make a difference if an adult-and-mother subject-position, and not mainly a daughter subject-position would be cherished in an analytical process?

We would never know in the case of Sylvia Plath. Plath committed suicide, and I respect *the sovereignty of her own subjectivity* over *her final act*. I wouldn't reduce the dignity and integrity of her decision, I wouldn't attribute it to a particular cause, I wouldn't suggest that someone else can speak in her place to "explain" her act. Nor would I suggest that of necessity another kind of therapy could have saved her from taking her destiny in her hands in this way. However, I do wish to point at a major lacuna in the analytical thinking concerning the maternal and the matrixial so well accounted for in her account of her own "case history" in the *Journals*. In SP's *Journals* and in her poetry her shocks of maternality are echoed. They boulverse me. Adulthood-motherhood so desired still came to SP as a shock—not only to the poetic subject but also to the literary persona of the poet as described by herself, to the person-poet, to the poet-woman. Art-as/is-life, life as/is-art bleeding. Ashes accumulated. The girl-daughter's position remained, it became even more and more attractive at moments. The poetic persona of Sylvia Plath is often that of the child-girl that detests the mother-moon-medusa and loves and adores (and then also hates) the father-dead or father-nazi. When Plath enters the mother-position in life she embodies and inhabits the symbolic space of crone-moon-medusa. Embodied fidelity to the child-girl person, persona, and position returns. It is reflected in a desire to die young and to dis-mother herself (Ettinger, 2014).

Growing into adulthood and (non-)motherhood demands the revitalization of the matrixial sphere by the *Eros of borderlinking* that is involved in the trauma of birthing and the phantasies of rebirthing. I suggest that in analysis it is possible to articulate threads that reflect the feminine space and the matrixial-maternal eros that had brought just the living infant into life and is thus inscribed in each of us. Analysis benefits from the archaic trust in this Eros of love. A revised psychoanalysis in this twenty-first century will attend to the subject as informed by the love-and-shock of the maternal and the trauma of *birthing*. When monster-medusa-subject non-I is interwoven with monster-medusa I in the *subject*, carriance becomes a source of support for each effort toward psychic and symbolic passage from psychic trauma (that feels as non-life) to yet another (phase in) life.

The archaic father is matrixially linked to the infant too. Son-mother, son-father, daughter-mother, daughter-father are matrixially linked. Early admiration for maternal figures is irrelevant to sexual object-*choice* and is gender-free. Mother is sometimes non-mother, as the gesture of Baubo reminds Demeter in one moment in the classical Myth. With major fatal tears in her original matrixial web: the death of the father and the imaginary diminishing of her mother in her psyche, SP goes through miscarriage, operation, birthing, and a second birthing soon followed by separation from her husband. When she intends to commit suicide, killing the mother that she now is merges with killing the mother in herself to paraphrase her own expression in her account of her therapy. Plath writes a poem in which she uses the same imagery that she used in her *Journals* when she was younger. As she unmothers herself she orphans her own children from her own mother-self in the real like she orphaned herself in the Imaginary when she *dis*mothered her future self. But she is actually already a mother now. To dis-mother herself and unbirth her children is like turning her skin inside-out, becoming like Lot's wife a perfected marble, frozen like barren white moon. In a poem, the tomb she goes into is the womb into which she enfolds her phantasmatic dead children-roses to unbirth them to a non-life *before* birthing, to reach her non-life whose name, for the now-mother-bee once-a-rose, is death. Dead mother-bee leaves a *red scar in the sky*. When she lines like a womb the gas-oven-grave with soft towels it's as if she desires to be reborn into death and return to a mother-tomb-womb space-home in dying. In an early mythology described in Plath's *Journals*, the young poet herself was a Demeter that returns her infants to her womb. It is interesting how this myth reappeared in one of her very last poems that announced, expressed, predicted a suicidal poet-I. The red tulips (children), says the poet, took away the air she (mother) needs to breathe. The infant (I, or non-I) is suffocating; and still the mother (I, non-I) loves. Could a Demeter's love have brought Persephone a relief? Perhaps. It takes a trusting in it though. What is a Persephone-without-Demeter? Under the shock of maternality SP realizes how one can love *and* suffocate, desire to give birth *and* be shocked. Will she have compassion for herself as Mother? The discovery that the figure of the mother (herself now) is sexual and desiring can be known in advance by compassion and awe. As young mother who is sexually desiring yet already a potential future-Demeter and even crone, Persephone is in anguish. SP hurts in the rejected Mother-*object*, yet, great artist that she is, she succeeds exquisitely to subjectify and give to the daughter-monster-subject and mother-monster-*subject* a poetic voice—a voice of her own, for us all.

SP's daily life began to resemble her mother's, a kind of life she not only wished to avoid but also came to loath. In her last poems, after putting her Dead Father to symbolic death inside herself, the poet desires pre-maternal non-life. In nestling in the gas-oven and, like that ill newborn bird that Ted and she had to kill by pity with the gas tube, surrendering body and soul to the Tenebrae of the gas cave-womb-tomb ceremoniously prepared, she shapes her last real-symbolic space. A womb-tomb of her own.

In matrixial analysis, the *passage* from non-life to life can distinguish itself from the *schism* of death where a symbolic *orphanization* is not desired by the analyst. The analyst carries the matrixial tissue into which she enters. The equation "her hateful—me lovable" expressed by "my" self is sometimes necessary (the object is always destroyed), but such an expression by a significant Other (analyst) is not. Individuation needs metramorphic re-attunement. The becoming-Demeter when you are a Persephone needs the compassionate carriance of a Demeter in the transferential bordertime. Caring for the maternal shocks is humanizing.

According to this mythology told by Robert Graves, that Sylvia Plath was reading with her husband the poet Ted Hughes, Persephone is both the younger self of Demeter and one of the three guises of the Triple Goddess—Kore (the youngest, the maiden, signifying green young grain), Persephone (the nymph, the maiden, signifying the ripe grain waiting to be harvested), and Hecate (the eldest, the crone, the harvested grain). To admire them is a path to being initiated by them—a creative healing force in the direction of consolidating solidarity between different life phases and different generations. Here, SP-Proserpine (Persephone, a daughter desiring a man) lost Ceres (Demeter, a mother) inside and outside herself but still longed for a m/Other: in herself, outside of herself. When she took death to be that non-life she has longed for, the idea of a real-symbolic return to a mother who became a hole in her matrixial sphere insists, the feeling of a tragic re-search for a symbolic space of her own which will embrace the enigma of a mother-woman now her-self.

A letter was written in-between the first period of hospitalization (where electric shocks were operated on Plath) and the late period of therapy (taken up with the same therapist): November 22, 1955:

> ...the hungry cosmic mother sees the world shrunk to embryo again and her children gathered sleeping back into the dark, huddling in bulbs and pods, pale and distant as the folded beanseed to her full milky love which freezes across the sky in a crucifix of stars. / so it costs ceres all that pain to go to gloomy dis and bargain for proserpine again. we wander and wait in november air as rat fur stiffened with frozen tears, endure, endure [...] / artificial fires burn here: leaping red in the heart of wineglasses [...] crackling crimson in the fairytale cheeks of a rugged jewish hercules hewn fresh from the himalayas and darjeeling to be sculpted with blazing finesse by a feminine pygmalion whom he gluts with mangoes and dmitri karamazov fingers blasting beethoven out of acres of piano and striking scarletti to skeletal crystal. (Plath, 2000, p. 191).

Hinting on resurrection before committing suicide, Plath points *with Ceres and Proserpine* to her urgent quest concerning maternal love and its partial and total loss.

17.5 Countertransference Psychosis: From *Hallucination à Deux* to Trauma

In quite a number of "case histories" *after* Freud I observe a systematic fixating of the mother in some kind of a monster-crone-*object* (mother dry of sexuality) position or a medusa-*object* (mother saturated with aggressive and sexual connotation) position. During this fixating process, the affective investment by way of trust *as such* is damaged, though trust in the analyst at this point does grow. How will an internalized mother figure continue to nourish Persephone (daughter or son) from withing in each new passage from non-life to life if trust in her is in the process of diminishing? It even seems that if for some reason the paternal figure has failed, the rejection of the mother (by an analyst parent-figure) appeals even more to analytical semiotic mechanism.

Winnicott's patient, a boy—for example—enacts sadomasochistic phantasies in front of the eyes of his indifferent father. Winnicott suggests as cause the maternal absences, in denial of what seems to me the sexual aspects of the boy's symptoms which manifest an intensive questioning of paternal sexuality and plays to his possible sadism manifested by the child's scribbles and by his words: "whip, whop... another crop, another whip" (*Playing and Reality*, pp. 16–17). Winnicott, in my view, translates a real paternal failure into an imaginary and symbolic maternal fault.

The collapse into psychosis described in a case-study by Christopher Bollas (1987, pp. 173–188) is connected to an analytical process that in my view could have contributed to psychosis by the expression of direct countertransferential remarks and by a systematic symbolic and imaginary rejection of the patient's original early transformational figures. Their care-taking is named "psychopathic," (Bollas, 1987, p. 187), the beloved mother is characterized as "maddening," her absences identified as "devastating" and the patient's condition is conceived and described as "madness" (Bollas, 1987, p. 188).[1] A patient, Jonathan, reveals that the different transformational figures for him are the most precious things in his life. The moments where the other "can transform" him are "the most glorious moments of his life, because they fill him with a 'transcendental' sense of 'exquisite harmony'" (Bollas, 1987, p. 40). Jonathan describes his basic experiences as aesthet-

[1] A note to the reader. In faire disclosure: my interest in the case study is intllectual and professional, and my analysis and critique of this text are part of an ongoing philosophical engagement and research in psychoanalysis. However, I also have a personal stake concerning its author.

ical; his object-other is source of wonder and hope. The patient shares with his analyst his space of dreams as aesthetical (Bollas, 1987, pp. 73–77). The analyst describes what in my view is his patient's aesthetic-artistic *vision* as a manifestation of "aesthetic problems" (Bollas, 1987, p. 77). Jonathan associates mother with "warmth, soft clothing and tranquility" (Bollas, 1987, p. 40) and his father with grace, dignity, ancient muses, philosophy, and history. For the analyst this mother was "maddening" and both parents were "traumatizing primary objects" (Bollas, 1987, p. 188). In my reading, Jonathan and George, two figures in the book, appear as one and the same figure at different moments during the same analytical process. In both cases different versions of the same "cause" of "madness" was offered: the mother who placed the infant in the care of few persons. The patient was "placed with a nanny who looked after him while his mother attended classes and worked" (Bollas, 1987, p. 130), the parents opted for "a division of the care-taking function amongst several people" (Bollas, 1987, p. 178); "she hired a nanny, and the infant was passed from one figure to another, from mother to nanny, from nanny to mother" (Bollas, 1987, pp. 39–40). "Madness and catastrophe in the transference," infers the analyst, are the enactment of the maddening "unidentifiable" reality from unremembered infantile past where the patient as baby alternated between frustrating presences and maternal "devastating absences" (Bollas, 1987, p. 188). The maternal figure through this proposed cause is reduced to a ready-made mother-monster object-cause of "madness." Such ready-made mother-"cause" is recognized by its repetition. When the mother is thus rejected, is it not the rejection of the patient's emerging self which is inseparable in fact from its primordial transformational object? Is it not the basic creative-aesthetic mode of its being which is rejected? The rejection of the parental figures hits, in my view, the archaic reality where the I dwelled and will always dwell with its non-I(s). This psychic entity is shared. Like Jonathan's, so is George's case: "George was in fact a staunch defender and protector of his mother, and he rarely talked about her except in glowing terms during the first year of his analysis. Nevertheless these positive feelings suddenly collapsed quite dramatically" (Bollas, 1987, p. 128). An analyst's symbolic-emotional (countertransferential) rejection of the patient's primary transformational and conservative object might push to this regression to a "basic fault." Freud suggests that signs of anger are to be understood and interpreted in the transferential here-and-now as caused by it. Bollas suggests that if his own feeling in the countertransference is so intolerable then the patient's admired parents must have been maddening and provided a "psychopathic" "care-taking." (Bollas, 1987, p. 187). A retroactive "cause" is established. Jonathan's "absent parents" and mainly mother are supposed to account not only for the patient's current symptoms during analysis but also for *murderous plans* developed *during* many analytical sessions where an unwarned other is in danger; plans of the kind that, in the tradition of Winnicott are considered as never too far from suicidal intentions. Like Jonathan so George: "As an infant he had been separated from his mother on several occasions and she left him in the care of a series of people" (Bollas, 1987, p. 224). "Over the years, however, I have managed to find a way to live inside the environment he creates, and I have done so by analyzing him even when he threatened to murder me if I didn't shut up [...] I was saying to myself, 'Oh what's the use? The son of a bitch is hopeless'." (Bollas, 1987, p. 223) "[T]he fact that I had not personally resisted his created environment" writes the analyst "had left him [George] feeling doomed and monstrous" (Bollas, 1987, p. 225). How can we tell the analysand's unconscious productions from the analyst's projections here as well as in what is described (in the case of Jonathan) as a "countertransference psychosis" (Bollas, 1987, p. 184)? The analyst describes his "hallucination à deux" with his patient (Bollas, 1987, p. 181). He also writes that analysands might "invite the analyst into a pathological transferential relations [...] in order to compel the analyst to misunderstand them" (Bollas, 1987, p. 29, and see Chap. 14 for more). But is it not one of the analyst's functions by definition? Is this function not structured by the analytical setting and invited in the process?

For Jacques Lacan, negative countertransference is the sum-up of the analyst's misunderstanding. In other words, the analyst has to take care and responsibility over his own countertransference. The analyst is not supposed to indulge in the transferential relationships or share his countertransferential impressions. The Lacanian analyst doesn't operate with transference–countertransference interpretations. The clinical interventions take another path. Bollas' choice is to expresses to the patient a "direct countertransference comment" even when he recognizes it to be "intellectualized" and "explanatory" and thus serves the analyst's needs (Bollas, 1987, p. 225).

The subject's relations of love to his primordial objects are precious for the psychic-aesthetical apparatus. The subject's poetic structure is linked to its capacity for wonder, admiration and primal love. The original objects are at the heart of the subject's aesthetic-poetic core. And yet a script concerning the failure of the mother-environment is already written in the collective psychoanalytic consciousness. Starting with Winnicott and down his theoretical lineage, could any patient have, in the eyes of his analyst, a "good-enough" mother? Is not the ready-made mother-monster a part of the meaning-donation mechanism itself? For Winnicott, ideally, the mother is *silent* unless she fits her baby's subjective ideation of an object-mirror: "Shall we stop trying to understand human beings? The answer might come from mothers who do not communicate with their infants except in so far as they are subjective objects" (Winnicott, 1963, p. 192). "What does the baby see when he or she looks at the mother's face? [...] himself or herself," when "[T]he mother's face is not then a mirror" this is a catastrophic blow (Winnicott, 1971, p. 151). It was Winnicott, however, who also remarked, briefly, that the output of the analytical processes of subjectivization needs to be understood in terms of *waste disposal*. "The next task for a worker in the field of transitional phenomena is to restate the problem in terms of disposal" (Winnicott, 1971, p. 123 *footnote*). When the mother is instrumentalized to serve as waste-disposal her dehumanization is a part of the process: any toxic waste material can be channeled to her. When absence due to structural lack is mistaken for absence due to loss, resentment and revenge flourish. In the reconstruction of one's personal past special attention is also called to the possibility that traits of a present object can come to stand for and represent *a lack* (in the structure) or *a* different *loss* in reality, thus transforming the present object into a cause for the suffering. In other words, upon the subject's (patient's) attempts at destroying her object (mother), the analyst will remember that the "good-enough" mother is always re- and re-destroyed, for no other reason than the process of subjectivizing in-itself: "the object is in fantasy always being destroyed" (Winnicott, 1971, p. 125). "While I am loving you I am all the time destroying you [...] here fantasy begins for the individual" (Winnicott, 1971, p. 120) when the object has autonomy though it belongs to a "'shared' reality."

In the psyche, by virtue of being humanly-born and transconnected to female-maternal body-psyche, the link to maternality persists. According to Freud, death is not represented in the Unconscious as such. Whether we agree with this statement or not, *non-life as pre-life-coming-into-life*—that passage between non-life and life through female corpo-reality—does look for imaginary and symbolic outlets. This passage shouldn't be amalgamated with or translated into the notion of death.

The archaic (m/)Other as subject both participates and eludes the narcissistic mirror. Her openness to the other subjectivizes our creative and aesthetic core. The secret of wonder and trust is rooted in this possibility of love, which I suggest as supplementary to the routes of love mapped by Freud in "On Narcissism" (Freud, 1914). The *non-I* doesn't only *reflect* the *I* when it *participates* in its emergence in love. After birth, the maternal-matrixial Eros continues to seduce the *I* into life inasmuch as the *I* enters the contact with a figure—(be it female or male, be it the mother of pregnancy or another mother-figure, known and unknown) on sensitive, tactile, visual, and other levels—in vulnerable trust-wonder.

The analyst of a daughter-patient can easily triumph over the real mother, use her potency and potentiality and hide traces of this use *even-though* the transference is nourished by this. Only when the analyst recognizes itself as joining the joys and sorrows of the earlier webs *a caring strike grows, the strike of non-betrayal.* Persephone (daughter) tries to differenc/tiate herself not against but with-in Demeter. A new *loving* engagement in the matrixial sphere would rather work not to split the patient-subject from the archaic Love sources. A mother-figure can love her child and be *both* transconnected *and* shocked on the level of individual subjectivity, suffer from the loss of rhythms of her individual life, suffocate in contracting the new psychic breathing, feel invaded by reality, by new needs, by new tasks.

In his "The Analyst's Murder of the Patient" Peter Rudnytzky writes: "Of the radical and innovative ideas put forward by Ferenczi during his last years none is perhaps more startling than the suggestion in his 1932 *Clinical Diary* that although the analyst "may take kindness and relaxation as far as he possibly can, the time will come when he will have to repeat with his own hands the act of murder previously perpetrated against the patient" (1998, p. 52). In what follows I propose to use the *Diary* to explore not only the theoretical and clinical implications of this idea but also its autobiographical dimension and its bearing on Ferenczi's relationship to Freud.

It must be said immediately that the murder of which Ferenczi speaks is not literal, but rather emotional or psychic. As he goes on to explain, "analytic guilt consists of the doctor not being able to offer full maternal care, goodness, self-sacrifice; and consequently he again exposes the people under his care, who just barely managed to save themselves before, to the same danger, by not providing adequate help" (pp. 52–53). Once this is understood, it becomes clear that Ferenczi is referring to the way in which the inevitable imperfections and limitations of the analyst trigger the memory of childhood traumas experienced by the patient, which must be relived during analysis in order to be exorcised [...] this model of the psychotherapeutic process proposed by Ferenczi is very similar to that articulated independently by D. W. Winnicott in his posthumously published paper "Fear of Breakdown," where he sets forth the way that agony of the patient "experienced in the transference, in relation to the analyst's failures and mistakes," enables the patient to recollect "the original failure of the facilitating environment" (1974, p. 91). Even from this brief summary, it is evident that the view of psychoanalysis held by Ferenczi and Winnicott stresses the need for humility on the part of the analyst" (Rudnytsky, 1998, p. 345). However, it is not enough to recognize the analyst's regressive tendency for psychic murder for which the Oedipus Complex doesn't give proper parameters. With the Laius Complex, Laius' impulse is to be recognized starting from adult, not infantile, subjectivity. There are clinical indications to follow in order to counterbalance this countertransferential tendency. The analyst's rejection of the archaic paternal figures is in my view a tool in the service of Laius. When, contrary to this splitting tendency, the (m)other's values, the trauma she had to go through, and her vulnerability are valued by the analyst (in his paternal position during regression), a healing different/ciation will most probably follow.

17.6 The Medusa's Stings: Sylvia Plath (II)

> Axes / After whose stroke the wood rings, / And the echoes / [...] The sap / Wells like tears, like the / Water striving / To re-establish its mirror / Over the rock / That drops and turns / A white skull [...] Years later I / Encounter them on the road—— / Words dry and riderless / [...] While / From the bottom of the pool, fixed stars / Govern a life. (from "Words," Plath, 1965, p. 86)

Traces of love are hidden within the archaic aesthetic sphere; they are to be embraced and recognized even (and especially) when they are hidden behind the *Mother-phantasies of* Devouring, Abandonment, and Not-enoughness, which are primary, necessary, and must appear whether or not a real trauma has occurred.

The shocks of maternality are primal *even though* they appear for the first time in adulthood, not infancy: they ignite new psychic traumatic starting-points, new anxieties, and new responsibilities. Imprints of the shocks of maternality include traces of the intimate other's non-life-coming-into-life, imprints of the non-I's death or risk of dying with-in me (these losses, even when they are desired, are also painful and require mourning), the process of life-giving and finally of birthing. With a language to talk about these zones of shock, we can struggle against laws that appropriate the female body through censure, taboo, shame, guilt, and against the silencing of experiences related to femaleness. Unrecognized, shocks and the space related to the female body turn traumatic.

In her poetry, Sylvia Plath gives voice to shocks of maternality even where their subjectivizing processes fail as the "mother" is objectified and rejected both outside and inside of the self:

> The tulips are too red in the first place, they hurt me [...] I could hear them breathe / Lightly, through their white swaddlings, like an awful baby. / Their redness talks to my wound [...] A dozen red lead sinkers round my neck [...] And I have no face, I wanted to efface myself. / The vivid tulips eat my oxygen [...] Before they came the air was calm enough [...] Then the tulips filled it up like a loud noise [...] They concentrate my attention, that was happy / Playing and resting without committing itself [...] The tulips should be behind bars [...] And I am aware of my heart [...] / Its bowl of red blooms out of sheer love of me [...] ("Tulips," Plath, 1965, pp. 21–23)

She aches in her trans(sub)jective core—in her abjected I and abjected non-I. I is a red rose (daughter-mother) and tulip (daughter/infant) at the same instant or in a different time-space; red scar and dark ashes. I and non-I change places in-between different crystallizations of unborn-yet/new-born/girl/adult/(m/)Other clusters.

Shocks of maternality may be envisioned from the perspective of a matrixial bordertime, where a Persephone is already a virtual facet of a Demeter, where the now-daughter needs to create a respectful space-time for her possible futurities, for her own future old-age croneness. Deprived of the potency of her archaic-mother when her own mother-monster is as object abjected, the daughter's rebellion might work inside herself as a death wish that hides from her that she is languishing, longing to re-enter anew the passage from non-life to life.

> God's lioness / How one we grow / [...]—The furrow / Splits and passes [...] / Black sweet blood mouthfuls, / Shadows, / Something else / Hauls me through air—— / The child's cry / Melts in the wall. / And I / Am an arrow, / The dew that flies / Suicidal, at one with the drive / Into the red / eye [...] ("Ariel," Plath, 1965, pp. 36–37)

> You house your unnerving head—Godball,/ Lens of mercies / [...] Did I escape, I wonder? / My mind winds to you / Old barnacled umbilicus, Atlantic cable / [...] In any case, you are always there, / [...] touching and sucking / [...] I didn't call you at all / [...] You steamed to me over the sea, / Fat and red, a placenta. / [...] Overexposed like an X-ray. / Who do you think you are? [...] I shall take no bite of your body / Bottle in which I live [...] / Off, off eely tentacle! / There is nothing between us. ("Medusa," Plath, 1965, pp. 45–46)

And what now, when *she* is *her* kids' medusa, how does such a "*nothing* between us" function, does it bring any solace? Who is the infant then? Who is the mother? Spinning in a mother-abjection loop, the suffocated I tears holes in its matrixial web. When the hate toward medusa awakens, a poem's female body (of her mother? of her self as mother?) is fragmented; part body objects like mouth and breasts evade the pregnant body-home transformed into *female without embryo*. The poem reclaims an I through repulsion-dissection-fragmentation of a female body which bleeds in her red flower—one moment her infant, one moment her self-as-infant. Tulips push the mother-re-becoming-a-maiden to repulse them—and also herself, a now-mother always-still-an-infant.

The psychoanalytical idea that to complete individuation one must dissect each parent out ("castration") fails the subject as such. In "Medusa," connected through an "Old barnacled umbilicus," the poet-speaker rebirths herself by purging the connecting cable. Her triumph is: "There is nothing between us." Soon enough though she suffers *in her cable.* In such a triumph the I joins the rejected non-I envoided; the matrixial web is torn. The cable's tears burn. Pure red flame. A lioness flies bleeding. Aren't the wonderful queen-bee and the old bee a *one-with-in-one*?

> Is there any queen in it? / If there is, she is old, / Her wings torn shawels / [...] Poor and bare and unqueeny and even shameful. / [...] Is she dead, is she sleeping? Where has she been, / With her lion-red body, her wings of glass? / Now she is flying, / More terrible then she ever was, red / Scar in the sky, red comet / Over the engine that killed her [...] ("Stings," Plath, 1965, pp. 65–67)

> Perfection is terrible, it cannot have children. / Cold as snow breath, it tamps the womb / Where the yew trees blow like hydras, / The tree of life and the tree of life / Unloosing their moons, month after month, to no purpose. / The blood flood is the flood of love, / The absolute sacrifice. ("The Munich Mannequins," Plath, 1965, p. 74)

Each poem gives a voice to a mother's shock. Each poem a hair's breath between shock and trauma, between trauma and beauty.

A poem expresses a delirium-like desire of a mother to return her children to pre-life and non-life in her womb, the same womb whose infertility and menstruation was not so long ago deeply lamented. Death wishes appear as a desire to *dis*-mother and a *dis*birth the infant, to de-mother and unmother the mother.

The subject doesn't ask why she should go on living. She asks *why have I been born?*This is a trace of the cry of the *enigma of the primal scene*, the quest concerning not only what was the sexual desire between the parental figures but also what was, and therefore what is love. When Sylvia Plath becomes a mother she hurts as a potential becoming-crone for *her* daughter:

> The woman is perfected / Her dead Body wears the smile of accomplishment / [...] Each dead child coiled, a white serpent, / One at each little / Pitcher of milk, now empty, / She has folded / Them back into her body like petals / of a rose close when the garden / Stiffens its odours bleed / From the sweet deep throats of the night flower. ("Edge," Plath, 1965, p. 85)

> A gift, a love gift / Totally unasked for / By a sky / [...] O my God, what am I / That these late mouths should cry open / in a forest of frost [...] ("Poppies in October," Plath, 1965, p. 29)

17.7 Postface

A few pregnancies and two child-birthings revealed to me the shocks of maternality. The early periods of motherhood were moments where painting resisted me. I struggled to find voice for my silenced experiences for some decades to come. In becoming mother for the first time I m-othered myself through drawing and painting. My womb-and-skull shapes refused to be transformed to a human face. How this space form resisted me! How I couldn't draw in it a mouth! The heart of my hand refused, my heart-hand signed what I could hardly admit, a gapping void in the space-subject-matter. No mouth, no voice. Silence pronounced itself as a voice, like in my childhood. Lost in my experiences of child-birthing and early motherhood I painted faces without mouth, then destroyed the paintings (not all of them).

The passage from shock through trauma to full blown testimony might take 40 years. It demands a language. I will never really know where the shock hurts, since it hurts in me and in my non-I(s), the living and the dead. I became mother to a daughter abandoned by her father. This contributed to my thoughts about shocks of maternality. When in Paris I was pregnant with my second child (from my second partner), a boy, my ex-husband—father of my first daughter—committed suicide in London on May 24, 1988. I remember his mother's shock. I remember his father's shock. Secrets invaded our space. As I was lying in bed with contractions, navigated between home and hospital, hospital and home, I started to transform my fragmented notes into a theoretical writing. I desired some coherence. And I instantly knew that from now on, painting all day and writing all night, my life will be swallowed by painting-drawing-theorizing-painting-painting-theorizing-drawing-painting - - -

17.8 Note

Different versions of the chapters on Sylvia Plath were given as conference papers in 2012. (1) "Red Scar in the Sky. Ashes of *I & Non-I*—Nobody's Roses" and "Shocks of Maternality and Demeter-Persephone Complexity." Lectures at *IFPP Clinical Conference (Ibid)*. Dublin, 24 March 2012. (2) Symposium: *Com-passion and/as Self-fragilization: Thinking Art-Theory-Ethics with Bracha L. Ettinger and Rosi Braidotti.* [In *Fragilizing the Self, Resisting the System*, A Four part Event.] Utrecht University 13 April, 2012. (3) *Ettinger Masterclass.* "Matrixial Trans-subjectivity and the Subject: Fragilization and Resistance." and "Shocks of Maternality, Demeter-Persephone Complex and the Journal of Sylvia Plath." Utrecht University, 16 April, 2012. (4) "Red scar in the sky, Purple scar in our selves.

Resisting the self, Resisting endless fragmentation." Seminar-lecturing-performance in Solo installation: Seminar/*Room*. Casco, Utrecht, 18 April 2012.

Chapter V is reprint from different passages from: "Demeter-Persephone Complex, Entangled Aerials of the Psyche and Sylvia Plath." *ESC Journal,* 40.1: *Hysteria Manifest*. 2014. Some passages from the present chapter III appear also in ESC 40.1, 2014.

Different versions of the chapters on Laius Complex were given as conference papers in 2015. (1) "Shocks of Maternality, Laius Complex, Trust and Carriance. Franz Kafka and Sylvia Plath". Visiting Artist Masterclass. Seminar: *Fragilizing the Self: The Matrixial Borderspace*. Netherland Institute for Cultural Analysis (NICA). Faculty of Arts, Leuven, Belgium. 29 May 2015. (2) "Shocks of Maternality, Laius Complex, Trust and Carriance. Franz Kafka and Sylvia Plath". Conference: *Motherhood and Creativity*. Centre for Media and Culture Research, School of Arts and Creative Industries, London South Bank University. 1 June 2015. (3) "Carriance, Copoiesis and the Subreal", and "Laius Complex (with Franz Kafka) and Shocks of Maternality (with Sylvia Plath.)" Reading Seminar. *Istanbul in/+Leeds* series of events. The Tetley, Leeds. 4 June 2015.

Chapters I and II were read as "Laius Complex. Son's Sacrifice after Kafka, Benjamin, Delueuze-Guattari, Derrida." EGS Public Lecture. 2015.

References

Balint, M. (1954). *Primary love and psycho-analytic technique*. London: Hogarth Press.

Benjamin, W. (2007). Franz Kafka. *Illuminations*. (H. Zohn, Trans.). New York: Schocken Books.

Bion, W. R. (1977). *Two papers. The Grid and Caesura* (p. 1989). London: Karnac.

Bollas, C. (1987). *The shadow of the object*. London: Free Association.

Deleuze, G., & Guattari, F. (1986). An exaggerated Oedipus. In *Toward a minor literature* (pp. 9–15). (D. Polan, Trans.). Minneapolis: University of Minnesota Press.

Derrida, J. (1996). *The gift of death*. Chicago: University of Chicago Press.

Ettinger, B. L. (2005). On the fascinum—The freezing and killing gaze. And on the fascinance—The gaze as continual encounter that evokes a creative event [Hebrew]. In *Proceedings of History and Theory*, Bezalel. Online Web Journal. http://bezalel.secured.co.il/zope/home/he/1126095346/1127749237

Ettinger, B. L. (2006a). *The matrixial borderspace*. London: University of Minnesota Press.

Ettinger, B. L. (2006b). Fascinance. The woman-to-woman (Girl-to-m/Other) matrixial feminine difference. In G. Pollock (Ed.), *Psychoanalysis and the image* (pp. 60–93). Oxford: Blackwell.

Ettinger, B. L. (2006c). Antigone with(out) Jocaste. Compassionate co-response-ability and matrixial tear. In S. E. Wilmer & A. Zukauskaite (Eds.), *Interrogating Antigone* (pp. 212–228). Oxford: Oxford University Press. 2010.

Ettinger, B. L. (2007). Diotima and the matrixial transference: Psychoanalytical encounter-event as pregnancy in beauty. In C. N. Van der Merwe & H. Viljoen (Eds.), *Across the threshold: Explorations of liminality in literature* (pp. 105–132). New York: Peter Lang & Potchefstroom. Literator.

Ettinger, B. L. (2010). (M)Other Re-spect. Maternal Subjectivity, the ready-made mother-monster and the ethics of respecting. *Mamsie—Studies in the Maternal, 3*, e-Journal. London: Birkbeck University. http://www.mamsie.bbk.ac.uk/mother_respect.html

Ettinger, B. (2013). Rethinking subject through theology, psychoanalysis and Levinas. EGS Public Lecture. 2013. Lecture in video on youtube https://www.youtube.com/watch?v=hlSxiM_6918

Ettinger, B. L. (2014). Demeter-Persephone complex, entangled Aerials of the Psyche, and Sylvia Plath. *English Studies in Canada, 40*(1), 123–154.

Freud, S. (1914). On Narcissism: An introduction. In *The standard edition of the complete psychological works of Sigmund Freud* (Vol. XIV, pp. 73–102). London: Hogarth Press. 1957.

Freud, S. (1926). Inhibitions, symptoms and anxiety. In *The standard edition of the complete psychological works of Sigmund Freud* (Vol. XX, pp. 87–169). London: Hogarth Press. 1959.

Kafka, F. (1966). Letter to his father: Brief an den/Franz Kafka; translation by Ernst Kaiser and Eithne Wilkins. New York: Schocken Books.

Lyotard, J.-F. (1996). *The differend. Phrases in dispute*. (G. Van Den Abbeele, Trans.). Minneapolis: University of Minnesota Press.

Plath, S. (1965). *Ariel*. London: Faber and Faber.

Plath, S. (2000). *The Journals of Sylvia Plath 1950–1962*. (K. V. Kukil (Ed.)). London: Faber and Faber.

Rudnytsky, P. L. (1998). The analyst's murder of the patient. *American Imago, 55*(3), 349–359.

Winnicott, D. W. (1949). Birth memories, birth trauma and anxiety. In *Collected papers: Through pediatrics to psychoanalysis*. London: Karnac. 1992.

Winnicott, D. W. (1963). Communicating and not communicating. In R. Winnicott (Ed.), *Lesly Caldwell and Angela Joyce*. London: Routledge. 2011.

Winnicott, D. W. (1971). *Playing and reality*. London: Routledge.

Winnicott, D. W. (1974). Fear of breakdown. *International Review of Psycho-Analysis, 1*, 103–107.

18 Fear, Trauma, and Posttraumatic Stress Disorder: Clinical, Neurobiological, and Cultural Perspectives

Mikael Rubin, Maya Neria, and Yuval Neria

18.1 Introduction

Fear is key to animal and human experience and function. It evokes a clear behavioral response, and has traditionally been considered a biologically "basic" emotion (Adolphs, 2013; Ekman, 1992), directly linked to exposure to threat. Because effective response to threat (i.e., detecting danger and responding appropriately) is regarded as crucial to survival, the mammalian brain has developed an excellent fear detection networks capable of tracking and monitoring threats and determining suitable responses (Öhman & Mineka, 2003; Öhman, 2005).

The most commonly characterized fear response is "fight or flight," motivated by a threatening encounter. The imperative to respond to threat relates primarily to self-preservation, although for humans other factors, such as the ethical or moral, may play a role that potentially mitigates the very *response* to fear, though pointedly not the feeling of fear itself. Furthermore, there is a third option that is not as frequently discussed, known as freezing (or tonic immobility). The response of freezing is characterized primarily as "playing dead," and can be effective in situations where there is no apparent possibility of escape; this response also involves a certain degree of physiological numbing (Nijenhuis, Spinhoven, Vanderlinden, van Dyck, & van der Hart, 1998). The feeling of fear, the fight or flight response, and freezing all occur contextually—in situations of imminent threat.

Imminent threat, if severe, may constitute a psychological trauma (e.g., physical and/or sexual assault, wars, and natural disasters). Yet the primary difference between fear and trauma is that fear is a *response* to an event, while trauma is the *event* itself; moreover, fear may be a response to a traumatic event, but this is not always the case. This distinction has become blurred as the *response* to an event has become increasingly connected with the *event* itself. This leads to the somewhat ambiguous definition of trauma. As is increasingly the case in contemporary discourse, the term trauma can both refer to the time of the traumatic event (the event itself), as well as the psychosocial and cognitive ramifications of experiencing intense fear during a traumatic event (the result of the event).

To clarify this distinction, in this chapter we explore the multiple relationships between fear and trauma and examine how they intertwine in

M. Rubin, M.A.
Psychology Department, University of Texas at Austin, Austin, TX, USA

M. Neria, B.A.
Middlebury College, Middlebury, VT, USA

Y. Neria, Ph.D. (✉)
Columbia University Medical Center and the New York State Psychiatric Institute, New York, NY, USA
e-mail: ny126@cumc.columbia.edu

Y. Ataria et al. (eds.), *Interdisciplinary Handbook of Trauma and Culture*,
DOI 10.1007/978-3-319-29404-9_18

the context of their most relevant psychopathology—posttraumatic stress disorder (PTSD).

PTSD is characterized by persistent fearful responses to cues that are related to the event directly or peripherally. In either case, a cue can trigger memories of past traumatic event(s). Symptoms of this disorder include reexperiencing, increased arousal (e.g., hypervigilance), and efforts to avoid threat-related cues (e.g., attentional avoidance). Overall, PTSD results in severe functional impairments, as well as psychological and physical health issues. Reports have consistently confirmed that those who suffer from PTSD tend to have lower life satisfaction, poorer health, are more likely to be unemployed, and struggle with interpersonal difficulties (Kessler, Sonnega, Bromet, Hughes, & Nelson, 1995; Kimble & Kaufman, 2004). In other words, in PTSD, a traumatic experience leads to an impairment of the fear network (e.g., a difficulty in extinguishing fear memories) that results in a number of emotional, behavioral and cognitive impairments.

Current understanding of the fear network involves interaction between several brain regions, hypothesized to govern emotional response—both at "higher" functions towards the front of the brain, and "lower" functions (where higher/lower refer to evolutionary sequence, with higher function appearing later), which include the hippocampus, amygdala, and prefrontal cortex—broadly considered the "fear circuit" (Knight, Smith, Cheng, Stein, & Helmstetter, 2004; Öhman 2005). The fear network is also intimately connected to neurochemical interactions of dopamine and serotonin, the brain's main neurotransmitters related to mood and affective disorders, among others, centered around mediation from the hypothalamic–pituitary–adrenal axis (Vermetten & Bremner, 2002). A basic response to a fearful event involves a series of psychological and neurochemical cascades that are also reflected physiologically. While a fear of a specific thing, such as a snake, represents a fairly linear response-activation pattern, in PTSD the fear response is not necessarily directly related to a specific memory cue. In other words, the resultant fear from PTSD may interact and intersect with activities of daily life—it is not necessarily a fear of a specific thing (like a snake), but a more general, more difficult to define fear, that permeates experience more broadly.

So that while a fear of snakes can severely impact a person's functioning, it does so primarily in response to the phobia-specific stimulus. PTSD however, which emerges from the traumatic experience, is linked to the memory of the event, but not necessarily to a feeling of fear *about* the event. Thus, the difference is that regardless of how much fear is felt by an individual *during* a traumatic event, what emerges as the root of the development of PTSD is the individual's relationship to the *memory* of the event. And while, as with a phobia, there can be stimuli specific triggers that induce a fear response, there are also broader implications of the disorder, affecting functioning across a range of domains (from attention to sleep).

The critical domain that is linked most to both the symptomology and treatment of PTSD is intrusive memories. It is, more specifically, that these memories interfere with an individuals daily functioning, while awake and even while asleep. The most well-studied and effective treatments of PTSD aim to completely and thoroughly treat the disorder by addressing the root of the fear, which is essentially related to memory. What is significant for the discussion here is that the memory of the trauma, in the experience of intrusion, manifests in both psychological and physiological symptoms of distress. Unfortunately, since the effect of memory on psychopathology is not fully understood, it is difficult to determine the precise mechanisms that interrelate memory with fear and how this can influence an individual in so many ways.

As PTSD represents one kind of involuntary change in fear processing and response, culture itself exerts a diametrically opposed response to fear—and, in many cases, to trauma—one in which the response of fear becomes loaded with social implications that are divorced from the emotional experience of fear itself. Within contemporary culture, the very concept of fear has shifted away from the neurobiological and evolutionarily necessary understanding of fear as an important, appropriate, survival-driven emotional response to events that may be fundamentally threatening. Instead, acceptable fear has broadened beyond an individual's scope of experience—fear exists instead as an abstract (the fear of crime, for instance). Hypocritically, actual fear experienced by an individual, or individuals, in the context of trauma has become largely characterized as a weakness. Culturally biased perspectives of fear not only characterize individual fears as poor, but also exacerbate trauma-related psychopathology by minimizing the effect of traumatic events. In the course of providing an overview of the neurological and sociological effects of fear and their interaction with trauma, we argue that it is imperative that psychological treatments focus on the consequences of fear in individual as well as social realms, and their interaction with trauma-related psychopathology.

18.2 The Evolutionary Basis of Fear

Survival is dependent on the ability to detect threat and successfully cope with it. The chosen detection and coping mechanism is dependent on a host of factors including fear learning and fear extinction (i.e., the ability to learn potential associations between threat and related cues and as well as to extinguish those associations if they do not predict threat). Although the basic capacity to detect and respond to a threat is present in the simplest organisms, changes in scope and complexity of these responses and the development of the "emotional brain" that includes a well-devised fear network have been refined in the mammalian brain (LeDoux, 2012). Hence, the evolution of a more complex symptomatology associated with fear has both saved and plagued the human race; hence, reexperiencing, increased arousal (e.g., hypervigilance, facilitated attention), and efforts to avoid threat-related cues (e.g., attentional avoidance) are the cornerstones of fear- and trauma-related psychopathologies.

18.3 The Development of Fear

While most fear *processing* is unconscious, involving basic processes of learning (mainly fear conditioning and fear extinction), the *experience* of fear is conscious. When the exposure to a threatening object is ongoing and repeated, the emotion of fear is distinctly conscious and at times overwhelming. While most fear-related behaviors are well justified, human beings of all ages can be haunted by anxiety, lack a sense of safety, and have feelings of vulnerability. This chronic presence of fear, specifically in a typically safe context, can be characterized as symptomatic of PTSD. Additionally, one of the key characteristics of PTSD is an impaired ability to effectively distinguish between safe and dangerous conditions. Furthermore, and with regard to attention deficits, trauma-exposed individuals often exhibit heightened reactivity to natural stimuli associated with a traumatic event, even in the absence of real danger. A soldier returning from combat, for example, may react to a loud sound, such as a car backfiring, as though it were an exploding bomb, with a level of physiological and emotional arousal more appropriate to a war zone than to a suburban street. Indeed, overgeneralization of fear is common among trauma-exposed people and is a significant component of the clinical presentation of PTSD symptoms.

18.4 Fear Takes a Pathologic Turn

Exposure to severe trauma is common. More than three-quarters of the general population of the USA is likely to be exposed to at least one traumatic event in their lifetime. Additionally, more than one-third of people are exposed to severe traumas—wars, disasters, and assaults—and are subsequently at high risk of developing a significant psychopathology, such as PTSD (Galea, Nandi, & Vlahov, 2005; Glover, Olfson, Gameroff, & Neria, 2010). While surveys have consistently shown that most people exhibit resilience after being exposed to trauma, those who develop trauma-related psychopathology, particularly PTSD, suffer from a considerable health burden, psychosocial dysfunction, suicidal behaviors, and increased utilization of health services (Kessler, Chiu, Demler, & Walters, 2005; Shvil et al., 2013; Bonanno, Westphal, & Mancini, 2011). Further, reports have consistently confirmed that those who suffer from PTSD tend to have lower life satisfaction, poorer health, are more likely to be unemployed, and struggle with interpersonal difficulties (Kessler et al., 1995; Kimble & Kaufman, 2004; Neria, Nandi, & Galea, 2008).

18.5 The Diagnosis of PTSD

The diagnosis of PTSD, as defined in the *Diagnostic and Statistical Manual of Mental Disorders* (DSM) used by health professionals in the USA to diagnose mental disorders based on a checklist of symptoms, has undergone several important transformations in the last few decades. Initially, the diagnosis of PTSD in the DSM-3 assumed a stressor beyond an ordinary event (e.g., combat, torture, sexual assault). Such stressors became the primary criteria (Criterion A) for the diagnosis of PTSD (APA 1980). However, further clinical and scientific developments in PTSD research indicated that better characterization of the potentially traumatic events was needed. Consequently, Criterion A(1) of PTSD was refined to be more specific regarding types of traumas experienced and another facet was added: Criterion A(2), to specify that the individual's response to the trauma needed to involve fear, helplessness, or horror (APA 1994). Interestingly, less than 20 years later, the DSM-5 Criterion A(2) was removed (APA 2013), following accumulating evidence that the experience of fear at the time of the traumatic event did not necessarily play a predictive role for PTSD following exposure to trauma. This point is especially important with regard to the discussion of the role of trauma (e.g., chronic fear related to a traumatic event) versus fear (e.g., intense fear versus lack of fear during a trauma event) in determining psychopathology.

Nevertheless, fear plays a central role in defining a number of criteria across the five symptom clusters outlined in the DSM-5, including within Criterion B (intrusion symptoms), Criterion D (negative alterations in cognition and mood), and Criterion E (alterations in arousal and reactivity). What the diagnostic shifts over these iterations of the DSM perhaps indicates is an increasing understanding that PTSD involves a dysfunctional fear response and that this response is not necessarily involved in the initial experience of the trauma itself and instead may be related more broadly to the aftermath and the course of the processing of a traumatic event.

The physiological symptoms related to fear (e.g., sweating, pupil dilation, and increased heart rate and respiration) normally only last a few seconds in response to a startling event (Bradley, Lang, & Cuthbert, 1993). For individuals suffering from PTSD, however, a mild startling sound may elicit a heightened and extended response. Instead of subsiding after a few seconds, the response may take minutes to resolve itself and lead to further psychosocial complications (Vaidyanathan et al. 2009); the very activation of a fear response may have a titrating effect, triggering a host of other symptoms intimately related to the feeling of fear that generates a reminder of the traumatic event (Hetzel-Riggin 2010). What fundamentally distinguishes the diagnosis of PTSD from a "typical" fear response is that the behavioral reactions are normal responses—e.g., being startled by a loud sound—but the intensity, duration, and frequency of the responses are significantly heightened, and may sometimes manifest themselves in situations unrelated to a "normal" potentially threatening event. Related to this phenomenon, another symptom listed in the DSM-5 of Criterion E (alterations in arousal and reactivity) involves vigilance. Again, while it is acceptable and expected that one is cautious in a dangerous neighborhood at night, being constantly vigilant in a safe environment, such as at work or home, suggests that a feeling of fear pervades the relatively mundane—that is, fear transcends context and manifests in a more continuous way. Such hypervigilance is a cornerstone of PTSD and can result in severe functional attentional impairments.

Many people have, at least once, woken from a nightmare sweating or gasping for breath. Experiencing nightmares night after night, however, constitutes one of the Criterion B symptoms for intrusion in the diagnosis of PTSD. While other reexperiencing symptoms include intrusive thoughts or memories of the event(s) or flashbacks, because they occur during waking life and because they directly represent the memory of the event that is thought to be at the root of the PTSD, they are frequently the main targets in treatments for PTSD. However, a question remains: How is it possible to target dreams in treatment, that is, to control one's dreams? What if, even after someone feels generally better in his or her daily life, he or she still experiences recurring nightmares? The answer seems to lie in the hypothesis that the nightmares that individuals with PTSD experience are related to intrusive memories—similar to what individuals with PTSD experience while awake (Coalson, 1995). Furthermore, even when an individual reports general symptom amelioration after treatment, they may still have nightmares related to the traumatic event. This suggests that there is an imperfect understanding of how memory is related to fear and that, in turn, treatments that focus on targeting this significant but not exclusive feature of PTSD do not necessarily utilize a comprehensive approach—though we recognize that this may be less a question of the treatments themselves and more an issue with the understanding of memory itself.

Gaps in treatment, however, may have as much to do with the lack of an understanding of precisely how fear and memory lead to PTSD. It is important, then, to emphasize that psychological trauma is not only a neurological, psychological, and physiological phenomenon, but that the experience of fear is also closely tied to a shared cultural understanding of what should be feared. Hence, to examine fear in its cultural milieu, both broadly, and more narrowly within the military, offers a contrast to the biological predisposition of fear, and the pathological turn of fear in PTSD, and from this we then turn to perspectives on treatment—incorporating the social considerations along with the biological and psychopathological.

18.6 Fear: The Sociocultural Domain

To understand the role of fear in present-day society, and as a key factor in the modification of an individual's psychology and behaviors, it is necessary to place special emphasis on its temporal nature. Today, the object of fear cannot simply be defined as a presently threatening agent; rather, it is the expectation that a negative outcome will arise from that threatening agent (Barbalet, 1998). The perception of danger in the future constitutes a present state of fear, which is both socially mediated by external factors (the environment, social discourse, individual biases, anxiety levels, trauma history, etc.) (Tudor 2003).

In attempting to examine fear macroscopically, Tudor (2003) outlined six parameters of fear: environments, cultures, social structures, bodies, personalities and social subjects. "The object of fear is not adequately conceptualized as a threatening agent who or which should be avoided. Rather the object of fear is an expectation of negative outcome" (Tudor 2003, p. 240). While this informs the primary psychopathology discussed above, a critical consideration of the social contextual elements that inform a new (post)modern etiology of fear is required.

1. *Environments*: Converging evidence suggests that, across species, fear guides behaviors associated with coping with and navigation through dangerous environments. Considered a mode of institutional fear, the environment consists of the physical attributes of one's surroundings. For example, the presence of a threatening object or feature plays a large role in the mediating the evocation of fear. More indirectly, there may be a particular quality or trait about a specific place that is suggestive of a future threat (perhaps due to a past traumatic/fearful event or due to a cultural understanding of "scary" or potentially threatening places), thereby instigating a fear in response to a potential danger.
2. *Cultures*: Our cultures teach us what should be feared. During the Cold War between the Soviet Union and the USA, for example, there was a very real sense of fear over the perceived threat of communism. Today, such fear is by and large absent from our everyday thinking. Historically, fear has been associated with a clear object of threat: the threat of death, whether by enemy, predator, or starvation.

Today, however, the *experience* of fear itself is feared (Furedi, 1997). In particular, human consciousness has developed and advanced in such a way that the biological basis for fear has been psychosocially surpassed, and the emotion has become farther removed from its evolutionary roots. The feeling of fear indirectly determines the actions of our society. The fear of crime, for example, is in many ways viewed as a serious problem both distinct from and potentially more debilitating than the physical acts of crime themselves (Bannister & Fyfe, 2001). This idea constitutes the "culture of fear," recently acknowledged by many sociologists, that dictates everyday behaviors and contributes to society's institutional structures (Tudor 2003). As prominent sociologists observe, the fear of crime is viewed as a distinct societal problem, which has led to institutional and political changes aimed at reducing fear levels, rather than reducing crime itself (Garland, 2001).

3. *Social structures*: Sociologists have echoed the growing discourse of fear in modern-day society. Cultural perspectives of fear play a large role in creating and changing this discourse. In reflecting upon modern-day society, sociologists have pointed to the fact that evaluation of everyday activities and society as a whole has shifted towards a consideration of safety (Furedi, 1997). The idea behind surveillance and safety measures is to minimize the feeling of fear surrounding a future danger, serving as calming force to decrease the destabilizing effect of fear on everyday functioning rather than resolving the danger itself.
4. *Bodies*: According to psychologists and neurobiologists, fear, and more specifically fear-processing, serves a key function in human survival. Historically, three components of fear have been elucidated: physiological arousal, subject reactivity, and behavioral avoidance (Lang, 1970). The physical symptoms of fear have been extensively investigated, especially with regard to "fight or flight" reactions and the activation of the parasympathetic and sympathetic branches of the autonomic nervous system. For example, psychophysiological and endocrine measures of fear in humans include skin-conductance response, increased heart rate and respiration, the presence of salivary cortisol (associated with long-duration arousal and stress), and dilated pupils.
5. *Personalities*: the role that fear plays in present-day society is largely defined in contrast to courage. Fear, perceived as a "basic" emotion, is frowned upon and carries a negative association, especially if it results in cowardice. Further, in certain cultures, particularly among societies at war, fear is regularly persecuted in trials that may even result in the death penalty. On the other hand, acts of courage in the same war-ridden societies may lead to recognition and widespread public support for individuals who have acted courageously in the face of fear. However, fearlessness, seemingly quite similar to courage, is frequently considered foolish or ignorant. The line separating courage and fearlessness, therefore, carries significant importance because both appear to function in opposition to fear. The distinction between courage and fearlessness lies in the presence or absence of fear. Courageous behavior can be defined as persistence in dealing with a subjectively dangerous situation (i.e., a soldier advancing towards an enemy) despite physiological and psychosocial signs of fear. Fearlessness, in contrast, is persistence in dealing with a potentially dangerous situation in the absence of the aforementioned indicators of fear (Rachman, 2004). Some psychologists claim that with routinized behavior, courage may transform into fearlessness. In a study conducted on skydivers, for example, researchers concluded that successful practice of a fearful act (e.g., jumping out of the plane and landing)—noted as competence—and increased self-confidence contribute to courageous performance, leading to a decrease in subjective fear and ultimately, a state of fearlessness surrounding the act (Rachman, 2004). Henceforth, overcoming acts that are fear-inducing, whether they be related to combat (e.g., facing an enemy) or daring activities (e.g., skydiving),

may first be viewed as courageous, though once habituated to, may result in fearlessness and be redefined as foolish.

6. *Social subjects*: Studies conducted on soldiers and skydivers reveal that there are several factors that contribute to the performance of courageous and fearless acts, one of which is support from a cohesive group (Rachman, 2004). In the case of a soldier, the knowledge that a lack of display of courage may lead to a court sentence, however, is frightening in and of itself. Though accounts of camaraderie between and within troops are widespread and well known, the support from the greater social system—our society, the judicial system, etc.—is virtually nonexistent. Court trials are made public; soldiers become aware of the possibility of judicial punishment. Such sentiment is then enveloped into the discourse of army troops, with commemoration of all those who have proven to be courageous, and profound humiliation for those who let fear incapacitate them.

With regard to Tudor's parameters of fear, the first group (environments, cultures, and social structures) macroscopically transcend an individual's agency. The second group (bodies, personalities, and social subjects) is centered on the involvement of individual agents that are subjective and have greater experience-based flexibility. All six parameters interact in different ways to produce distinctive types of fear related to a variety of circumstances. The temporal component of fear relates primarily to the dynamic nature of fear where the individual and social environments interact over time to continually generate distinct conceptualizations of fear. For instance, the fear of communism has basically subsided and is now attributed to the historical period of the cold war, whereas terrorism is a very present fear in contemporary society; moreover, the way that an individual experiences fear fundamentally interacts with extant fear of the sociocultural environment they are situated in. "Fear, then, is a product of interlocking relations between…the 'modes of institutional fearfulness' (given by the structuring environments) and the 'modes of individual fearfulness' (deriving from the formations of individual identity)" (Tudor 2003, p. 251).

The juxtaposition of the biological basis of fear and the persecution of fear, especially during times of war and under the umbrella of "cowardice," reveals an opposition between biological and social imperatives, and more specifically on the interaction between fear and trauma. To examine this distinction more closely we examine to a specific case that introduces fear of persecution as a fear that lies at an intersection of the conflict between biological response and social expectations, and that soldiers must overcome during times of war.

In 2003, a US Army Green Beret soldier, Sergeant Pogany, faced charges of cowardice, of being "too scared to do his duty," as an interrogator in Iraq (Gettleman, 2003a). During the investigation, the army contended that the soldier was guilty of "cowardly conduct as a result of fear," pointing to his response to a violent act he witnessed, where he experienced uncontrollable violent shaking and vomiting. In response to the charge, the soldier countered that he was only guilty of a panic attack that resulted in his inability to function. If he had been found guilty, Pogany could have faced the death penalty. The indictment of cowardice relates to the inability to function in the face of fear; that is, the inability to act "courageously." The juxtaposition between a soldier's response to fear and a civilian's response to fear illuminates the conflicting definitions of courage and fearlessness. Had a civilian had a panic attack witnessing the disembodiment of another human, his or her response would have been expected (and lack of a response might have been considered abnormal). But Pogany's fear led to widespread humiliation and, ultimately, a legal battle.

During investigations of cowardice, military officials emphasize the role that fear plays in such charges: being scared is "not enough to be charged with cowardice" (Gettleman, 2003a). Rather, what leads to a conviction is misbehavior stemming from fear. Specifically, the Manual for Courts-Martial defines cowardice as "misbehavior motivated by fear" (as cited in Gettleman, 2003a).

Further, the Military Judges' Benchbook defines cowardly conduct as "the refusal or abandonment of a performance of duty" before or in the presence of the enemy "as a result of fear" (as cited in Gettleman, 2003a). In reflecting upon military settings, as well as in social setting more broadly, the persecuted soldier claimed, "coward is a pretty big stigma to carry around" (Gettleman, 2003b). Courage, so highly esteemed during times of conflict and in military settings, is regarded as the ability to continue a behavior despite feeling a high degree of subjective fear and/or unpleasant bodily sensations. Hence, the inability to act due to fear is considered the individual's failure in the context of a broader social prerogative (such as war—or more specifically in Pogany's case, interrogation).

18.7 Implications for the Treatment of PTSD

Cultural and social expectations have muddied the distinction between fearfulness (i.e., the experience of fear) and "cowardice" (i.e., not being able to cope with fear). More significantly, fear—as a "basic" emotion that cuts across species, with a true evolutionary prerogative in the neurobiological and evolutionary sense, where it represents a functional and necessary emotion—lacks any sort of social or cultural significance for the individual (except when it is used by institutions to manipulate populations along political, economic or religious lines, but this is, also, not really the kind of fear we are discussing here). The onset of fear results in behavioral modifications within an organism, specifically the modulation of memory coding and retrieval, the redirection of attention, and the performance of vigilant or avoidant behaviors. In this sense, fear goes hand-in-hand with adaptation, encouraging the modification of cognitive and behavioral responses to increase individual fitness (Adolphs, 2013). Put simply, Western culture has emphasized fear as "bad," as an emotion that interferes with healthy functioning. Such a viewpoint ultimately makes PTSD patients, such as clinically traumatized war veterans, perceived as having failed in some fundamental way.

In addition to a contradictory characterization of fear as an irrational emotion (as compared to its evolutionary definition as both necessary and valuable), society has an overwhelming tendency to blame the victim of a trauma. Hence, fear-related psychopathology has become something that is frequently delegitimized, and patients are forced to suffer from both the symptoms of trauma(s) as well as symptoms related to society's perceptions of them as sufferers of trauma(s).

The idea that the survivor is responsible for the trauma leads to a cycle of self-blame, where the event is a failure of the individual's prerogative—what he or she could have said and/or done differently, and indeed what he or she can *do* differently. In some cases, an overwhelming sense that the survivor should no longer bear the experience of the trauma in the public sphere assumes control, this leads to the belief that the survivor should bury his or her fear, because an inability to keep it suppressed represents another kind of weakness, another form of fear.

Outright blame as well as self-blame of people suffering from PTSD is largely due to societal reinforcements that the feeling of fear is something to be embarrassed about. The group and/or community that the victim of a trauma belongs to generally facilitates stigmatization of said victim. For example, the victim may be seen as causing or deserving of the trauma. Further, the community may wish to maintain a view of the just/moral world they live in; that is, they wish to see the world as predictable, orderly, and controllable and overall without threatening or trauma-inducing agents. As Holloway and Fullteron (1994) point out, the sense of an ethical world is retained at the cost of blaming the victim. This phenomenon is commonly internalized by the victim and is manifested as self-blame. Brewin, MacCarthy, and Furnham (1989) found that greater posttrauma self-blame was associated with greater social withdrawal, reinforcing the cycle of societal-enhanced posttrauma symptomatology.

The majority of current treatments are not adequately addressing this pervasive issue. Prolonged Exposure (PE) therapy, considered a first line treatment for PTSD, involves imaginal exposure sessions in which patients describe the traumatic event in the present tense while attempting to integrate as much detail as possible into the retelling (Foa, Rothbaum, Riggs, & Murdock, 1991). Additionally, it has elements of cognitive reformulation that address self-blame and cultural impetus, providing an opportunity to reframe and rename experiences in order to make them less guilt-oriented. Trauma-focused Cognitive Behavioral Therapy (CBT) and Eye Movement Desensitization and Reprocessing (EMDR) have been shown to be equally effective (Jeffries & Davis, 2013), and are generally considered to be similarly effective as PE (Powers, Halpern, Ferenschak, Gillihan, & Foa, 2010). These three treatments (and numerous variations on these treatment modalities) all emphasize engaging with the feared experience and working to overcome it. It is interesting to note, however, that Interpersonal Psychotherapy (IPT), which does not involve exposure to reminders of the trauma, was recently shown to be as effective as PE for treating PTSD (Markowitz et al., 2015). Indeed, IPT is systematically focused on interactions with human networks, engaging in activities, accomplishing newly defined life goals, and overcoming guilt, shame and self-defeat. Thus, while treatments of PTSD necessarily engage with *emotions* arising from the experience of the trauma—including, but not exclusively fear—part of their effectiveness may stem from a consideration of the role emotions play, not just in an individual context, but a social one.

While there are a number of different factors, like socioeconomic status, that may contribute to the development of psychological disorders in general, and PTSD specifically (McEwen & Gianaros, 2010; Wadsworth & Achenbach, 2005) psychological treatment in Western contexts is considered to be treatment of the individual. So that even though some highly effective psychotherapies do focus more generally on social implications of PTSD, there remains at issue the idea of a broader approach to mental health that seeks to work at a social level. In PTSD a fearful response is not evoked intentionally, or deliberately; indeed, it is not desired. But because, broadly, psychological distress is not necessarily taken seriously, and more specifically because individuals with PTSD sometimes have a fearful response to a relatively benign event, there is concern over lack of support for the individual who suffers as the result of a traumatic event. The socialized unacceptability of a fearful response, the stereotyping/mockery/denigration that ensues at the expression of fear, means that current treatments must act to a greater or lesser extent as insulation from the unfavorable sociocultural atmosphere. And this is doubly problematic: first, because it means an individual with PTSD is either forced to hide or minimize their distress and second, because treatment is forced to address, in many cases, not only the traumatic event and its response, but others' (i.e., social) response, particularly when it is negative, to the event(s). The primary, and very simple, idea this paper concludes with is that a compassionate attitude towards individuals who experience fear can have a positive influence. Because fear is a basic biological function that everyone experiences, recognizing and accepting fear as an emotion in oneself and others has the potential to positively influence the recognition and treatment of PTSD, even outside of treatment itself.

References

American Psychiatric Association. (1980). *Diagnostic and statistical manual of mental disorders: DSM-III* (3rd ed.). Arlington, VA: American Psychiatric Publishing, Inc.

American Psychiatric Association. (1994). *Diagnostic and statistical manual of mental disorders: DSM-IV* (4th ed.). Arlington, VA: American Psychiatric Publishing, Inc.

American Psychiatric Association. (2013). *Diagnostic and statistical manual of mental disorders: DSM-V* (5th ed.). Arlington, VA: American Psychiatric Publishing, Inc.

Adolphs, R. (2013). The biology of fear. *Current Biology, 23*(2), R79–R93.

Barbalet, J. M. (1998). *Emotion, social theory, and social structure: A macrosociological approach.* Cambridge: Cambridge University Press.

Bonanno, G. A., Westphal, M., & Mancini, A. D. (2011). Resilience to Loss and Potential Trauma. Annual Review of Clinical Psychology, 7(1), 511–535. http://doi.org/10.1146/annurev-clinpsy-032210-104526.

Bannister, J., & Fyfe, N. (2001). Introduction: Fear and the city. *Urban Studies, 38*(5–6), 808.

Bradley, M. M., Lang, P. J., & Cuthbert, B. N. (1993). Emotion, novelty, and the startle reflex: habituation in humans. *Behavioral Neuroscience*, *107*(6), 970–80. Retrieved from http://www.ncbi.nlm.nih.gov/pubmed/8136072

Brewin, C. R., MacCarthy, B., & Furnham, A. (1989). Social support in the face of adversity: The role of cognitive appraisal. *Journal of Research in Personality, 23*(3), 354–372. doi:10.1016/0092-6566(89)90007-X.

Coalson, B. (1995). Nightmare help: Treatment of trauma survivors with PTSD. Psychotherapy: Theory, Research, Practice, Training, 32(3), 381–388. http://doi.org/10.1037/0033-3204.32.3.381.

Ekman, P. (1992). An argument for basic emotions. *Cognition Emotion, 6*, 169–200.

Foa, E. B., Rothbaum, B. O., Riggs, D. S., & Murdock, T. B. (1991). Treatment of posttraumatic stress disorder in rape victims: A comparison between cognitive-behavioral procedures and counseling. *Journal of Consulting and Clinical Psychology, 59*(5), 715–723.

Furedi, F. (1997). *The culture of fear risk taking and the morality of low expectations*. London: Cassell.

Garland, D. (2001). *The culture of control; crime and social order in contemporary society* (p. 10). Oxford: Oxford University Press.

Galea, S., Nandi, A., & Vlahov, D. (2005). The epidemiology of post-traumatic stress disorder after disasters. *Epidemiologic Reviews, 27*, 78–91. doi:10.1093/epirev/mxi003.

Gettleman, J. (2003a, November 6). Soldier accused as coward says he is guilty only of panic attack. *The New York Times*. http://www.nytimes.com.

Gettleman, J. (2003b, November 7). Reduced charges for soldier accused of cowardice in Iraq. *The New York Times*. http://www.nytimes.com.

Glover, K., Olfson, M., Gameroff, M. J., & Neria, Y. (2010). Assault and mental disorders: A cross-sectional study of urban adult primary care patients. *Psychiatric Services, 61*(10), 1018–1023. doi:10.1176/appi.ps.61.10.1018.

Holloway, H., & Fullteron, C. (1994). The psychology of terror and its aftermath. In *Individual and community responses to trauma and disaster: The structure of human chaos* (pp. 31–45). New York: Cambridge University Press.

Jeffries, F. W., & Davis, P. (2013). What is the role of eye movements in eye movement desensitization and reprocessing (EMDR) for post-traumatic stress disorder (PTSD)? A review. *Behavioural and Cognitive Psychotherapy, 41*(3), 290–300. doi:10.1017/S1352465812000793.

Kessler, R. C., Sonnega, A., Bromet, E., Hughes, M., & Nelson, C. B. (1995). Posttraumatic stress disorder in the National Comorbidity Survey. *Archives of General Psychiatry*, *52*(12), 1048–60. Retrieved from http://www.ncbi.nlm.nih.gov/pubmed/7492257

Kessler, R. C., Chiu, W. T., Demler, O., & Walters, E. E. (2005). Prevalence, severity, and comorbidity of 12-month DSM-IV disorders in the National Comorbidity Survey Replication. Archives of general psychiatry, 62(6), 617–627.

Kimble, M., & Kaufman, M. (2004). Clinical correlates of neurological change in posttraumatic stress disorder: An overview of critical systems. *The Psychiatric Clinics of North America, 27*(1), 49–65. doi:10.1016/S0193-953X(03)00108-4.

Knight, D. C., Smith, C. N., Cheng, D. T., Stein, E. A., & Helmstetter, F. J. (2004). Amygdala and hippocampal activity during acquisition and extinction of human fear conditioning. *Cognitive, Affective, & Behavioral Neuroscience, 4*(3), 317–325.

Lang, P.J. (1970). Stimulus control and the desensitization of fear. In D.J. Lewis (Ed.), Learning approaches to therapeutic behavior change. Chicago: Aldine.

LeDoux, J. E. (2012). Evolution of human emotion. A view through fear. *Progress in Brain Research, 195*, 431–442. doi:10.1016/B978-0-444-53860-4.00021-0.

Markowitz, J. C., Petkova, E., Neria, Y., Van Meter, P. E., Zhao, Y., Hembree, E., et al. (2015). Is exposure necessary? A randomized clinical trial of interpersonal psychotherapy for PTSD. *The American Journal of Psychiatry, 172*(5), 430–440. doi:10.1176/appi.ajp.2014.14070908.

McEwen, B. S., & Gianaros, P. J. (2010). Central role of the brain in stress and adaptation: Links to socioeconomic status, health, and disease. *Annals of the New York Academy of Sciences [Internet], 1186*:190–222. Retrieved from http://onlinelibrary.wiley.com/doi/10.1111/j.1749-6632.2009.05331.x/full

Neria, Y., Nandi, A., & Galea, S. (2008). Post-traumatic stress disorder following disasters: A systematic review. *Psychological Medicine, 38*(4), 467–480. doi:10.1017/S0033291707001353.

Nijenhuis, E. R., Spinhoven, P., Vanderlinden, J., van Dyck, R., & van der Hart, O. (1998). Somatoform dissociative symptoms as related to animal defensive reactions to predatory imminence and injury. *Journal of Abnormal Psychology, 107*, 63–73.

Öhman, A. (2005). The role of the amygdala in human fear: Automatic detection of threat. *Psychoneuroendocrinology, 2005*, 953–958.

Öhman, A., & Mineka, S. (2003). The malicious serpent. *Current Directions in Psychological Science[Internet], 12*:5–9. Retrieved from: http://cdp.sagepub.com/content/12/1/5.abstract\nhttp://cdp.sagepub.com/content/12/1/5.full.pdf

Powers, M. B., Halpern, J. M., Ferenschak, M. P., Gillihan, S. J., & Foa, E. B. (2010). A meta-analytic review of prolonged exposure for posttraumatic stress disorder. *Clinical Psychology Review, 30*(6), 635–641. doi:10.1016/j.cpr.2010.04.007.

Rachman, S. J. (2004). Fear and courage: A psychological perspective. *Social Research, 71*(1), 149–176 (CR – Copyright © 2004 The New School. http://doi.org/10.2307/40971664).

Shvil, E., Rusch, H. L., Sullivan, G. M., & Neria, Y. (2013). Neural, psychophysiological, and behavioral markers of fear processing in PTSD: a review of the literature. Current psychiatry reports, 15(5), 1–10.

Tudor, A. (2003). A (macro) sociology of fear? *The Sociological Review, 51*(2), 238–256. http://doi.org/10.1111/1467-954X.00417.

Vaidyanathan, U. (2009). Reinterpreting Comorbidity Among Common Mental Disorders Using Latent Class Analysis (Doctoral dissertation, University of Minnesota).

Vermetten, E., & Bremner, J. D. (2002). Circuits and systems in stress. I. Preclinical studies. *Depression and Anxiety, 15*(3), 126–147. doi:10.1002/da.10016.

Wadsworth, M. E., & Achenbach, T. M. (2005). Explaining the link between low socioeconomic status and psychopathology: Testing two mechanisms of the social causation hypothesis. *Journal of Consulting and Clinical Psychology, 73*, 1146–1153.

Part III

Case Studies of Collective Trauma

19 Some Reflections on Transmitting the Memory of the Holocaust and its Implications, Particularly in Israel

Saul Friedländer

19.1 Introduction

On March 2, 1988, the then director of the Van Leer Institute, the late professor Yehuda Elkana, published an article in *Haaretz*, a leading Israeli newspaper, under the title "The Need to Forget" (Elkana, 1988). He was referring to forgetting the Holocaust (hereafter, Shoah the Hebrew name of the holocaust will be used). Yehuda's motivation was undoubtedly complex, as he himself survived Auschwitz, but the essential thrust of his argument was moral or moral-political. He argued that the frequent references to the Shoah in all aspects of Israeli life had become a justification for policies of domination imposed on the Palestinians and for the defiant nationalism that has become familiar. Yehuda's impassioned plea closed with the following lines: "I do not see any more important political or educational stance for our leaders than to stand up for life… rather than deal, day and night, with symbols, ceremonies and lessons of the Holocaust." And he added: "The rule of historical remembrance must be uprooted from our lives" (cited in Segev, 1993).

Yehuda's forceful statements, representing a sentiment shared at that time by only a minority of Israelis, was written during the first Intifada (1987) in light of reports about the brutality of Israeli soldiers in the occupied territories; but his argument was a matter of principle that aimed well beyond the immediate circumstances. In the final part of this chapter, I return to Yehuda's moral injunction.

My aim in this chapter is to raise a few questions and to point to rarely evoked issues while reminding readers of some basic facts. Throughout, memory is considered here as that of traumatic events. Let me start by mentioning briefly the difference between the transmission of individual trauma and that of collective trauma. I then turn specifically to the memory of the Shoah in Israel, where, as we shall see, the difference between individual and collective trauma has paradoxically faded. Finally, I venture some comments on present developments in Israel, which seem to point to two thoroughly opposed positions regarding the transmission of the memory of the Shoah.

19.2 Two Modes of Transmission of Traumatic Memory

On the face of it there is a fundamental difference between the transmission of individual and collective trauma. Both my personal experience and numerous encounters with Holocaust survivors suggest that a traumatized individual has little control over the multiple ways in which his or her

S. Friedländer, Ph.D. (✉)
Chair in Holocaust Studies, History Department, UCLA, Los Angeles, CA, USA
e-mail: friedlan@history.ucla.edu

Y. Ataria et al. (eds.), *Interdisciplinary Handbook of Trauma and Culture*, DOI 10.1007/978-3-319-29404-9_19

experience is transmitted. And, obstinate silence transmits the memory of trauma just as powerfully as cries and whispers.

Furthermore, a traumatized individual cannot efface the psychological traces of his or her experience; the faintest trigger may induce a massive reaction. Thus, although individual memory of traumatic events tends to become a well organized, often repeated, perfectly coherent narrative, any unexpected circumstance such as may occur in everyday life or in the course of a lengthy interview—once the interviewers are forgotten and the interviewee loses his or her inhibitions—often brings to the surface a sudden surge of an underlying "deep memory" in its natural chaotic state (Langer, 1991). In principle, there should be no surge of "deep memory" at the collective level.

Whereas the transmission of individual trauma usually takes place within a relatively closed emotional field, mainly between the parent and child, the transmission of collective trauma takes place within a very different dynamic, which depends entirely on the *social function* it fulfills. Such social functions may include bolstering national or religious cohesion or, on a subnational level, feeding partisan enthusiasm and so on. This collective transmission lasts as long as a necessary social function is fulfilled; it vanishes when the function loses its significance. And, whereas on the individual level the memory of transmitted trauma often does not find resolution but rather disappears over time, on the collective level, trauma is mostly integrated into a wider, coherent narrative and thus transformed from a negative and incomprehensible occurrence into a positive and empowering mandate for the community.

A case in point is the memory of a quintessential traumatic event of modern pre-Holocaust times: the "Great War," i.e., the First World War. The primary function in all belligerent countries was to create a narrative that would give significance to the sacrifice of millions of lives. "The aim," in George Mosse's words, "was to make an inherently unpalatable past acceptable, important … above all for the justification of the nation in whose name the war had been fought. The reality of the war experience came to be transformed into what one might call the 'Myth of the War Experience,' which looked back upon the war as a meaningful and even sacred event" (Mosse, 1990, p. 7).

The overall meaning turned rapidly into political narratives, sanctified by the sacredness of it all. In France, for example, every village, every town erected its *monument aux morts* carrying the names of the local inhabitants fallen on the battlefield. And, on each November 11, at least two opposed ceremonies took place: on the one hand, a nationalist commemoration, on the other, a pacifist one—both invoking the same dead and including local flag-carrying crowds, generating emotional speeches and emotional responses. Such opposite ceremonies punctuated the political life of most European countries during the twenties and thirties, functioning, in each political camp, as essential carriers of lofty ideals whereby the memory of the dead prodded the living towards very different political horizons.

World War Two did not extinguish the memory of the "Great War" but it put an end to its function in the political landscape of postwar Europe: nowadays the sacredness of the "Nation" is disappearing and with it the compelling meta-narratives of the two world wars. Commemorations still take place but they have turned into rituals attended by diminishing numbers of participants. In the USA the change of emphasis from the "nation" to the "individual" is reflected on "Memorial Day": The Arlington memorial to the dead of the Vietnam War—where the names of the fallen are engraved on black marble plaques—constitutes the main site of commemoration; but, it must be added, most Americans mainly celebrate Memorial day sales at department stores and malls.

How long can the memory of traumatic events be socially transmitted? Indefinitely—if its function remains collectively essential. The most telling example in Jewish history is the ever lasting memory of the destruction of the Temple, the essential archetype for the integration and acceptance in religious consciousness of every new catastrophe and thus of the hope for messianic redemption. In a thoroughly different context, the French Revolution became, according to François Furet, part of ordinary history only at about its two hundredth anniversary.

Silence about or avoidance of a traumatic event can fulfill as significant a function for the community as the evocation of it. A notorious example is, of course, the quasi-amnesia regarding the Holocaust in West Germany, from the late forties to the late sixties. The same was true in other European countries. In each country the context of growing awareness was different, but it generally took two or three decades before some confrontation with the past emerged.

During these decades of silence, the absence of memory transmission also fulfilled an essential social function: preserving a self-image usually bolstered by tales of "resistance" or, in the case of Germany, by fictions of ignorance and/or individual acts of help to the victims. As the national self-image became less and less dependent on the war years, the change slowly took place. Instead of national meta-narratives, Western countries create in our day a variety of socially determined conversations about the most shameful years of their past.

19.3 A Few Remarks on the Transmission of the Memory of the Shoah in Israel

The memory of trauma is still massively present in contemporary Jewish society in Israel. The "meaning" given to the Shoah became integrated into several narratives that, as we shall see, only partially fulfilled their aim. Presently, a segment of Israeli society is questioning, even rejecting these narratives while the other part, probably the majority, is reenforcing them. Let me attempt in this section to offer a short outline of that evolution and of some of its paradoxical aspects.

During the immediate post-war period, three ideological choices competed for the commemoration date of the Shoah: The DPs in the European camps wanted to commemorate the Shoah on the day of the liberation of Auschwitz, the Orthodox sector in Eretz Yisrael opted for a date close to "Tish'a be-Av" and the Zionist parties chose a date related to the rebellion at the Warsaw ghetto. The Zionist option prevailed.

The memory of the Shoah in Israel was successively integrated into two major meta-discourses. First, during the so called "statist" era ("Mamlakhtiut"), the official discourse remained ambivalent, as in one of the founders and the first prime minister of state of Israel, Ben-Gurion's view, the passivity of the Jewish masses was hard to integrate into the Zionist ethos. The commemoration of the millions of supposedly passive victims could not represent the reborn nation built by the fighting spirit of the "New Jew." Thus, the official discourse turned Shoah into *Shoah ve-Gevurah* ("Holocaust and Heroism Remembrance) in choosing the date of the commemoration as close as possible to the date of the Warsaw ghetto uprising.

The official ambivalence towards the Shoah found its expression in the location of Yad Vashem—Israel's official memorial to the Jewish victims of the Holocaust (established in 1953). While the tombs of the great names of the National revival (from Herzl on) face Jerusalem, Yad Vashem, the memorial of the Shoah, has been built with its back to the city; in fact it is slightly hidden in the hills. This may be an excessive interpretation and the location of Yad Vashem may simply be due to the land available in the fifties; but it may also represent the reticence regarding the Shoah at the time, albeit allegorically.

Simultaneously, however, independent of Ben Gurion's ambivalence, public memory of the Shoah found its place in the religious theodicy of *Hurban ve-Geulah* (Destruction and Redemption) already mentioned and accepted by a significant sector of the population. For the majority, the religious interpretation of the Shoah has mutated into a secular paradigm. *Hurban ve-Geulah* became the matrix of *Shoah ve-Tekuma* (Shoah and Revival), that is, of the founding myth of post-Shoah Zionism: Israel became the quasi-messianic outcome of the Shoah, notwithstanding Ben Gurion's hesitations.

In any case, for Ben Gurion, Ben Zion Dinur—the all influential education minister and first chairman of Yad Vashem—and for most Zionist ideologues and intellectuals, it was Exile that had led to Catastrophe; it was Israel that meant safety and redemption. As Gershom

Scholem wrote in 1961: "The establishment of the State of Israel is for now the first positive consequence of the Shoah… both events are after all two sides of one immense historical process" (cited in (Kenan, 2000, p. xxi)).

These intertwined narratives—the religious and the secular—created a representation of the traumatic past that for two, even three generations evoked, within a context entirely different from that of the Nazi years, a sense of isolation and threat, even a possibility of physical eradication. Such transposition skewed the self-perception and collective identity of many Israelis and affected their relation to the world. All of this does not, of course, exclude the *reality* of surrounding threat and the evocation of the Shoah is meant to mobilize national energy, under the slogan "never again!"

Such mobilization should have been utilized during the War of Independence, mostly in May–June 1948, before the first truce, when the new State was in a dire situation. Yet, as a matter of fact, the Shoah was hardly referred to under Ben Gurion's leadership, for the reasons already mentioned. Thus, paradoxically, during the early years of Israel, when the Jewish State was at its weakest, the call upon the memory of the Shoah remained minimal both in the educational system and in the army (this of course was unrelated to the violent internal political controversies about the German reparations and around the Kastner affair).[1] And, when war came again, with the 1956 Sinai campaign, the references to "Munich" or to the "Genocide" were more frequent in the statements of French Prime Minister Guy Mollet than in those of Ben Gurion or Moshe Dayan.[2]

However, the entire discourse changed with the Eichmann trial (1961). Incidentally, it is not entirely clear, to me at least, why Ben Gurion, the leader who ordered Eichmann's abduction and who stood behind the staging of the trial, decided on a move that—he knew—would transform the perception of the extermination among young Israelis and put the victims at center stage, thus moving the public reference from *Gvurah (heroism)* to *Shoah*. Whatever Ben Gurion's reasoning may have been, the trial triggered a profound change in the understanding of the Shoah among many and it is at this point that a paradoxical series of events occurred.

During the Six-Day War, following the official reinstatement of the Shoah as Israel's "foundational myth," and its key traumatic memory—by now also transmitted to the second generation—certainly functioned as an energizing topos for the majority. But during the "waiting period" of the 1967 Six Day War, it also became an omen of potential catastrophe. Thus, while the fear of doom helped energize a majority of Israelis, it simultaneously overwhelmed part of the population.

During the days following October 6, 1973 the Shoah was not publicly mentioned, but it is hard to believe that it was not associated in the minds of many with the widespread sense of doom, all the more so because it surfaced again in 1990, during the Gulf War. In other words, instead of fulfilling an energizing function—as the collective transmission of a traumatic event in the life of a group is supposed to do—the memory of the Shoah, in a segment of the population at least, repeatedly became the root of a dysfunctional experience, similar in that sense to the eruption of individual traumatic "deep memory"; the hypothetical difference between the two processes—postulated at the outset of this chapter—simply faded. In other words, in 1967, and probably in 1973 and 1990, a segment of the Jewish population in Israel experienced a kind of collective posttraumatic stress disorder.

The first (very simplistic) explanation is the presence—within Israeli society—of a significant number of people who had been directly traumatized during the Shoah and had transmit-

[1] Rudolf Israel Kastner (1906—March 15, 1957) was an Austro-Hungarian-born Jew, Zionist activist, journalist and lawyer. He became known for facilitating the 'Blood for goods' proposal which was supposed to help Jews escape Nazi-occupied Hungary during the Holocaust. He was assassinated in 1957 after an Israeli court accused him of having collaborated with the Nazis

[2] Moshe Dayan was the Chief of Staff of the Israel Defense Forces (1953–58) and the Defense Minister during the Six-Day War (1967).

ted their fears and anxieties to a second generation. A part of this group did not and could not hide its reawakened sense of looming disaster.

A more convincing explanation is, to my mind, the impact of the force-feeding of the Israeli public with images of the Shoah; be it during high-school or army units' visits to Yad Vashem, during the "March of the Living" and so on. Such concrete confrontations with stark representations of the past may indeed have mobilized the fighting spirit of the participants in such rituals on the one hand, but also brought up anxiety and dark premonitions, on the other.

Although such educational methods, ceremonies and rituals have remained as present as ever during the past few decades, the official metanarrative of *Shoah ve-Tekuma* has been put in question from the mid-1980s on, mostly on the Liberal-Left. We are all familiar with the criticism leveled at the official Shoah narrative in post Zionist historiography. The core argument of a number of major Israeli writers including Tom Segev, Idit Zertal, and Moshe Zuckerman has been the same: Israeli leadership, at different times, has exploited the fate of Shoah survivors and later the traumatic memory of the extermination for political aims, including the establishment of the State and, later, for financial support, be it from the USA, from Germany, or from Jews in the Diaspora. Such historiography contributed—at least slightly—to the revision of the official Zionist discourse, the more so that historians of the war years have questioned the will of the Yishuv (a term referring to the body of Jewish residents in Palestine, before the establishment of the State of Israel) leadership to assist European Jewry in any possible way. Suffice it to mention Antek Zuckerman's bitter comment towards the end of Claude Lanzmann's film "Shoah": "If you could lick my heart, you would be poisoned."

And yet, in some cases, I would not be such a harsh a critic: When, in 1983, during the attack on Beirut, the writer Amos Oz reminded the prime minister Begin that Hitler was dead, he did not understand that the then prime minister, who had abandoned his family and the *Beitarim* (Betar Movement is a Revisionist Zionist youth movement founded in 1923 in Riga, Latvia, by Vladimir [Ze'ev] Jabotinsky) of whom he was responsible in Poland, was living in the shadow of the extermination that he could not dispel.

While Yigal Loussin's 1981 seminal TV production "Amud ha-Esh" (Pillar of Fire)[3] was probably the last widely seen Zionist metanarrative integrating the Shoah as *Shoah ve-Tekuma*, telling indications of change, apart from historiography, surfaced in literature, particularly in fiction, in the 1980s and 1990s. The destructive impact of the traumatic memory of the Shoah upon the second generation found a particularly forceful expression in two novels: Yoram Kanyuk's *Bito* (*His Daughter, 1987*) and in Michal Govrin's *HaShem* (*The Name, 1995*). In both cases, daughters of the second generation whose real (Kanyuk) or imagined (Govrin) mother, died in the Shoah or was mentally destroyed by it, are unable to escape from the grip of those mothers who, in different ways, ruin their lives. These widely read novels could be seen as expressions of individual problems of the second generation or, more plausibly so, as allegories of the Shoah's dramatic influence on important segments of Israeli society.

19.4 Present Debates and Perspectives

Almost 24 years have gone by since the Gulf War—that is since the latest retraumatization of part of the Israeli public by the imagined threat of extermination. In the meantime, the country has undergone a huge transformation both demographically and in its level of modernization. Is the memory of the Shoah as deeply ingrained in present-day Israel as it was two decades ago? Not to mention in the late eighties when Elkana published his plea. The official [mis]use of the Shoah by political parties has not changed, the ceremonies and rituals have not changed either, and

[3]A miniseries documentary of the Israel Broadcasting Authority (IBA), named after the Pillar of Fire which presents the history and narrative of Zionism from the late nineteenth century until the establishment of the state of Israel in 1948

some of their manifestations are more excessive than ever. I am referring to the 2003 overflight of Auschwitz by the present commander of the Air Force, General Amir Eshel and his interview about it. From the interview, I gathered that the overflight was meant to remind ourselves of the world's passivity in the spring of 1944 when allied overflights of Auschwitz took place in the midst of the deportation of Hungarian Jews and not a single bomb was dropped on the gas chambers. Unfortunately, General Eshel seems to have forgotten the passivity of the Yishuv throughout the entire period of the Shoah. Moreover, the *bravado* one can sense in the interview reminds one of the atmospheres that permeated the political and defense establishment after the Six Day War and that led straight to the Yom Kippur War.

Several elements have changed on the Israeli scene, however, and the first of these, naturally and drastically so: the proportion of survivors of the Shoah in Israeli society is rapidly diminishing and the second generation that bore the brunt of the trauma transmission during childhood is, for the most part, far away from these difficult beginnings. I suggest that this overall demographic and temporal factor is, of necessity, lowering the sensitivity level of Israeli society in general to the evocation of the Shoah.

There is more. Shulamit Aloni (Minister of Education 1992–1993) and Amnon Rubinstein (Minister of Education 1993–1996) introduced universal, humanist contents in relation to the teaching of the Shoah in high schools (including the interpretation given to the "March of the Living"). More generally, the emphasis on exceptionalism is probably weakening as a result of the country's symbiosis with European and American culture and values. Finally, meta-narratives as such are disappearing from western thought and such shifts may have found some echo in Israel.

And yet, notwithstanding the changes I just mentioned, it seems that the tendency is to strengthen the misuse of the Shoah, as illustrated by General Eshel's interview and by repeated references to the Shoah by the Prime Minister Benjamin Netanyahu, who still dominates the Israeli public landscape. I mentioned the danger of retraumatization within segments of Israeli society, I alluded to the *hubris* we experienced on the path to the Yom Kippur War, and I cannot but sense a skewed pride in *Am Levado* (the lone people?) facing, in isolation, the supposedly existential threat represented by our neighbors. Watchfulness does not demand reference to extermination, a reference that may lead to a misperception of the danger scale and to catastrophic initiatives: our national narrative has to change. This brings me back to Yehuda Elkana's plea.

In March 1988, when Yehuda published his article, I was visiting the USA and do not remember having reacted to it either then or in later conversation. I understood the circumstances that convinced him to write this piece and shared his political views; but I disagreed with the general thrust of his text: "the rule of historical remembrance must be uprooted from our lives" (Elkana, 1988). Yehuda probably meant that the State-staged rituals had to be cancelled and State-encouraged education about the Shoah abolished as it fanned nationalism, hatred for the Palestinians and brutality against them under the pretext that our sufferings granted us special rights. In a part of the text that I have not quoted, Yehuda compared our practice of mobilizing the past for our national ambitions to the very similar exploitation of the past by fascist states for their aggressive policies (Elkana, 1988). But every State on the planet mobilizes glorious or catastrophic moments of its past to serve as a justification of the present and a guidance for the future. And even if modes of commemoration are modified and the meaning of commemorating is changed, commemoration as such cannot be eradicated from any society.

Sooner or later the dangerous trend previously mentioned will reach a turning point: the moment will arrive when no direct personal memory of the Shoah will exist anymore; the extraordinary memoir that Dov Kulka (2013) published recently is most probably the last of its kind. The second generation is not likely to transmit its anxieties to a third one or, let us say, not in most cases. Thus, on the collective level, the commemoration of the Shoah will probably call for a more universalist discourse, as the memory of the world wars did in Western imagination.

Differently from Western practice, however, the memory of the Shoah in Israeli and Jewish historical consciousness will likely to remain *alive*. This will be true for the orthodox religious sector and its belief in a messianic theodicy. It will also be true for many secular Israelis, as the Shoah remains the most important event in Jewish history together with, but not linked to, the creation of the Israeli State. There is no mystery regarding the ways in which this memory will be transmitted: by historical research, by art, by literature and—ultimately—by considering and reconsidering the nature of Evil.

References

Elkana, Y. (1988 (republished online Oct. 13, 2012)). From "The Need to Forget". *Haaretz*. http://www.haaretz.co.il/opinions/1.1841380.

Kenan, O. (2000). *Between memory and history*. Los Angeles: University of California.

Kulka, O. D. (2013). *Landscapes of the metropolis of death: Reflections on memory and imagination*. (R. Mandel, Trans.). London: Allen Lane.

Langer, L. (1991). *Holocaust testimonies: The ruins of memory*. New Haven: Yale University Press.

Mosse, G. L. (1990). *Fallen soldiers: Reshaping the memory of the world wars*. New York: Oxford University Press.

Segev, T. (1993). *The seventh million*. New York: Hill and Wang.

Placing Collective Trauma Within Its Social Context: The Case of 9/11 Attacks

20

Emily Joyner, Katharine Reiner van der Hoorn, Ari Platt, Mikael Rubin, Erel Shvil, and Yuval Neria

20.1 Introduction

It has been 14 years since the September 11, 2001 (9/11) attacks, and their aftermath has yet to be fully explored. The unprecedented scope and magnitude of these attacks in the USA set off a tide of distress and uncertainty among millions of people who were both directly and indirectly affected by the violence. The almost constant television coverage of the events on 9/11 throughout the world allowed others to experience the events from thousands of miles away, with potentially dramatic trauma responses for those who had already experienced either direct or familial exposure to traumatic circumstance before (Neria & Sullivan, 2011). As these attacks occurred in one of the largest, most diverse cities in the world, the trauma was experienced collectively by millions of people. Indeed, Updegraff, Silver, and Holman (2008) aptly described the 9/11 attacks as a "collective cultural upheaval" (p. 709). When those planes hit the twin towers, the devastation extended not only to individuals, but also to communities, neighborhoods, and families. This was an attack that interacted with cultures so profoundly that it elucidated how our social world abides in the face of unthinkable tragedy.

Immediately after and in the months following the 9/11 attacks, the likelihood that Americans would develop an acute stress response or posttraumatic stress disorder (PTSD) as a result skyrocketed (Neria, DiGrande, & Adams, 2011). Several studies reported elevated rates of PTSD among American civilians who experienced 9/11 indirectly by as much as 17%, although later research called those numbers into question (Breslau, 2009; Neria & Sullivan, 2011; Silver, Holman, McIntosh, Poulin, & Gil-Riva, 2002). PTSD is a debilitating mental illness that arises after direct or indirect exposure to a traumatizing event and leaves sufferers with symptoms such as intrusive memories, flashbacks, nightmares, physiological and emotional hyperactivity, avoidance, and negative emotions and mood (American Psychiatric Association, 2013).

While the events of 9/11 represent a significant tragedy, they have also provided an opportunity to examine sociocultural responses in the context of both global and local man-made disasters. In order to analyze this collective trauma through a culturally sensitive lens, we begin by clarifying why we are doing so in the first place. Consistent with Arthur Kleinman's formulation

E. Joyner, M.A. • K.R. van der Hoorn, M.A.
A. Platt, B.A. • E. Shvil, Ph.D. • Y. Neria, Ph.D. (✉)
Columbia University Medical Center and the New York State Psychiatric Institute, New York, NY, USA
e-mail: ejoyner28@gmail.com; ny126@cumc.columbia.edu

M. Rubin, M.A.
Psychology Department, University of Texas at Austin, Austin, TX, USA

Y. Ataria et al. (eds.), *Interdisciplinary Handbook of Trauma and Culture*,
DOI 10.1007/978-3-319-29404-9_20

that "illness is shaped by cultural factors governing perception, labeling, explanation, and valuation of the discomforting experience" (Kleinman, Eisenberg, & Good, 2006, p. 141), we similarly recognize that mental illnesses do not occur independently. Rather, illnesses, including PTSD, are mediated by components that are culturally constructed (Kleinman et al., 2006) and associated with cultural identity.

The term cultural identity is somewhat amorphous and challenging to define. However, for the purposes of this chapter, cultural identity mainly refers to ethnicity, but is also grounded in and influenced by socioeconomic status, religion, migration, geography, gender, sexual orientation and various processes such as oppression, racism, and (McGoldrick, Giordano, & Garcia-Preto, 2005). These factors intersect and combine in order to compose a cultural context. When a tragedy such as 9/11 strikes, various factors related to cultural identity—such as ethnicity, race, gender, and socioeconomic status—may place individuals and communities at a higher risk for developing psychopathologies such as PTSD (Breslau, 2009; DiGrande, Neria, Brackbill, Pulliam, & Galea, 2011; Galea et al., 2002; Neria, Nandi, & Galea, 2008; Roberts, Gilman, Breslau, Breslau, & Koenen, 2011). However, some aspects of culture can also act as adaptive and protective mechanisms that promote mental health (Constantine, Alleyne, Caldwell, McRae, & Suzuki, 2005; Seirmarco et al., 2012). In this chapter we explore both approaches.

20.2 Culture and PTSD in Psychiatric Research and Diagnosis

Until recently, psychiatric research has historically excluded culture from its discourse, relegating it to a separate field of "cross-cultural" psychology (Betancourt & Lopez, 1993). This tendency is exemplified by the prior dearth of information on culture in the Diagnostic and Statistical Manual of Mental Disorders (DSM), the manual regarded as the standard for the classification of disorders in the USA. In the development of the fourth version, much of the authors' work on culture was removed from the published manual, and the "culture-bound" syndrome section excluded disorders seen as primarily North American disorders (for example, anorexia nervosa and chronic fatigue syndrome) from the glossary in order to restrict the section to problems of "ethnic minorities" (Lopez & Guarnaccia, 2000; McGoldrick et al., 2005). Recently, the publication of the newest version of the Diagnostic and Statistical Manual for Mental Disorders (DSM-5) demonstrates an unprecedented effort to include culture in the diagnosis of mental disorders (Aggarwal, 2013). This newest effort reflects a shift in the field of psychiatry toward the acknowledgement of culture in diagnosis and underlines the importance of thinking about culture when developing new interventions.

The question of the inherent relevance of a PTSD diagnosis for a cross-cultural population is an important one to address. Some researchers have made the case that certain PTSD criteria, including flashbacks, are a phenomenon exclusive to the western culture (Jones et al., 2003). Others have argued that because certain symptoms only effect certain populations, PTSD is not a truly cross-culturally valid diagnosis. For example, in a study of Latino psychiatric outpatients in the Boston area, Salvadoran women between the ages of 20 and 62 who developed posttraumatic symptoms suffered from responses to the trauma outside the realm of DSM diagnoses; namely *nervios* which includes several dysphoric and somatic effects such as physical pain, shaking, and trembling, and often *calor* (a sensation of intense heat that may rapidly spread throughout one's entire body) (Jenkins & Valiente, 1994). As described in Janis H. Jenkins chapter, *Culture, Emotions and PTSD*, the element of *calor* often occurs in response to a threat to one's physical integrity or safety, to a threatening or violent event, or to a life threatening illness (Jenkins, 1996). Because of the lack of overlap of symptoms between Western and Salvadorian responses to a traumatic event, the cross-cultural applicability and validity of a PTSD diagnosis to this population seems somewhat questionable. With this caveat addressed, however, other studies have found PTSD to be cross-culturally valid. A study of Cambodian refugees living in the USA found high levels of Diagnostic and Statistical Manual (DSM) symptoms, as well as significant relationships between each symptom measure and the amount of trauma experience, both similarly observed in US trauma survivors (Carlson & Rosser-Hogan, 1994). In addition, a more recent review of the DSM-IV PTSD diagnosis has cross-cultural validity, although several recommendations were made to improve and expand the definition to have more applicability, such as the incorporation of cultural differences in the meaning of traumatic events, and the expansion of acceptable symptom dimensions (Hinton & Lewis-Fernández, 2011). For the purpose of exploring cultural responses to trauma, as they are related to PTSD, this chapter assumes that PTSD is a valid cross-cultural diagnosis, while acknowledging the need for the criteria to be more inclusive of the diversity of symptoms and trauma criteria that impact different cultures on different levels.

20.3 Cultural Risk Factors for the Development of PTSD

Current research has yet to identify the exact mechanisms through which cultural factors are associated with mental health response to trauma, although accumulating research has identified risk factors for PTSD following exposure to a traumatic event. Accordingly, factors including belonging to a minority group, being a woman, and having a low socioeconomic status have been found to be strongly associated with PTSD (Breslau, 2009; DiGrande et al., 2011; Galea et al., 2002; Neria et al., 2006, 2008; Roberts et al., 2011).

Consideration of this knowledge in the context of national disasters such as 9/11 may enhance highly needed awareness of the impact of culture and social status on survivor's mental health and may be central to efforts to develop effective community responses. More research to inform community responses is needed. As McGoldrick et al. (2005)) states, "We must incorporate cultural acknowledgment into our theories and into our therapies, so that clients not of the dominant culture will not have to feel lost, displaced, or mystified."

20.4 Ethnicity and Risk for PTSD After 9/11

As previously mentioned, ethnicity is one of the cultural variables that can elevate the risk of developing PTSD. The concept of conditional risk for the development of PTSD refers to the likelihood of developing PTSD after experiencing a potentially traumatic event (Roberts et al., 2011). It is worthwhile to make the distinction between prevalence of PTSD and conditional risk for developing PTSD. The prevalence of PTSD refers to the amount of people who are diagnosed with the disorder, while conditional risk refers to the likelihood of someone within a certain group of developing PTSD if a traumatic event is experienced. Previous studies have demonstrated modest differences in lifetime prevalence of PTSD between Latinos (4.4–7.0 %), non-Latino Blacks (8.6–8.7 %), and non-Latino Whites (6.5–7.4 %) (Alcántara, Casement, & Lewis-Fernández, 2013; Alegría et al., 2008). However, when focusing on conditional risk for developing PTSD, the risk of developing PTSD found to be clearly higher among Latinos as compared to other ethnic groups (e.g., Neria et al., 2008).

20.5 9/11 PTSD Among Latinos

Several studies on PTSD onset and persistence have demonstrated that Latinos have a higher conditional risk than non-Latino whites to meet criteria for PTSD after a traumatic event (DiGrande et al., 2008; Galea et al., 2002, 2004; Norris, Perilla, Ibañez, & Murphy, 2001; Perilla, Norris, & Lavizzo, 2002; Williams et al., 2008). Furthermore, after September 11th, Latino status was one of the most cited risk factors for the development of the disorder (Bowler et al., 2010; Galea et al., 2002; Neria et al., 2008 Schuster et al., 2001). Bowler and colleagues (2010) observed elevated rates of PTSD among Latino male first responders after the 9/11 attacks. Additionally, Neria et al. (2006) in a study of urban primary care observed that Latina females were at the highest risk for developing PTSD, reflecting an intersection of gender and ethnicity, which we will explore in more detail later.

Symptoms of PTSD among Latinos were found to persist well after the attacks of 9/11. There was a higher rate of probable PTSD onset among Latinos relative to non-Latino Whites or the combined non-Latino group at 5–8 weeks following the WTC attack (Galea et al., 2002) and 6 months after the attack (Galea et al., 2004). This finding of PTSD among Latino's post-9/11 continued for at least 2 years after the attacks. For example, in a population-based prospective study after the attacks of 9/11, Galea et al. (2008) found that the ethnic identification of Latino was consistently related to PTSD at each of three time points over a 2-year period. PTSD among Latinos was found even while excluding the endorsement of panic symptoms in the hours following the World Trade Center attack, as well as whether respondents were directly affected by 9/11 (i.e., injured during attack, lost possession or property, friend/relative killed, involved in rescue effort, or lost job as a result of attack) (Alcántara et al., 2013; Galea et al., 2008). Similarly, in another study, Latino ethnicity was associated with symptoms of PTSD 2–3 years post-9/11 among a representative sample of Manhattan residents living south of Canal Street (Adams & Boscarino, 2006).

This abundance of information regarding prevalence and probable PTSD among Latinos after 9/11 begs the question of why this particular ethnic group was more vulnerable to PTSD than others. What sociocultural factors place Latinos at a higher conditional risk for developing PTSD? Social disadvantage, emotional reactions to trauma, expressive style, familism/fatalism, and acculturation have all been identified as potential reasons for this differential (Alcántara et al., 2013; Galea et al., 2004; Lewis-fern, Turner, Marshall, Turse, & Dohrenwend, 2008; Perilla et al., 2002).

Social disadvantage (e.g., low educational attainment, work problems, and low income) has been shown to increase the likelihood for Latinos to develop PTSD (Adams & Boscarino, 2006; DiGrande et al., 2008; Galea et al., 2004). This makes sense since it has been well established that the poor and less educated are more likely to live in at-risk areas that are less safe and desirable, with fewer resources (Quarantelli, 1997). Notwithstanding, when considering the Latino population as a grouping category, one must take into account that it encompasses individuals from various different countries with different cultural backgrounds. Presently, many studies of Latinos tend to lump all Latinos into a homogenous ethnic group, without taking different countries of origin into account. Among a representative sample of Latinos in the New York metropolitan area, Galea et al. (2004) examined within-group differences in Latinos after 9/11 and found that Hispanics of Dominican and Puerto Rican descent were more likely to report symptoms of PTSD after 9/11 than Latinos of other origins. Social disadvantage played a large role in this difference, as Dominicans and Puerto Ricans were found to have lower socioeconomic positions, fewer years of education, and lower incomes.

Another factor that was found to affect risk of PTSD among Latinos was the concept of emotional reactions to trauma. These reactions include cultural idioms of distress such as "ataque de nervios," which describes "a loss of control in emotional expressions, sensations, and actions in Hispanics," and has "been shown to be associated with panic disorder, post-traumatic stress, and depression" (Galea et al., 2004, p. 526). Galea et al. (2004) found that "ataque de nervios" was particularly pertinent among Dominicans, leading to a heightened risk for developing PTSD after 9/11, compared with those from other Latino groups. Another traumatic reaction to a trauma is dissociation, defined as experiencing an altered state of consciousness at the time of trauma, and has been shown to be a strong predictor of PTSD (Ozer, Best, Lipsey, & Weiss, 2008). Dissociation has been identified as a "culture-bound" syndrome in Latin America (Pole, Best, Metzler, & Marmar, 2005). Consequently, this leads one to wonder if higher levels of dissociation among Latinos can account for some of the elevated levels of PTSD. A few studies examined whether higher rates of PTSD among Latinos could be explained by an expressive nature of Latino culture, which would suggest over-reporting of symptoms (Ortega & Rosenheck, 2000). Lewis-fern et al. (2008) analyzed data from the National Vietnam Veterans Readjustment Study subsample of Latino male Vietnam veterans interviewed by clinicians using a standard diagnostic interview. The researcher did not find evidence of over-reporting, which offers evidence to counter the idea that the development of PTSD might be related to being overly expressive.

Another concept that may have contributed to higher levels of PTSD among Latinos post 9/11 is coping style. Perilla et al. (2002) examined whether adherence to and maintenance of cultural values of fatalism and familism may have had an effect on the rate of PTSD among Latinos in the wake of Hurricane Andrew, another collective trauma. Fatalism, defined as a "predisposition to attribute high causal power to external forces and minimal causal power to personal forces" (Perilla et al., 2002, p. 23) is a characteristic associated with Latino culture and is related to negative mental health outcomes. Familism reflects a collectivistic conception of Latino culture, and that familial obligations are of the utmost importance (Perilla et al., 2002). Higher levels of familism were related to higher levels of distress, possibly due to the difficulty of seeking help from outside the family, as well as stress due to familial obligations. Similarly, fatalism was associated with higher levels of distress. Fatalism and familism as ways of coping may have contributed to the higher levels of PTSD among Latinos (Perilla et al., 2002).

20.6 Racism After 9/11

Several studies have found that ethnic minorities exhibited particularly high rates of PTSD after the events of 9/11 (Abu-Ras & Abu-Bader, 2008; Galea et al., 2002; Neria et al., 2008), but how ethnicity, race and religion play into response to traumatic experience is a nuanced and multifaceted area yet to be explored. For the purposes of this chapter, we consider these identifiers not only in terms of how particular groups responded to the traumatic events of 9/11, but also how others responded to and behaved towards members of these groups after those events and whether any significant change was experienced. Specifically, for many men and women of Arab descent or Muslim practice, there was a twofold trauma; not only the events that occurred on the day, but the growing intensity of racism and anti-Islamist discrimination that occurred after (Abu-Ras & Abu-Bader, 2008).

Islam is one of the fastest growing religions in the USA, with estimates ranging from two to seven million Muslims living in the USA, or up to 2% of the US population (Johnson, 2011). Muslims are reported to have first entered what is now USA in 1312, and American Muslims come from almost every race and nation and are not limited to any particular ethnic group (Haque, 2004). The number of Arab-Americans—described here as those persons whose heritage is from countries where the primary language is Arabic, including Algeria, Bahrain, Djibouti, Egypt, Iraq, Jordan, Kuwait, Lebanon, Libya, Morocco, Oman, Palestine, Qatar, Saudi Arabia, Somalia, Sudan, Syria, Tunisia, the UAE, and Yemen (Pupcenoks, 2011)—is estimated to be between 1.5 (Asi & Beaulieu, 2013) and 3.7 million (Foundation, 2012). The exact number is unclear for a number of reasons, one being that members of the Arab-American community may be reluctant to identify themselves, due to fear of negative societal response (Abu-Ras & Abu-Bader, 2009).

Many Arab Americans and Arab immigrants are no strangers to traumatic events. For many, trauma had become an integral part of their personal identities, and the events of September 11th may have retriggered those memories. As one Muslim person described "Every time we overcome one trauma, we find ourselves struggling with another one, leaving us with no room to breathe and reflect on what happened earlier, until we become numb" (Abu-Ras & Abu-Bader, 2008).

Racism towards American Arabs and Muslims has been exhibited since long before the events of September 11th. Discrimination was both blatantly evident in public opinion polls in the 1970s and 1980s and present in more subtle areas, such as in high school social studies textbooks (Jarrar, 1983). Media, such as television and film, often depicted Arabs as being obsessed with wealth or power, as sex maniacs, as terrorists and as radicals (Shaheen, 2003). However, following 9/11, Arab and Muslim Americans became pronounced targets of suspicion, hostility, and fear, and many experienced a heightened level of fear as a result (Abu-Ras & Abu-Bader, 2009). Reported hate-crimes, including mosque burnings, bomb threats, physical assaults, verbal assaults, and employment discrimination against Muslims rose 21 % after 9/11 from the year before (FBI, 2001; Rippy & Newman, 2006), and it is probable that many more subtle forms of targeted abuse were not reported, such as the yelling of disparaging remarks regarding foreignness at Arab Americans, or in one instance, the pulling off of a head scarf of an observant Muslim woman (Scurfield, 2002). White Americans often reported fear or a heightened sense of awareness when around people of Arabic or Middle Eastern descent (Hall, 2005). Arabs and Muslim Americans, in spite of a long history of discrimination, are not immune to the pain of being discriminated against, nor is any group impervious to the mental and emotional difficulties that may arise following such persecution.

In a study examining the reaction of refugees to the events of 9/11, those who expressed the greatest outrage at the events—Somalis, Cambodians, Vietnamese, Laotians, and Bosnians—were those in the Muslim community, who saw the act as a desecration of Islamic ideology and feared the response from Westerners towards all Muslims (Kinzie, 2005). In addition to the increased fear and sense of threat that Muslims and Arab Americans often experienced after 9/11, they may also have suffered more from a lack of social support, as many migrated from interdependent cultures that put a high value on social support systems. Several studies have indicated lack of social support as a predictor of PTSD development after a trauma (Besser & Neria, 2010; Kaniasty & Norris, 2008). As described by Abu-Ras and Abu-Bader (2009), when Arab and Muslim immigrants in the USA find themselves without the support systems in which they were raised, the resultant isolation and loneliness they experience can increase vulnerability to stress reactions after trauma. Additionally, for Muslims, the American lifestyle can present challenges in nearly every arena of human experience, from something as basic as food (pork and alcohol are not permissible in the religion), to dress, to religious and cultural beliefs. This, combined with the lack of social support, as well as the common misconceptions and fear of Islamic and Arabic culture among many others, may contribute to the high psychosocial vulnerability in this group (Haque, 2004). Indeed, in a study of New York Muslim men and women post 9/11, the vast majority scored high on all items on list of common responses to trauma adapted from the measure created by Foa, Riggs, Dancu, and Rothbaum (1993), with 94 % exhibiting at least one symptom of PTSD, such as increased arousal. Another interesting finding was that the events of 9/11 brought more anxiety to non-Arab Muslims than to Arab Muslims (86 % as opposed to 64.4 % for Arab Muslims) (Abu-Ras & Suarez, 2009). Racism and discrimination from Westerners towards foreigners may be generalized to superficial standards, such as to those wearing different dress and hairstyle, than due to an actual understanding of whether they are genuinely Muslim or not. In the weeks and months following 9/11, Sikhs (a pacifistic religion of mainly Indian descent, in which men wear turbans and uncut hair) were discriminated against in ways varying from verbal attacks by strangers, to racial profiling at airlines, to 800 reported hate crimes perpetuated against Sikhs after 9/11 (Ahluwalia & Pellettiere, 2010). Taken together, Arab-Americans and Muslims were targeted in the aftermath of September 11th and were forced to grapple with increased discrimination and racism in the USA, which appears to have contributed to the high incidence of trauma related symptomology among these populations.

20.7 Immigration and PTSD Following the 9/11 Attacks

The process of migration can become an integral part of one's culture. The promise of a sense of security and comfort is among one of the most common reasons for which people immigrate to the USA (Rumbaut & Portes, 2001). The swift and irrevocable damages, including mass fatalities, of September 11th shattered, for many, this notion of security.

The Latino population represents the largest ethnic minority group in the USA, which continues to rapidly grow (Lopez, 2009). A feature that distinguishes the Latino population from other ethnic groups in the USA is its large proportion of immigrants (Caplan, 2007). Surveys and interviews conducted after September 11th have shown that Latino immigrants were a particularly vulnerable group to symptoms of PTSD after the attacks of September 11th, 2001 (Galea et al., 2002; Pantin, Schwartz, Prado, Feaster, & Szapocznik, 2003). Spanish-speaking immigrants, in particular, have been shown to develop higher rates of PTSD following a disaster (Perilla et al., 2002).

Pantin et al. (2003) demonstrated this higher incidence by surveying Hispanic immigrants in Miami, Florida 3 months after the terrorist attacks of 9/11. Miami, nearly 1000 miles from New York City, is a city with many Latinos who have emigrated from countries such as Cuba, Colombia, and Honduras, where traumas from exposure to violence from guerilla warfare and natural disasters are not uncommon. Though they lived nearly 1000 miles away from the attacks, many Latino individuals exhibited PTSD symptoms including intrusive reexperiencing of the attacks, as well avoidance. The greater the number and severity of prior traumatic events experienced in their home countries, the more severe their PTSD symptoms were likely to be (Pantin et al., 2003).

Immigrants from other cultural groups, especially those who experienced unspeakable traumas in their own countries, are susceptible to developing anxiety and PTSD after reexposure to trauma. In a study that took place at the Boston Center for Refugee Health and Human Rights at Boston Medical Center, patients who were either refugees or asylum seekers from 18 countries were interviewed (Piwowarczyk & Keane, 2007). The majority either survived torture themselves or were family members of those who had. After 9/11, all 63 participants were more fearful of immigration-specific threats, such as deportation, arrest, detention, imprisonment, and discrimination. Some participants made changes to hide their cultural identity, such as changing how they dressed or socialized in order to fit in better (Piwowarczyk & Keane, 2007).

In another clinical study of Vietnamese, Cambodian, Laotian, Bosnian, and Somali refugees at the Intercultural Psychiatric Program at Oregon Health & Science University, patients with preexisting PTSD had the strongest responses to the events of 9/11. Refugees had a varying decrease in their feeling of security after 9/11; Somalis indicated the greatest decrease, while Cambodians indicated the least decrease. The authors theorize that the muted response of the Cambodians may be partly due to prevalence of Buddhist practice in Cambodia, at the core of which is a belief in fatalism and acceptance (Kinzie, Boehnlein, Riley, & Sparr, 2002).

Another study conducted with the same population found that indirect exposure to the events, even via television, was enough to retrigger PTSD symptoms, including recurrent nightmares, intrusive memories, depressed mood, and a sense of lack of safety. Clinically, patients returned to their pre-9/11 levels of symptoms after 2–3 months (Kinzie, 2005). The same community of refugees also noticed a strong and often negative community response, particularly towards traditionally dressed women, who were occasionally told to dress "like Americans" (Kinzie, 2005). These findings suggest the importance of considering immigrant mental health in the context of community disasters.

20.8 Gender and 9/11

After the attacks of September 11th, several investigators began large-scale phone and internet-based surveys to observe trends in the development of PTSD. These researchers found that women were at a higher risk for the development of PTSD after 9/11 (Adams & Boscarino, 2006; Breslau, 2009; Galea et al., 2002; Schuster et al., 2001; Silver et al., 2002). Generally, despite some conflicting findings, it has been established that there are gender differences related to the development of PTSD, such that women are more likely to develop PTSD (Breslau, 2009; Kessler, Sonnega, Bromet, Hughes, & Nelson, 1995). Interestingly, it has been shown that while men are more likely to be exposed to trauma, women are more likely to develop the disorder after experiencing a traumatic event (Breslau, 2009). Research has also shown that women exhibited reduced levels of resilience after the attacks of 9/11 (Bonanno, Galea, Bucciarelli, & Vlahov, 2007).

Bowler et al. (2010) found that the prevalence of probable PTSD was significantly higher among female police responders than male responders in the World Trade Center attacks. In another study of PTSD prevalence after 9/11, researchers collected data in-person from a primary care facility in Lower Manhattan, close to where the attacks occurred (Neria et al., 2006; Weissman et al., 2005). The people interviewed were primarily low-income Hispanic immigrants who lived just a few miles north of the tragedy. Though the female participants had significantly less direct exposure to the attacks, they exhibited higher rates of PTSD. Many of the women interviewed were divorced or separated, and the researchers concluded that divorced or separated women are even more likely than are other women to develop PTSD. Other research has found that a lack of social support makes one more susceptible to PTSD symptoms (Besser & Neria, 2010; Kaniasty & Norris, 2008). If marriage is taken to be a measure of social support, these findings further emphasize this claim.

Furthermore, in the context of 9/11, risk factors for developing PTSD reflect intersections of different cultural identities such as gender and ethnicity. For example, Latina women had a uniquely higher likelihood of developing posttraumatic stress disorder after September 11th when compared with women of other ethnicities or men (Neria et al., 2006). This effect of intersectionality has been observed in other research. Neria et al. (2006), in the aforementioned study in urban primary care, found that unmarried Latino women had the highest prevalence of PTSD. This intersectional effect has been found in response to other community disasters. In a study of Hurricane Andrew in South Florida, Norris et al. (2001) found that Mexican women had elevated rates of PTSD in relation to non-Latino whites. When the study evaluated PTSD diagnosis without considering gender, rates of PTSD in Latinos and non-Latino Whites were similar.

20.9 Culture and Coping Methods After 9/11

Though thus far we have focused on the pathology of post trauma responses, research has shown that most people are generally resilient after experiencing a trauma. While most people will experience at least one potentially traumatic event in their lives, only a small percentage of those people will develop symptoms of PTSD (Kessler et al., 1995). While it is important to research the differences in pathological response to traumatic experience among those from different cultures, it is arguably just as vital to learn from cultures how they cope and grow after disastrous experiences. Bonanno (2004) defined resilience as,

> The ability of adults in otherwise normal circumstances who are exposed to an isolated and potentially highly disruptive event such as the death of a close relation or a violent or life-threatening situation to maintain relatively stable, healthy levels of psychological and physical functioning … as well as the capacity for generative experiences and positive emotions. (20–21)

This definition of resilience not only addresses the ability for those faced with trauma to continue functioning, but it also highlights growth and positive emotions that can surface after a traumatic event. There exists a breadth of research on coping strategies after trauma within a Western context; however, research has tended to neglect other potential coping tools that reflect more collectivistic, interdependent, and communal value orientations that may be more relevant to ethnic minorities (Cross & Vick, 2001).

After 9/11, while Muslims often experienced negative changes to their quality of life, they also reported positive changes in their religious belief, self-knowledge, and coping skills (Abu-Ras & Suarez, 2009). Muslims used both religious and nonreligious coping methods in the time after 9/11, relying on a secure relationship with God and a sense of spiritual connectedness with others, as well as increased religious practices such as prayer and fasting. Additionally, nonreligious methods included reaching out to other Muslims and Americans of other religions for support, educating other people about Islamic practices and beliefs, and encouraging interfaith dialogue. The people who engaged in these behaviors showed more posttraumatic growth, while those who used an isolative coping strategy experienced more depression and anger (Abu-Raiya, Pargament, & Mahoney, 2011).

As previously mentioned, Sikhs were frequent targets of discrimination and hate crimes due solely to their appearance. It was found that Sikh men use active coping, such as problem solving, more frequently than support-seeking or avoidance strategies (Liang, Alvarez, Juang, & Liang, 2009). Although many Sikhs turned to their religion and scriptures for support and strength, many others chose to discard outward symbols of their faith, considered central to their practice, such as cutting their hair and no longer wearing Turbans (Ahluwalia & Pellettiere, 2010). Many Sikhs also felt the need to show that they were patriotic Americans, covering their places of worship with American flags and even wearing red, white, and blue turbans (Ahluwalia & Pellettiere, 2010; Puar & Rai, 2002).

An influx in religiosity and spirituality was also found among Latinos and non-Latino Blacks post 9/11 compared with non-Latino Whites (Seirmarco et al., 2012). Previous studies have found that decreased importance of religion is associated with PTSD (Falsetti, Resick, & Davis, 2003). As such, the finding of increased religiosity and spirituality suggest a potential protective cultural mechanism against PTSD. After conducting qualitative interviews among New York City residents after 9/11, Constantine et al. (2005) also found that Latinos and African Americans reported going to church in order to cope with the tragedy more frequently than other ethnic groups. One Latina respondent stated:

> I went to [a Catholic] church every day after 9/11 for almost a month. I brought my husband and kids with me and we lit candles in memory of [the people who died in the 9/11 attacks]. Our pastor was so helpful to the parishioners during this time. I think [going to church] really helped me and my family to realize that we're not in control of a lot of things that go on in our life. (300)

This use of religion as a coping strategy appeared to promote resilience after the attacks of 9/11. McIntosh et al. (2011) found spirituality predicted fewer infectious ailments, more cognitive intrusions, and a faster decline in intrusions in response to a collective trauma.

It has also been found that there are gender differences in forms of coping. Among young adults, Wadsworth et al. (2004) found that young women were more likely to engage in emotion-based coping strategies such as reflective journaling and seeking contact with other people. In addition, females have been shown to use crying as a coping mechanism in dealing with 9/11 more than males (Constantine et al., 2005).

20.10 Conclusion

The events of September 11th, 2001 shattered the tranquility of the USA with a terrorist attack of unprecedented scope—in terms of shock, loss of life, and aftermath—in the nation's history. That the attacks centered on New York City, one of the most populous as well as culturally and economically diverse cities in the world, means that it is crucial to consider how the city's diversity has influenced the trajectory of trauma related mental health in the past decade and a half. Western psychology has tended to focus on the way that an event influences an individual, without taking into consideration how community praxis is, in some cultures, critical to the healing of trauma. We have considered how research indicates that there are cultural indices critical to both the development of trauma related disorders and to its amelioration; moreover, that cultural responses vary widely, even within specific Ethnic groups, and that the tendency to homogenize categories intended to describe facets of difference may obfuscate critical internal differences within proscribed group circumscriptions. Furthermore, we have considered research that shows how other kinds of group identity, such as sex and socioeconomic status, also play a role in the development of trauma related disorders. Further, these groups intersect (such as ethnicity and sex in the case of Latino women) to implicate a higher preponderance of trauma related disorders.

With 9/11 and the collective traumatization of a huge number of people, focus of treatment on the individual threatens to miss important group factors that implicate a variety of influences (beyond, but connected with, the individual's personal experience) in terms of the etiology and treatment of trauma related disorders such as PTSD. In the future, we suggest that mental health care efforts might be developed specifically to be sensitive to individuals from diverse backgrounds on many different levels. Mental health interventions clearly need a high consideration of cultural implications and diversity, which should account not only for treatment modality but also for the assessment of trauma related disorders, so that they can be applied with the greatest efficacy.

References

Abu-Raiya, H., Pargament, K. I., & Mahoney, A. (2011). Examining coping methods with stressful interpersonal events experienced by Muslims living in the United States following the 9/11 attacks. *Psychology of Religion and Spirituality, 3*(1), 1–14. doi:10.1037/a0020034.

Abu-Ras, W., & Abu-Bader, S. H. (2008). The impact of the September 11, 2001, attacks on the well-being of Arab Americans in New York City. *Journal of Muslim Mental Health, 3*(2), 217–239. doi:10.1080/15564900802487634.

Abu-Ras, W., & Abu-Bader, S. H. (2009). Risk factors for depression and posttraumatic stress disorder (PTSD): The case of Arab and Muslim Americans post-9/11. *Journal of Immigrant & Refugee Studies, 7*(4), 393–418. doi:10.1080/15562940903379068.

Abu-Ras, W. M., & Suarez, Z. E. (2009). Muslim men and women's perception of discrimination, hate crimes, and PTSD symptoms post 9/11. *Traumatology, 15*(3), 48–63. doi:10.1177/1534765609342281.

Adams, R. E., & Boscarino, J. A. (2006). Predictors of PTSD and delayed PTSD after disaster: The impact of exposure and psychosocial resources. *The Journal of Nervous and Mental Disease, 194*(7), 485.

Aggarwal, N. (2013). Cultural psychiatry, medical anthropology, and the DSM-5 field trials. *Medical Anthropology, 32*(5), 393–398. doi:10.1080/01459740.2013.776047.

Ahluwalia, M. K., & Pellettiere, L. (2010). Sikh men post-9/11: Misidentification, discrimination, and coping. *Asian American Journal of Psychology, 1*(4), 303–314.

Alcántara, C., Casement, M. D., & Lewis-Fernández, R. (2013). Conditional risk for PTSD among Latinos: A systematic review of racial/ethnic differences and sociocultural explanations. *Clinical Psychology Review, 33*(1), 107–119. doi:10.1016/j.cpr.2012.10.005.

Alegría, M., Canino, G., Shrout, P. E., Woo, M., Duan, N., Vila, D., et al. (2008). Prevalence of mental illness in immigrant and non-immigrant U.S. Latino groups. *The American Journal of Psychiatry, 165*(3), 359–369.

American Psychiatric Association. (2013). *Diagnostic and statistical manual of mental disorders, 5th edition (DSM-5). Diagnostic and statistical manual of mental disorders 4th edition TR.*

Asi, M., & Beaulieu, D. (2013). *Arab households in the United States: 2006–2010* (p. 4). http://www.census.gov/prod/2013pubs/acsbr10-20.pdf.

Besser, A., & Neria, Y. (2010). The effects of insecure attachment orientations and perceived social support on posttraumatic stress and depressive symptoms among civilians exposed to the 2009 Israel–Gaza war: A follow-up cross-lagged panel design study. *Journal of Research in Personality, 44*(3), 335–341. doi:10.1016/j.jrp.2010.03.004.

Betancourt, H., & Lopez, S. R. (1993). The study of culture, ethnicity, and race in American psychology. *American Psychologist, 48*(6), 629.

Bonanno, G. A. (2004). Loss, trauma, and human resilience. *American Psychologist, 59*(1), 20–28.

Bonanno, G. A., Galea, S., Bucciarelli, A., & Vlahov, D. (2007). What predicts psychological resilience after disaster? The role of demographics, resources, and life stress. *Journal of Consulting and Clinical Psychology, 75*(5), 671.

Bowler, R. M., Han, H., Gocheva, V., Nakagawa, S., Alper, H., DiGrande, L., et al. (2010). Gender differences in probable posttraumatic stress disorder among police responders to the 2001 World Trade Center terrorist attack. *American Journal of Industrial Medicine, 53*(12), 1186–1196.

Breslau, N. (2009). The epidemiology of trauma, PTSD, and other posttrauma disorders. *Trauma Violence Abuse, 10*(3), 198–210. doi:10.1177/1524838009334448.

Caplan, S. (2007). Latinos, acculturation, and acculturative stress: A dimensional concept analysis. *Policy, Politics, & Nursing Practice, 8*(2), 93–106.

Carlson, E. B., & Rosser-Hogan, R. (1994). Cross-cultural response to trauma: A study of traumatic experiences and posttraumatic symptoms in Cambodian refugees. *Journal of Traumatic Stress, 7*(1), 43–58. http://www.ncbi.nlm.nih.gov/pubmed/8044442.

Constantine, M. G., Alleyne, V. L., Caldwell, L. D., McRae, M. B., & Suzuki, L. a. (2005). Coping responses of Asian, Black, and Latino/Latina New York City residents following the September 11, 2001 terrorist attacks against the United States. *Cultural Diversity & Ethnic Minority Psychology, 11*(4), 293–308. doi:10.1037/1099-9809.11.4.293.

Cross, S. E., & Vick, N. V. (2001). The interde- pendent self-construal and social support: The case of persistence in engineering. *Personality and Social Psychology Bulletin, 27*, 820–832.

DiGrande, L., Neria, Y., Brackbill, R. M., Pulliam, P., & Galea, S. (2011). Long-term posttraumatic stress symptoms among 3,271 civilian survivors of the September 11, 2001, terrorist attacks on the World Trade Center. *American Journal of Epidemiology, 173*(3), 271–281. doi:10.1093/aje/kwq372.

DiGrande, L., Perrin, M. A., Thorpe, L. E., Thalji, L., Murphy, J., & Wu, D., et al. (2008). Posttraumatic stress symptoms, PTSD, and risk factors among Lower Manhattan residents 2–3 years after the September 11, 2001 terrorist attacks, *21*(3), 264–273. doi: 10.1002/jts.

Falsetti, S. A., Resick, P. A., & Davis, J. L. (2003). Changes in religious beliefs following trauma. *Journal of Traumatic Stress, 16*(4), 391–398.

FBI. (2001). *Hate crime reporting*. http://www.fbi.gov/about-us/cjis/ucr/hate-crime/2001/hatecrime01.pdf.

Foa, E. B., Riggs, D. S., Dancu, C. V., & Rothbaum, B. O. (1993). Reliability and validity of a brief instrument for assessing post-traumatic stress disorder. *Journal of Traumatic Stress, 6*, 459–473. doi:10.1007/BF00974317.

Foundation, A. A. I. (2012). *Demographics of Arab Americans* (p. 1).

Galea, S., Ahern, J., Resnick, H., Kilpatrick, D., Bucuvalas, M., Gold, J., et al. (2002). Psychological sequelae of the September 11 terrorist attacks in New York City. *The New England Journal of Medicine, 346*, 982–987. doi:10.1056/NEJMsa013404.

Galea, S., Ahern, J., Tracy, M., Hubbard, A., Cerda, M., Goldmann, E., et al. (2008). Longitudinal determinants of posttraumatic stress in a population-based cohort study. *Epidemiology, 19*(1), 47–54.

Galea, S., Vlahov, D., Tracy, M., Hoover, D. R., Resnick, H., & Kilpatrick, D. (2004). Hispanic ethnicity and post-traumatic stress disorder after a disaster: Evidence from a general population survey after September 11, 2001. *Annals of Epidemiology, 14*(8), 520–531.

Hall, J. M. (2005). Responses of adults in the Southeast to events of September 11: Six months later. *Issues in Mental Health Nursing, 26*(4), 415–432. doi:10.1080/01612840590922443.

Haque, A. (2004). Religion and mental health: The case of American Muslims. *Journal of Religion and Health, 43*(1), 45–58. http://link.springer.com/article/10.1023/B:JORH.0000009755.25256.71.

Hinton, D. E., & Lewis-Fernández, R. (2011). The cross-cultural validity of posttraumatic stress disorder: Implications for DSM-5. *Depression and Anxiety, 28*(9), 783–801. doi:10.1002/da.20753.

Jarrar, S. A. (1983). The treatment of Arabs in US social studies textbooks: Research findings and recommendations. In E. Gareeb (Ed.), *Split vision: The portrayal of Arabs in the American media* (pp. 369–380) Washington, DC: American-Arab Affairs Council.

Jenkins, J. H. (1996). Culture, emotion and PTSD. In A. Marsella, M. Friedman, E. Gerrity, & R. Scurfield (Eds.), *Ethnocultural aspects of posttraumatic stress disorder* (pp. 165–182). Washington, DC: American Psychological Association.

Jenkins, J. H., & Valiente, M. (1994). Bodily transactions of the passions: El calor among Salvadoran women refugees. *Embodiment and Experience: The Existential Ground of Culture and Self, 2*.

Johnson, T. (2011). *Muslims in the United States. Council on Foreign Relations*.

Jones, E., Vermaas, R. H., McCartney, H., Beech, C., Palmer, I., Hyams, K., et al. (2003). Flashbacks and post-traumatic stress disorder: The genesis of a 20th-century diagnosis. *The British Journal of Psychiatry: The Journal of Mental Science, 182*, 158–163. doi:10.1192/bjp.182.2.158.

Kaniasty, K., & Norris, F. H. (2008). Longitudinal linkages between perceived social support and posttraumatic stress symptoms: Sequential roles of social causation and social selection. *Journal of Trauma Stress, 21*(3), 274–281. doi:10.1002/jts.20334.

Kessler, R. C., Sonnega, A., Bromet, E., Hughes, M., & Nelson, C. B. (1995). Posttraumatic stress disorder in the National Comorbidity Survey. *Archives of General Psychiatry, 52*(12), 1048–1060.

Kinzie, J. D. (2005). Some of the effects of terrorism on refugees. Journal of Aggression, Maltreatment & Trauma, 9(3-4), 411–420. doi:10.1300/J146v09n03.

Kinzie, D (2005). Some of the Effects of Terrorism on Refugees, *Journal of Aggression, Maltreatment & Trauma, Volume 9*, Issue 3-4, 411–420. doi: 10.1300/J146v09n03_12J.

Kinzie, J. D., Boehnlein, J. K., Riley, C., & Sparr, L. (2002). The effects of September 11 on traumatized refugees: Reactivation of posttraumatic stress disorder. *The Journal of Nervous and Mental Disease, 190*(7), 437–441. doi:10.1097/01.NMD.0000022443.69161.0A.

Kleinman, A., Eisenberg, L., & Good, B. (2006). Culture, illness, and care: Clinical lessons from anthropologic and cross-cultural research. *FOCUS: The Journal of Lifelong Learning in Psychiatry, 4*(1), 140–149.

Lewis-fern, R., Turner, J. B., Marshall, R., Turse, N., & Dohrenwend, B. P. (2008). Elevated rates of current PTSD among Hispanic veterans in the NVVRS: True prevalence or methodological artifact? *21*(2), 123–132. doi: 10.1002/jts.

Liang, C. T. H., Alvarez, A. N., Juang, L. P., & Liang, M. X. (2009). The role of coping in the relationship between perceived racism and racism-related stress for Asian Americans: Gender differences. *Asian American Journal of Psychology*. doi: 10.1037/1948-1985.S.1.56.

Lopez, M. H. (2009). *Latinos and education: Explaining the attainment gap*. Washington, DC: Pew Hispanic Center.

Lopez, S. R., & Guarnaccia, P. J. (2000). Cultural psychopathology: Uncovering the social world of mental illness. *Annual Review of Psychology, 51*(1), 571–598.

McGoldrick, M., Giordano, J., & Garcia-Preto, N. (Eds.). (2005). *Ethnicity and family therapy*. New York: Guilford Press.

McIntosh, D. N., Poulin, M. J., Silver, R. C., & Holman, E. A. (2011). The distinct roles of spirituality and religiosity in physical and mental health after collective trauma: A national longitudinal study of responses to the 9/11 attacks. *Journal of Behavioral Medicine, 34*(6), 497–507.

Neria, Y., DiGrande, L., & Adams, B. G. (2011). Posttraumatic stress disorder following the September 11, 2001, terrorist attacks: A review of the literature among highly exposed populations. *American Psychologist, 66*(6), 429.

Neria, Y., Gross, R., Olfson, M., Gameroff, M. J., Wickramaratne, P., Das, A., et al. (2006). Posttraumatic stress disorder in primary care one year after the 9/11 attacks. *General Hospital Psychiatry, 28*(3), 213–222.

Neria, Y., Nandi, A., & Galea, S. (2008). Post-traumatic stress disorder following disasters: A systematic review. *Psychological Medicine, 38*(4), 467–480. doi:10.1017/S0033291707001353.

Neria, Y., & Sullivan, G. M. (2011). Understanding the mental health effects of indirect exposure to mass trauma through the media. *Journal of the American Medical Association, 306*(12), 1374–1375.

Norris, F. H., Perilla, J. L., Ibañez, G. E., & Murphy, A. D. (2001). Sex differences in symptoms of posttraumatic stress: Does culture play a role? *Journal of Traumatic Stress, 14*(1), 7–28.

Ortega, A. N., & Rosenheck, R. (2000). Posttraumatic stress disorder among Hispanic Vietnam veterans. *American Journal of Psychiatry, 157*, 615–619.

Ozer, E. J., Best, S. R., Lipsey, T. L., & Weiss, D. S. (2008, August). Predictors of posttraumatic stress disorder and symptoms in adults: a meta-analysis. In *Annual Meeting of the International Society for Traumatic Stress Studies, 14th, Nov, 1998, Washington, DC, US;* This article is based on a paper presented at the aforementioned meeting. (Vol. 1, p. 3). Educational Publishing Foundation.

Pantin, H. M., Schwartz, S. J., Prado, G., Feaster, D. J., & Szapocznik, J. (2003). Posttraumatic stress disorder symptoms in Hispanic immigrants after the September 11th attacks: Severity and relationship to previous traumatic exposure. *Hispanic Journal of Behavioral Sciences, 25*(1), 56–72.

Perilla, J. L., Norris, F. H., & Lavizzo, E. A. (2002). Ethnicity, culture, and disaster response: Identifying and explaining ethnic differences in PTSD six months after Hurricane Andrew. *Journal of Social and Clinical Psychology, 21*(1), 20–45.

Piwowarczyk, L. A., & Keane, T. M. (2007). Impact of September 11 on refugees and those seeking asylum. *Transcultural Psychiatry, 44*(4), 566–580. doi:10.1177/1363461507083897.

Pole, N., Best, S. R., Metzler, T., & Marmar, C. R. (2005). Why are Hispanics at greater risk for PTSD? *Cultural Diversity and Ethnic Minority Psychology, 11*(2), 144.

Puar, J. K., & Rai, A. S. (2002). Monster, terrorist, fag: The war on terrorism and the production of docile patriots. *Social Text, 20*, 117–148.

Pupcenoks, J. (2011). Race and Arab Americans before and after 9/11: From invisible citizens to visible subjects. *International Migration Review*. doi:10.1111/j.1747-7379.2010.00845.x.

Quarantelli, E. L. (1997). Ten criteria for evaluating the management of community disasters. *Disasters, 21*(1), 39–56.

Rippy, A. E., & Newman, E. (2006). Perceived religious discrimination and its relationship to anxiety and paranoia among Muslim Americans. *Journal of Muslim Mental Health, 1*(1), 5–20. doi:10.1080/15564900600654351.

Roberts, A. L., Gilman, S. E., Breslau, J., Breslau, N., & Koenen, K. C. (2011). Race/ethnic differences in exposure to traumatic events, development of post-traumatic stress disorder, and treatment-seeking for post-traumatic stress disorder in the United States. *Psychological Medicine, 41*(1), 71–83. doi:10.1017/S0033291710000401.

Rumbaut, R., & Portes, A. (2001). *Ethnicities: Children of immigrants in America*. Berkeley: University of California Press.

Schuster, M. A., et al. (2001). A national survey of stress reactions after the September 11, 2001, terrorist attacks. *New England Journal of Medicine, 345*(20), 1507–1512.

Scurfield, R. M. (2002). Commentary about the terrorist acts of September 11, 2001: Posttraumatic reactions and related social and policy issues. *Trauma, Violence, & Abuse, 3*(1), 3–14. doi:10.1177/15248380020031001.

Seirmarco, G., Neria, Y., Insel, B., Kiper, D., Doruk, A., Gross, R., et al. (2012). Religiosity and mental health: Changes in religious beliefs, complicated grief, posttraumatic stress disorder, and major depression following the September 11, 2001 attacks. *Psychology of Religion and Spirituality, 4*(1), 10–18. doi:10.1037/a0023479.

Shaheen, J. G. (2003). Reel Bad Arabs: How Hollywood Vilifies a People. *The ANNALS of the American Academy of Political and Social Science, 588*, 171–193.

Silver, R. C., Holman, E. A., McIntosh, D. N., Poulin, M., & Gil-Rivas, V. (2002). Nationwide longitudinal study of psychological responses to September 11. *The Journal of the American Medical Association, 288*, 1235–1244.

Updegraff, J. A., Silver, R. C., & Holman, E. A. (2008). Searching for and finding meaning in collective trauma: Results from a national longitudinal study of the 9/11 terrorist attacks. *Journal of Personality and*

Social Psychology, 95(3), 709–722. doi:10.1037/0022-3514.95.3.709.

Wadsworth, M. E., Gudmundsen, G. R., Raviv, T., Ahlkvist, J. A., McIntosh, D. N., & Kline, G. H., et al. (2004). Coping with terrorism : Age and gender differences in effortful and involuntary responses to September 11th, *8*(3), 143–157.

Weissman, M. M., Neria, Y., Das, A., Feder, A., Blanco, C., Lantigua, R., et al. (2005). Gender differences in posttraumatic stress disorder among primary care patients after the World Trade Center attack of September 11, 2001. *Gender Medicine, 2*, 76–87.

Williams, A. E., Smith, W. R., Starr, A. J., Webster, D. C., Martinez, R. J., Vojir, C. P., et al. (2008). Ethnic differences in posttraumatic stress disorder after musculoskeletal trauma. *Journal of Trauma-Injury, Infection, and Critical Care, 65*(5), 1054–1065.

21 Masculinity, Spirituality, and Male Wartime Sexual Trauma

R. Ruard Ganzevoort and Srdjan Sremac

Religion itself faces a trauma, a shock which dissolves the link between truth and meaning, a truth so traumatic that it resists being integrated into the universe of meaning.

Slavoj Žižek 2012, p. 155

21.1 Introduction

In wartime sexual and gender-based violence is widespread and fueled by ethnic, religious, and political hatred (Eriksson-Baaz & Stern, 2013; Leatherman, 2011; Roth & Rittner, 2012; Smith, 2005). Sexual violence includes any violence, physical or psychological, carried out through sexual means. It can include rape, various unwanted sexual and paraphilic acts, genital mutilation, total and partial castration, injuries to the testes with blunt objects, and harassment or degrading treatments liked forced public wearing of the other gender's underwear (Human Rights Watch, 2003). In order to understand Conflict Related Sexual Violence (CRSV) we need to be aware of the social, religious, and gender realities that underlie this type of violence. Sexual violence is not simply the act of one individual against another, but is embedded in group-based performances aiming at the disempowerment of the enemy. In conflict zones, different nations use militarized masculine norms to elucidate national (and religious) superiority, whilst simultaneously ascribing subordinate characteristics of the masculinities (e.g., effeminate, homosexual) to the other ethnic groups (Trošt-Pavasović & Slootmaeckers, 2015). In this way, the demasculinization and homosexualization of the ethnic other is used as a political strategy or war technique. The primary inducement of wartime violence is ethnicity, and the particular forms of sexual violence are intersectionally informed by religion and culture, gender (or more specifically masculinity), and heteronormativity (Žarkov, 2011, p. 109). This chapter examines the relationships between CRSV, masculinity, and meaning. To understand the occurrence and aftermath of CRSV, we need to look at the cultural and religious meanings attributed to gender, sexuality, and violence. This chapter will therefore explore the following: (1) the relationship between trauma and CRSV and its impact on psychological well-being; (2) the roles of cultural (often religiously bolstered) gender norms in sexual traumatization, and (3) the connections between masculinity and posttraumatic growth and spirituality (we use the term "religious" for the sociocultural traditions referring to the sacred and "spiritual" for the personal experiences, meanings, and practices). Recommendations and implications for reconciliation processes in post-conflict societies and effective interventions for traumatized male survivors/victims will be discussed.

R.R. Ganzevoort, Ph.D. (✉) • S. Sremac, Ph.D.
Amsterdam Centre for the Study of Lived Religion, Faculty of Theology, Vrije Universiteit Amsterdam, De Boelelaan 1105, Amsterdam, HV 1081, The Netherlands
e-mail: r.r.ganzevoort@vu.nl; s.sremac@vu.nl

Y. Ataria et al. (eds.), *Interdisciplinary Handbook of Trauma and Culture*,
DOI 10.1007/978-3-319-29404-9_21

Available data suggest that CRSV is not uncommon. In many armed conflicts acts of sexual violence are used to humiliate and dehumanize the enemy. During the conflict in Bosnia and Herzegovina (1992–1995) for example, an estimated 20,000 women and girls were raped in the period of 3 years, in the 4 months of the 1994 genocide in Rwanda between 250,000 and 500,000 Tutsi women and girls were raped, and in the Sierra Leona civil war 64,000 women became victims of sexual violence between 1991 and 2001 (cited in Brouwer, 2005, p. 9). Although conflict-related sexual violence (CRSV) has typically been defined as a subject affecting women and girls, there are also reports of substantial sexual violence against men and boys. Throughout the armed conflict in Yugoslavia, for example, 6000 cases of male victimization have been reported including rape, mass sterilization, and genital mutilation (Lewis, 2009). In the Congo conflict 23.6 % of men reported being sexually abused (Johnson et al., 2010) while in El Salvador 76 % of political prisoners reported being subjected to at least one form of sexual torture (Agger, 1989). Similar numbers can be found in other Latin American countries that experienced armed conflicts between 1987 and 2007: Colombia, Guatemala, Nicaragua, Argentina, and Peru. This indicates that CRSV against men and boys may commonly be underreported or may vary in frequency from one context to another.

Because many conflicts and wars concern ethnic and cultural group boundaries, CRSV functions as a military and political strategy that targets the ethnic or cultural Other. The direct purpose is to destroy the individual's dignity through his or her body and mind. Ultimately, however, it serves to annihilate, demoralize, terrorize, dehumanize, and eventually humiliate the entire population (Kaitesi, 2014, p. 17). Scarry (1985) describes how torture uses the body in pain to establish a power relation and turn the body into an enemy of the victim by making it speak the language of the oppressor. Cooey (1994) clarifies how the body is both a "site" of power conflicts and a "sign" of contested cultural and religious meanings. Olujic (1998) rightly points out that in wartime, individual bodies become the metaphoric representatives of the ethnic and/or religious body, and raping a body symbolizes seizing and overpowering the victim's ethnic and/or religious group. CRSV thus ethnicizes the human body and defines the body as a national, cultural, and possibly religious territory (Drezgić, 2010, p. 958).

In the case of CSRV against men and boys, the impact of sexualized violence is intensified by the cultural and religious taboos on (homo) sexuality. In many cultural systems only the receptive role in sexual activity between males counts as homosexual, effeminate, and weak, which leaves the victim of male-to-male sexual violence with the stigma of a sexually polluted and depersonalized body. The perpetrator then acquires masculine power by sexually overpowering another man, while the victim is culturally emasculated. When masculinity and heterosexuality are considered to be intrinsically connected and culturally and religiously sanctioned, the stigma of sexual victimization becomes unbearable.

This stigma serves to keep the trauma hidden and reduce the chances of intervictim solidarity because every victim survives in shame. The Human Rights Watch report *We'll Kill You If You Cry* (2003, p. 42), for example, notes that "[d]ue to the stigma attached to [receptive] homosexuality in Sierra Leone, male victims of rape feared they would be perceived as homosexuals and therefore few boys were willing to report it." Some researchers even speculate that societal pressure can produce denial of rape or may even hinder encoding, storage, or retrieval of such memories (Elzinga & Bremner, 2002). In addition, one of the major reasons for the failure to identify male survivors of sexual torture is internalization of traditional gender role stereotypes (males as perpetrators, females as victims) that further leads to nonresponsive service provision (Donnelly & Kenyon, 1996). The problem of male sexual violence in conflict zones for those reasons remains a public secret, "hidden topic" (Sivakumaran, 2013, p. 81) and the "forgotten method of torture" (UNOCHA, 2008, p. 1).

Although admittedly the line between these motives may be thin, CRSV is not primarily an expression of sexual lust or erotic interest. Rather, it must be understood as an exertion of power, violence, and aggression (Žarkov, 2007, p. 33). It is motivated by violent intentions to disempower and humiliate others, often based on race and/or ethnicity. CRSV is therefore regarded as an element of the crime of torture and considered to be a crime against personal dignity. Recent debates claim that wartime rape and sexual torture are the ultimate humiliation of the victim and must be regarded as one of the most serious crimes against humanity (cited in Hirschauer, 2014). For victims, it is an ontological crisis in which the person is forced to negotiate the contamination of self-narrative in the face of severe psychological, somatic, and social consequences. It completely overshadows the victims' lives and calls into question their individuality, sexuality, social acceptance, and identity. Its main characteristics of hopelessness, emptiness, loss of meaning in life, often perceived feelings of being abandoned by others and ultimately by God, lack of self-esteem and worth, stigma, and shame, all indicate a level of distress that clearly has ontological and spiritual connotations. The traumatic event destroys the person's faith in a metaphysical order and destabilizes the symbolic order the person dwells in (Janoff-Bulman, 1992). As Žižek (2014, p. 120) puts it, the traumatic encounter of extreme violence destabilizes our entire horizon of meaning. Trauma casts us into a state of ontological and/or existential crisis. CRSV as a terror tactic thus touches on fundamental aspects of identity, sexuality, spirituality, and culture. This existential dimension may be further triggered by complex physical consequences; many victims of sexual violence contract sexually transmitted diseases, including HIV/AIDS, hepatitis C, and suffered genital and anal mutilation or enforced sterilization (including castration).

21.2 Trauma and Conflict-Related Sexual Violence Against Males

Before we explore the intersections of masculinity and sexual trauma in more depth, we introduce several cases of male sexual brutality during the civil war in Bosnia and Herzegovina. These cases will provide examples of the ideas introduced later in the essay. Narratives provide unique and deeply disturbing insights into the ethical deadlock of male sexual violence in armed conflicts. Some of these testimonies have been accessed via the website of the International Criminal Tribunals for the Former Yugoslavia (ICTY). The ICTY was the first tribunal to prosecute wartime rape.

The examples come from the Čelebići and Omarska Detention Camps during the Bosnian War. These camps were used to detain prisoners of war arrested during military operations. Prisoners were subjected to extreme forms of human cruelty and brutality such as torture, sex-based atrocities, forced homosexual contact with other prisoners, beatings, killings and other physical and psychological abuse. In the Mucić et al. "Čelebići Camp" case witness *S.G.* testified about two detained brothers who were forced to perform fellatio on each other. The perpetrators did not engage in the sexual activities themselves, but used forced sexual contact for the purpose of humiliation:

> Sometime in mid July they brought in two young men, whom I knew very well, because I was their teacher in Bradina. They were two brothers. They were singled out by Zenga for torture. He beat them and then they had to slap each other's face, for instance, and if the slaps were not strong enough, then he would show them how it's really done. One day they had to suck each other's penis. (Mucić et al., IT-96-21; Trial Transcripts pp. 1450–1451)

A second example from one of the eyewitnesses in the Omarska Prison Camp testifies to the genital violence and mutilation that took place. He recalled that 1 day a member of the Serbian forces ordered *G.* and *H.* to lick *F.H.*'s buttocks and genitals and then to sexually mutilate him. *H* covered *F.H.*'s mouth to silence his screams and *G.* bit off one of his testicles:

> I saw when H. was holding, I cannot quite say whether it was E.K. or somebody else, by the hands, when he was holding him by the hands, G. had to bow down in his crutch and it was ordered to him that he must bite the genital. When I looked up the second time, in those moments there were screams. When the second time I looked, G. got up with his mouth full. (Persecutor vs. Dusko Tadić, Trial Transcript, IT-94-1-T, p. 3986)

Several narratives give evidence of cultural or religious dimensions in these cases of sexual violence, especially in how the body and person of the Other are defined. One victim remembered his experience in the Omarska Camp with these words:

> They were hitting me, as well as others, in the testicles, using metal hampers, metal bars, kicking with the boots. My testicles were swollen, the size of oranges. The number of tortures varies from one [or] two to twenty or more… They were deliberately aiming their beatings at our testicles saying, "you'll never make Muslim children again." (Instituting Proceedings, 1993)

In her book, *The Body of War*, Žarkov (2007, p. 159) refers to the testimony of a Catholic priest who was sexually assaulted by the Serbian soldiers: "I was covered in blood. They took off all my clothes and poured cold water on me. They were suffocating me with water, mocking my nakedness and continuing to beat me with whatever they had around." In their empirical research among 60 male rape survivors from the Yugoslav civil war, Loncar, Henigsberg, and Hrabac (2010, p. 197) report how cases of semi-castration were performed either by cutting the victim's scrotum or penis or by tying up the penis with rope or wire, followed by pulling the rope by hand. The Croatian research team further revealed how the perpetrators were placing different objects such as glass bottles in the victims' anuses and then forcing the victims to sit on these objects (Loncar et al., 2010, p. 198).

There is much evidence of the potential psychosocial harm of sexual violence, especially in the more brutal shapes of rape or sexual torture. Several studies have confirmed major similarities between male and female survivors of rape as described in the rape trauma syndrome (RTS). Rape trauma syndrome has been described as a complex posttraumatic stress disorder (PTSD) that manifests itself in the somatic, emotional, cognitive, and interpersonal behavior of the rape victim. Kessler, Sonnega, Bromet, Hughes, and Nelson (1995) and others argue that rape is among the traumatic experiences most highly correlated with the development of PTSD. The feelings of shame, guilt, loss of trust, lack of self-esteem and worth, the loss of honor, feeling of isolation and estrangement, self-harming behaviors (including suicidal tendencies and substance abuse), sexual dysfunction, vulnerability, and embarrassment indicate a level of existential distress that verges on spiritual crises. However, the connection between men's psychological health and sexual violence they experienced often remains hidden.

A number of studies suggest that it is not the rape itself but the social exclusion and stigmatization in the aftermath that constitutes the deepest trauma (cited in Johnson et al., 2010; Sivakumaran, 2013). This aftermath is influenced by the cultural meanings attached to the event and by the response from the victim's social context. Recognition or the lack thereof, stigmatization, and ostracization are powerful factors. The common view of men as sexually inviolable and the "myth of male invulnerability" is a case in point. Scholars of male sexual victimization, therefore, have paid close attention to rape's function in the victim's construction of masculinity, femininity, and (homo)sexuality (Ganzevoort, 2002). Due to culturally embedded and often religiously fortified patriarchal stereotypes, male-by-male rape is experienced as indicative of homosexuality, not only because both victim and perpetrator are usually male, but more so because of the notion of feminization or emasculation. These cultural stereotypes are clearly gendered: through penetration the raped male body becomes a feminized body: weakened, subordinated, and homosexualized. The rapist, on the other hand, underscores his masculinity through this act. According to Butler (2008, p. 17) we have to understand sexual torture as "the actions of a homophobic institution against a population that is both constructed and targeted for its own shame about homosexuality…" All this makes it less likely for male rape victims to seek counseling and increases the risk of more severe psychological consequences. As Fuchs notes (2004, p. 94), "society is reluctant to accept the idea that a "real man" could be reduced to such a sexually passive role, and when a man attempts to report his assault, he is often ridiculed."

21.3 Masculinities and Sexual Traumatization

Given these powerful social discourses and internalized norms, Sivakumaran (2005) argues that male rape victims' suffering includes being made weak and effeminate. This subordinates the victim's status, making him inferior as a man by social norms that are present mostly in the male-dominated and homophobic societies (which seems to be the case in many war dominated countries). At the same time, the acts of sexual violence bolster the sense of masculinity in the perpetrator: when the Other is made weak and powerless, the perpetrator gains hypermasculinity. In many contexts, to overpower another man sexually does not invoke notions of homosexual desire but of strong masculinity; it is only the victim that becomes stigmatized as homosexual. In this respect Wood (2013, p. 145) refers to societies in war that develop norms that instill aggressive "militarized masculinity." In this way, a "cult of masculinity" functions as sociopolitical supremacy in order to masculinize and *empower* the perpetrator and feminize and *disempower* the victim. In other words, the cultural meanings of violence are produced through dominant discursive structures of masculinity, power, and heteronormativity. Referring to castration in the Balkan context, Žarkov argues that dominant notions of manhood (or masculinity) in patriarchal societies are inseparable from norms of heterosexuality. She claims that:

> [t]he embodiment of that dominance is the penis, and its symbolic equivalent is the phallus. In that light, castration and the cutting of a man's penis are acts of physical as much as symbolic emasculation, because the lack of a penis symbolizes the lack of phallic power. Žarkov (2007, p. 165)

According to Žarkov, sexual torture like genital mutilation or rape uses homosexualization and feminization of the victim in a struggle for power, social control, humiliation, and dehumanization of the ethnic and/or religious Other. For Žarkov (1997, p. 144) this phallic aggression against men is "making a man into a non-man. It is not in itself an act of a perverted homosexual desire; it is an act of perverted desire for power [...] A victimized man is not a man." Therefore, to rape a man is to symbolically emasculate and feminize him in order to humiliate his physical, moral, and social integrity (MacKinnon, 1997).

The sexual violation victims have experienced is, thus, much more than a violation of the body; it implies a fundamental threat to core ideas about masculinity and therefore challenges one's legitimate position in society. The objectified body is rendered passive and vulnerable and is used as a means to dehumanize and emasculate the person. At the same time, the sexual torture or penetration of the body—either sexually or as physical harm—undermines the self-evident boundary between the self and the other. The double meaning of objectified powerlessness and forced loss of boundaries makes the traumatic experience the ultimate denial of masculinity that it is construed as in many cultural contexts.

One of the more frequent responses to traumatization in males, then, is to aim at a restoration of the old paradigms of masculinity or even hypermasculinity. This sometimes results in "acting out," because traumatized males may engage in self-destructive and aggressive behaviors like substance abuse or violence. Our previous research on the role of spiritual transformation in the religious therapeutic outcomes among recovering drug addicts has shown that male sexual childhood trauma can be an important factor contributing to drug abuse (Sremac, 2013; Sremac & Ganzevoort, 2013). Many of these participants disclosed a history of sexual or physical abuse. This kind of traumatic experience had a long-term and profound impact on the participants' sense of self and identity. The participants frequently reported powerful long-term effects of sexual trauma, engendering self-destructive behavior, aggression, depression, anxiety, and a sexual identity crisis later in their lives. For many of them substance use functioned as a coping mechanism for their trauma by anesthetizing the painful memories of early sexual abuses and the agonizing emotions that resulted.

Notwithstanding individual variation, sexually traumatized men tend to be more prone to acting out, whereas traumatized women tend towards developing depression (Solomon et al., 2005; Stewart & Harmon, 2004). Even though there are certainly more factors involved, one of the reasons for this difference may be found in the different gender messages men and women encounter. For men, the threat to masculinity inherent to the traumatic experience may compel them to develop compensatory behavior, which includes intimacy avoidance, emotional distancing, and power restoration.

Psychological conditions of male survivors of rape are further complicated by the refusal of men to disclose rape trauma due to the cultural stigma they feel they might endure. The shame and humiliation that flows from societies' responses can thereby increase psychological harm and bring about a multitude of individual losses such as loss of identity and self-esteem. This can further isolate male victims from the real world and potentially intensify the effects of their traumas. Some male victims said that the horrors they experienced were more than they could endure, noting that they had no words to describe and articulate the residual trauma (cited in Andersen, 2008). Franke (1998) explains how male victims during the Bosnian conflict were not able to conceptualize and verbalize their sexual assaults at the tribunal in The Hague. Significantly, the majority of testimonies about sexual violence against men at the ICTY came from witnesses and not from the direct victims. It was only after rape was reconsidered as a weapon of war and a form of torture—instead of an individualized sexual act—that male victims were able to articulate their deeply disturbing traumatic experiences of sexual torture. The reframing of rape as an instrument of war may serve as a preventative and/or coping mechanism. This reminds us of how Judith Butler (1997, p. 36) refers to the encoded traumatic memory that "lives in language and is carried in language."

The sexual dimension of these acts of violence includes issues regarding the possible experience of involuntary erections or ejaculations within the context of nonconsensual sex (cited in Bullock & Beckson, 2011; Lewis, 2009). Although these are direct biological responses that do not indicate sexual pleasure, they may lead the victim to question his sexual orientation (Sivakumaran, 2005, pp. 1290–1291). In homophobic societies with a strong cultural and religious bias against homosexuality, this leaves the male victim betrayed by his own body and vulnerable to further stigmatization and shame.

21.4 Masculinities, Trauma, and Culture

The exploration above already indicates how masculinity plays a central role in defining the relationship between CRSV and cultural and religious meaning. The term "masculinity" is not taken here in an essentialist sense as referring to certain innate qualities of male-bodied individuals, but in a constructionist sense as the messages and meanings that are projected onto a person because of his male body (and in an indirect sense onto female-bodied persons, which represent a negative model). The masculine identity is constructed out of individual experiences and longings, idiosyncratic models and contexts, and the (sub)cultural meanings attributed to this complex, resulting in prescriptions of what it is to be a man. This is for every person a specific configuration of meanings. Masculinity consists of the "messages men hear" (Harris, 1995). The central question we are exploring is which messages are conveyed to men in the context of trauma (more specifically CRSV), recovery, and religion.

We will describe these messages in a heuristic model—admittedly broadly overgeneralizing—as mathematical vectors in an interplay of forces. The matrix in which we describe these forces consists of two axes. The vertical axis is about power and powerlessness, the horizontal axis about isolation and boundlessness (Ganzevoort

& Veerman, 2000). On both axes, the ideal point is in the middle. Too much power can be just as problematic as too little power, because both distort the relation of the person to significant others as well as to the vicissitudes of life that are fundamentally beyond our control. If a person lives his or her life with too much power, an illusion of complete autonomy is confirmed that jeopardizes the person's openness to the uncontrollable exterior world (Winnicott's illusion of omnipotence). In the case of powerlessness, the person develops too little autonomy and becomes a plaything of others and of external forces. On the horizontal axis, too much isolation is negative, because it leaves the person deprived of significant relations and closes him or her in. Too much openness, as is the case in boundlessness, means that the person has no choice whether or not to admit others to his or her private life. Boundless people are unable to protect their individual space. Ideally, at the center of the matrix, the person has adequate control over her of his own life and is able to acknowledge external influences. He or she is able to relate to other people and to protect the hidden sphere of their personal identity. This ideal center point, however, is difficult to realize because of the various forces at play in the case of sexual traumatization. The force lines our model describes are the influences that move the person away from the ideal center.

The first vector or force line regards implicit and explicit gender messages. It is a vector that distinguishes between men and women and offers them opposite criteria or values by which to order their lives. Generally, it is about domination versus submission, rationality versus emotion, hard versus soft, sexually active versus sexually receptive, and so on. Especially in patriarchal contexts, men are expected to be strong, self-sufficient, and autonomous. In our matrix they will score high on both power and isolation. Accounting for subcultural and individual differences, specific norms of masculinity may be found according to different patterns, like the standard bearer, the worker, the lover, the boss, or the rugged individual (Harris, 1995). In these patterns, the axes of power and isolation are represented differently, but the general image remains that men should be strong and self-sufficient, and even if they connect to others they do so from their position of power, caring for others or fighting with them. In various ways, then, this message of power and isolation is a powerful aspect of masculinity, a standard that men need to try to live by, so that they will be recognized by others and by themselves as "real men." Contexts of war and violence often intensify these hypermasculine gender messages, especially in patriarchal cultures that cherish machismo.

The second vector is the impact of sexual traumatization. The message inherent in this traumatization is one of loss of autonomy and forced boundlessness. As a result, many victims experience a damaged capacity to guard the borders of their identity and as a result have difficulty negotiating this border in encounters with others. This can result in either too much or too little openness. Although this vector of meanings is basically the same for men and women, the combination with the gender-messages results in a different kind of conflict. One could say—more or less cynically—that sexual traumatization is a radical endorsement of patriarchal notions of femininity and an equally radical denial of masculinity. Victimization is not something that fits in the canonical stories of masculinity, leaving the victim with a serious threat to his gender-identity: "If men aren't to be victims, then victims aren't men" (Lew, 1988). To own up to experiences of sexual traumatization, then, activates fundamental gender ambivalences: to object to the patriarchal gender system present in the acts of sexual violence is to place oneself outside the cultural system; to accept the gender system is to validate the violence. In both cases the victim fails to meet the ideals of masculinity and is thus culturally emasculated. When sexual traumatization occurs in the hypermasculine context of war, the impact may be even more focused on gender issues. CRSV then is very threatening to the messages that many men hear in western societies, if not in all societies with a patriarchal inheritance.

The third vector regards the aftermath of sexual violence, including the cultural meanings, social responses, and individual coping strategies.

Survival strategies include a tendency to withdraw from others out of shame, protection, and/or fear of intimacy (Fischer & Good, 1997), which strengthens the sense of isolation. Gender differences are especially relevant on the axis of power. Men more often seem to develop survival strategies that restore their power and autonomy, sometimes in dysfunctional or self-destructive ways. Women seem to tend towards strategies that involve less power and consequently more servitude. In their own ways, both incorporate the presumed gender messages in their own coping strategies. For men, these coping strategies are consonant with the gender messages. In fact, one could argue that the primary purpose of these strategies is to restore masculinity. Thus, the interaction between coping and gender sometimes leads to dysfunctional hypermasculinities that reiterate the violence.

The final vector describes the impact of religious messages. The general message of the dominant religious traditions in patriarchal contexts summons the believer to surrender him or herself to God. This means abandoning one's autonomy and instead opening up and surrendering. For women, this message can be associated with gender messages that tell them to be subservient, but for men it is contradictory to gender messages telling them to be autonomous and powerful. Here C.S. Lewis' (1946, p. 316) dictum—"What is above and beyond all things is so masculine that we are all feminine in relation to it"—is indicative of the contradictions in religious gender messages. In more traditional religious groups, this threat to masculinity is countered by the power that is unequally delegated to men, especially in ecclesial office. For victims of CRSV who face the threats of emasculation and feminization, this empowerment may be less accessible, leaving religious messages on the side of the messages of traumatization. At least in some shapes, religious messages deprive the person of an affirmed masculinity. The messages of religion carry at least some degree of feminization, leaving little room for self-affirmation, strength, and pride. Of course, this may be a healthy counterbalance to damaging messages of hypermasculinity, but in the case of victims of CRSV, it may strip these men of their last suggestion of masculinity. In sum, religious gender messages in a patriarchal context bolster the position of those in positions of power and undermine the position of the powerless. This masculinizes the perpetrators and further emasculates the victims.

If we apply this heuristic model to the concrete context of the war in former Yugoslavia, from which we drew our examples, we see that conflict related sexual violence reflects the patriarchal gender system that is supported by social, religious, ethnic, and cultural power relationship (the vertical axis). In such a context, and especially after traumatization, a victim fails to meet the ideals of masculinity and is thus culturally emasculated (the horizontal axis). Žarkov (2007, p. 167) shows, in her analysis of sexual violence against men in the Balkans war, that the tortured male bodies are defined as the multiple Other—"through race, religion, and culture as much as through masculinity and sexuality." The body of the male other becomes a national, cultural, and possibly religious territory as well as a site of violence.

As we stated earlier, the coping mechanism of male victims depends on dominant notions of masculinity and the norms of heterosexuality in a particular cultural, religious, and political space. Consequently, we cannot fully comprehend the intersection of religion and coping without understanding its relationship to masculinity and heteronormativity. However, solid empirical investigations of religious coping and sexual torture among male victims are rare. In a framework where masculinity is inseparable from norms of control and power, it seems that religion has less potential to function in coping and transformation. We will address this issue later in the chapter.

21.5 Posttraumatic Growth and Spirituality

The relation between religion or spirituality and trauma is complex. There is convincing research to date that shows that traumatization is not always detrimental to spirituality but may even enhance the person's spiritual engagement and growth. Some of these studies focus on posttraumatic growth among war survivors. Başoğlu and colleagues (2005) found that war survivors in the former Yugoslavia had a stronger faith in God compared with the control group. Carmil and Breznitz (1991) investigated long-term consequences of the Holocaust and found that survivors and survivors' offspring expressed greater belief in God and greater belief in a better future. Other studies have shown that survivors of torture had more posttraumatic growth and practice their religion more than survivors of "general trauma" (Kira et al., 2006).

The concept of posttraumatic growth (PTG) has emerged in the last two decades to account for the observation of positive life changes as a result of a trauma or life crisis (Linley & Joseph, 2004). According to Christopher (2004), growth instead of pathology is in fact the normal outcome of traumatic stress. Congenial to "positive psychology," researchers into posttraumatic growth are interested in health promoting factors that may be called upon in coping with traumatizing events, in order to support coping efforts and resilience (Wilson, 2006). According to Ai and Park (2005), mental health research into trauma and related fields would benefit from the complementary approaches of stress-related growth, positive psychology, and the recognition of the role of spirituality and religion. Fontana and Rosenheck (2004) found that guilt and weakened religious faith are central to the prolonged use of mental health services and concluded that questions of meaning and spirituality deserve more attention in the treatment of PTSD. Summarizing these insights, Linley (2003) notes three dimensions of "wisdom" that support posttraumatic growth: the recognition and management of uncertainty, the integration of affect and cognition, and the recognition and acceptance of human limitation.

The observations that led to the development of concepts like posttraumatic growth or posttraumatic spirituality are not that new. Especially when it comes to the intersection with meaning, spirituality, or religion, there is a long tradition of writing and research that explores something like spiritual growth following negative life events (Howe 1988; Shandor Miles & Brown Crandall, 1986). Boisen (1970) noted that crisis periods may be times of new interpretations because people tend to focus their mental activities on what is immediately necessary, they will tend to contemplate the meanings of life only when they are challenged. That does not mean that every individual will show a change in terms of the importance or meaning of religion to them (Croog & Levine, 1972; Ganzevoort, 1994), but it stresses the fact that these meanings may be considered more in times of stress, crisis, or trauma. This points to the inherent relationship between religion and coping with crisis, which is evident in the theoretical framework of Pargament's (1997) *Psychology of Religion and Coping*. He describes coping as a search for significance in times of stress and religion as a search for significance in ways related to the sacred. The shared notion of a search for significance supports the view that crises or traumatic events may give way to semantic innovation and thus growth.

21.6 Masculinities and Spirituality

As we near the end of this chapter we explore one approach towards posttraumatic growth at the intersection of masculinity and spirituality (Krondorfer 1996). A seminal text in this field has been James Nelson's (1992) *Male Sexuality, Masculine Spirituality*, in which he describes two types of masculine spirituality, both offering a positive view of body and sexuality grounded in theological notions of incarnation and resurrection. The first, often associated with traditional masculinity, can be termed "phallic." It is symbolized by the erect male organ and can carry meanings of power, dominance, and penetration. Nelson notes, however, that the male organ is erect only from time to time, separated by much longer periods of flaccidity. This symbolizes the second type of masculine spirituality that Nelson calls "penile." Penile masculinity is like the theological *Via Negativa* characterized by receptivity rather than penetration, creating space for others rather than dominating them. In penile masculinity, touch, passivity, and intimacy are welcomed, while it is highly ambivalent in phallic masculinity.

Nelson's distinction directly relates to the issues discussed earlier in this chapter. The ambivalences about male sexuality are intensified by the context of war and violent traumatization. The psychological impact of sexual torture can be interpreted in light of a forced passivity that could fit well within a penile masculinity but is unacceptable in a phallic masculinity. The context of war and violence itself, however, is defined by hyperphallic masculinities and it is precisely for that reason that CRSV carries the meaning of emasculation. Penile masculinity, when forced upon a person through violence and oppression then becomes a threat rather than a possible source of new meaning.

In coping with the aftermath of sexual traumatization, many men tend towards withdrawal, touch avoidance, and restoration of phallic masculinity, but it comes at the price of foreclosing intimacy and connectedness with others and with one's own body. This defensive response buys into traditional notions of phallic masculinity that were more or less destructive from the beginning. Instead of critiquing these notions, they are bolstered as if they are part of the solution. The response of receptive or penile masculinity seems counterintuitive for many, because it allows the destruction of precisely the type of masculinity that is threatened. This seems like accepting the message that one does not live up to the criteria for masculinity, that one is not a real man. This is clearly a paradoxical outcome: the natural attempt to restore phallic masculinity leads to foreclosure, whereas the acceptance of receptive, penile masculinity seems unmasculine but creates space for a new way of living.

It is not too strong to call this a posttraumatic spiritual transformation. Ganzevoort (2008) uses the metaphors of scars and stigmata when addressing the interaction between trauma and identity. The former recognizes trauma as an "alien" intrusion that calls for resistance. The latter recognizes trauma as integral to identity development. The harmful and painful touch that figures in the wounds or scars inflicted on the body can be transformed into stigmata that carry spiritual significance. This suggests a need for a dialectical response. If one only stresses the touch avoidant response to trauma, phallic masculinity is preserved and the wounds remain alien to the self. If one only stresses the receptive response to trauma, the phallic masculine self is given up and penile suffering is accepted uncritically. Spiritual transformation of scars into stigmata comes from the audacious effort to refuse either extreme (Ganzevoort, 2008) and keep the phallic and penile dimensions together in a dialectical connection. It is a fragile balance, but it results in a deconstruction and not just destruction of masculinity. For spiritual caregivers it is necessary to resist the temptation to succumb to and restore hegemonic notions of masculinity, but also the escape of explaining away the menace to masculinity. Keeping open the area between these two positions can support spiritual transformation.

In the interplay of trauma and spirituality, coping and gender are important factors. Posttraumatic spirituality belongs to the realm of coping strategies and coping outcomes. Posttraumatic spirituality can be either functional and support a satisfying life, or it can be dysfunctional and contribute to self-harm or violence. The gender messages for men are contradicted by both traumatization and religion, which makes it more difficult to integrate them in a posttraumatic spiritual identity. Spiritual counseling of male victims of CRSV should therefore address the issues of masculinity much more explicitly.

21.7 Recreating Victimized Identity

One of the major problems in the treatment of CRSV has been the lack of sufficient caregivers qualified and willing to attend to survivors' stories of atrocities. Medical caregivers and recovery-oriented practitioners are often emotionally unprepared to listen to the horrifying experiences of survivors of sexual violence (Goldfeld, Mollica, Pesavento, & Faraone, 1988). Consistent with a narrative approach, a primary path to recovery is through the telling of the trauma stories to an empathic audience. Caregivers should take seriously the narrative features of psychological functioning of male rape trauma survivors to help them to develop a new narrative identity, foster spiritual growth and address significant concerns. Ganzevoort (2010) identifies three conditions to do this: (1) the person should be viewed as a potential author of narratives; someone with stories to tell; (2) the work of pastoral "intervention" should be sensitive to the power of narrative in religious traditions in the accomplishment of its aims, and (3) pastoral counseling and care should be enhanced by the understanding that its activity consists of the negotiation of mutual meanings through joint or cooperative story-making. For Ganzevoort two distinct dimensions are at stake here: the first is the construction of a meaningful story, the second is the exchange of stories between a narrator and her or his audience. In other words, the first is about the *narrative product* and the second is about the *narrating process* (Ganzevoort 2010, p. 332). Religious traditions can play a role here in offering symbols, language, images, stories, and supportive environments that may evoke a transformation of meaning. This supportive environment helps the individual to create a new story and to find an audience where they can perform a new narrative identity. In this way, the care seeker is "taken seriously as a unique narrator with the right and capacity to find new meanings in old stories and with an audience that accepts, invites and challenges" (Ganzevoort 2010, p. 339). The spiritual caregiver facilitates the creation of a space in which a trauma survivor's story intersects with the story of a supportive community. In this regard, an empathic audience, to whom trauma stories are told and retold, will have deep influence on the reaffirmation of narrative identity and the removal of stigma attached to (homo) sexual victimization.

In a similar vein, Mollica (2006) notes that people who have been (sexually) tortured do not want to be treated primarily as torture survivors. Instead, they prefer a holistic approach that addresses their current reality in a culturally sensitive way. For Mollica (2006) the "trauma story" has four elements: (1) a factual recounting of the traumatic experience; (2) the cultural meaning of the trauma; (3) an opportunity to make distance ("put the past behind them") from the intensity of the trauma; and (4) a sharing of the story to an enthusiastically listener who is willing to learn from the storyteller. Furthermore, Mollica (1988, p. 312) argues that the significance of the trauma changes over time: "The new story that emerges is no longer a story about powerlessness … no longer about shame and humiliation—it becomes a story about human dignity and virtue."

It would be helpful to victims of CRSV if post-conflict societies would address male sexual victimization more explicitly in order to foster healing, rebuild lives and create positive legacies to pass on to future generations. Facing the past is a painful process in which culture, spirituality, and wartime trauma play an important role. It is a journey of reconciliation, justice, peace, and healing. As Tombs (2014) points out: the omission and taboos of CRSV remains a significant obstacle for any individual that seeks to reconcile with and face a painful, traumatic past.

Acknowledgements Parts of this chapter were presented by R. Ruard Ganzevoort at the international colloquium on Christian Religious Education in Coping with Sexual Abuse, Montreal, Canada (2006) and at the conference *Noli me tangere*, Leuven, Belgium (2009). Other parts were presented by Srdjan Sremac at the international conference Religion, Reconciliation and Transitional Justice, Sarajevo, Bosnia and Herzegovina (2013).

References

Agger, I. (1989). Sexual torture of political prisoners: An overview. *Journal of Traumatic Stress, 2*, 305 318.

Ai, A. L., & Park, C. L. (2005). Possibilities of the positive following violence and trauma: Informing the coming decade of research. *Journal of Interpersonal Violence, 20*(2), 242–250.

Andersen, T. H. (2008). Speaking about unspeakable: Sexually abused men striving toward language. *American Journal of Men's Health, 2*(1), 25–36.

Başoğlu, M., Livanou, M., Crnobarić, M., Francisković, T., Suljić, E., Durić, D., et al. (2005). Psychiatric and cognitive effects of war in former Yugoslavia. *The Journal of the American Medical Association, 294*(5), 580–590.

Boisen, A. T. (1970). Crises in personality development. In W. A. Sadler (Ed.), *Personality and religion* (pp. 191–205). New York: Harper & Row.

Brouwer, A.-M. (2005). *Supranational criminal prosecution of sexual violence*. Antwerpen: Intersentia.
Bullock, M. C., & Beckson, M. (2011). Male victims of sexual assault: Phenomenology, psychology, physiology. *The Journal of the American Academy of Psychiatry and the Law, 39*, 197–205.
Butler, J. (1997). *Excitable speech*. London: Routledge.
Butler, J. (2008). Sexual politics, torture, and secular time. *The British Journal of Sociology, 59*(1), 1–23.
Carmil, D., & Breznitz, S. (1991). Personal trauma and world view: Are extremely stressful experiences related to political attitudes, religious beliefs, and future orientation? *Journal of Traumatic Stress, 4*(3), 393–405.
Christopher, M. (2004). A broader view of trauma: A biopsychosocial-evolutionary view of the role of the traumatic stress response in the emergence of pathology and/or growth. *Clinical Psychology Review, 24*(1), 75–98.
Cooey, P. M. (1994). *Religious imagination and the body: A feminist analysis*. Oxford: Oxford University Press.
Croog, S. H., & Levine, S. (1972). Religious identity and response to serious illness: A report on heart patients. *Social Science and Medicine, 6*, 17–32.
Donnelly, D. A., & Kenyon, S. (1996). Honey, we don't do men: Gender stereotypes and the provision of services to sexually assaulted males. *Journal of Interpersonal Violence, 11*, 441–448.
Drezgić, R. (2010). Religion and gender in the context of nation-state formation: The case of Serbia. *Third World Quarterly, 31*(6), 955–970.
Elzinga, B. M., & Bremner, J. D. (2002). Are the neural substrates of memory the final common pathway in posttraumatic stress disorder (PTSD)? *Journal of Affective Disorders, 70*(1), 1–17.
Eriksson-Baaz, M., & Stern, M. (2013). *Sexual violence as a weapon of war? Perceptions, prescriptions, problems in the Congo and beyond (Africa now)*. London: Zed Books.
Fischer, A. R., & Good, G. E. (1997). Men and psychotherapy: An investigation of alexithymia, intimacy, and masculine gender roles. *Psychotherapy, 34*(2), 160–170.
Fontana, A., & Rosenheck, R. (2004). Trauma, change in strength of religious faith, and mental health service use among veterans treated for PTSD. *Journal of Nervous and Mental Disease, 192*(9), 579–584.
Franke, M. K. (1998). Constructing heterosexuality: Putting sex to work. *Denver University Law Review., 75*(4), 1139–1180.
Fuchs, F. S. (2004). Male sexual assault: Issues of arousal and consent. *Cleveland State Law Review, 51*(1), 93–121.
Ganzevoort, R. R. (1994). *Een cruciaal moment: Functie en verandering van geloof in een crisis*. Zoetermeer: Boekencentrum.
Ganzevoort, R. R. (2002). Common themes and structures in male victims' stories of religion and sexual abuse. *Mental Health, Religion & Culture, 5*(3), 313–325.
Ganzevoort, R. R. (2008). Scars and stigmata: Trauma, identity, and theology. *Practical Theology, 1*(1), 19–31.
Ganzevoort, R. R. (2010). Minding the wisdom of ages: Narrative approaches in pastoral care for the elderly. *Practical Theology, 3*(3), 331–340.
Ganzevoort, R. R., & Veerman, A. L. (2000). *Geschonden lichaam: Pastorale gids voor gemeenten die geconfronteerd worden met seksueel geweld*. Zoetermeer: Boekencentrum.
Gardner, R., Wills, S., & Goodwin, J. M. (1995). The Io myth: Origins and use of a narrative of sexual abuse. *Journal of Psychohistory, 23*(1), 30–39.
Goldfeld, B. H., Mollica, R. F., Pesavento, B. H., & Faraone, S. V. (1988). The physical and psychological sequelae of torture: Symptomatology and diagnosis. *American Medical Association Current, 259*(18), 2725–2729.
Harris, I. M. (1995). *Messages men hear: Constructing masculinities*. London: Taylor & Francis.
Hirschauer, S. (2014). *The securitization of rape: Women, war and sexual violence*. New York: Palgrave Macmillan.
Howe, L. T. (1988). Crises and spiritual growth. *Pastoral Psychology, 36*(4), 230–238.
Human Rights Watch. (2003). *We'll kill you if you cry*. New York: Human Rights Watch.
Instituting Proceedings. (1993). Application of the convention of the prevention and punishment of the crime of genocide, Bosnia and Herzegovina v. Yugoslavia (Serbia and Montenegro), general list no. 91. http://www.icj-cij.org/docket/files/91/7199.pdf.
Janoff-Bulman, R. (1992). *Shattered assumptions: Towards a new psychology of trauma*. New York: Free Press.
Johnson, K., Scott, J., Rughita, B., Kisielewski, M., Asher, J., Ong, R., et al. (2010). Association of sexual violence and human rights violations with physical and mental health in territories of Eastern Democratic Republic of Congo. *Journal of American Medical Association, 304*(5), 553–562.
Kaitesi, U. (2014). *Genocidal and sexual violence*. Antwerpen: Intersentia.
Kessler, R. C., Sonnega, A., Bromet, E., Hughes, M., & Nelson, C. B. (1995). Posttraumatic stress disorder in the National Comorbidity Survey. *Archives of General Psychiatry, 52*, 1048–1060.
Kira, I. A., Templin, T., Lewandowski, L., Clifford, D., Wiencek, P., Hammad, A., et al. (2006). The effects of torture: Two community studies. *Peace and Conflict: Journal of Peace Psychology, 12*(3), 205–228.
Krondorfer, B. (Ed.). (1996). *Men's bodies, men's gods: Male identities in a (post-) Christian culture*. New York: New York University Press.
Leatherman, L. J. (2011). *Sexual violence and armed conflict*. Cambridge: Polity.
Lew, M. (1988). *Victims no longer: Men recovering from incest and other sexual abuse*. New York: Nevraumont.

Lewis, C. S. (1946). *That hideous strength*. New York: Macmillan.

Lewis, D. (2009). Unrecognized victims: Sexual violence against men in conflict settings under international law. *Wisconsin International Law Journal, 27*(1), 1–49.

Linley, P. A. (2003). Positive adaptation to trauma: Wisdom as both process and outcome. *Journal of Traumatic Stress, 16*(6), 601–610.

Linley, P. A., & Joseph, S. (2004). Positive change following trauma and adversity: A review. *Journal of Traumatic Stress, 17*(1), 11–21.

Loncar, M., Henigsberg, N., & Hrabac, P. (2010). Mental health consequences in men exposed to sexual abuse during the war in Croatia and Bosnia. *Journal of Interpersonal Violence, 25*(2), 191–203.

MacKinnon, A. C. (1997). Oncale v. Sundowner Offshore Services Inc., 96-568, *Amici Curiae* brief in support of petitioner. *UCLA Women's Law Journal, 8*(1), 9–46.

Mollica, R. F. (1988). The trauma story. The psychiatric care of refugee survivors of violence and torture. In F. Ochberg (Ed.), *Post-traumatic therapy and victims of violence* (pp. 295–314). New York: Bruner/Mazel.

Mollica, R. F. (2006). *Healing invisible wounds: Paths to hope and recovery in a violent world*. Orlando: Harcourt.

Mucić et al. (IT-96-21) *"Čelebići Camp." Witness: Witness F & Mr. Stevan Glogorevic, trial transcripts* (pp. 1450–1451). http://www.icty.org/x/cases/mucic/trans/en/970327ed.htm.

Nelson, J. B. (1992). *The intimate connection: Male sexuality, masculine spirituality*. London: SPCK.

Olujic, B. M. (1998). Embodiment of terror: Gendered violence in peacetime and wartime in Croatia and Bosnia and Herzegovina. *Medical Anthropology Quarterly, 12*(1), 31–50.

Pargament, K. I. (1997). *The psychology of religion and coping: Theory, research, practice*. New York: The Guilford Press.

Persecutor vs. Dusko Tadić, Omarska, Trial Transcript. (IT-94-1-T). *Witness: Mehmend Alić*, (p. 32986).

Roth, K. J., & Rittner, C. (Eds.). (2012). *Rape: Weapon of war and genocide*. Minnesota: Paragon House.

Scarry, E. (1985). *The body in pain: The making and unmaking of the world*. New York: Oxford University Press.

Shandor Miles, M., & Brown Crandall, E. K. (1986). The search for meaning and its potential for affecting growth in bereaved parents. In R. H. Moos (Ed.), *Coping with life crises: An integrated approach* (pp. 235–243). New York: Plenum.

Sivakumaran, S. (2005). Male/male rape and the "taint" of homosexuality. *Human Rights Quarterly, 27*, 1274–1306.

Sivakumaran, S. (2013). Prosecuting sexual violence against men and boys. In A.-M. Brouwer, C. Ku, R. Römkens, & L. van den Herik (Eds.), *Sexual violence as an international crime: Interdisciplinary approaches* (pp. 79–97). Intersentia: Antwerpen.

Smith, A. (2005). *Sexual violence and American Indian genocide*. New York: South End Press.

Solomon, Z., et al. (2005). Is terror gender-blind? Gender differences in reaction to terror events. *Social Psychiatry and Psychiatric Epidemiology, 40*(12), 947–954.

Sremac, S. (2013). *Addiction and spiritual transformation*. Münster: LIT Verlag.

Sremac, S., & Ganzevoort, R. R. (2013). Addiction and spiritual transformation: An empirical study on narratives of recovering addicts' conversion testimonies in Dutch and Serbian contexts. *Archive for the Psychology of Religion, 35*(3), 399–435.

Stewart, D., & Harmon, K. (2004). Mental health services responding to men and their anger. *International Journal of Mental Health Nursing, 13*(4), 249–254.

Tombs, D. (2014). News media, conflicted-related sexual violence and reconciliation in the Balkans. In D. Valić-Nedeljković, S. Sremac, N. Knežević, & D. Gruhonjić (Eds.), *The role of media in normalizing relations in the Western Balkans* (pp. 31–47). Novi Sad: University of Novi Sad Press.

Trošt-Pavasović, T., & Slootmaeckers, K. (2015). Religion, homosexuality and nationalism: The role of religious institutions in defining the nation. In S. Sremac & R. R. Ganzevoort (Eds.), *Religious and sexual nationalisms in Central and Eastern Europe: Gods, gays, and governments* (pp. 154–180). Leidel/Boston: Brill.

UNOCHA (2008). *The nature, scope and motivation for sexual violence against men and boys in armed conflict. Use of sexual violence in armed conflict: Identifying gaps in research to inform effective interventions* (pp. 1–13). Brussels: Unocha.

Wilson, J. P. (Ed.). (2006). *The posttraumatic self: Restoring meaning and wholeness to personality*. London: Routledge.

Wood, J. E. (2013). Multiple perpetrator rape during war. In M. Horvath & J. Woodhams (Eds.), *Handbook on the study of multiple perpetrator rape: A multidisciplinary response to an international problem* (pp. 132–159). London: Routledge.

Žarkov, D. (1997). War rapes in Bosnia: On masculinity, feminity, and power of the rape victim identity. *Tijdschrift voor Criminologie, 29*(2), 140–151.

Žarkov, D. (2007). The body of the other man. In D. Žarkov (Ed.), *The body of war: Media, ethnicity and gender in the break-up of Yugoslavia* (pp. 155–169). Durham: Duke University Press.

Žarkov, D. (2011). Exposures and invisibilities: Media, masculinities and the narratives of wars in an intersectional perspective. In H. Lutz, M. T. Herrera Vivar, & L. Supik (Eds.), *Framing intersectionality* (pp. 105–120). Farnham: Ashgate.

Zawati, H. M. (2008). Impunity or immunity: Wartime male rape and sexual torture as a crime against humanity. *Torture Volume, 17*(1), 27–48.

Žižek, S. (2014). *Event*. London: Penguin.

Žižek, S., & Gunjević, B. (2012). *God in pain: Inversions of apocalypse*. New York: Seven Stories Press.

Killing the Killer: Rampage and Gun Rights as a Syndrome

22

Kirby Farrell

This essay examines the Sandy Hook school rampage in Newtown Connecticut (Dec. 14, 2012) and the subsequent radical firearms advocacy voiced by the National Rifle Association (NRA) as a traumatic syndrome. I foreground Adam Lanza's slaughter of 26 primary school children and personnel at the Sandy Hook school because it caused exceptional shock and an impassioned reconsideration of firearms policies: "no story received more public attention" (Pew Research Center, 2013a, May 7) than the debate over gun control that followed 2 months later. In addition, Adam Lanza's behavior leading up to his rampage shows symptoms of traumatic stress that were mirrored in the positions of radical gun rights advocates.

Although rampage killings "accounted for less than 1 % of all homicide deaths from 1980 to 2008," the attacks "are a matter of great public interest and concern" (Pew Research Center, 2013a, May 7). There have been two attacks per year on average since 1982. "Yet, 25 of the 62 cases we examined have occurred since 2006. In 2012 alone there have been seven mass shootings, and a record number of casualties" (Follman et al., 2013). A Harvard study concludes that "the rate of mass shootings in the United States has tripled since 2011" (Cohen et al., 2014).

The Sandy Hook killings (December 14, 2012) took place during this escalation of mass shootings, and in the months afterward, as headlines reported, gun sales "surged." Anxious parents bought $200 bulletproof backpacks for school children; some gun shops sold out their stock of ammunition (Pisani, 2012). Calls for more tightly regulated access to firearms were countered by the NRA, which outspent opponents and successfully lobbied for more permissive gun policies, including sale of military-style weapons designed for mass killing. Driving the NRA's policy was a conviction that only a comprehensively armed populace can stop a rampage killer. In the slogan repeated by the NRA's Wayne La Pierre, "The only thing that stops a bad guy with a gun is a good guy with a gun" (Lichtblau & Rich, 2012). This formula reduces the principals to abstract forces with no inner life. But it also masks affinities between the vigilante behavior of the "good guy with a gun" and the rampage violence it seeks to control, since the formula embraces a fantasy solution that, in many particulars, mirrors the killer's. The symmetry is not simply a matter of moral stance, but a function of traumatic stress.

Traumatic events "involve threats to life or bodily integrity, or a close personal encounter with violence and death. They confront human beings with the extremities of helplessness and

K. Farrell, Ph.D. (✉)
Department of English, University of Massachusetts, Amherst, MA 01003, USA
e-mail: kfarrell@umass.edu

Y. Ataria et al. (eds.), *Interdisciplinary Handbook of Trauma and Culture*,
DOI 10.1007/978-3-319-29404-9_22

terror, and evoke the responses of catastrophe" (Herman, 1992, p. 32). *The Comprehensive Textbook of Psychiatry* defines the core experience as one of "intense fear, helplessness, loss of control, and threat of annihilation" (Andreasen, 1985, p. 919). Death anxiety is ubiquitous in the background of everyday life and managed by denial (Becker, 1973); it becomes traumatic and produces post-traumatic sequelae when shock or stress overcomes psychic defenses and the terror of annihilation threatens the integrity of the self.

Trauma symptoms cluster around depressive and aggressive behaviors. One person may be immobilized, another panicked, while a third may become enraged or berserk. As the psychiatrists say, much depends on how you are wrapped, which in turn depends partly on your neurological makeup, and partly on how you interpret your experience, since how you understand what is happening to you affects your particular symptoms (Farrell, 1998).

Aggressive responses to traumatic stress make headlines as rampage killings in a war zone, a workplace, or a school. Under stress, feeling the self imperiled by real or imagined forces, killers seek to destroy the threat: in combat by attacking enemies and in the workplace or school by attacking others who expose them to failure and social death. In the buildup to a rampage, killers seethe, fantasizing about violence and vindication that can substantiate them. The unreality of this project confuses heroism and infamy. It exposes the would-be hero to suicide or police fire, which makes the idea of compelling the world's attention, even in infamy, an immortality fantasy as well as a solution to psychic turmoil.

At age 20, Adam Lanza was suffering from the core symptoms of trauma and fixated on an act of supreme violence as a way to end his distress. Since his experience can help us to understand some of the disquieting responses to rampage, it deserves a closer look.

We have enough evidence to make out the rough outlines of Adam Lanza's motivation. Despite a relatively happy childhood, he had trouble processing experiences. "A doctor diagnosed sensory-integration disorder, and Adam underwent speech therapy and occupational therapy in kindergarten and first grade. Teachers were told to watch for seizures" (Solomon, 2014 p. 37). That he did not speak until he was three and "always understood many more words than he could muster" (Solomon, 2014 p. 37) is symptomatic of cognitive difficulties that grew into a feeling of being overwhelmed, trapped in an incoherent body, unable to respond effectively to life. This helps to explain why in fifth grade he said he "did not think highly of himself and believed that everyone else in the world deserved more than he did" (Sedensky, 2013, p. 33). This despair may have reflected the child's and the family's anxieties over his disabilities, as well as his awareness that he was not fitting in.

In fifth grade, Adam and another boy "wrote a story called 'The Big Book of Granny,' in which an old woman with a gun in her cane kills wantonly. In the third chapter, Granny and her son want to taxidermy a boy for their mantelpiece. In another chapter, a character called Dora the Berserker says, 'I like hurting people … Especially children'" (Solomon, 2014, p. 38). The story suggests that Adam felt pressured to live up to mainstream expectations. Like Granny, Adam's mother Nancy was experienced with guns. Since she was determined to help her son succeed despite his disabilities, it makes sense that Adam identified with the "trophy" boy mummified for Granny's mantelpiece, and felt pressured into a lifeless ideal. Already he was aware of the word "berserker": someone who goes on a cold-blooded rampage. The book was likely a complaint that the child couldn't put into words.

Although he could be voluble when happy and had "a sharp sense of humor" (Solomon, 2014, p. 38), Adam began to lose his equilibrium in adolescence. Noisy, crowded corridors between classes at school upset him. "Many people with autism speak in a flat tone, and avoiding eye contact is common, too, because trying to interpret sounds and faces at the same time is overwhelming" (Solomon, 2014, p. 39). In seventh grade, the child who felt undeserving and fantasized about a mummified trophy boy on a mantel was fantasizing about warfare. A teacher described Adam as "intelligent but not normal, with antisocial issues. He was quiet, barely spoke and did not want to participate in anything. His writing assignments obsessed about battles, destruction and war, far more than others his age. The level of violence in the writing was disturbing. At the same time, when asked to write a poem, he was able to write a beautiful one and presented it in public" (Sedensky, 2013, p. 34). Adam could mask his anger, even as he was identifying with representations of warfare that, on paper at least, made him a force to be reckoned with.

By the time he was diagnosed with Asperger Syndrome in 2005, at age 13, Adam "was described as presenting with significant social impairments and extreme anxiety. It was also noted that he lacked empathy and had very rigid thought processes" (Sedensky, 2013, p. 34).[1] Additional diagnoses included emotional and/or pervasive developmental disorder (PDD) spectrum behaviors and obsessive compulsive disorder (OCD), which became progressively disabling (Sedensky, 2013, p. 35). He suffered panic attacks so severe that one day, as he started eighth grade, his mother took him to a hospital emergency room, telling doctors that he was wracked by anxiety (Griffin & Kovner, 2013a, 2013b).

Reflecting, his father now says, "It was crystal clear something was wrong." He added, "The social awkwardness, the uncomfortable anxiety, unable to sleep, stress, unable to concentrate, having a hard time learning, the awkward walk, reduced eye contact. You could see the changes occurring" (Solomon, 2014, p. 38).

After Adam's initial success taking college courses at age 16, the demands of schoolwork became too much for him. Like many conflicted teenagers, he compensated for buffeted self-esteem with unrealistic ambitions that tormented him when reality fell short. At a time when he was cutting classes and failing courses, his mother reported, "I have the feeling when he said he would rather be homeless than to take any more tests, he really meant it" (Solomon, 2014, p. 42). To be homeless, abandoned, and forgotten is social death, and Adam's threat suggests that he was imagining a kind of play-death that would allow him to be at once in and out of the world. Time would show the suicidal character of his despair to be more than adolescent bravado.

By 2010, when high school students ordinarily graduate, Adam was seriously isolated, prone to "meltdowns," and also developing "his private obsession with killing. He started editing Wikipedia entries on well-known mass murderers," although there were still no outward signs of violence (Solomon, 2014, p. 41). He announced that he was going to enlist in the military when he turned 18, planning to join the elite Army Rangers yet subject to prolonged weeping fits that proved the futility of his wishes.

On the threshold of adulthood, Adam was at home neither in society nor in his own mind. A few of the materials he left behind—music, comedy videos, and videos of him dancing to DDR (the Dance Dance Revolution video game)—imply a healthy outlook. But the intensity of his inner conflict is evident in the many materials relating to his obsessions: firearms, the military, politics, suicide, and mass murder. The hours he spent practicing difficult dance moves (DDR) could be evidence that part of him resisted the drive to isolation and violence, although the dance game is solitary and may signal the awkward adolescent's dream of commanding admiration as much as any sociable inclination.

Caught between impossible social fulfillment and fantasies of violence, Adam looked to the prestige and legitimate violence of the soldier as a compromise. His admired uncle had been an army Ranger; his mother gave him guns and trained him to shoot. By definition, soldiers magnify human force and fight for a heroic, gut conviction of "what's right," which offered Adam a means of validating his "very rigid thought processes" and mastering his inner turmoil. To the soldier, what Adam's father described as "the arrogance that Aspies [Aspberger's syndrome] can have" (Solomon, 2014, p. 39) is command and dominance. The tragedy is that in

[1] At the Yale Child Study Center, in 2006, Dr. Robert A. King concluded that Adam "displayed a profound autism spectrum disorder with rigidity, isolation and a lack of comprehension of ordinary social interaction and communications" (Griffin & Kovner, 2013b, Dec. 28).

military guise, arrogance can also become a "messianic-grade superiority complex" such as Eric Harris demonstrated, and for Adam, the wish to enlist would eventually harden into the role that the forensic psychiatrist Park Dietz has called the "pseudocommando"—the rampage killer (Dietz, 1986, p. 477). Whatever its cause, even the most desperate rage follows one model rather than another, and warrior ideation is a compelling model for young men and a strong determinant of the direction their violence will take.

The State Attorney concluded "that the shooter had significant mental health issues that affected his ability to live a normal life and to interact with others, even those to whom he should have been close. As an adult he did not recognize or help himself deal with those issues" (Sedensky, 2013, p. 3). Though conventional wisdom depends on it as a black box to contain what we cannot understand, the label "mental health issues" explains little. Like "pseudocommando," "autism," and "adult," it names a mystery in hopes of taming it—which is how imagination routinely copes with a world that is ultimately beyond our control.

"As an adult," says the report, Adam "did not recognize or help himself deal with those issues." Yet we know that Adam felt trapped in himself and tried to make sense of his psychic distress. To one of his few acquaintances in his last years, he "indicated that he had an interest in mass murders and serial killing. They never spent a lot of time discussing them, but it would be a topic of conversation" (Sedensky, 2013, p. 47). "Other topics of discussion included human nature, perception, judgment, morality, lack of control, prejudice, empathy, suicide, mental illness, existential crisis, urban exploration of abandoned areas, hiking and cookies" (Sedensky, 2013, p. 32). The topics center on anxiety about alienation and feeling ungrounded; they also explicitly bring up the rampage themes of suicide and mass murder. As he withdrew from social experience, Adam's fantasy of "urban exploration of abandoned areas" suggests an unconscious concern for the abandoned parts of his personality and anxieties about the ground of personality aroused by his withdrawal. In a treatment session at the Yale Child Study Center, at the time of the autism diagnosis (2005–2006), Adam "would ask [the clinician] about schizophrenia and obsessive compulsive disorders but would never elaborate about whether he was experiencing any of the symptoms" (Griffin & Kovner, 2013b).[2]

From this perspective the "autistic adult" was afraid of being overwhelmed not only from the outside, but also from within. This is the terror of losing a coherent self. Suicide offers an escape, but arouses the terror of annihilation, which is the root of traumatic stress (Andreasen, 1985). Given the pressure of that threat, Adam was not only role-playing a "pseudo"-soldier, he was actually experiencing the sort of do-or-die, dead-end psychic emergency that triggers a soldier's berserk outbreak.

In his last months Adam stayed in his bedroom, in disembodied Internet chat, with black trash bags over the windows, researching rampage killings. In effect, he was immersing himself in a subculture that substantiated—made "real"—his obsessions. Investigators later found

"Three photographs of what appear to be a dead human, covered in blood and wrapped in plastic; the book *Amish Grace: How Forgiveness Transcended Tragedy* by Donald B. Kraybill, et al.; two videos showing suicide by gunshot; commercial movies depicting mass shootings; the computer game titled 'School Shooting' where the player controls a character who enters a school and shoots at students; screen shots (172) of the online game 'Combat Arms'; images of the shooter holding a handgun to his head; images of the shooter holding a rifle to his head; five-second video (dramatization) depicting

[2] Alaine Griffin and Josh Kovner, "Lanza's Psychiatric Treatment Revealed in Documents," *Hartford Courant*, Dec. 28, 2013. Adam's father suspected that Adam's Asperger's could be masking schizophrenia (Solomon, 2014, p. 40), which might accord with a symptom of schizophrenia described by Louis Sass: hyperrationality and an anxious preoccupation with the core or ground of identity. See "Introspection, Schizophrenia, and the Fragmentation of the Self," in *Representations* 19 (Summer 1987).

children being shot; images of shooter with a rifle, shotgun, and numerous magazines in his pockets; documents on weapons and magazine capacity; a document showing the prerequisites for a mass murder spreadsheet; a spreadsheet listing mass murders by name and information about the incident; large amount of materials on firearms; amount of materials relating to Columbine shootings and documents on mass murders" (Sedensky, 2013, p. 26).

Brooding over these themes, rehearsing possible plans, Adam must have had moments of relief and terrifying doubt. Binge killing promises to command spectacular attention, but it also reveals the futile nothingness of the self. The warrior can only exist in fantasy, in secret, until the instant of open fury. Just as the wannabe Army Ranger suffered weeping fits, at times the warrior assassin must have seemed to Adam a frightening illusion. Hence the urge to collect more and more rampage materials and the hours spent testing his resolve and firming up the reality of the warrior role.

Despite his individual disabilities, Adam's rampage fits a familiar pattern.[3] The killer seethes, caught between self-aggrandizement and self-destruction, wanting to settle scores, building toward an outburst. The force behind that seething is moral aggression. The berserk soldier kills to avenge dead buddies. For Adam, "what's right" crystallized in the murder—the execution—of his mother Nancy. His mother gave him conflicted messages, urging him toward mainstream achievement even as she indulged his dependency and his retreat from reality. She seems to have emphasized her own tough-minded independence.[4] In teaching Adam to shoot and keeping guns in an unlocked case, she believed that she was encouraging his self-confidence and independence, not tempting him to act out ghastly fantasies. Yet in the end she was unable or unwilling to stand up to his bullying and moods, overlooking the role-playing in their relationship. "The mother took care of all the shooter's needs" (Sedensky, 2013, p. 30). As Adam became increasingly unstable, she was making his care the central purpose in her life: a heroic project in otherwise mundane suburban affluence.

Mother and son were both trapped in their conflicts. The mother who had had to rescue him from panic attacks in school "did the shooter's laundry on a daily basis as the shooter often changed clothing during the day. She was not allowed in the shooter's room, however, even to clean. No one was allowed in his room" (Sedensky, 2013, p. 30). His demands implied that he was the dominant figure, even as they confirmed his childlike neediness. He exaggerated his difficulties with coordination, for example, to elicit his mother's help. The element of role-playing came out when his father told her that Adam "had to pause to retie his shoes on a hike. Nancy responded in astonishment, 'He tied his own shoes?'" (Solomon, 2014, p. 41).

As his personality constricted, Adam needed his mother more than ever, yet the would-be warrior hated his dependency.[5] As a voice of parental

[3] Perpetrators of "autogenic" rampages, says P. E., Mullen, "tend to share common social and psychological disabilities. They are isolates , often bullied in childhood, who have rarely established themselves in effective work roles as adults. They have personalities marked by suspiciousness, obsessional traits, and grandiosity. They often harbor persecutory beliefs, which may occasionally verge on the delusional. The autogenic massacre is essentially murder suicide, in which the perpetrators intend first to kill as many people as they can and then kill themselves" (Mullen, 2004, p. 311). Cf. Katherine S. Newman, *Rampage: The Social Roots of School Shootings* (also 2004), which emphasizes social forces leading to isolation and infamy.

[4] In her e-mail exchanges with Marvin LaFontaine, Nancy Lanza humorously (?) bragged that her Green Beret brother had taught her lethal self-defense moves. See "Nancy Lanza in her own words." The clinician Adam saw at the Yale Child Study Center described her as "non-compliant" because she refused to continue Adam's medication (Celexa) and terminated the sessions (Griffin & Kovner, 2013b, Dec. 28).

[5] "Matricide is usually committed by overprotected boys—by a son who wishes, as one study puts it, 'with his desperate act, to free himself from his state of dependency on her, a dependency that he believes has not allowed him to grow up.' Another study proposes that, in each case examined, 'the mother-child relationship became unusually intense and conflict-laden,' while the fathers 'were uniformly passive and remained relatively uninvolved.' The state's attorney's report says that when Nancy asked Adam whether he would feel sad if anything happened to her, he replied, 'No.' A Word document called 'Selfish,' which was found on Adam's computer, gives an explanation of why females are inherently selfish, written while one of them was accommodating him in every possible way" (Solomon, 2014, p. 43).

conscience, she regularly reminded him of the need to make his way in the world, yet she could not relieve his anxiety and depression.[6] Adam "disliked birthdays, Christmas and holidays. He would not allow his mother to put up a Christmas tree. The mother explained it by saying that the shooter had no emotions or feelings. Adam's judgment was equally aggressive: 'A person who knew the shooter in 2011 and 2012 said the shooter described his relationship with his mother as strained because the shooter said her behavior was not rational'" (Sedensky, 2013, p. 30).

Like Kip Kinkel, who murdered his parents and high school students in Oregon (May 20, 1998), Adam turned against the family that mediated his painful connection to the social world. As his father observed, "With hindsight, I know Adam would have killed me in a heartbeat, if he'd had the chance. I don't question that for a minute. The reason he shot Nancy four times was one for each of us: one for Nancy; one for him; one for [his brother] Ryan; one for me" (Solomon, 2014, p. 43).

Why did Adam target Sandy Hook schoolchildren? The answer probably overlaps with his rage toward his family. The murders of enviable "trophy" children punished parents whose trophy children "Granny" had taxidermied in Adam's fifth grade story, even as the killing acted out envy. But there is another, ambivalent dimension to his motivation to consider. Among Adam's effects were "Materials regarding the topic of pedophilia and advocating for rights for pedophiles (not child pornography)" (Sedensky, 2013, p. 26). Since his father remembers Adam being happy as a child at Sandy Hook (Solomon, 2014), an attraction to children would be a logical expression of memories of an idealized lost happiness. By extension, it may be that, having decided on suicide, Adam wanted to kill that memory too. In this respect, the murders may have been in part Adam's effort to fulfill and suppress what he recognized as taboo pedophilia in himself. Like the materials justifying pedophilia, his behavior was striking out at strong adult taboos. And finally, more strategically, the wannabe soldier who wept could attack children and be sure that they would not fight back and humiliate him. He had no need to fear children or feel inadequate around them.

A consideration of Adam's motives needs to take account of his mental state as well. The cold-blooded fury in Adam and the Columbine killers resembles the "icy" rage in soldiers who run amok under traumatic stress (Shay, 1994). The paradox is crucial. Adam and the Columbine killers were systematic about running amok; they knew what they were doing. But both rampages had a copycat dimension. Harris and Klebold code-named their rampage "NBK," after the movie *Natural Born Killers*. Like a parable, the film and the acronym condensed all the irrationality and complicated logistics of their plan into a more manageable form. Likewise, Adam had his spreadsheet, his library of precedents, and his hours of rapt study. Seeking to outdo earlier atrocities, all three murderers were pumping themselves up for maximum impact. This mentality preconditions decisions at each stage, so that the action requires minimal thought, and it is already promoting abandon.

It might seem implausible to link murderous civilians with soldiers under fire, but the military fatigues and weapons—the role of pseudocommando—not only project a self-aggrandizing heroic reality for the civilian killers, but also work to block the guilt and doubt that could inhibit their aggression. The rampage killers seethe and then kill for revenge or vindication or some other form of what's right. But just as "combat trauma destroys the capacity for social trust" (Shay, 1994, p. 33), so rampage mentality strips away empathy and trust, concentrating emergency physiology and thinking on aggression against others and the self. No matter how fanatically moral or arrogant their motives, they are violating foundational taboos, and killers who

[6] In e-mail correspondence with Marvin LaFontaine (Frontline PBS, 2013), Nancy Lanza alluded to a potentially life-threatening inherited "time bomb" for which she underwent extensive medical tests, and about which she was secretive. It is unclear how this anxiety affected her behavior with her children ("Nancy Lanza in her own words") http://www.pbs.org/wgbh/pages/frontline/social-issues/raising-adam-lanza/nancy-lanza-in-her-own-words/.

survive may report that they "blacked out" or were "beside themselves," wondering what had "possessed" them.

Like soldiers facing imminent death, rampage killers are trapped in a dead end. Once in motion, they too are unable to retreat, knowing that they face police bullets, execution, or the living death of prison. In his mental state Adam saw the social world ahead (school, career, relationships) as a "dead" end as well; he felt trapped by his expectations, and the expectations of the world and his family. In Vietnam, many soldiers felt that a cynical war betrayed the conviction of "what's right" that they needed to justify their sacrifices and the damage they'd caused. In the name of survival and moral aggression, some retaliated by assassinating sleeping officers through "fragging" (murder by fragmentation grenade), as Adam murdered his mother. In Adam's eyes, his body, his family, women, doctors, schools, and the social world had all failed him.

Pumping up for their assault on Columbine high school, Eric Harris and Dylan Klebold gloated in anticipation of their "godlike revenge." Like a lynch mob, they were gripped by vigilante conviction. Feelings of revenge for imaginary slights mixed with "a messianic-grade superiority complex, out to punish the entire human race for its appalling inferiority" (Cullen, 2004). Yet fantasies of superiority usually compensate for dread of—and rage against—insignificance. The apotheosis of fantasy attempts to counter fears of social death.

In studying the Columbine massacre, Adam Lanza must have identified with this conflict. He could also see that Harris and Klebold were willing, even avid, to be consumed by their violence. Adam left behind images of himself holding a gun to his head, the way Harris and Klebold committed suicide. In Adam's photo, the godlike fantasy soldier could be executing the futile, tormented young man. The image shows him trying out a role, even as it demonstrates his magical thinking, since it acknowledges his suicidal end even as it compels a beholder's attention, as if that attention after his death, like the moment of global infamy to come at Sandy Hook, keeps him from really dying.

While disorders such as Asperger's syndrome undoubtedly played a part in Adam Lanza's rampage behavior, much of his suffering and alienation reflect the stress of ordinary American adolescence on a particularly vulnerable individual. What makes his crisis so horrifying is his traumatic effort to use cultural materials such as heroic command of death to keep himself from coming apart in terror.

The gratuitous deaths of defenseless children and the posterity they represent are traumatic, especially in a comfortable suburb such as Newtown. Efforts to cope generated debates about mental illness, autism in particular, and gun control. In the impassioned debate over firearms, the radical positions most clearly showed traumatic sequelae.

As in a traumatic freeze response, for example, one position in the debate wished guns severely regulated or banned and the threat of violence banished. The wish resonates with the radical gun advocates' fear that guns will be confiscated. Advocates of regulation proposed more strictly policed access to lethal weapons, on the assumption that individual self-control is at best provisional, unpredictable, and therefore always potentially dangerous (Pew 2013b, May 23). While their opponents, most prominently the NRA, shared this assumption, they maintain that a trained gun owner is always autonomous, responsible, and effective, even during an episode of violence. Hence they urged a paramilitary response: an armed populace, including guards in schools, hypervigilance, and vigilante reflexes. The dispute was heated, with partisans at times accusing each other of abetting murder, as when an NRA event "was briefly interrupted twice by individuals who stood up with banners and shouted that the NRA has 'blood on its hands' and is 'killing our kids'" (Memmott, 2012).

The systemic argument for gun control looks to social oversight to prevent accidents, predatory aggression, and survival panic. The NRA countered with a proposal organized around the idea of vigilante heroism. As the NRA's executive vice president Wayne LaPierre put it in a press conference a fortnight after Adam Lanza's rampage, "The only thing that stops a bad guy with a gun is a good guy with a gun." He went to elaborate: "our society is populated by an unknown number of genuine monsters—people so deranged, so evil, so possessed by voices and driven by demons that no sane person can possibly ever comprehend them. They walk among us every day. And does anybody really believe that the next Adam Lanza isn't planning his attack on a school he's already identified at this very moment?" (*Washington Post*, 2012).

The NRA vision replicates the do-or-die urgency of a rampage and the killer's fascination with guns and terror as the most potent instruments of social control. In the NRA theory, if everyone were armed and a potential vigilante, a rogue killer would be cowed—and if he did act, he would be gunned down. This prescription disregards the suicidal bent of most berserkers, just as it ignores the treacherous ambiguities of "good" and "bad." After all, Nancy Lanza was fatally deceived in thinking that responsible weapons training would bolster her son's self-esteem. Instead of creating a good guy, the weapons she bought tragically empowered a fantasy warrior with a hidden agenda. In a word, nobody can predict who, under stress, may be "good" or "bad." A study of 62 attacks since 1982, for example, found that:

> In not a single case was the killing stopped by a civilian using a gun. And in other recent (but less lethal) rampages in which armed civilians attempted to intervene, those civilians not only failed to stop the shooter but also were gravely wounded or killed… There is no evidence indicating that arming Americans further will help prevent mass shootings or reduce the carnage, says Dr. Stephen Hargarten, a leading expert on emergency medicine and gun violence at the Medical College of Wisconsin. To the contrary, there appears to be a relationship between the proliferation of firearms and a rise in mass shootings. (Follman et al., 2013)

A core problem is that the NRA formula exhibits many characteristics of the aggression it opposes. Like the killer, it focuses on killing as heroic vengeance against a despised enemy. It converts flight to fight: terror becomes rage against "monsters." By making the "good guy with a gun" the nation's savior, the prescription mirrors the self-aggrandizing, vindictive righteousness of killers such as Harris and Klebold, and the paranoid delusions of Jared Loughner, who thought he was delivering America from a sinister government conspiracy when he shot Rep. Gabrielle Giffords (January 8, 2011). In their use of militia symbols such as the musket and the flag, and their demands for military-style automatic weapons and large-capacity magazines, radical gun advocates role-play soldiers as the pseudocommando does.

In arguing their case, radical gun advocates resort to an embattled tone and sporadic death threats that mirror the rampage killers' seething anger. In a speech at the N.R.A.'s annual convention in 2000, [NRA president, Charlton Heston] brought the audience to its feet with a ringing attack on gun-control advocates. Paraphrasing an N.R.A. bumper sticker ("I'll give you my gun when you take it from my cold, dead hands"), he waved a replica of a colonial musket above his head and shouted defiantly, "From my cold, dead hands!" (Dao, 2000). The repetition of slogans echoes the self-intoxicating obsessiveness of killers such as Lanza, Harris, and Klebold. Like the killers, NRA advocacy relishes "a ringing attack" rather than negotiation or social solutions. What's more, the "good man with a gun" dictum prescribes intervention that is potentially as indiscriminate as the rampage it would prevent. In a chaotic situation, the good guy may accidently shoot another armed citizen or bystanders, or be mistakenly killed by police. The hypothetical vigilante is assumed to be on the edge of do-or-die hypervigilance, as ready to kill as a soldier in combat, but masterful and not susceptible to berserk impulse. And like the rampage killer, the vigilante may be influenced by all sorts of prejudices, including racism, that can warp judgment.

In good guys and bad guys alike, magical thinking leads to intoxicating, totalized language. The Columbine teenagers envisioned themselves as "godlike" judges. In a mirror reflection, Wayne LaPierre claimed that "our society is populated by an unknown number of genuine monsters—people so deranged, so evil, so possessed by voices and driven by demons that no sane person can possibly ever comprehend them. They walk among us every day. And does anybody really believe that the next Adam Lanza isn't planning his attack on a school he's already identified at this very moment?" (*Washington Post,* 2012).

This is the language of the supernatural. If "no sane person can possibly ever comprehend" the killer, the hero must have exceptional resources to kill him. As in the climax of countless Hollywood thrillers, the formula assumes that the vigilante brings uncanny instincts to the scene. If, like a soldier amok, the good guy acts on reflexes, he would be mirroring the killer, who also has a hair-trigger mindset. Still more confounding: if "our society is populated by an unknown numbers of genuine monsters," the call for armed guards in every school presents the near-certainty that some of them would be monsters.

Like rampage fantasies, NRA conceptions of the gun fuse self-aggrandizement and annihilation. In the formula, the larger-than-life good guy annihilates demonized bad guys as Elliot Rodger vowed to do before he ran amok in Isla Vista California (May 24, 2014): "Humanity is a disgusting, wretched, depraved species. If I had it in my power I would stop at nothing to reduce every single one of you to mountains of skulls and rivers of blood and rightfully so" (Medina, 2014).

But just as Rodger's vision culminated in predictable suicide, so the NRA fight for guns mounts a suicidal threat display: "I'll give you my gun when you pry it from my cold, dead hands." The slogan can imply martyrdom, a fight to the last man, but the threat to stop at nothing also amounts to maximum intimidation (Farrell, 2011).

The core theme is traumatic: not constitutional rights but survival terror. Yet the faith in do-or-die shootouts turns emergency behavior into a style that can be a routine tool and readily copied, as in the death threats that proliferated during the gun debates. For example, "James Yeager, CEO of Tactical Response, a Tennessee company that trains people in weapon and tactical skills, claimed in a video posted on YouTube and Facebook that he would 'start killing people' if President Barack Obama decides to take executive action to pass further gun control policies, Raw Story reports. In a frenetic address to the camera, Yeager puts a call out to other gun rights advocates to 'load your damn mags' and 'get ready to fight' in what he claims will turn into a 'civil war' if gun control measures in the country get any stricter" (*Huffington Post,* 2013).

Modeled on partisan radio rant and militia slogans ("lock and load!"), Yeager's call to arms *uses* threat display as a style. He projects a life-or-death showdown on the edge of control, yet he is cagey enough to avoid prosecution by making his threat conditional ("if … then"). With all of its absurd ironies—the weapons "trainer" unhinged—his outcry is at once an advertising stunt for his training business, an ideological pitch for supporters, and a threat of a rampage. This style of double-think allows Yeager and the NRA to promote the ideal of the citizen as tacit military-hero, honoring the Second Amendment right of a militia to own and bear arms while resisting the government oversight denoted by the qualifier "well regulated."

Like the NRA's crisis rhetoric, Yeager's rant expresses an ideology that has evolved over a decade or more. But the traumatic resonance of the Sandy Hook massacre and the gun control debate sharpened ideology into a fight-or-flight paroxysm. It can be difficult to evaluate such behavior because trauma is an injury that has to be interpreted. As a result, the idea of trauma can be used to rally morale or evoke compassion; it can also be an explanatory tool, a marketing ploy, or a cry for help (Farrell, 1998). Even the denial of trauma can be a symptom. In Connecticut, for example, a "truther" stole a 50-pound peace sign from a playground memorial to one of the Sandy Hook victims, and telephoned to tell her mother that her daughter "never existed," because "Sandy Hook 'truthers' believe that the Newtown shooting never occurred or was part of a 'false flag' operation designed to open the door to the confiscation of all guns by the government" (Boggioni, 2014). The fantasy transforms the actual source of terror—the threat of annihilation the caller feels—into a government conspiracy to strip him of his defenses, a narrative that gives him a monstrous enemy to fight.

The interpretive dimension of trauma can buffer its terror, but it can also make its terrors more contagious. In his address after the Newtown murders, Wayne La Pierre simultaneously reassures us that guns dispel menace even as he inflames the threat:

> How can we possibly even guess how many [more killers there are], given our nation's refusal to create an active national database of the mentally ill? And the fact is, that wouldn't even begin to address the much larger and more lethal criminal class: Killers, robbers, rapists and drug gang members who have spread like cancer in every community in this country. (*Washington Post,* 2012)

Like many rampage killers, including Adam Lanza, the speaker simplifies the world into totalizing abstractions (the "criminal class") and fantasy tools ("a database for the mentally ill"). This style of thinking sees mysterious evil everywhere, even as it forces people into reassuring stereotypes. It assumes that criminals are "cancerous," but also intentionally evil and therefore legitimate targets for a good guy to kill. The mentally ill can be even more of a threat because they may move between categories: they are ordinary citizens one minute, mass killers the next. At once they are stereotypes and yet unfathomable monsters. They can be vicious child killers and yet also sympathetic victims of illness, with caring families and a school such as Sandy Hook. Paradoxically, unless captured in "an active national database"—as if that could identify potential killers—the unpredictable mentally ill are more like ordinary people than the good-guy/bad-guy stick figures of the NRA formula.

This is as close as NRA rhetoric gets to recognizing the inherent terror and violence in firearms and in the irreducible human personality. And this paradox opens into another: the partisans' rigid abstractions understandably fuel a compensatory belief in totalized "freedom" and in freedom's "enemies"—government and an enforced social contract. Accordingly, guns are fetishistic for militias and like-minded groups. They stand for "freedom," but also for the fantasy power to overcome death.

As the ripples from the primary shock expand, the psychocultural effects of trauma can have subtle but devastating effects. As "stand-your-ground" laws have foregrounded gun ownership and personal insecurity they have been accompanied by a number of tragic deaths in which good guys with a gun turn out to be lethally on edge. In a climate of vigilante alarm they have killed unarmed black teenagers, disoriented Alzheimer's patients, motorists seeking directions, movie theater patrons, and teens pilfering from an open garage.

Firearms are a peculiarly potent tool of denial. As in cyborg fantasies such as James Cameron's *Terminato*r films or *Robocop*, guns extend, and magnify, the power of body parts. Before his rampage in Tucson (January 8, 2011), Jared Loughner had himself tattooed with bullets, as if to transform himself into a fearsome weapon the way Mesoamerican warriors overcame fear and pumped up ferocity by wearing jaguar masks and soldiers today still identify with tigers, wolves, and other predators. This is the meaning of Adam Lanza's fascination with firearms. After buying the first of the pistols he would use in his rampage (May 24, 2014), Elliot O. Rodger exulted that he "felt a new sense of power" and demanded, "who's the alpha male now?" (Medina, 2014).

Conventional wisdom frames such boasts in cultural terms, as signs of competition between males. But the boast is also a fantasy solution to the terror of social death and psychic annihilation. On the threshold of adulthood, neither Rodger nor Adam Lanza could bear to be in society or in his own tormented mind. Adam's final withdrawal had qualities of suicide, while his imaginative escape from terrifying futility focused on spectacular killing, as Elliot Rodger did. Beset by traumatic suffering, both young men found the tragic, expedient, and certain relief of gunfire.

References

Andreasen, N. C. (1985). Post-traumatic stress disorder. In H. I. Kaplan & B. J. Sadock (Eds.), *The comprehensive textbook of psychiatry* (pp. 918–924). Baltimore, MD: Johns Hopkins University Press.

Becker, E. (1973). *The denial of death*. New York, NY: Free Press.

Berkvist, R. (2008, April 6). Charlton Heston, Epic Film Star and Voice of N.R.A., Dies at 84. *New York Times*.

Boggioni, T. (2014, May 12). Sandy Hook truther steals memorial sign, tells victim's mother her child never existed, *Raw Story*. Retrieved from http://www.rawstory.com/rs/2014/05/12/sandy-hook-truther-steals-memorial-sign-tells-victims-mother-her-child-never-existed/

Cohen A. P., Azrael, D., & Miller, M. (2014, October 15). Rate of mass shootings has tripled since 2011, Harvard Research Shows. *Mother Jones*.

Cullen, D. (2004, April 20). The depressive and the psychopath. *Slate*.

Dietz, P. E. (1986). Mass, serial and sensational homicides. *Bulletin of the New York Academy of Medicine, 62*, 477–491.

Dao, J. (2000, May 21). N.R.A. leaders cast Gore as arch-enemy. *New York Times*.

Farrell, K. (1998). *Post-traumatic culture: Injury and interpretation in the 90s*. Baltimore, MD: Johns Hopkins University Press.

Farrell, K. (2011). *Berserk style in American culture*. New York, NY: Palgrave.

Follman, M., Aronsen, G., and Pan, D. (2013, February 27). A guide to mass shootings in America. *Mother Jones*. Retrieved from http://www.motherjones.com/politics/2012/07/mass-shootings-map?page=2

Frontline, PBS. (2013, February 19). *Raising Adam Lanza*. Retrieved from http://www.pbs.org/wgbh/pages/frontline/raising-adam-lanza/

Gettys, T. (2014, May 13). FL cops fired 377 rounds at unarmed men in deafening barrage that killed suspect, friend. *The Raw Story*. Retrieved from http://www.rawstory.com/rs/2014/05/13/fl-cops-fired-377-rounds-at-unarmed-men-in-deafening-barrage-that-killed-suspect-friend/

Griffin, A., & Kovner, J. (2013a, June 30). Adam Lanza's pediatric records reveal growing anxiety. *Hartford Courant*.

Griffin, A., & Kovner, J. (2013b, December 28). Lanza's psychiatric treatment revealed in documents. *Hartford Courant*.

Herman, J. L. (1992). *Trauma and recovery*. New York, NY: Basic Books.

Huffington Post (2013, January 10). Tactical Response CEO Threatens 'To Start Killing People' Over Possible Obama Gun Measure. *Huffington Post*. Retrieved from http://www.huffingtonpost.com/2013/01/10/james-yeager-start-killing-people-obama-gun-policy_n_2448751.html

Langman, P. (2014). *Dylan Klebold's Journal and other writings, transcriptions of Jefferson County Sheriff's Office (JCSO) Columbine documents*. Retrieved from http://www.schoolshooters.info/dylan-klebold-journal.pdf

Lichtblau, E., & Rich, M. (2012, December 21). NRS Envisions 'a Good Guy With a Gun' in Every School. *New York Times*.

Luscombe, R. (2014, February 7). Michael Dunn murder trial under way in Florida echoes Trayvon Martin case. *The Guardian*. Retrieved from http://www.theguardian.com

McNally, R. (2003). Progress and controversy in the study of posttraumatic stress disorder. *Annual Review of Psychology*. doi:10.1146/annurev.psych.54.101601.145112.

Medina, J. (2014, May 25). Even in a state with restrictive gun laws, gunman amassed weapons. *New York Times*.

Memmott, M. (2012, December 21). Only 'A Good Guy With A Gun' Can Stop School Shootings, NRA Says. *National Public Radio*. Retrieved from http://www.npr.org/blogs/thetwo-way/2012/12/21/167785169/live-blog-nra-news-conference

Miniter, F. (2012, August 23). What the left won't tell you about the boom in U.S. gun sales. *Forbes*. Retrieved from http://www.forbes.com/sites/frankminiter/2012/08/23/what-the-left-wont-tell-you-about-the-boom-in-u-s-gun-sales/

Mullen, P. E. (2004). The autogenic (self-generated) massacre. *Behavioral Sciences and the Law, 22*(3), 311–323.

The Nation (2003, April 15). Heston to Step down as NRA President.

Newman, K. S. (2004). *Rampage: The social roots of school shootings*. New York, NY: Basic Books.

Pew Research Center. (2013a, May 7). *Gun homicide rate down 49% since 1993 peak; Public Unaware*. Retrieved from http://www.pewsocialtrends.org/2013/05/07/gun-homicide-rate-down-49-since-1993-peak-public-unaware/

Pew Research Center. (2013b, May 23). *Broad support for renewed background checks bill, skepticism about its chances*. Retrieved from http://www.people-press.org/2013/05/23/broad-support-for-renewed-background-checks-bill-skepticism-about-its-chances/

Pisani, J. (2012, December 29). Gun sales surge in wake of Newtown shooting as panicked enthusiasts rush to stock up. *Huffington Post*. Retrieved from http://www.huffingtonpost.com/2012/12/29/gun-sales-surge_n_2380738.html

Sass, L. A. (1987). "Introspection, Schizophrenia, and the Frangmentation of the Self." *Representations* 19.

Sedensky III, S. J. (2013, November 25). Report of the State's Attorney for the Judicial District of Danbury on the Shootings at Sandy Hook Elementary School and 36 Yogananda Street, Newtown, Connecticut on December 14, 2012. OFFICE OF THE STATE'S ATTORNEY JUDICIAL DISTRICT OF DANBURY. Retrieved from http://www.ct.gov/csao/lib/csao/Sandy_Hook_Final_Report.pdf

Shay, J. (1994). *Achilles in Vietnam*. New York, NY: Atheneum.

Solomon, A. (2014, March 17). The father of the Sandy Hook killer searches for answers. *New Yorker*, pp. 36–45.

Washington Post. (2012, December 21). Wayne LaPierre (Speaker). Remarks from the NRA press conference on Sandy Hook school shooting (Transcript). Retrieved from http://www.washingtonpost.com/politics/remarks-from-the-nra-press-conference-on-sandy-hook-school-shooting-delivered-on-dec-21-2012-transcript/2012/12/21/bd1841fe-4b88-11e2-a6a6-aabac85e8036_story.html

Loss, Traumatic Bereavement, and Mourning Culture: The Israel Example

23

Eliezer Witztum, Ruth Malkinson, and Simon Shimshon Rubin

23.1 Introduction

In this chapter, we address conceptual issues regarding traumatic bereavement and culture in Israel. We begin by first addressing the terms trauma and bereavement. Next we put forth a frame of reference, the Two-Track Model of Bereavement assessing functioning and the relationship to the deceased, which underlies any culturally sensitive approach to traumatic bereavement. It delineates and clarifies a way of conceptualizing, assessing, and intervening following traumatic bereavement. We then turn our attention to the cultural frameworks that are most involved with traumatic bereavements in Israel—deaths related to combat and to terror. After describing the way national bereavements in the military have changed over time, we turn to two cases of cultural disconnect. The first involves Russian immigrants who were bereaved due to terror attacks and the second considers the case of Ethiopian families whose loved ones die during military service. We conclude with recommendations regarding how to approach/manage culturally sensitive attention to the points of contact between trauma, bereavement, and culture. Done properly, this facilitates appropriate regard for biopsychosocial functioning and the relationship to the deceased.

23.2 Trauma, Loss, Bereavement, and Traumatic Bereavement

The terms trauma and bereavement are often used together, both in common speech and in mental health discussion. The frequent use of the terms in combination is present in the professional literature where there is growing attention to a category of loss referred to as "traumatic bereavement" or "traumatic grief" (Malkinson, Rubin, & Witztum, 2000; Prigerson & Jacobs, 2001). This may seem to imply that there is also a distinct type of nontraumatic bereavement to be sharply separated from the traumatic kind. Although we have used the terms traumatic and nontraumatic loss and bereavement (Malkinson et al., 2000), we believe that bereavement and trauma interact to form a mixture whose psychological and behavioral expression is difficult to predict. When bereavement occurs under external

E. Witztum, M.D. (✉)
Division of Psychiatry, Faculty of Health Sciences, Ben-Gurion University of the Negev, Be'er Sheva, Israel
e-mail: wtztu@yahoo.com

R. Malkinson, Ph.D. • S.S. Rubin, Ph.D.
International Center for the Study of Loss, Bereavement and Human Resilience, University of Haifa, Haifa 3498838, Israel
e-mail: ruti.malkinson@gmail.com; Rubin@psy.haifa.ac.il

Y. Ataria et al. (eds.), *Interdisciplinary Handbook of Trauma and Culture*, DOI 10.1007/978-3-319-29404-9_23

conditions of threat to life, it brings together the causal events, as well as the life experiences, physiological responses, and varied symptomatic responses that vary in their manifestations (Rubin, Malkinson, & Witztum, 2012).

Traumatic bereavement refers to the interaction between the event and the enduring experience of grief: it is the interaction between the sudden traumatic circumstances of the event of death and the bereaved person's traumatic experience of grief (Pearlman, Wortman, Feuer, Farber, & Rando, 2014).

For clinicians and clients alike, it is useful to specify the location of the trauma in a context of bereavement. "What here is traumatic?" is the relevant question to be asked. Sometimes this is almost self-evident and reflects the objective external trauma surrounding or accompanying the bereavement. One instance of this would be when the bereaved witnesses death under terrible circumstances. Alternatively, bereavement that stems from a death that was not directly witnessed, but involving particularly violent and unusual events, would fall under this category as well (Rynearson, 2001). Terror attacks, suicides, homicides, and natural disasters all generate a type of loss that is intertwined with external trauma—without regard to whether the bereaved were themselves present or not. Not all individuals are bereaved similarly, but it is clear that the external circumstances of horror to which the deceased and/or the bereaved were exposed increase the risk for dysfunction and symptomatic difficulties in the bereavement response (Neria et al., 2007; Rynearson, 2001).

23.3 Bereavement, Trauma, Culture, and the Two-Track Model of Bereavement

The Two-Track Model of Bereavement (Rubin, 1999) is a perspective that is well suited to considering the interface between bereavement and trauma. Succinctly, this perspective assumes that assessment of the relationship to the deceased other is a central axis for understanding the bereavement response at any time following the loss. The significance of how the bereaved is functioning, is living his or her life, from the perspective of the biopsychosocial framework, is critical to assessing and understanding the magnitude of how individuals respond to threat and change. Yet it is along the parallel and often covert axis of the relationship to the deceased that bereavement assumes some of its unique aspects as a life event. The Two-Track Model of Bereavement allows specification and focuses on multiple dimensions of response to loss as an indication of the state of the bereaved's adjustment and adaptation to loss. It combines important aspects associated with the stress and trauma perspective on life events, assessed in the biopsychosocial domain of Track I of the model, as well as important features central to the interpersonal relationship to the deceased at the very heart of the loss experience in Track II.

The assessment of biopsychosocial functioning and response to loss in the model focuses on features of behavioral, cognitive, and physiological aspects of the traumatic response to loss. Indeed, one of the dimensions assessed on Track I directly examines the degree and duration of traumatic responses for various disorders as seen in full-blown PTSD or acute stress disorder, as well as their sub-threshold manifestations.

Historically, the stress and trauma literatures highlighted the notion that loss could trigger persistent or permanent changes in personality (Rubin, 1999). The empirical focus and rigor of this approach, of the response to major life events, are basic to the understanding of the impact of major negative life events, and bear forcefully on the person experiencing the trauma of loss. By itself, however, this perspective underemphasizes the uniqueness of interpersonal relationships and their implications for the organization of self as well as the self in relationship to significant others. In contrast, the concentration on the interpersonal relationship basic to the bereavement experience has been the focus of the psychodynamic and attachment theory literatures (Rubin, Malkinson, & Witztum, 2000). Concentration on the emotional investment in the relationship with the bereaved, and the need to reorganize that relationship in the internal psychological world of the deceased, is fundamental to that approach. Although rich in clinical application, the empirical study of the "reworking" of the relationship to the deceased following death has been quite limited among many of those studying the interface of traumatic bereavement (Rubin, Malkinson, & Witztum, 2003).

Ultimately, the melding of the two perspectives advocated by Rubin became the Two-Track Model of Bereavement (Rubin, 1999). The multidimensional focus on "functioning" in the biopsychosocial realm included the affective, cognitive, interpersonal, somatic homeostasis, psychiatric/PTSD indicators, and organization of meaning structure. This multidimensional analysis made Track I a broad-based evaluation of response to loss in much the same way one would study the response to other forms of highly stressful life events. Similarly, the examination of the ongoing cognitive and emotional relationship to the deceased, encompassing associations, imagery, memories, and the gamut of emotions associated with the deceased as experienced by the bereaved, was the core of Track II. In addition, examining how the story of the death affected the experience of the relationship is highly significant and particularly relevant in cases of trauma associated with loss.

With this parallel focus on biopsychosocial functioning on the one hand and the ongoing relationship to the deceased on the other, the field remains open and attentive to the unique interpersonal nature of the loss event and bereavement response. This occurs without neglect of the myriad ways in which dysfunction can be manifest in the response to loss, grief, trauma, and mourning. With this dual approach it is much easier to revisit the phenomena of "traumatic bereavement" with the goal of assessing the response of bereavement as well as designing interventions when necessary. With the Two-Track Model of Bereavement, both the individual's biopsychosocial response and the complex manner in which the deceased is represented, remembered, and experienced are being considered. In this way, one takes into account the symptoms of dysfunction classified as acute stress disorder, post-traumatic stress disorder, and other symptomatic expressions of difficulty, without neglecting the specific relational aspects of the loss of the living interpersonal relationship that must be modified to adapt to the reality of death. The end of the lived behavioral relationship and the need to reorganize that relationship into one that is primarily experienced from within are often the major features of the bereaved individual's experience of what is going on in his or her life during the experience of acute grief and mourning.

The significance of adopting the dual approach central to the Two-Track Model of Bereavement is that it tracks both functioning and the status of the relationship to the deceased. This is done without presupposing the predominance of either of the tracks as the more significant. In terms of conceptual, empirical, and clinical work, both tracks remain the focus of concern and attention (Rubin et al., 2003).

In the case of traumatic bereavement which is the focus of this chapter, a number of negative responses warrant particular consideration. These include the assault on the meaning structure and world view of the traumatically bereaved, often manifesting itself in the questioning of national, spiritual, religious, and other guiding belief systems; the re-experiencing of the death imagery, whether as a result of having been a witness to it or in one's own imagination, which can interfere with the return to life and the management of somatic homeostasis; further, in connection with deaths that are perceived as particularly "senseless," there are often impediments to finding meaning to the loss which also serves to interfere with the successful adaptation to the death of a valued or loved individual significant relationship (Pearlman et al., 2014). When the death was the result of violence or other difficult circumstances, there is often a ruminative preoccupation with the degree of suffering the deceased experienced at the time of death and many times these thoughts are associated with pronounced feelings of guilt and remorse. From the perspective of the Two-Track Model of Bereavement, these responses are an amalgam often representing both a disruption in biopsychosocial functioning (Track I) and in the ability to rework the relationship to the deceased and to integrate their death story (Track II). When the ongoing attachment to the deceased is not a source of difficulty but of solace and when the openness to living a full life that is associated with the biopsychosocial domain is well represented, we are speaking of a well-balanced response to dealing with traumatic bereavement (Witztum, Malkinson, & Rubin, 2001).

23.3.1 Adding the Lens of Culture to Traumatic Bereavement

People from different cultures often display wide variations in the ways in which they express patterns of grieving. The study of bereavement patterns across cultures shows very different ways of reacting to loss; Western concepts of "normal" reactions or "healthy" ways of coping emerge as ethnocentric constructions (Rosenblatt, 2008). Cultural approaches to dealing with death are embedded in larger and well-articulated aspects of culture and society. Each culture and even subculture has its own approach to dealing with loss. To understand each culture's way of dealing with death may require extensive knowledge of its history, social structure, economic, and politic. Beliefs and practices concerning death and mourning should be thought of not as a matter of taste but as an extremely important part of a person's life. In many societies, death rituals are far more elaborate and protracted than those prevalent in Western societies. To outsiders, they may require actions that seem pointless and even destructive or unpleasant (Witztum et al., 2001). In Israel, the two poles of the cultural response to loss reflect Jewish tradition and the cultural construct of bereavement at the national level.

23.4 Collective and Individual Bereavement Responses in Israel and Military Losses

While every country deals with loss and bereavement, in Israel, deaths related to military service and terrorist attacks are particularly significant in the collective consciousness. We would like to consider a number of important variables that serve to exacerbate the bereaved individual's experience of loss. The losses we wish to address would be considered traumatic bereavements in any context, but a combination of the response of the individual and the collective simultaneously heightens the shock, trauma, and sense of dislocation involved so as to constitute an almost independent source of trauma.

Israel has undergone numerous changes in its 65-year history in terms of how loss is discussed and assimilated, both in the public and private spheres. The trends and changes that have taken place are most notable in their impact on secular Israeli culture and identity. The manner in which the continued impact of loss and traumatic bereavement are experienced has been particularly affected by the transition from a collective society to a much more individualistic one. These processes took place in a society assimilating successive waves of Jewish immigrants whose language and subculture of origin impacted their new country even as they were themselves changed by their joining the Israeli state and culture. During these years, for a large proportion of the population the meaning of what it was to be Jewish and Israeli shifted from an identity in dialogue with—or opposition to—traditional religious society and observance to an identity revolving around identification with a modern state with a mix of some traditional Jewish characteristics as well as a radical reforming of what it meant to be a "new Israeli Jew."

As a result of these processes, part of what was being shed was the expectation that traditional and religious mourning rituals would continue to define how to deal with death and mourning (Rubin, 2014–2015). In their place, the emerging Israeli experience sought to create rituals and structures that would assist the bereaved families and the bereaved society to deal with the losses of the Holocaust and those of the Arab-Israeli conflict (Barel, Van Ijzendoorn, Sagi-Schwartz, & Bakermans-Kranenburg, 2010).

Loss and bereavement in the public space of Israeli society are particularly salient in the short period of time in which Holocaust Memorial Day, Memorial Day, and Independence Day follow each other. Both on Holocaust Memorial

Day and on Memorial Day for Fallen Soldiers (now expanded to include civilian victims of terrorism), the local print and electronic media are heavily focused on stories of loss: regarding what happened, to whom it happened, and how this affected family and friends left behind. In addition to a heavy emphasis on the memorialization of Holocaust victims and fallen soldiers in public schools on these dates, there are many public ceremonies, visits to gravesites and memorial sites, and public markings of the tragedies (Bilu & Witztum, 2000; Malkinson & Witztum, 2000). One of the more striking examples of the far-reaching participation in these memorial services is the sounding of sirens throughout the country; the entire population stands for 2 min of silence on these memorial days (Ephratt, 2008).

While Israeli consciousness of the Holocaust is highly developed, it is the loss of young soldiers in Israel that is the predominant influence on the conceptualization and public discourse of loss and bereavement in this country. Over the years, with the growing number of fallen soldiers in wars, a "culture of bereavement" has emerged reflecting the importance Israeli society places on the death of its young people. It views these deaths as a sacrifice. The sense of heroism associated with such a death confers existential meaning on the national-social level. The term "family of the bereaved" embodies this concept. Memorialization and commemoration give concrete expression to this concept on different levels through a variety of means, such as monuments and memorial ceremonies. The various frameworks give expression to the collective representations the Israeli society has developed as part of the meaning attached to the trauma loss and death of its children in combat. These forms of commemoration and memorialization play an important role in both the national and the personal mourning process (Ben-Amos & Bet-El, 1999; Malkinson & Witztum, 2000).

Historically, in Israel there has always been a link between personal and collective bereavement. On the personal level, it seems reasonable to assume that the bereaved are moved by anguish and distress over their painful loss. But even if expressions of their emotions appear universal and innate, ethnographic evidence suggests that its articulation is bound to cultural construction and is consequently highly variable (Bilu & Witztum, 2000).

The milestones and catalysts most strongly affecting these changes are associated with the Yom Kippur War of 1973, which led to the shattering of the myths of invincible Israel and a sociopolitical revolution in Israel, and the 1982 war in Lebanon, in the aftermath of which voices were raised, particularly by bereaved parents, questioning the necessity of the war and its attendant costs in human life. The sounds of personal grief were heard in full force—anger and blame that were no longer "cloaked" (i.e., sublimated) under the mantle of meaning related to the needs of the Israeli collective. On the contrary, for the first time, protest, fury, and pain were expressed out loud and publicly. There was, however, a certain ambivalence in the protest since the heroism and mythic status related to death in combat serves as an important source for support in coping with personal grief. Precisely because of the special significance accorded it by society, there are innumerable ways in which these losses are valued and the families of the fallen honored and supported in Israeli society. Thus, the response to military loss in Israel has lost much of its monolithic regimentation and self-censorship—and individuals' grief has moved to center stage.

Attempts to honor and remember those who fell in the struggle to establish and defend the State of Israel are reflected by the evolution over the years of burial and memorial ceremonies. Six decades after the establishment of the State, there is a fixed pattern and tradition to mark the loss of a soldier. Following death during military service, the deceased's family is notified and the army steps in to organize the proceedings. The military is responsible for arranging the funeral, organizing the religious ceremony for its Jewish soldiers, and seeing to the erection of the gravestone in a uniform military style. The army has taken responsibility for organizing the rites of mourning for the individual soldiers and for establishing the annual day of remembrance for the fallen soldiers. In a variation marking the anniversary of the death of the individual, the military has instituted special annual remembrance days for the different army units to mark the deaths of their members (Malkinson & Witztum, 2000). At the same time, the Ministry of Defense has established a special wing for memorializing the deceased and caring for the families of the bereaved with economic, therapeutic, and social support. A third source of support for militarily bereaved families is the Yad Labanim Organization (memorializing children and siblings) and the IDF Widows and Orphans Organization, which honor the memories of the deceased. The existence of these supportive agencies provides the bereaved family with levels of assistance that aid in the working through of the traumatic bereavements that the death of soldiers in combat inevitably results in.

In recent years, and particularly with the wave of suicide bombing and civilian casualties, the meaning structure and embrace of the nation have been sought for victims of terror. The families' political struggle for recognition was successful and in 1998 the national day of mourning was renamed to include those civilians who died as a result of terror. Today the families of those who died as a result of terror or during military service are found across the political spectrum, and their voices are given particular attention because of the family's special status as those bereaved in the national struggle (Yom Hazikaron, 2014).

The roles that the government—working through the Army, Ministry of Defense's Memorial division, and with NGO agencies—has taken on reflects continued support for the families of the bereaved. But what happens when the supports present in society fail to adapt to the social and cultural demands of more recent immigrants to Israel?

23.4.1 Death and Mourning in a Russian Immigrant Community

Against the backdrop of the bereavement culture in Israel for military and terror bereavement, it is important to consider how procedures and customs that are associated with respectful caring for the deceased and the bereaved can become something quite different for those not part of the dominant culture. For some of the recent immigrants to Israel, their unique cultural norms were ignored with disastrous results in a number of cases of what were already "traumatic bereavements" in and of themselves. Here we bring two examples that illustrate how the norms of immigrant communities differed from those of the predominant culture and how these differences were ignored with the result that they became their own source of the traumatic experience.

In Israel today, for Jewish burials, the rites of ritual purification, burial rituals, and the graveyards themselves are part of the services provided to citizens. By law, these services are handled by local burial societies, known as the "Hevra Kadisha," and these are generally staffed by ultra-orthodox members of society. In recent years, secular burial has been legislated by the Knesset, but the number of persons using this or the private secular burial services is quite limited. The limited utilization of secular burial serves to limit the awareness among the population that this is a realistic option to be considered. In addition to the many who do not know of this option, the expense of private secular burial is prohibitive for most new immigrants to Israel. When the local burial society undertakes the burial of a member of these subgroups, the cultural gaps sometimes yawn very widely. In the case of traumatic bereavement, the gap between the burial society expectations and behaviors and that of the immigrant subculture can produce highly negative outcomes.

23.4.2 Traumatic Bereavement in the Terror Attack at Tel Aviv's Dolphinarium (2001)

On June 1st, a suicide bomber took the lives of 21 young adults, most of whom were from families that had recently immigrated to Israel from the former Soviet Union. Many of the families experienced the events subsequent to the deaths as particularly upsetting and as contributing to the experience of trauma in the context of the traumatic bereavements. The print and electronic media captured what transpired and showed how the response of the established burial services failed to assist the parents.

The following reports are taken from print media (Givertz & Mosogaviya, 2001). The first failure that occurred was in the notification of the bereaved families. In many cases, newspaper and other media persons were already waiting for the bereaved families upon their return from identifying the bodies at the Pathology Institute where this work is carried out. The media journalists set out to interview them in the midst of their acute grief, even as the family members were suffering from shock and confusion. Many described this as overwhelming and contributing to the trauma of the experience. On top of this, the public intrusion into their lives in the guise of political and media persons resulted in dramatic public exposure for people who came from a culture with greater adherence to privacy, especially in the context of exposure of painful emotions and economic hardship. Often limited in their mastery of Hebrew, and fearful of the stigma and negative stereotyping that they encountered, they were additionally concerned about how they would be portrayed in the media which further added to the stress they experienced.

A particularly poignant example of miscommunication in the encounter between the bereaved and those handling the bereavement is illustrated in the following case.

A. was one of the victims in the terror bombing. Her father had died 10 years previously. The mother, a physician, only immigrated to Israel in 1999. A. received the first funeral. Expecting to encounter a casket with the remains of her daughter, the mother was overwhelmed and re-traumatized to see the body of her daughter wrapped only in simple shrouds lying on a stretcher. In her native Russia, the dead were brought for burial in a casket with only the upper portion open for viewing. This form of presentation of the dead was so foreign to her that she had trouble believing her daughter was in the "sack" she saw. "It's not her" she cried, "show me her face, her eyes" and broke out wailing. The fact that no one had prepared the families for the traditional Israeli Jewish burial customs made what was often perceived as a reassuring accompaniment to "permanent rest" into a traumatizing experience instead. In funeral after funeral, this experience repeated itself where the customs of the dominant Jewish culture were too different and too "foreign" for the immigrant families. Many of the Russian immigrants had come to Israel only a few years earlier, and were still new to the language and to the customs. At the funeral, there were additional issues as well. They feared the cutting instruments that were produced at the funeral to make the ritual tear in their own clothes, they were fearful and shouted when the stretchers bearing the deceased were placed in the grave, and they feared that the shrouds would fall away and their loved ones would be cruelly exposed. Watching the burial team standing in the grave, they objected to their loved ones being trod upon. They did not understand what the rabbi recited nor his reference to the victims having been killed by "bnai avlah (literally sons of evil)." They did not know that they were expected to answer Amen when required. No one translated or transliterated the Kaddish prayer into Russian.

The way in which the deceased is interred and the manner in which the community serves to support the bereaved in the earliest stages of bereavement are extremely important. In the case we described above, the mismatch between cultures was so pronounced as to make the experience of the burial and the community response traumatic in the extreme. The traumatic bereavements described here ultimately required that the way in which the families experienced the response of the dominant culture became its own trauma, requiring additional working through. From the perspective of the Two-Track Model of Bereavement, the nature of the relationship to the deceased and the story of the manner of death and the subsequent handling by the community were two critical areas related to the working through of bereavement.

23.4.3 Bereavement Customs, Grief, and Rituals Among Ethiopian Immigrants to Israel

In their homeland, mourning and burial for Ethiopians who are Jewish are regulated according to special cultural codes that have been well established historically. Mourning and burial ceremonies are not uniform and may vary according to the type of death. According to custom, when a Jew belonging to Beta Israel does not die in his/her home but in a hospital for example, a message is delivered to one of the neighbors who serve as a middleman, and who is always a male, according to the Ethiopian tradition. He first brings the bad news to the elders who then tell the close relatives. This is done usually in the morning or the afternoon, but before nightfall when people return from work. According to Ethiopian Jewish customs, it is unacceptable that the tragic news be delivered directly to the immediate family, but rather must be mediated by the middleman volunteer who takes on the difficult mission of transmitting the sad news himself. The middleman will thus be the first to be informed. These are people who are close to the bereaved but not so close that they would be themselves emotionally involved in the bereavement itself or with those in the first circle of close family or friends.

With the Ethiopian immigration to Israel there has frequently been a lack of awareness of the proper, culturally sensitive way to break tragic news. The culturally insensitive announcement of a death in this community has been associated with complications of what is already a traumatic grief. This is stated best in the words of the mother of a fallen soldier, who stated bitterly: "We were killed twice—once when our beloved son died, and then when we were informed in the wrong way" (Grisaru, Malkinson, & Witztum, 2008, p. 115). In other cases, when families of a fallen soldier of Ethiopian origin were informed directly of his death without attention to cultural norms (as was customary in the Israeli army), strong emotional and behavioral responses were often observed. "In such incidents the shocked bereaved family members fainted, wailed, and screamed vigorously" (Grisaru et al., 2008, p. 114).

When the cultural norms of a community are ignored, the assimilation of the news and the supportive elements of the communities cultural buffering are diminished. From the perspective of the Two-Track Model of Bereavement, the reworking of the relationship to the deceased and how the death story is integrated suffer when the notification of death becomes itself a traumatic feature beyond the circumstances of the death. We find that the traumatic features of a "traumatic bereavement" can be found in the manner in which the bereaved are informed of the death, and the manner in which the community modes of responding to death are mishandled by the dominant culture.

23.5 Adopting Culturally Sensitive Practices

In the years following the Dolphinarium terrorist attack, many of the mutual misunderstandings between the immigrants from other countries and the general Israeli secular and religious culture have been moderated. The expectations for what constitutes the Israeli burial and mourning rituals are now familiar to these new immigrant Israelis. Organizations such as SELAH focusing on working with bereaved immigrants from the former Soviet Union have been extremely successful in reaching out to the bereaved families who lost loved ones to terror (Pardess, 2013; Shalev, 2009).

On the other hand, the need to adapt to the special needs of the Ethiopian community whose members serve in the armed forces remains a challenge. Following a number of few serious incidents such as those described above, the Military Psychology Department of the Israel Defense Forces decided to create a special team for informing Ethiopian families in cases of loss (Grisaru et al., 2008) in order to make culturally sensitive notification and support available. The team includes an Ethiopian as a permanent member whose task is to recruit the Ethiopian elders, and to make sure that the "right" relatives can be present while breaking the bitter news. The Ethiopian team member is expected to translate discreetly and in a culturally sensitive manner the officer's official announcement in appropriate Ethiopian language, whether in Amharinya or Tigrinya. Although the Ethiopian member and cultural broker who is always a male may embrace a male grieving parent, he is not allowed to embrace a grieving female parent due to strictures of religious law and practice (Grisaru et al., 2008).

In the interest of avoiding traumatization and complications of grief in the process of informing, burying, and memorializing the deceased, the need to display cultural consideration extends even further. It is also important to understand the significance of the custom of community participation in the funeral and at death anniversaries. This participation is crucial even for second- and third-degree relatives. The value of this custom is in its cohesiveness and preservation of cultural identity. When "distant relatives" are not allowed to attend these bereavement ceremonies, as is often the case for soldiers serving in the army or for employees at many places of work, the cultural "insensitivity" is highly problematic. Firstly, for these members of the community of the bereaved, they are thrust into a severe conflict between the obligation to honor the deceased as is the custom in their community and the formal demands of their work or the army. When they honor their community commitments without "permission" or leave, the action is often regarded as breaking the rules and can lead to discharge from work or facing a military court for absence without leave (Grisaru et al., 2008). And in those cases where they bow to the requirements of army or work, they are themselves emotionally conflicted. Their absence in the communal response to bereavement in turn affects the entire community, and impacts the grief and mourning of all concerned.

23.6 Concluding Remarks

In this chapter, we considered traumatic loss and the significance of the sociocultural context of such losses. We approached traumatic loss via the Two-Track Model of Bereavement which emphasizes that the mourning process proceeds along two primary axes. Track I addresses the biopsychosocial functioning of the bereaved while Track II is concerned with the ongoing relationship to the deceased and the assimilation of the death story. The death story includes how the death occurred, and also a variety of aspects immediately preceding and following the death. For the latter, the manner in which the bereaved are informed, the sensitivity and appropriateness of those entrusted with assisting in the handling of the death and burial, and the immediate aftermath extending to the very early hours and days of the response to loss are part of the death story (Rubin et al., 2012). Culturally sensitive means of responding to loss are central to the process of assisting the bereaved adapt to loss and serve to ease the pain of bereavement (Malkinson & Witztum, 2000; Witztum, 2004). By adopting culturally appropriate modes of response to the traumatically bereaved, the community and caregivers minimize the risks of adding additional anguish to individuals and communities already facing a horrible situation.

Our examples in this chapter were drawn from Israeli society beginning with the cultural practices regarding those who fell in the military service of their country. Cultural norms for the society have evolved dramatically over the decades of Israel's existence with current practices particularly accepting of individual differences in the expression of grief and mourning. From there, we focused on Israeli society's dealing with traumatic bereavement in two immigrant communities. Although Israel has been absorbing new immigrants for many years, the manner in which traumatic bereavements were handled in the examples we brought up illustrates the gap between the mourning rituals and expectations of the majority culture and that of the newcomers. This misalignment further complicates the already difficult traumatic bereavements described and becomes a quasi- or semi-independent source of trauma for the bereaved.

Thus, when the circumstances of death are traumatic, the manner in which the bereaved are informed of the loss and the degree to which the ritual needs and expectations are culturally adapted to the community have great importance. When the notification of death and the rituals surrounding the burial and communal support are not handled in ways that are culturally sensitive and familiar to the bereaved minority, the resultant dissonance can exacerbate the traumatic nature of the loss. In addition to the painful experience of bereavement, the manner in which the majority culture and its representatives behaved appeared disrespectful of the uniqueness of the "other" and the manner in which grief and mourning are dealt with by them. These elements become additional components of what is experienced as an almost multiple trauma and exacerbate the pain, bewilderment, and shock inherent in the transition to becoming bereaved. As a result, both Track I biopsychosocial functioning and Track II reworking of the relationship to the deceased and the death story are negatively affected. The grief and mourning of the bereaved become a process requiring them to adjust to the trauma of the loss of their loved one and the circumstances of his or her death and the trauma of how they experienced the initial response of a support system which did not work for them and their subculture and instead made things worse.

When the significance of the culturally sensitive encounter with the bereaved is understood and realized in actions by the majority culture, the supportive functions of the manner in which the burial ceremony, ritual actions, and community supports begin to assist in realizing the assuagement of the traumatic bereavement. Under appropriate conditions, the process of adaptation is facilitated and the sense of being supported emotionally is present from the earliest moments of dealing with loss.

References

Barel, E., Van Ijzendoorn, M. H., Sagi-Schwartz, A., & Bakermans-Kranenburg, M. J. (2010). Surviving the Holocaust: a meta-analysis of the long-term sequelae of a genocide. *Psychological Bulletin, 136*(5), 677–698.

Ben-Amos, A., & Bet-El, I. (1999). Holocaust Day and Memorial Day in Israeli schools: Ceremonies. *Education and History Israel Studies, 4*(1), 258–284.

Bilu, Y., & Witztum, E. (2000). War-related loss and suffering in Israeli society: An historical perspective. *Israel Studies, 5*, 1–31.

Ephratt, M. (2008). The functions of silence. *Journal of Pragmatics, 40*(11), 1909–1938.

Givertz, Y., & Mosogaviya, N. (2001). Unpeaceful rest. *Yedioth Ahronoth* (*Hebrew*).

Grisaru, N., Malkinson, R., & Witztum, E. (2008). Bereavement customs, grief and rituals among Ethiopian immigrants to Israel. *Illness, Crisis, & Loss, 16*(2), 111–123.

Malkinson, R., Rubin, S. S., & Witztum, E. (2000). *Traumatic and nontraumatic loss and bereavement: Clinical theory and practice*. Madison, CT: International University/Psychosocial Press.

Malkinson, R., & Witztum, E. (2000). Commemoration and bereavement: Cultural aspects of collective myth and the creation of national identity. In R. Malkinson, S. S. Rubin, & E. Witztum (Eds.), *Traumatic and non-traumatic loss and bereavement: Clinical theory and practice*. Madison, CT: International University/Psychosocial Press.

Neria, Y., Gross, R., Litz, B., Maguen, S., Insel, B., Seirmarco, G., et al. (2007). Prevalence and psychological correlates of complicated grief among bereaved adults 2.5–3.5 years after September 11th attacks. *Journal of Traumatic Stress, 20*(3), 251–262.

Pardess, E. (2013). *Fostering a sense of belonging in the face of adversity-An attachment framework*. Paper presented at the International Conference: Migration and Well-Being: Research Frontiers at Tel Aviv University.

Pearlman, L. A., Wortman, C. B., Feuer, C. A., Farber, C. H., & Rando, T. A. (2014). *Treating traumatic bereavement: A practitioner's guide*. New York, NY: The Guilford Press.

Prigerson, H., & Jacobs, S. (2001). Traumatic grief as a distinct disorder: A rationale, consensus criteria, and a preliminary empirical test. In M. Stroebe, W. Stroebe, R. O. Hansson, & H. Schut (Eds.), *Handbook of bereavement research: Consequences, coping, and care* (pp. 613–637). Washington, DC: American Psychological Association.

Rosenblatt, P. C. (2008). Grief across cultures. In M. S. Stroebe, R. O. Hansson, H. Schut, & W. Stroebe (Eds.), *Handbook of bereavement research and practice: Advances in theory and interventions* (pp. 207–211). Washington, DC: American Psychological Association.

Rubin, S. S. (1999). The Two-Track Model of Bereavement: Overview, retrospect and prospect. *Death Studies, 23*(8), 681–714.

Rubin, S. S. (2014–2015). Loss and bereavement in the Jewish tradition. *Omega, 70*(1), 79–98.

Rubin, S. S., Malkinson, R., Koren, D., Mor Yosef, S., & Witztum, E. (2011). Military bereavement and combat trauma. In S. Ringel & J. R. Brandell (Eds.), *Trauma: Contemporary directions in theory, practice, and research*. Thousand Oaks, CA: Sage.

Rubin, S. S., Malkinson, R., & Witztum, E. (2000). An overview of the field of loss. In R. Malkinson, S. S. Rubin, & E. Witztum (Eds.), *Traumatic and nontraumatic loss and breavement: Clinical theory and practice*. Madison, CT: International University/Psychosocial Press.

Rubin, S. S., Malkinson, R., & Witztum, E. (2003). Trauma and bereavement: Conceptual and clinical issues revolving around relationships. *Death Studies, 27*(8), 667–690.

Rubin, S. S., Malkinson, R., & Witztum, E. (2008). Clinical aspects of a DSM complicated grief diagnosis: Challenges, dilemmas, and opportunities. In M. S. Stroebe, R. O. Hansson, H. Schut, & W. Stroebe (Eds.), *Handbook of bereavement research and practice: Advances in theory and intervention* (pp. 187–206). Washington, DC: American Psychological Association Press.

Rubin, S. S., Malkinson, R., & Witztum, E. (2012). *Working with the bereaved: Multiple lenses on loss and mourning*. New York, NY: Routledge.

Rynearson, E. K. (2001). *Retelling violent death*. New York, NY: Psychology Press.

Shalev, R. (2009). *Bereaved parents: Change of self, future orientation, functioning and adaptation to loss*. Unpublished doctoral dissertation, University of Haifa.

Witztum, E. (2004). *Soul, loss and bereavement*. Tel Aviv: Ministry of Defense Publication.

Witztum, E., Malkinson, R., & Rubin, S. S. (2001). Death, bereavement and traumatic loss in Israel: a historical and cultural perspective. *The Israel Journal of Psychiatry and Related Sciences, 38*(3-4), 157–170.

Yom Hazikaron (2014). *Wikipedia*. http://en.wikipedia.org/wiki/Yom_Hazikaron. Accessed 16 November 2014.

24 Fear and Silence in Burma and Indonesia: Comparing Two National Tragedies and Two Individual Outcomes of Trauma

Robert Lemelson and Seinenu M. Thein-Lemelson

24.1 Introduction

On a sweltering August day in 2013, in Burma's[1] former capital city of Yangon,[2] exactly 25 years after government troops massacred thousands of civilians in the street, several thousand of those who survived gathered at a large convention center in order to commemorate the anniversary of the 1988 demonstrations, pay tribute to the heroes of the Uprisings, and honor the memory of those who perished. For three extraordinary days, paintings, photography, and poetry lined the walls of a temporary gallery that had been constructed on the grounds of the convention center, documenting the experiences of dissidents under the military dictatorship, including the imprisonment, torture, and deprivation that many endured.

Inside the main auditorium, scenes from 1988 of troops shooting at unarmed civilians flashed onto a screen as the tune from a 1970s pop song "Dust in the Wind" blasted from loudspeakers with new Burmese lyrics: "Oh … fallen heroes of the democracy movement … History written with our blood … corpses lying on the roads … this is the country where martyrs live." The halls of the convention center thundered as the entire audience clapped, pumped their fists, and sang along. Speaker after speaker took to the podium, talking at length about their memories of the massacres of 1988 and the years of struggle that followed, addressing an audience that included parliamentarians, former political prisoners, activists, university students, school children, housewives, military officers, and members of the monastic order. The speeches were impassioned, the mood celebratory—this was a fete, rather than a somber memorial.

In Jakarta, that same year, almost 50 years after Indonesian military and paramilitary brutally slaughtered hundreds of thousands of civilians in what was framed as an anti-communist purge, a group of survivors sat with community members during an event that was meant to commemorate these tragic events. The atrocities committed in 1965 were discussed at length in front of an audience that consisted largely of students too young to

[1] In 1989, Burma was renamed the Republic of the Union of Myanmar. There has not been uniform adoption of the name Myanmar. Because the change in name was an arbitrary decision on the part of the military junta, many prodemocracy activists within the country, as well as other nation-states, have not officially adopted the new name. Others have argued that the name Myanmar is more inclusive, because Burma references only the dominant ethnicity (the Bamar or Burman).

[2] In 1989, Rangoon was renamed Yangon.

R. Lemelson, Ph.D
Department of Anthropology, University of California, Los Angeles, USA
e-mail: lemelson@ucla.edu

S.M. Thein-Lemelson, Ph.D (✉)
Institute of Personality and Social Research (IPSR), University of California, Berkeley, USA
e-mail: seinenu@ucla.edu

Y. Ataria et al. (eds.), *Interdisciplinary Handbook of Trauma and Culture*,
DOI 10.1007/978-3-319-29404-9_24

remember the massacres. Neither of the two experts speaking that day had personally lived through the atrocities of 1965 and the event itself had been organized by outsiders not personally impacted by the killings.

As part of the event, a film, made by the first author about the 1965 killings and their aftermath, was screened. *Genjer, Genjer*, a song that had been a rallying cry for the Indonesian communist party, was part of the soundtrack for the film. As the song played, a small group of survivors, now well into their 80s and 90s, quietly sang along to the lyrics, while some sobbed silently. The mood inside the auditorium was somber. More than 50 years had passed since the mass killings in Indonesia and only now were survivors coming forward and breaking their silence, albeit cautiously and in small numbers.

The fundamental difference between the two scenes depicted above lies in the response of both survivors and the general population to historically situated political atrocities and state attempts to prevent their memorialization. In Indonesia, a state-sponsored imposition of silence with regard to the events of 1965 appeared to be largely successful, with survivors remaining silent for decades. In Burma, the opposite was the case. Just a short time after the military purportedly ceded control to democratic rule in 2011, survivors of the 1988 massacres were coming forward in astounding numbers, relating their narratives to the larger society, exposing past human rights violations, and publically confronting those who committed the atrocities. The events of 1988 were emerging as integral to the public discourse on human rights, democratization, identity, and nationhood.

What accounts for these differences in remembering, discussing, or even confronting past historical traumas? What might these differences mean about how survivors in these two societies experience, understand, and regulate fear, anxiety, sadness, and other emotions implicated in traumatic experience? What might these differences mean for the overall course of posttraumatic responses in the individuals who experience political atrocities?

24.2 Overview of Chapter

An attempt to situate traumatic experience in relation to culture is a complex undertaking, requiring multiple levels of analyses (Hinton & Good, 2015; Hinton & Hinton, 2014; Hinton & Kirmayer, 2013; Hinton & Lewis-Fernandez, 2011; Hinton & Simon, 2015; Kirmayer, Lemelson, & Barad, 2007; Rechtman, 2000). Universalizing accounts that explain trauma at the foundational level of the neurobiology of fear have been productive in providing an understandable model for posttraumatic experience and formulating a diversity of treatment modalities (Dias, Banerjee, Goodman, & Ressler, 2013; Foa & Kozak, 1998; Powers, Halpern, Ferenschak, Gillihan, and Foa (2010); Shin and Liberzon (2012); see also LeDoux, 2014 on the concept of fear in current neuroscience research). However, explanations that rely upon neurobiological models of fear are incomplete unless individual experiences of trauma and posttraumatic response are situated at more complex levels that account for the unique political, historical, and psychocultural contexts in which they occur. This is particularly true in relation to the study of individual outcomes. While there is a robust literature that indicates that individuals often do respond to traumatic experience with resilience, it is not clear what specific factors facilitate recovery (Bonanno, 2004).

This chapter explores the relationship between the personal experience of trauma and larger cultural and political processes that can shape individual outcome by examining two historic national tragedies in Southeast Asia: one in Burma, and the other in Indonesia. We will utilize a comparative case analysis of two individuals—one Indonesian, and one Burmese—who underwent significant traumas that were part of historically situated political atrocities. By exploring these two case studies in detail, we hope to illuminate the complex interplay of psychocultural, social, political, and even religious variables that frame traumatic exposure and the cultural models that orient trauma survivors to interpret their individual experiences in particular ways. We hope especially to highlight that individual outcome to traumatic experience is not only determined by neurobiology and personality, but that resiliency and recovery can be impacted both by immediate social factors and larger structural ones that reflect the politics, culture, religion, and history of a particular society.

24.3 Comparing Two National Tragedies of Trauma: Burma and Indonesia

Indonesia and Burma have had similarly troubling modern political histories: both countries had opposition movements that posed a significant enough threat to the ruling regime that they were brutally suppressed, resulting in the death and imprisonment of several thousand individuals in Burma (Lintner, 1990) and upwards of a million in Indonesia (Robinson, 1995). Both nations are also marred by a history in which a state military and police apparatus, through violent and nonviolent measures, including imprisonment, censorship, propaganda, intimidation, social control, and manipulation of cultural narratives, attempted to silence survivors of these atrocities and hide the reality of their traumas.

In Burma, we will focus on the 1988 Uprising and subsequent massacres as seen through the eyes of a former student activist who was a long-term prisoner of conscience. In Indonesia, we will focus on the events that led up to the 1965 massacres, as narrated by a farmer who witnessed and survived the mass violence in Bali in late 1965. We then explore the commonalities and differences in the psychocultural, familial, social, historical, religious, and political factors that shaped both traumatic experiences and subsequent outcomes in Burma and Bali.[3]

[3]Due to the scope of this chapter, we will not be able to explore potential genetic predispositions, developmental life course issues, or other psychobiological factors that would predispose either of these subjects to developing post-traumatic stress disorder.

24.3.1 Historical Context in Indonesia: The September 30th Movement and Mass Killings

Up until 1965, the communist party of Indonesia (or *Partai Komunis Indonesia*-PKI) was one of the largest political parties in the country. According to official accounts put forth by the Indonesian Government, on September 30th, 1965, a "communist conspiracy" within the military resulted in the murder of seven high-ranking military officials. The September 30th Movement, as purportedly enacted by the communist party, was the justification for a wave of mass killings instigated by General Suharto that spread throughout Indonesia in 1965 and that culminated in the deaths of hundreds of thousands of civilians (Anderson, 1987; Cribb, 2004; Roosa, 2006; Wardaya, 2006; Wertheim, 1979). The primary victims of the violence were actual or alleged PKI members and others accused of being sympathetic to the communist cause, including members of artist communities and women's organizations (Dwyer, 2004; Pohlman, 2004, 2008, 2014). Perpetrators of the violence were primarily military and paramilitary forces, though some civilians also participated in the killings, either voluntarily or under coercion.

Estimates for the number of people killed nationwide are somewhere between 500,000 and 1 million. On the island of Bali between 80,000 and 100,000 (approximately 5–8 % of the population) were killed between December 1965 and March 1966 (Cribb, 1990; Dwyer & Santikarma, 2003; Robinson, 1995). Thousands more were imprisoned and subjected to torture, forced labor, and other harsh conditions, with many prisoners being held for decades (Fuller, 2000).

24.3.2 History of Political Repression Following the 1965 Mass Killings

The events of 1965 had reverberations for decades, as the "New Order" regime of former president Suharto (1966–1998) led a campaign to frame the events of 1965 in ways that stigmatized the communists and those perceived as supporting them (Lemelson, Supartini, & Ng, 2010; Rochijat & Anderson, 1985). The state was devoted to weeding out internal dissent by continuing the purge, control, and surveillance of supposed communists. Families of former and alleged PKI members became the target of discriminatory laws which limited their civil rights: they were prevented from entering the military, teaching, and working for the government, and deterred from any other occupation deemed socially significant. Their ability to travel both in the country and abroad was severely restricted.

Furthermore, the New Order regime put forth a monolithic state narrative regarding the events of 1965 that hid the atrocities committed by military and paramilitary and framed the events of 1965 as the Indonesian nation-state protecting itself from communists (Anderson, 2012; Heryanto, 2012). The state-built museum at the site of the murder of the military officers reinforced this narrative, as did the yearly memorials attended by Suharto himself, and mandatory annual screenings of a film portraying the communists as vicious killers.

Any public discussion of the events of 1965 that was at variance with this official state version was forbidden and those who engaged in it were jailed or "disappeared." The enforced silence affected every level of Indonesian society, from family relationships to village life, large-scale social organizations, all the way up to national politics, only beginning to crack after the fall of the Suharto regime in the wake of the Asian economic crisis of 1998 (Dwyer, 2009; Dwyer & Santikarma, 2006; Zurbuchen, 2002, 2005).[4]

24.3.3 Historical Context in Burma: The 1988 Uprising and Subsequent Massacres

In September 1987, the Burmese Government demonetized the national currency and the savings of hundreds of thousands of families were wiped out. The demonetization, public outcry over the death of a student killed during a protest (the Phone Maw incident), as well as the deepening poverty and despair born out of 26 years of economic mismanagement by General Ne Win's military-run socialist regime were the catalysts for a growing opposition movement led largely by university students (Fink, 2009; Lintner, 1990).

This student-led movement culminated in several protests throughout the spring and summer of 1988—which were all brutally crushed by government authorities. Particularly noteworthy is what is now known as the Red Bridge incident (Lone, 2014). On March 16th, 1988, military and paramilitary officers attacked thousands of students who had gathered for a protest near Inya Lake in Yangon. Eyewitness accounts report that both male and female students were beaten with clubs and chased into the lake, with paramilitary holding students' heads under water until they drowned.[5,6] At least 49 students suffocated in a military van; for others, atrocities began once they were taken into custody. There were reports of brutality and torture inflicted in the interrogation rooms and prisons, including the rape of female students by military, police, and paramilitary officers (Lintner, 1990).

The most remarkable set of protests came on August 8th, 1988—what came to be known as the *8888 Uprising*. Whereas previous demonstrations had been largely confined to the capitol city of Yangon, this protest spread to major cities throughout Burma and included members of the monastic order, university students, government employees, school children, laborers, dockworkers, housewives, and even members of the mili-

[4] It is perhaps not coincidental that the two documentary films that have explored the 1965 tragedy from the perspective of the victims have "silence" in their titles ("40 Years of Silence" Lemelson 2008; "The Look of Silence" Oppenheimer 2014).

[5] Interviews conducted with former 1988 activists, Yangon, May 2014.

[6] Interviews conducted with former Yangon University students, Sydney, February 2014.

tary. In response to the protests, troops opened fire on unarmed civilians in almost all major cities. The killings continued for several days and it is estimated that more than a thousand were killed just in Yangon.

Immediately following the bloodshed of the 8888 demonstrations, Sein Lwin stepped down as head of government.[7] For a few weeks in August and September, after this announcement, it seemed that the military had withdrawn from public life. The withdrawal was short-lived, however, because in late September members of the military reasserted themselves through a coup. Once again, the killings began and it is estimated that at least 10,000 perished in just 2 days (Lintner, 1990).

24.3.4 History of Political Repression Following the 1988 Uprising

After the massacres of 1988, the state continued to impose silence on dissidents, their families, and the population at large. From the earliest days of the movement, the worst atrocities were employed in interrogation centers and prisons, where victims were psychologically and physically tortured, starved, and dehumanized. Some prisoners were kept in cells meant for military dogs for months at a time, some were left in solitary confinement for several years at a time, and others were used as forced labor. Many perished from injuries or other diseases (Assistance Association for Political Prisoners, 2005; Fink, 2009; Lemere & West, 2011).[8]

The prison system was intertwined with the vast military intelligence system. The Burmese state surveillance system required household registries for every family, with the military conducting surprise inspections in the middle of the night. Any overnight guests and any travel had to be registered with the local authorities. Military intelligence organized a vast neighborhood surveillance network (Fortify, 2015; Pitman & Htusan, 2015; Slow, 2015).[9]

State attempts to prevent protests led to strict prohibition of public meetings. Universities were closed down for months, sometimes years at a time (Fink, 2009). The university system was restructured into new regional campuses, such that if large-scale protests did occur, the military could swiftly and easily crush any dissent.

This explicit repression was matched by state control of the media. The military government put forth the prevailing narrative that the democracy movement in 1988 had plunged Burma into chaos and violence, and it was only the military that could restore the nation. From the outset, the military regime called themselves the "State Law and Order Restoration Council" as part of this rhetoric. After 1988, the government built several military museums in order to further this myth and signify their own glory. Total censorship of international magazines, newspapers, television news programs, the Internet, and other media completed the silence and control (Fink, 2009; Skidmore, 2003).

We now turn to how these complex histories framed and were reflected in two individual narratives of survivors of these national traumas.

24.4 Indonesia Case Study: Kereta[10]

Nyoman Kereta, born in the mid-1940s, is a poor rice farmer in rural central Bali. In early 1966 Indonesian military and paramilitary forces entered his village looking for suspected communists. The

[7] General Ne Win, Burma's dictator from 1962 to 1988, had officially stepped down as president and chairman of the Burmese Socialist Programme Party (BSPP) after public outcry over the Red Bridge incident and Sein Lwin had been appointed both party chair and president in July of 1988.

[8] Interviews conducted with former political prisoners and their families, San Francisco, Los Angeles, New York, Sydney, Yangon, Mandalay, June 2014 to April 2015.

[9] Interviews conducted with former political prisoners and their families, San Francisco, Los Angeles, New York, Sydney, Yangon, Mandalay, June 2014 to April 2015.

[10] Nyoman Kereta's case study is also explored in the ethnographic films: "Shadows and Illuminations" and "40 Years of Silence: An Indonesian Tragedy" by the first author and discussed at length in the following publications: Lemelson and Suryani (2006), Lemelson and Tucker (2012), and Lemelson (2014).

troops singled out a number of villagers and marched them to a local cemetery. Although a PKI member himself, Kereta escaped this roundup, but followed the villagers to the cemetery, and from a hiding place in a tree witnessed them being hacked to death with machetes. Local members of the PKI were also forced to participate in these mass killings, as a way of proving their loyalty to the new regime. The next evening, Kereta's cousins colluded in his father's murder, luring him out of his compound to be set upon by paramilitary members, some of whom were Kereta's neighbors. Kereta watched as his father was brutally tortured and killed.

It was after these traumatic events that Kereta began to experience both social withdrawal and fear. He began to experience an "inner pressure" weighing down on his body, as well as heart palpitations. For months after the massacre he had difficulty eating, lost weight, and began looking gaunt. He had difficulty sleeping, experiencing nightmares. He was easily startled, and his mind would go blank for extended periods of time. Perhaps, most striking, given the very dense nature of Balinese social relationships, was that Kereta withdrew socially and stopped participating in community work projects.

Kereta eventually married and his wife gave birth to a son and then a daughter. Their daughter, however, died immediately after birth. Kereta describes this as the most difficult time in his life. He cried continuously. It was at this time that Kereta began seeing small, black figures, which he believed to be spirits known as the *wong samar*, a commonly recognized form of potentially dangerous spirits in Bali. He reported that these spirits would enter his body and take possession of him. When possessed by these spirits, Kereta would avoid social contact by hiding in solitary places, such as the rice fields and canyons. His experiences with the *wong samar* caused him to withdraw even further from village life, and avoid social contact, with even his own family. Sometimes he refused to leave his room at all.

Over the years Kereta's experiences with spirit beings waxed and waned. In 2002 and 2003, when Indonesia held its first democratic elections, he experienced a relapse of symptoms. He reports that this time the spirits were asking him to rejoin the PKI. Kereta began wearing a camouflage military jacket and helmet, believing that this prevented the spirits from entering his body and causing him to become a communist.

Although Kereta's family is largely supportive of him, there has been no dialogue about the death of his father or the massacre of the other villagers. It was only at the end of the first author's 2-year fieldwork, after having interviewed him multiple times, that Kereta confided that he had experienced this trauma. Neither he nor his family mentioned it in any other contexts. Even then, he would not fully disclose all aspects of what he had witnessed until a number of years later. Kereta had literally remained silent about 1965 for 40 years.

From a psychiatric perspective, Kereta has the cardinal features of chronic post-traumatic stress disorder (PTSD) with psychotic features, according to the fifth edition of the *Diagnostic and Statistical Manual of Mental Disorders* (DSM-5; American Psychiatric Association [APA] 2013, pp. 271–280). From the time of witnessing the murders to the present, he has had persistent symptoms of increased arousal and associated physiological reactivity, as indicated by tachycardia, difficulty concentrating, confusion, and dizziness, and he has had nightmares and other persistent sleep disturbances. He experienced both numbing and flooding/flashback states.

24.5 Burmese Case Study: Thura[11]

Thura's first experience with trauma was in 1988 when he took part in a student protest that culminated in the Red Bridge incident. Thura, along with hundreds of other students from Rangoon University, began marching from their campus towards Inya Lake. The group was soon surrounded by paramilitary troops (the *Lone Htein*

[11] A pseudonym is used in order to protect the identity of the subject. In arriving at a pseudonym, the authors selected a name that is common among the Burmese majority population in order to avoid references to ethnic identity. Other minor details are also altered in order to further protect the identity of the subject (please see Skidmore, 2003).

or riot police) on all sides, who ordered them to disperse. The students resisted and began to sing songs, including the Burmese national anthem. Thura approached the head officers to negotiate with them, but the negotiations were unsuccessful and the troops eventually stormed the students, killing some and brutally beating many more. Many students were also arrested, illegally detained, and brutalized inside the prisons. Thura managed to escape that day but witnessed violence inflicted on other students.

Following these events, Thura continued to organize and participate in protests. On August 8th, 1988, Thura witnessed the military fire into the crowds near the Shwedagon Pagoda. Some time during the protests, Thura narrowly escaped being shot. He recalls a bullet flying so close to his head that he could feel how much heat it was radiating. Even with atrocities all around him, Thura remained focused on his goals, possessing a larger sense of purpose. After the military had seemingly withdrawn following August 11th, he began traveling to other parts of Burma in order to organize representatives from different townships.

After the military coup was announced on September 18th, Thura realized that he could not safely return home again and relied on friends to remain in hiding. Even while in hiding, he continued to communicate with others and organize dissident acts, including passing out newsletters, putting up banners, and holding secret meetings. Thura was eventually captured. Soldiers surrounded him on the street as he was walking to a friend's home during the evening hours, put a hood over his head, bound his hands and feet, and took him to an interrogation center, where he was deprived of adequate food, drink, and sleep for several days, and tortured.

After several days of interrogation, the intelligence officers asked him to sign a statement denouncing his activities. He refused and was almost immediately transferred to a prison. Once he arrived at the prison, he realized that he would be there for a long time. His thoughts turned to survival and how he could make the best of his situation.

Thura was imprisoned for over a decade, during which time he was deprived of basic needs on a daily basis, including adequate food, drink, medicine, and sanitation and was subjected to physical violence and other forms of torture. He was kept in solitary confinement for months at a time. Rather than falling into depression or despair, he tried to maintain as normal a routine as possible. He made a habit of remaining awake during the daylight hours, occupying himself with completing various goals, such as memorizing English vocabulary words. Because he did not sleep in the daytime, he was typically able to fall asleep right away at night.

After he was released from prison, he eventually began to reconnect with other dissidents who had also been imprisoned. There was a sense of solidarity that had emerged in the prisons that made former rivalries that had existed during their student days recede. He eventually married. Thura continues his political work to this day. Like other democracy activists of his generation in Burma, Thura always wears white in order to commemorate his time as a political prisoner (prisoner's uniforms during his time of imprisonment were white). He goes into work each day and continues to act in ways that are proactive, engaging in advocacy, conducting meetings with activists and foreign dignitaries, teaching, and writing. Much of the social activities that he engages in are within the community of tight-knit democracy activists, many of whom were also involved in the 1988 movement and have spent time in the prisons.

Although he is familiar with the discourse on trauma, Thura has not sought treatment all these years and appears to be functioning well without intervention. From a psychiatric perspective Thura has almost none of the diagnostic features of PTSD, according to DSM-5 (APA 2013, pp. 271–280). While he obviously remembers distinctly the multiple trauma inflicted on his body and mind, analysis drawn from ethnographic interviews indicates that almost none of his experiences fit into the psychiatric model of PTSD.[12]

[12] Please note that there are narratives of 1988 and life in Burmese prisons whereby survivors report symptoms that fit the clinical model of PTSD [please see Lemere and West (2011)].

Rather than remaining silent, he talks often and energetically about politics and his entire life is devoted to furthering democracy in Burma.

24.6 The Psychocultural Context of Fear and Silence: Contrasting *Ngeb* and *Abhaya*

Kereta and Thura's strategies for coping with their trauma are shaped by localized understandings of fear in relation to human suffering, existential meaning, and desired forms of personhood. While there are no definitive cultural explanatory models that map directly onto the Western clinical explanatory model of PTSD in either Indonesia or Burma, there are numerous descriptors related to fear in both languages that resemble the Western concept of psychological trauma. We will focus on two models of fear—one in Burma and one in Bali—that situate trauma and posttraumatic responses in their cultural context.

In Bali, fear and trauma can be seen as culturally translated and encapsulated by the concept of *ngeb* (Lemelson, 2014; Lemelson & Suryani, 2006; Lemelson & Tucker, 2012). *Ngeb* is understood specifically as an illness that emerges when one has witnessed something horrific, frightening, or bizarre. As a result of these frightening experiences, sufferers of *ngeb* put themselves in a self-imposed exile, being characterized by *membisu*, meaning muteness or lack of participation in the social world. The concept of *ngeb* is also resonant with the Balinese practice of *puik*, which can be translated as intentional silence and social avoidance (Geertz, 1973; Bateson & Mead, 1942; Santikarma, 1995).

Kereta described himself as suffering from *ngeb*, believing that this "illness" began after witnessing the massacres in his village (Lemelson, 2014; Lemelson & Suryani, 2006; Lemelson & Tucker, 2012). It is interesting to note that Kereta has several neighbors who are similarly characterized as *ngeb*. Since *ngeb* can be viewed as a means of mute political protest, Kereta and others from his village who are seen as suffering from *ngeb* can be thought of as silent witnesses to the atrocities that were committed in 1965 (Lemelson & Tucker, 2012). Moreover, because *ngeb* can also be translated as a fear of resisting cosmological authority, in Bali this political culture of silencing was also reinforced by a set of cosmological beliefs that, likewise, served to suppress social memory.

In contrast to Bali where silence and withdrawal are seen in some ways as being an expected, although undesirable, response to intense fear, in Burma, fear is seen as an emotion to be tamed and overcome. The Buddhist mantra *abhaya* ("fear not") is often privately and publically invoked in relation to fearful situations, with the goal of dispelling and containing the fear, rather than avoiding the fearful stimulus by withdrawing.

Thura does not talk about fear in relation to the events of 1988, his time in prison, or his life afterwards. This is not for lack of an adequate vocabulary because Burmese descriptors for fear-like states commonly occur in everyday discourse (Skidmore, 2003). His preference not to dwell on fear cannot be taken as an attempt to avoid painful memories because Thura talks freely about his experiences during 1988 and while in prison. While he is willing to commemorate and bear witness to the past, a large part of his coping appears to involve downregulating negative emotions like fear.

Buddhist concepts such as *abhaya* have been adopted into the language and discourse of the Burmese prodemocracy movement of which Thura is a part. In a series of now-famous essays, Burma's most well-known dissident and political prisoner, Aung San Suu Kyi, wrote that one of the main tasks facing Burma is achieving "freedom from fear." She states that fear is "not a natural state for civilized man" (Kyi, 2010, p. 184) and that the defining characteristic of those engaged in the Burmese democracy movement is that they have faced their fears again and again, over decades (Mackay, 2011). For Thura and other activists their commitment to the political cause that has defined their lives is equated with their degree of fearlessness.

This adoption of the Buddhist concept of *abhaya* by the Burmese prodemocracy movement is interesting in light of the fact that there are many tenets within Therevedan Buddhism that bear a resemblance to emotional and social withdrawal (Obeyesekere, 1985). While a prevalent discourse within Buddhism encourages disengagement, prodemocracy activists have chosen to emphasize the opposite (e.g., bearing witness, effecting change) while still evoking Buddhist concepts such as fearlessness (Kyi, 1992). Thura never invokes less agentic Burmese Buddhist notions such as *kan* (fate) nor emphasizes his *dukkha* (suffering) in relating his experiences, which stands apart from what has been observed to be common practice in Burma (Spiro, 1982).

It is significant that although both *abhaya* and *ngeb* have both spiritual and political connotations, the two subjects do not employ both sets of meanings to their experiences. Kereta's understanding of his experiences is almost entirely cosmological. This stands in contrast to Thura, whose explanations of his experiences are almost entirely political.

24.7 The Familial and Social Context of Fear and Silence: Embeddedness Versus Isolation

A main feature of Kereta's response to the experience of trauma has been the extent to which he is socially avoidant. Kereta's withdrawal into the spirit world can be regarded in some ways as a rejection of a human world that he viewed as untrustworthy (Lemelson & Tucker, 2012). The focal area of this basic distrust is the family system (Wikan, 1990) and local hamlet. Kereta's own cousin encouraged the paramilitary to kill Kereta's father and one of Kereta's sisters is now married to a paramilitary officer, who participated in the 1965 killings. It is common for victims and survivors of 1965 to remain in the same villages as perpetrators, hence forced to see them on a day-to-day basis. Survivors were forced to remain silent about past atrocities in order to maintain social harmony—a quality valued in the socially dense world of the Balinese village, where families traditionally rely on one another in order to carry out communal work projects.

Rather than being socially avoidant, Thura is deeply embedded in a tightly knit community of political dissidents. His embeddedness within this community started in the early days of the democracy movement and continues to the present. Student dissidents relied on each other to both further the movement and ensure their own safety. They often hid with one another, sleeping in the same beds, and eating communally.[13]

Prison life often increased their sense of solidarity to one another, because they were reliant on one another for solace, safety, company, and even caregiving in times of sickness or food scarcity.[14] Thura reported feeling concerned about what life would be like in prison on the car ride over, but once he realized how many other political prisoners there were in his cellblock and how many of them he already knew, he felt more at ease. Although there were rules that prohibited the prisoners from speaking to one another, they found ways in which they could communicate surreptitiously and older, more educated prisoners would often tutor the younger student activists.

Thura, along with his friends in the democracy movement, regularly and diligently enacts many practices, including commemorating multiple events throughout the year to honor the memory of 1988. The community of dissidents possesses a shared vocabulary, consistently referring to those who were massacred or perished as "fallen martyrs." This stands in contrast to Indonesia, where those who were killed are referred to as "victims" at best, and more commonly thought of as despised PKI members.

After his release, Thura began wearing white (the color of prison uniforms) in order to memorialize his time in prison. His actions stand in complete contrast to those of Kereta, who actually resorted to wearing a military uniform (a green camouflage jacket and helmet) on a daily basis in order to "protect" himself from spirit

[13] Interviews conducted with former political prisoners, San Francisco, Los Angeles, New York, Sydney, Yangon, Mandalay, June 2014 to April 2015.

[14] Interviews conducted with former political prisoners, San Francisco, Los Angeles, New York, Sydney, Yangon, Mandalay, June 2014 to April 2015.

beings whom he claims try to entice him to join the communist party. Kereta's donning of the uniform worn by his perpetrators is a stark example of the hegemony of the cultural narrative put forth by the Indonesian Government surrounding the events of 1965. Kereta's own psyche was usurped by those attempting to subordinate him to such an extent that, even 40 years after the atrocities had taken place, he seeks solace through the donning of a uniform that his perpetrators were wearing the day they enacted the killings and inflicted the trauma.

Thura's relationships with others in the activist community was forged over many years of shared goals, shared pain, and shared privations as they worked towards a common cause. Thura took pledges with other students during the earliest days of the 1988 Uprising that they would continue on with the movement until they were able to reach their goals. This loyalty not only to a cause, but also to fellow activists, stands in contrast to the isolation that Kereta experienced.

24.8 The Political and Societal Context of Fear and Silence: Coherence Versus Fragmentation

Burma and Indonesia have similar geopolitical histories. In both countries, the military was an ever-present part of day-to-day life. In both nations, the military sought to safeguard and consolidate its power through the employment of paramilitary forces.

However, there are also crucial differences in these histories that have clearly impacted how individual citizens processed and coped with the traumatic experience of state violence. In Indonesia, recruited members of the paramilitary were often integrated into local village life, which meant, in the wake of violence, perpetrators and survivors were forced to reside in the same villages for decades. Kereta's avoidance of village work projects is understandable in light of the fact that participation in such activities necessarily required that he interact with perpetrators and families of perpetrators—some of whom were in his own kinship network.

In Burma, it was often the case that there was much more of a physical and, hence, psychological separation between survivors and perpetrators. The 1988 democracy movement began amongst university students, the vast majority of whom were urban, middle class, and from well-educated families. Those who carried out the brutalities, including paramilitary, prison staff, and foot soldiers, were often from less educated families and lower rungs of the socioeconomic strata (Prasse-Freeman, 2012). Military families typically resided in separate compounds and military officers made their way through a system of education that stood apart from the university system from which the student movement had emerged. While there are cases of military and prodemocracy activists within the same extended family (Fink, 2009), it was rarely the case that they had to physically reside in the same compound as one another and it was almost never the case that a family member would be directly responsible for the death of another family member, as happened in Kereta's family. In Thura's case and in the case of many other political prisoners there was little opportunity for prolonged interaction between perpetrators and victims outside of the prisons and the interrogation rooms.

Although Burma and Indonesia have had large-scale police state apparatus in place, in Indonesia, in the period of reform inaugurated with the fall of the New Order in 1998, there was a diversifying of political parties, media outlets, and civil society organizations. After 1998 there was an increasing diversity in understanding of what happened in 1965, but running parallel to these new and alternative discourses was the very entrenched dialogue and continuation of the state narrative that framed communists as "enemies" of Indonesia and their elimination as justified. The entrenched fear of being affiliated with the communist party existed in an environment where many other aspects of civic life *resembled* diversity. This seeming diversity and the appearance of a society that was, on the surface, open to new ideas may have ironically made the manipulation of facts surrounding 1965 by the Indonesian Government more palatable and believable.

Kereta's own family and neighbors recapitulated the narrative put forth by the state, believing that Kereta was an instigator of the events of 1965. It was only in 2004 that Kereta's family and fellow villagers finally forgave him for causing the "disorder" of the events of 1965 (Lemelson & Tucker, 2012). More than anything, the propaganda put forth by the Suharto regime fragmented and disoriented survivors of 1965 such that they could no longer identify who were the true perpetrators.

This diversity stands in contrast to Burma, wherein the political apparatus and state surveillance up until recently were all encompassing, regulating every aspect of life. There was a bifurcation of institutions following the 1962 coup and the only two stable, viable societal bodies were the military-run government, with its vast bureaucracy, and the monastic order. This bifurcation of institutions, a nonexistent civil society, a centralized education system, and complete control of the media by the state ironically worked against the military in terms of gaining broader acceptance of the cultural narratives that they put forth about 1988.

In the face of a monolithic state entity that regulated virtually all aspect of information transfer, the Burmese populace often relied on what can be termed broadly as rumors (Skidmore, 2003). Rather than having veiled secrets locked away in an otherwise seemingly forward-moving society (as was the case in Indonesia, post-New Order), the Burmese populace was, itself, locked away. A Burmese colleague of the second author once compared Burma under military rule to the unhappy residents of Plato's cave—chained inside a dark cave and unable to emerge into the light, the Burmese were reliant on the flickers and shadows that fell on the cave wall to inform them of what lay beyond the cave, in the outside world, where true "reality" resided.

Thus, although the military bombarded the populace with propaganda after 1988, there was a shared understanding that there were other narratives and other realities. The propaganda that the military put forth was characterized by an obtuseness, a lack of sophistication, and, as such, never truly captured the imagination of the people. As university students, many of whom had fine arts background, student organizers of the 1988 movement were much more adapt at lending imagination to the longings of the people through the circulation of narratives. Thura's family, friends, and other civilians conveyed to the second author that they never believed that Thura or any of the young people involved in the 1988 Uprising were ever "enemies" of the state. Rather than recapitulating and internalizing the state-sponsored narrative about what occurred in 1988, they viewed Thura and other student activists as heroes. Thura's beliefs about himself, his own actions, and the ideals associated with the democracy movement, therefore, have a deep coherence not only with those in his immediate social environment, but also with the larger society.

24.9 Conclusion

Both Thura and Kereta lived through political violence and large-scale atrocities, but their long-term outcomes and journey through and, in Thura's case *beyond*, traumatic experience are vastly different. Their divergent trajectories illustrate the importance of contemplating the complex interaction of psychocultural, familial, social, political, spiritual, and historical factors that can either support individuals' strengths and resiliencies and allow them to sublimate traumatic experience and connect meaningfully with others or render them more vulnerable, increasing their sense of isolation and alienation from their social world.

Thura is deeply committed to a political movement and has deep cohesion with the world around him, even after having experienced what, to many others, would have been life-debilitating forms of violence and social control. Kereta withdrew into delusion as a compensatory measure in response to his experiences with political violence, having been, in almost all ways, permanently silenced as a social and political actor. Kereta remains alienated from those around him, even within the context of his own family, while Thura is deeply embedded within a large, supportive, network of dissidents and possesses a strong, active voice in the larger society.

Perhaps what is most fascinating about the two case studies in relation to trauma is that Kereta did not, himself, experience physical violence or torture. Kereta had witnessed the massacres of villagers without himself being physically harmed and without his body being broached in any way. Moreover, Kereta's exposure to trauma was contained in both time and space. He witnessed the atrocities within the boundaries of his village, over a matter of days. Thura, in contrast, was repeatedly exposed to various forms of physical and psychological trauma for almost his entire adult life, across many different collective and personal spaces. Rather than simply witnessing violence directed at others, he often had direct, bodily experience with violence, torture, and physical constraint.

Remarkably, it is Thura—the subject who has experienced, multiple, severe, and sustained traumatic exposure—who appears to have the better outcome. Key factors that contributed to his outcome are social support, coherence with the world around him, sense of meaning and purpose, a high sense of agency, continued communication with those around him (a lack of silence), an ability to self-regulate through goal setting, and cultural explanatory models that supported a productive engagement with fear. The very different trajectories of the two subjects help us understand how the social and political landscape, following traumatic events, can be shaped to allow victims of trauma to thrive, rather than recede into silence.

Shaping the political and social landscape such that it facilitates, rather than hinders, recovery from trauma remains complex issues in both Burma and Indonesia. After the fall of the New Order, artistic productions, biographies, autobiographies, documentary films, and even journalistic exposés covering aspects of 1965 mass killings became more common. Although, with each passing year, there are more and more of these efforts, and an increasingly open attitude in Indonesia towards exploring the truth of the events of 1965 (Schonhardt, 2012), movement towards a societal space that is safe and open for survivors has been unusually slow. Furthermore, efforts towards truth and reconciliation, in a judicial sense, appear to be a long way off and with the passing away of both survivors and perpetrators the prospects of holding tribunals or trials become increasingly unlikely.

Burma's journey towards national reconciliation and accountability is only now beginning. Strong leadership from activist groups such as the 88 Generation and the All Burma Federation of Student Unions (ABFSU), as well as the social, political, historical, and psychocultural factors highlighted in this chapter, contributed to an environment where there have been an astonishing number of survivors coming forward and narrating individual and collective experiences of the atrocities related to 1988, just a short while after the transition into a nominally civilian government.

Even with such seemingly rapid progress towards an open society, a long-term strategy is needed to ensure that an environment, where survivors of trauma feel safe coming forward with their stories, is maintained. More permanent infrastructures are needed to ensure that these narratives do not disappear after this generation of leaders and dissidents have passed away. Past atrocities need to be memorialized in such a way that they will become enduring aspects of national identity and so that they will be transformed from personal experience and the shared history of a small group of dissidents into the collective history of an entire nation.

Activists, journalists, students, and others who come forward with their stories continue to be brutalized, imprisoned, and killed (Kha, 2015; Nyein, 2015a, 2015b; Zaw, 2014). Continued advocacy is therefore needed to ensure that those exposing past and ongoing human rights violations on the part of the military and government are protected. This has been especially true in the months leading up to the 2015 elections (Mann, 2015). A particularly disturbing trend has been the brutal suppression and continued imprisonment of student activists affiliated with the All Burma Federation of Student Unions (ABFSU)—a group that was active during 1988 and whose current members constitute the younger generation of the tightly knit network of activists that came of age during 1988 (Mann, 2015; Nyein, 2015c; Weng, 2015; Weng & Snaing, 2015).

A recent legal memorandum summarized political atrocities and crimes against humanity committed by specific members of the Burmese army in military campaigns that were waged in Eastern Myanmar (Harvard & International Human Rights Clinic, 2014), but there has been no comparable studies done on human rights violations committed in 1988. As in Indonesia, the prospects of tribunals or trials for perpetrators appear to be a distant goal, but it will be interesting to note whether or not the Burmese prodemocracy movement eventually adopts the language of trauma to commemorate their history and to advocate for a social and moral order in which survivors and their families would be entitled to compensation and those who inflicted the trauma should be brought to justice.

Acknowledgements The authors thank Annie Tucker and Constance Cummings for comments on earlier drafts of this chapter. They also thank democracy activists in Burma and survivors of political atrocities in both Burma and Indonesia, who shared their narratives.

References

American Psychiatric Association. (2013). *Diagnostic and statistical manual of mental disorders* (5th ed.). Arlington, VA: American Psychiatric Publishing.

Anderson, B. (1987). How did the Generals die? *Indonesia, 43*, 109–134.

Anderson, B. (2012). Impunity. In J. T. Brink & J. Oppenheimer (Eds.), *Killer images: Documentary film, memory and the performance of violence* (pp. 268–286). New York, NY: Wallflower Press.

Assistance Association for Political Prisoners. (2005). *The darkness we see.* http://aappb.org/wp-content/uploads/2014/03/The-darkness-we-see.pdf

Bateson, G., & Mead, M. (1942). *Balinese character: A photographic analysis*. New York: Special Publications of the New York Academy of Sciences, Vol 2.

Bonanno, G. A. (2004). Loss, trauma, and human resilience: have we underestimated the human capacity to thrive after extremely aversive events? *American psychologist, 59*(1), 20.

Cribb, R. (Ed.). (1990). *The Indonesian killings of 1965–1966: Studies from Java and Bali.* Clayton, VIC, Australia: Centre of Southeast Asian Studies, Monash University.

Cribb, R. (2004). The Indonesian massacres. In S. Totten, W. S. Parsons, & I. W. Charny (Eds.), *Century of genocide: Critical essays and eyewitness accounts* (pp. 233–262). New York, NY: Routledge.

Dias, B. G., Banerjee, S. B., Goodman, J. V., & Ressler, K. J. (2013). Towards new approaches to disorders of fear and anxiety. *Current Opinion in Neurobiology, 23*(3), 346–352.

Dwyer, L. (2004). The intimacy of terror: Gender and the violence of 1965-1966 in Bali, Indonesia. *Intersections: Gender, History, and Culture in the Asian Context, 10.* http://intersections.anu.edu.au/issue10/dwyer.html

Dwyer, L. (2009). A politics of silences: Violence, memory, and treacherous speech in post-1965 Bali. In A. Hinton & K. O'Neill (Eds.), *Genocide: Truth, memory, and representations* (pp. 113–146). Durham, NC: Duke University Press.

Dwyer, L., & Santikarma, D. (2003). When the world turned to chaos: The violence of 1965-66 in Bali, Indonesia. In B. Keirnan & R. Gellately (Eds.), *The spectre of genocide: Mass murder in historical perspective* (pp. 289–306). New York, NY: Cambridge University Press.

Dwyer, L., & Santikarma, D. (2006). Speaking from the shadows: Memories of massacre in Bali. In B. Pouligny, S. Chesterman, & A. Schnabel (Eds.), *After mass crime: Rebuilding states and communities* (pp. 190–214). Tokyo: United Nations University Press.

Fink, C. (2009). *Living silence: Burma under military rule*. London: Zed Books.

Foa, E. B., & Kozak, J. J. (1998). Clinical applications of bioinformational theory: Understanding anxiety and its treatment. *Behavior Therapy, 29*, 675–690.

Fortify Rights (2015, March). *Midnight intrusions: Ending guest registration and household inspections in Myanmar.* Accessed April 30, 2015, from http://www.fortifyrights.org/downloads/FR_Midnight_Intrusions_March_2015.pdf

Fuller, T. (2000, March 15). Suharto's Gulag/The Buru Island Humanitarian Project: Former Prisoners Look Back on a Remote Tropical Hell. *The New York Times*. Accessed November 7, 2014, from http://www.nytimes.com/2000/03/15/news/15iht-jak.2.t_0.html

Geertz, C. (1973). *The interpretation of cultures.* New York: Basic Books.

Harvard University, International Human Rights Clinic. (2014, November). *Legal memorandum: War crimes and crimes against humanity in Eastern Myanmar.* Accessed April 30, 2015, from http://hrp.law.harvard.edu/wp-content/uploads/2014/11/2014.11.05-IHRC-Legal-Memorandum.pdf

Heryanto, A. (2012). Screening the 1965 violence. In J. T. Brink & J. Oppenheimer (Eds.), *Killer images: Documentary film, memory and the performance of violence* (pp. 224–240). New York, Chichester: Wallflower Press.

Hinton, D. E., & Good, B. J. (2015). *Culture and PTSD: Trauma in historical and global perspective.* Philadelphia, PA: University of Pennsylvania Press.

Hinton, D., & Hinton, A. (Eds.). (2014). *Genocide and mass violence: Memory, symptom, and recovery.* Cambridge, MA: Cambridge University Press.

Hinton, D., & Kirmayer, L. (2013). Local responses to trauma: Symptom, affect, and healing. *Transcultural Psychiatry, 50*(5), 607–621.

Hinton, D., & Lewis-Fernandez, R. (2011). The cross-cultural validity of posttraumatic stress disorder: Implications for DSM-5. *Depression and Anxiety, 28*(9), 783–801.

Hinton, D. E., & Simon, N. M. (2015). Toward a cultural neuroscience of anxiety disorders: The multiplex model. In L. J. Kirmayer, R. Lemelson, & C. A. Cummings (Eds.), *Re-visioning psychiatry: Cultural phenomenology, critical neuroscience, and global mental health*. New York, NY: Cambridge University Press.

Kha, K. (2015, March 16). Journalist detained, beaten by red armband thugs: Report. *The Irrawaddy*. Accessed April 30, 2015, from http://www.irrawaddy.org/burma/journalist-detained-beaten-by-red-armband-thugs-report.html

Kirmayer, L., Lemelson, R., & Barad, M. (Eds.). (2007). *Understanding trauma: Integrating biological, clinical, and cultural perspectives*. New York, NY: Cambridge University Press.

Kyi, A. S. S. (1992). In quest of democracy. *Journal of Democracy, 3*(1), 5–14.

Kyi, A. S. S. (2010). *Freedom from fear*. London: Penguin.

LeDoux, J. E. (2014). Coming to terms with fear. *Proceedings of the National Academy of Sciences of the United States of America, 111*(8), 2871–2878.

Lemelson, R. (2014). "The Spirits Enter Me to Force Me to Be a Communist": Political Embodiment, Idioms of Distress, Spirit Possession, and Thought Disorder in Bali. In D. E. Hinton & A. L. Hinton (Eds.), *Genocide and mass violence: Memory, symptom, and recovery* (pp. 175–189). New York, NY: Cambridge University Press.

Lemelson, R., Supartini, N., & Ng, E. (2010). *Anak PKI*: A longitudinal case study of the effects of ostracism, political violence, and bullying on an adolescent Javanese boy. In C. M. Worthman, P. M. Plotsky, D. S. Schechter, & C. A. Cummings (Eds.), *Formative experiences: The interaction of caregiving, culture, and developmental psychobiology* (pp. 378–389). Cambridge, MA: Cambridge University Press.

Lemelson, R., & Suryani, L. (2006). The Spirits, Ngeb, and the social suppression of memory: A complex clinical case from Bali. *Culture, Medicine and Psychiatry, 30*, 389–413.

Lemelson, R., & Tucker, A. (2012). Forty Years of Silence". In C. Rittner (Ed.), *Learn, teach, prevent-holocaust education in the 31st century: The Ethel Le Frak Holocaust Conference Proceedings*. Seton Hill: Seton Hill Press.

Lemere, M., & West, Z. (Eds.). (2011). *Nowhere to be home: Narratives from survivors of Burma's military regime*. San Francisco, CA: McSweeneys Books.

Lintner, B. (1990). *Outrage: Burma's struggle for democracy*. Bangkok: White lotus.

Lone, W. (2014, April 8). Red Bridge burns bright for student activists. *Myanmar Times*. Accessed June 16, 2015, from http://www.mmtimes.com/index.php/national-news/10110-red-bridge-burns-bright-for-student-activists.html

Mackay, J. (2011). *Abhaya: Burma's fearlessness*. Bangkok: Riber Books Co. Ltd.

Mann, A. (2015, April 2). Students freed after Letpadan could face trial for prior protests. *The Irrawaddy*. Accessed April 30, 2015, from http://www.irrawaddy.org/burma/students-freed-after-letpadan-could-face-trial-for-prior-protests.html

Nyein, N. (2015a, April 2). Letpadan detainees call for public trial, medical attention. *The Irrawaddy*. Accessed April, 2015, from http://www.irrawaddy.org/burma/letpadan-detainees-call-for-public-trial-medical-attention.html

Nyein, N. (2015b, April 3). Rights activist back to Insein on peaceful assembly rap. *The Irrawaddy*. Accessed April, 2015, from http://www.irrawaddy.org/burma/rights-activist-back-to-insein-on-peaceful-assembly-rap.html

Nyein, N. (2015c, April 6). Political prisoner count soars during months of arrests. *The Irrawaddy*. Accessed April, 2015, from http://www.irrawaddy.org/burma/political-prisoner-count-soars-during-month-of-arrests.html

Obeyesekere, G. (1985). Depression, Buddhism, and the work of culture in Sri Lanka. *Culture and depression*, 134–152.

Pitman, T., & Htusan, E. (2015, March 18). Burma's midnight inspections remnants of military rule. *The Irrawaddy*. Accessed April, 2015, from http://www.irrawaddy.org/burma/burmas-midnight-inspections-remnants-of-military-rule.html

Pohlman, A. (2004). Fragment of a story: Gerwani and Tapol experiences. *Intersections: Gender, History, and Culture in the Asian Context*, (10). Accessed December 7, 2014, from http://intersections.anu.edu.au/issue10/pohlman.html

Pohlman, A. (2008). Testimonial and telling women's narratives of genocide, torture and political imprisonment in post-Suharto Indonesia. *Life Writing, 5*(1), 47–60.

Pohlman, A. (2014). *Women, sexual violence and the Indonesian killings of 1965-66*. New York, NY: Routledge.

Powers, M. B., Halpern, J. M., Ferenschak, M. P., Gillihan, S. J., & Foa, E. G. (2010). A meta-analytic review of prolonged exposure for posttraumatic stress disorder. *Clinical Psychology Review, 30*(6), 635–641.

Prasse-Freeman, E. (2012, October). *Former political prisoners and patterns of re-subjectivisation*. Paper presented at the International Burma Studies Conference, DeKalb, IL.

Rechtman, R. (2000). Stories of trauma and idioms of distress: From cultural narratives to clinical assessment. *Transcultural Psychiatry, 37*(3), 403–415.

Robinson, G. (1995). *The dark side of paradise: Political violence in Bali*. Ithaca, NY: Cornell University Press.

Rochijat, P., & Anderson, B. (1985). Am I PKI or non-PKI? *Indonesia, 40*, 37–56.

Roosa, J. (2006). *Pretext for mass murder: The September 30th Movement and Suharto's coup d'état in Indonesia*. Madison, WI: University of Wisconsin Press.

Santikarma, D. (1995). *Koh Ngomong, the Balinese Tactic and Spirit of Resistance*. Paper presented at the Fourth International Bali Studies Conference, Sydney, Australia.

Schonhardt, S. (2012, January 18). Veil of Silence Lifted in Indonesia. *The New York Times*. Accessed December 7, 2014, from http://www.nytimes.com/2012/01/19/world/asia/veil-of-silence-lifted-in-indonesia.html?pagewanted=all&_r=0

Shin, L. M., & Liberzon, I. (2012). The neurocircuitry of fear, stress, and anxiety disorders. *Neuropsychopharmacology, 35*(1), 169–191.

Skidmore, M. (2003). Darker than midnight: Fear, vulnerability, and terror making in urban Burma (Myanmar). *American Ethnologist, 30*(1), 5–21.

Slow, O. (2015, March 20). Call for repeal of law enabling 'midnight' arrests. *The Myanmar Times*. Accessed April 30, 2015, from http://www.mmtimes.com/index.php/national-news/yangon/13639-call-for-repeal-of-law-enabling-midnight-arrests.html

Spiro, M. E. (1982). *Buddhism and society: A great tradition and its Burmese vicissitudes*. Berkeley, CA: University of California Press.

Wardaya, B. (2006). *Supersemar revealed! From the CIA to the creeping coup d'etat against Bung Karno*. Jakarta, Indonesia: Galang Press.

Weng, L. (2015, March 31). *Former political prisoner facing charges over Letpadan protest*. Accessed April 30, 2015, from http://www.irrawaddy.org/burma/former-political-prisoner-facing-charges-over-letpadan-protest.html

Weng, L., & Snaing, W. (2015, April 7). Authorities to transfer student court cases to remote the Irrawaddy district. *The Irrawaddy*. Accessed April 30, 2015, from http://www.irrawaddy.org/burma/authorities-to-transfer-student-court-cases-to-remote-tharawaddy-district.html

Wertheim, W. (1979). Whose plot? New light on the 1965 events. *Journal of Contemporary Asia, 9*(2), 197–215.

Wikan, U. (1990). *Managing turbulent hearts: A Balinese formula for living*. Chicago, IL: University of Chicago Press.

Zaw, A. (2014, October 28). Death of an activist-reporter. *The Irrawaddy*. Accessed December 7, 2014, from http://www.irrawaddy.org/commentary/death-activist-reporter.html

Zurbuchen, M. (2002). History, memory, and the "1965 Incident" in Indonesia. *Asian Survey, 42*(4), 564–581.

Zurbuchen, M. (Ed.). (2005). *Beginning to remember: The past in the Indonesian present*. Seattle: University of Washington Press.

Conclusion: Trauma and Culture: How Trauma Can Shape the Human Mind

Yuval Neria and Yochai Ataria

Exposure to violence is central to human development. Parental aggression and neglect, bullying, sexual abuse, torture, terrorism, and war trauma are all extremely prevalent, both across an individual's life-span and worldwide (Breslau et al., 1998; Kessler, Sonnega, Bromet, Hughes, & Nelson, 1995). Traumatic exposure can be life altering. Clinically, interpersonal violence is the worst form of trauma. More than other traumatic events, interpersonal traumas are often intentional, cruel, and painful. Studies have repeatedly shown that enduring interpersonal trauma, particularly in the form of violent relationships, disrupts human development, impairing sense of trust, justice, and fairness (Kessler et al., 1999; Yehuda, 2002). Moreover, violence may carry over across generations (i.e., transgenerational trauma, Schwab, 2010), as discussed in this book by Bartal (Chap. 7) and Zohar (Chap. 8). Some even suggest that people exposed to violence early in life may subsequently develop violent behaviors as adults. Moreover, some scholars speculated, based on the Freudian theory (Freud, 1939), that collectives (e.g., nations) exposed to organized trauma may themselves subject other collectives to a trauma once they become powerful enough (see LaCapra, 2001).

Numerous studies have shown that exposure to trauma has significant psychological and psychiatric consequences, including pathological anxiety, PTSD, and depression (American Psychiatric Association, 2013). The severity of these outcomes is often correlated with the severity of the trauma (Joyner et al., Chap. 20), particularly if the exposure is continuous and repeated (Herman, 1992). For example, many studies, including our own, among prisoners of war, suggest that torture and humiliation are detrimental to human physical and mental health (Ataria & Neria, 2013; Neria, Solomon, Ginzburg, Dekel, Enoch, & Ohry, 2000). Indeed, the injurious effects of confinement, isolation, and interpersonal cruelty may lead to mental "breakdowns" during imprisonment, and consequently severe mental health problems (Arthur, 1982). Importantly, exposure to extreme adversities may be associated with neurobiological impairments, including difficulties in fear processing, and accurate discrimination between safe and threatening stimuli (Shvil, Rusch, Sullivan, & Neria, 2013).

Yet, what this volume, in its entirety, proposed is that exposure to extreme trauma may also

Y. Neria, Ph.D. (✉)
Columbia University Medical Center and the New York State Psychiatric Institute, New York, NY, USA
e-mail: ny126@cumc.columbia.edu

Y. Ataria, Ph.D.
Department of Neurobiology, Weizmann Institute of Science, Rechovot, Israel

Y. Ataria et al. (eds.), *Interdisciplinary Handbook of Trauma and Culture*,
DOI 10.1007/978-3-319-29404-9

shape cultures. Such transformation may occur following exposure to large scale traumas which may alter core beliefs affecting traditions, and changing social values. As discussed in this book major events such as the Holocaust, the Vietnam War, and the 9/11 attacks have the potential to penetrate the core of societies, transforming basic ways of intellectual functioning, and overhauling their cultural infrastructures. Indeed, major traumas may have the awesome energy to shake entire social and political systems according to which people have lived their lives, undermining existing knowledge, replacing comfortable certainty with anxiety-provoking chaos, ambiguity, and fear (Bracken, 2001).

The book attempted to provide to the reader a number of examples of how religion (Chaps. 14 and 15), modern art (Chaps. 6, 8 and 10), film (Chap. 16), and philosophy (Chap. 11) are galvanized by violence and catastrophes. Furthermore, the chapters illustrate to what extent and how public traumas, via direct and indirect representations, may influence the public, affect its artistic expressions, and generate intense, often painful, social discourse.

Because modern wars and atrocities (e.g., 9/11 attacks) are widely and excessively reported live via multiple means of digital and social media, and transmitted to millions of spectators, traumas are increasingly becoming immediately available, highly public, and yet intrusive, repetitive, and eventually difficult to ever deny or forget. Moreover, current TV sets, through large industries of cables and satellites, can disseminate gruesome images of death and injury around the globe as never before, and indirectly traumatizing millions, even in remote places (Neria & Sullivan, 2011). Analyzing these phenomena, Rothe (Chap. 4) suggests that the concept of popular culture can be replaced, at least to some extent, with the concept of a popular trauma culture, and both Meek (Chap. 2) and Arav (Chap. 3) demonstrate how trauma becomes almost synonymous with high ratings.

Researchers and clinicians have played a critical role in transforming trauma from being a private event, often associated with shame and guilt, to the public domain. Initiated in the early 1980s a small group of highly dedicated and visionary clinicians and researchers, such as Robert Jay Lifton (1967, 1973, 1986), Bessel van Der Kolk (1987, 2014), Zahava Solomon (Solomon, 1990; Solomon & Benbenishty, 1986; Solomon, Weisenberg, Schwarzwald, & Mikulincer, 1987), Judith Herman (1992), among others, were able to effectively communicate the emotional toll of trauma to the public. During this time the consequences of severe psychological traumas such as wars, sexual abuse, and childhood adversities were clinically formulated and rigorously studied, opening the door for developing highly needed evidence-based therapies for PTSD (Foa et al., 2005; Markowitz et al., 2015; Schneier et al., 2012). Today, more than three decades later, while psychological trauma and its consequences are widely researched, what this book highlights is that more research is still needed to describe the interplay between culture and trauma. We hope that the chapters of this volume will elevate such efforts and energize future discussions, eventually contributing to a better understanding of the human reactions to human suffering.

References

American Psychiatric Association. (2013). *Diagnostic and statistical manual of mental disorders* (5th ed.). Arlington, VA: American Psychiatric Publishing.

Arthur, R. J. (1982). Psychiatric symptoms in prisoner of war and concentration camp survivors. In C. Friedmann & R. Faguet (Eds.), *Extraordinary disorders of human behavior* (pp. 47–63). New York and London: Springer.

Ataria, Y., & Neria, Y. (2013). Consciousness-body-time: How do people think lacking their body? *Humans Studies, 36*(2), 159–178. doi:10.1007/s10746-013-9263-3.

Bracken, P. J. (2001). Post-modernity and post-traumatic stress disorder. *Social Science & Medicine, 53*(6), 733–743. doi:10.1016/S0277-9536(00)00385-3.

Breslau, N., Kessler, R. C., Chilcoat, H. D., Schultz, L. R., Davis, G. C., & Andreski, P. (1998). Trauma and post-traumatic stress disorder in the community: The 1996 Detroit area survey of trauma. *Archives of General Psychiatry, 55*(7), 626–632.

Foa, E. B., Hembree, E. A., Cahill, S. P., Rauch, S. A., Riggs, D. S., Feeny, N. C., et al. (2005). Randomized trial of prolonged exposure for posttraumatic stress disorder with and without cognitive restructuring: outcome at academic and community c. *Journal of Consulting and Clinical Psychology, 73*(5), 953–964.

Freud, S. (1939). *Moses and Monotheism.* (K. Jones, Trans.) New York: Vintage Books.

Herman, J. L. (1992). *Trauma and recovery*. New York: Basic Books.

Kessler, R. C., Sonnega, A., Bromet, E., Hughes, M., Nelson, C., & Breslau, N. (1999). Epidemiological risk factors for trauma and PTSD. In R. Yehuda (Ed.), *Risk factors for posttraumatic stress disorder* (pp. 23–59). Washington: American Psychiatric Association.

Kessler, R. C., Sonnega, A., Bromet, E., Hughes, M., & Nelson, C. B. (1995). Posttraumatic stress disorder in the national comorbidity survey. *Archives of General Psychiatry, 52*(12), 1048–1060.

LaCapra, D. (2001). *Writing history, writing trauma.* Baltimore: Johns Hopkins University Press.

Lifton, R. J. (1967). *Death in life: Survivors of Hiroshima.* New York: Random House.

Lifton, R. J. (1973). *Home from the war.* New York: Simon & Schuster.

Lifton, R. J. (1986). *The Nazi doctors*. New York: Basic Books.

Markowitz, J. C., Petkova, E., Neria, Y., Van Meter, P. E., Zhao, Y., Hembree, E., et al. (2015). Does PTSD require exposure-based treatment? A randomized trial. *American Journal of Psychiatry, 175*(2), 430–440.

Neria, Y., Solomon, Z., Ginzburg, K., Dekel, R., Enoch, D., & Ohry, A. (2000). Posttraumatic residues of captivity: A follow-up of Israeli ex-prisoners of war. *Journal of Clinical Psychiatry, 61*, 39–46.

Neria, Y., & Sullivan, G. M. (2011). Understanding the mental health effects of indirect exposure to mass trauma through the media. *Journal of the American Medical Association, 306*(12), 1374–1375.

Schneier, F. R., Neria, Y., Pavlicova, M., Hembree, E., Suh, E. J., Amsel, L., et al. (2012). Combined prolonged exposure therapy and paroxetine versus prolonged exposure therapy and placebo in PTSD related to the world trade center attacks: A randomized controlled trial. *American Journal of Psychiatry, 169*(1), 80–88.

Schwab, G. (2010). *Haunting legacies: Violent histories and transgenerational trauma*. New York: Columbia University Press.

Shvil, E., Rusch, H. L., Sullivan, G. M., & Neria, Y. (2013). Neural, psychophysiological, and behavioral markers of fear processing in PTSD: A review of the literature. *Current Psychiatry Reports, 15*(5), 1–10.

Solomon, Z. (1990). Does the war end when the shooting stops? The psychological toll of war1. *Journal of Applied Social Psychology, 20*(21), 1733–1745.

Solomon, Z., & Benbenishty, R. (1986). The role of proximity, immidiacy and expectancy in front line treatment of combat stress reaction. *American Journal of Psychiatry, 143*(5), 613–617.

Solomon, Z., Weisenberg, M., Schwarzwald, J., & Mikulincer, M. (1987). Posttraumatic stress disorder among frontline soldiers with combat stress reaction: The 1982 Israeli experience. *The American Journal of Psychiatry, 144*(4), 448–454.

van der Kolk, B. A. (1987). *Psycological trauma.* Washington: Amrican Psychiatric Press.

van der Kolk, B. A. (2014). *The body keeps the score.* New York: Viking.

Yehuda, R. (2002). Posttraumatic stress disorder. *The New England Journal of Medicine, 346*(2), 108–114.

Index

Y. Ataria et al. (eds.), *Interdisciplinary Handbook of Trauma and Culture*,
DOI 10.1007/978-3-319-29404-9

CPSIA information can be obtained at www.ICGtesting.com
Printed in the USA
LVOW09*1402280916

506564LV00030B/395/P

9 783319 294025